Anatomy of
Orofacial Structures

A COMPREHENSIVE APPROACH

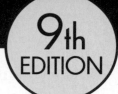

Anatomy of
Orofacial Structures

A COMPREHENSIVE APPROACH

Richard W. Brand, BS, DDS
Professor Emeritus
Washington University School of Medicine
St. Louis, Missouri

Donald E. Isselhard, BS, DDS, FAGD, MAGD, MBA
Private Practice
St. Louis, Missouri

Amy N. Smith, RDH, MS, MPH, PhD
Assistant Professor
Georgia State University Perimeter College
Dental Hygiene Program
Dunwoody, Georgia

ELSEVIER

Elsevier
1600 John F. Kennedy Blvd.
Ste 1800
Philadelphia, PA 19103-2899

ANATOMY OF OROFACIAL STRUCTURES:
A COMPREHENSIVE APPROACH, NINTH EDITION

ISBN: 978-0-323-79699-6

Previous editions copyrighted 2019, 2014, 2003, 1998, 1994, 1990, 1986, 1982, and 1977.

Senior Content Strategist: Kelly Skelton
Senior Content Development Manager: Kathryn M. DeFrancesco
Senior Content Development Specialist: Lisa M. Barnes
Publishing Services Manager: Deepthi Unni
Project Manager: Nayagi Anandan
Design Direction: Patrick Ferguson

Printed in India

Last digit is the print number: 9   8   7   6   5   4   3   2

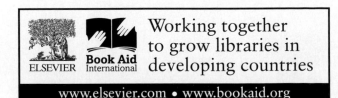

With heartfelt appreciation,
I dedicate this ninth edition to my co-author Richard Brand, DDS

Dr. Richard Brand spent a lifetime as a student advocate, teacher, and author.
He and I began the venture with this book over forty years ago.
He was my colleague, mentor, co-author, and best friend.
Richard was a kind and caring instructor who believed every
student deserved to be nurtured and motivated as well as protected and respected.
He was a man of great integrity and devotion.

Dr. Brand believed that if one worked hard enough, the rewards would follow.
To that end, if you want to honor him, put in the effort.
Perform the required amount of study time,
review your notes at the end of each class,
and answer the questions at the end of each chapter.
He would have loved to have been a part of your growth
and learning experience. Because of this book, he still can be.

Contributors and Reviewers

Reviewers

Warren F. Gabaree, Jr., DDS, MEd
Department Head/Instructor, Dental Programs
Coastal Carolina Community College
Jacksonville, North Carolina

Darlene Saccuzzo, CDA, CRDH, BASDH
Professor, Dental Education
South Florida State College
Avon Park, Florida

Bobby A. Sconyers, CDA, CPFDA
Dental Assisting Program Coordinator, Professor
South Florida State College
Avon Park, Florida

Therese L. Tippie, CDA, BS, MA, EFDA
Certified Dental Assistant
Adjunct Dental Assisting Instructor
South Florida State College
Avon Park, Florida

Kendra Velasco, RDH, MS
Program Director of Dental Hygiene
Cypress College
Cypress, California

Contributor

Julie Bencosme, RDH,MA
Professor
Dental Hygiene Unit
Eugenio Maria de Hostos Community College
Bronx, New York

Preface to the Ninth Edition

We wish to thank the many instructors for their ongoing input and suggestions. Their feedback has been extremely valuable in improving this and former editions of our book. We also want to thank all those students who have used this textbook over the years. From the very beginning, *Anatomy of Orofacial Structures* was written to assist learners with a complex subject matter in the most comprehensive manner.

This book has consistently been written for students who are beginning their study of the anatomic sciences relating to dentistry. We have endeavored to present content at a level that meets the needs of several types of dental programs, recognizing that some programs do not require as much detail as others. Although the subject matter presented here is intended to meet the needs of our students, we also recognize instructors will be discriminant in omitting or adding details in accordance to the requirements of their courses. This book covers three subjects: Oral Histology, Head and Neck Anatomy, and Dental Anatomy. It is our hope that by combining them into one book, we can help the student understand the correlation among subject matters and better comprehend their interrelationships.

Dr. Brand and I were excited about this ninth edition because with it we introduce Dr. Amy Nicole Smith as our co-author. Dr. Smith began her career as a dental assistant in the US Navy. She attended Montgomery County Community College and earned her A.A.S. in Dental Hygiene. She earned her Master's in Dental Hygiene and Master's in Public Health from Massachusetts College of Pharmacy and Health Sciences. She received her PhD in Curriculum and Instruction from Northern Arizona University where she was the lead instructor for Embryology and Oral Histology. She currently is on the faculty of Georgia State University.

The section on Oral Histology and Embryology has been enhanced by Dr. Smith. This section has been updated with new terminology and more concise descriptions for embryonic terms. Details about dental tissue development, formation, and composition have been simplified. There are new descriptions about principal fiber groups, mucosa, and the locations of these tissues.

Many new illustrations have been included to improve our book. Tables and charts have been added in this edition to aid students in clarifying the material presented. Every effort has been made to make this a more student-friendly textbook. We have maintained the general format of objectives at the beginning of the chapters and review questions at the end of the chapters. At the back of the book there are workbook questions for each of the chapters. At the end of each of the four main sections of this book, there are unit exams. The answers to the review questions in every chapter and the workbook questions for each chapter are placed on the Evolve companion site. This site also has the answers for the large unit exams that are found at the end of each of the four sections. We have bolded each important term and defined them in the glossary at the back of the book. Removable flashcards for dental and head and neck anatomy can be found on the last pages of this book. Past students have found them to be a valuable asset. Finally, there is an Index section to assist students in searching for additional information about a specific term or subject.

For instructors adopting this text, a variety of instructor's materials are available on the Evolve site, including a test bank, PowerPoint lectures, suggested activities, and color illustrations from the text. Be sure to ask your local sales representative for details.

We would like to recognize and thank the various people who have made this book possible. We would like to thank Kristen Wilhelm for her vision and support in this project. We also would like to thank Kelly Skelton for her direction, leadership, and constant support. She has helped guide us all the way through this ninth edition. We would like to thank Lisa Barnes, who assisted us through this edition and helped us with the illustrations, updating content, and staying on target. A special thank you to Nayagi Anandan for helping us do final edits, making this production as free from errors as possible. You will note our test bank and answers are much improved over any previous editions. A special thanks to John Tomedi for his assistance in final proof editing. We are also very grateful to Jason McAlexander who produced so many wonderful illustrations in this new edition of our book. We are indebted to many editors in past editions, and especially Brian Loehr for his work in past editions. We would also like to thank all those authors and publishers who have given us permission to use their illustrations in this ninth edition as well as in previous editions.

Finally, we have special thanks to Julie Bencosme who is a full time dental hygiene faculty member at Eugenio Maria de Hostos Community College for input and suggestions.

Donald E. Isselhard

Contents

UNIT 1

Introduction

1

Oral Cavity

As students of the dental profession, you will be concentrating your studies on the head and neck and, more specifically, on the structures that make up the oral cavity. It is imperative that you are extremely familiar with the normal makeup and structural components of this area. Therefore this chapter has been set forth to serve as an introduction to your studies of the head and neck region.

The oral cavity is the upper end and the beginning of the digestive system and at its posterior end forms a common pathway with the respiratory system. The oral cavity begins at the lips and cheeks and extends posteriorly to the area of the **palatine tonsils**, which are usually referred to as the *tonsils*. These lie on the sides of the throat between two folds of tissues, one in front and one in back, called the **tonsillar pillars**. Posterior to the tonsillar pillars the oral cavity ends and the **oral pharynx**, a pathway shared by the digestive and respiratory systems, begins. In the area from the oral pharynx to the **laryngeal pharynx**, the digestive system continues to share a common pathway with the respiratory system and then goes on to the esophagus to the rest of the digestive system. The respiratory system starts at the nasal cavity and includes the **nasal pharynx**, oral pharynx, and laryngeal pharynx (the last two of which are shared spaces with the digestive tract) and then continues into the larynx, trachea, bronchi, and lungs.

The oral cavity can be logically divided into two parts: the vestibule and oral cavity proper. The **vestibule** is the space or potential space that exists between the lips or cheeks and the teeth. In an edentulous person (one without teeth), it would extend between the lips or cheeks and the alveolar ridges where the teeth were at one time or will be if the person is an infant. The **oral cavity proper** is the area surrounded by the teeth or alveolar ridges back to the area of the palatine tonsils. This includes the region from the floor of the mouth upward to the hard and soft palates.

Vestibule

In considering the vestibular area, you should begin by examining the lips. The lips are the junction between the skin of the face, which is a dry tissue, and the mucosa of the oral cavity, which is a moist tissue. Between these two areas lies a transitional zone of reddish tissue known as the **vermilion zone** of the lip. It is along the border between the skin and the vermilion zone that one commonly encounters cold sores, which are generally caused by a herpesvirus. The skin of the upper lip has an indentation at the midline known as the **philtrum**, which is derived from the embryonic medial nasal processes (Fig. 1.1). It is at the lateral junction of this philtrum that a cleft lip might be formed.

Anterior and Posterior Borders

By elevating the mandible so that the teeth are in contact and then retracting the lips and cheeks, you can see the vestibule. It is bounded anteriorly by the lips (**labia**) and laterally by the cheeks (**bucca**). A finger placed in the posterior portion of the vestibule will be impeded by two obstacles, the bony anterior border of the ramus of the mandible and the soft tissue. The cheek is formed to a great extent by the buccinator muscle, which is covered with skin on the outside and moist mucous membrane on the inside. This muscle extends back from the corners of the mouth to join with the muscles of the upper throat wall. As it passes backward, it crosses in front of the mandibular ramus from a lateral position to a medial position, limiting the posterior extent of the vestibule. As you run your finger in the upper posterior vestibular space, you can feel the ridge of bone that is the beginning of the anterior part of the zygomatic arch (cheekbone). This is often referred to as the **zygomaticoalveolar crest**. Run your finger along the cheek area of the vestibule and note the landmarks and structures just mentioned.

Superior and Inferior Borders

The point at which the mucosa of the lips or cheeks turns toward the gingival or gum tissue is known as the *mucobuccal fold* or *mucolabial fold*. The mucosa lying against the alveolar bone is loosely attached and movable and known as the *alveolar mucosa*. This mucosa is generally reddish because of the presence of blood vessels underneath the relatively thin mucosa. The point at which it becomes tightly attached to the bone is the beginning of the gingiva. This is known as the mucogingival junction (Fig. 1.2). The normal color of the gingiva is pink because the mucosal layer is thicker; therefore the blood vessels do not impart as much color. In patients with darker skin color, generally some pigmentation to the gingiva is evident.

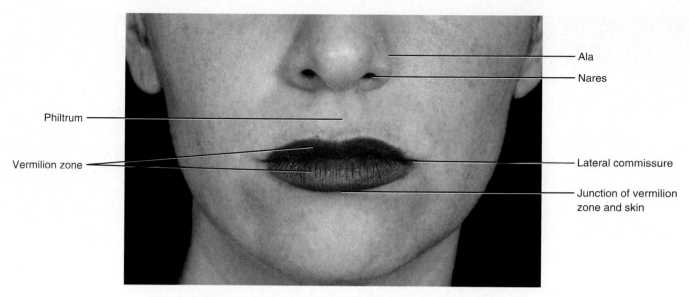

Philtrum

Vermilion zone

Ala

Nares

Lateral commissure

Junction of vermilion
zone and skin

• **Figure 1.1** Vermilion zone of lips and philtrum of the upper lip.

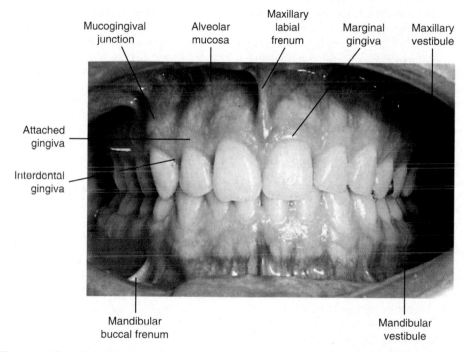

Mucogingival
junction

Alveolar
mucosa

Maxillary
labial
frenum

Marginal
gingiva

Maxillary
vestibule

Attached
gingiva

Interdental
gingiva

Mandibular
buccal frenum

Mandibular
vestibule

• **Figure 1.2** View of vestibule. A change in color at the mucogingival junction is noted. The maxillary labial frenum is more evident than the mandibular labial frenum. Mucobuccal folds are quite evident. (From Liebgott B. *The Anatomical Basis of Dentistry.* 3rd ed. St. Louis: Mosby; 2011.)

Pulling outward on the lips or corners of the mouth shows several areas in which the tissue is attached in folds to the alveolar mucosa. At the midline in both the upper and lower lips, a fold of connective tissue known as the **labial frenum** can be found. The frenum contains no muscle tissue and has only connective tissue. The upper frenum is usually more pronounced than the lower, but problems may occur with either one. The attachment of the upper (maxillary) frenum may extend to the crest of the alveolar ridge and even over the ridge. This band of tissue is so firm that the erupting central incisors might not penetrate it but may be pushed slightly aside so that a space exists between them. This space is known as a **diastema** (Fig. 1.3A). Correction of a diastema usually involves the surgical removal, or cutting, of the frenum tissue between the teeth. After this, the teeth will generally move together into normal contact. If they do not come back into normal contact, minor orthodontic treatment may be required. This procedure is best done when a child is 6 to 12 years old.

The mandibular labial frenum seldom extends up between the teeth, but it often extends close enough to the gingiva to contribute to gingival recession in that area by pulling downward on the

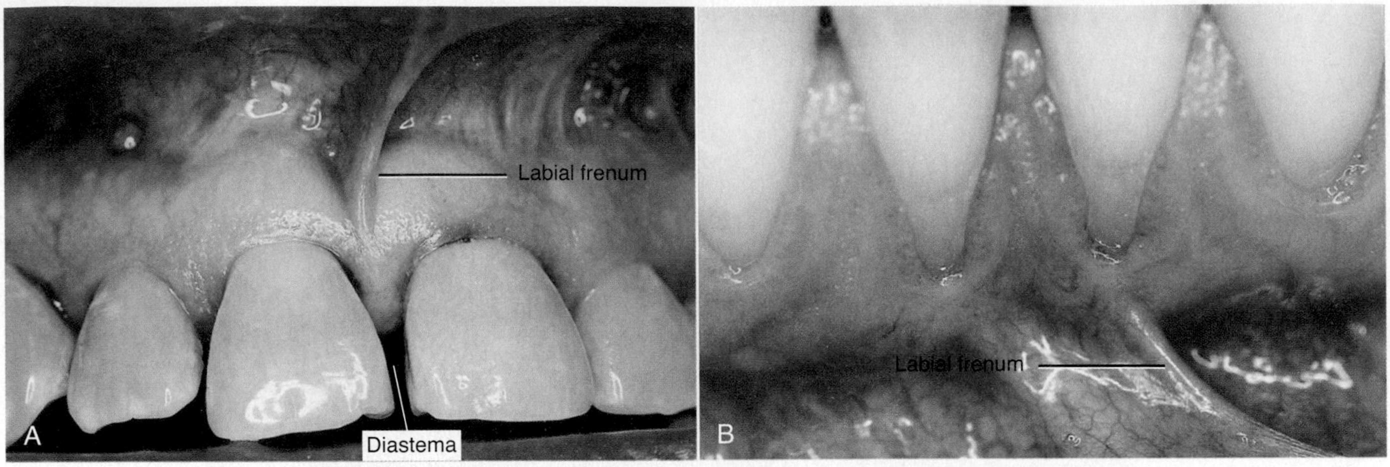

• **Figure 1.3** **(A)** Notice how the labial frenum extends between the maxillary teeth, causing separation or diastema. **(B)** Notice how the mandibular labial frenum attaches close to an area of gingival recession and contributes to that condition. (From Newman MG, Takei HH, Klokkevold PR, Carranza FA. *Carranza's Clinical Periodontology.* 11th ed. St. Louis: Saunders; 2012.)

tissue when the lip is tensed (see Fig. 1.3B). In this instance the frenum attachment needs to be incised with possible periodontal follow-up to restore the original gingival contours.

Less well-defined frena are evident in the maxillary and mandibular canine areas. These can be seen in Fig. 1.2, labeled mandibular buccal frenum, and in a similar area above it in the maxillary arch just superior and posterior to the area, labeled mucogingival junction. Although they are not as well developed, along with the midline frena they still have to be taken into consideration in the construction of a dental prosthesis. A space must be made in the dental prosthesis to make room for this frenum. Otherwise the appliance will be dislodged every time the frenum is pulled by the muscles, and the frenum itself will become ulcerated.

Coronoid Process

As we continue to consider the structure of the vestibule in relation to clinical dentistry, it is interesting to note what happens to the vestibule when the mouth is opened wide. Place the teeth together, with the lips and cheeks relaxed. Position your index finger in the posterior-superior part of the vestibule, adjacent to the maxillary third molar area, move your finger as far posteriorly as you can, and open the mouth wide. You can feel your finger being pushed anteriorly out of the area. This is happening because the **coronoid process** of the mandible is moving into that vestibular space.

Clinical Consideration

In radiology, for example, you can take two periapical films of the maxillary molar area: one using a **bisecting angle technique** with the mouth open and the patient holding the film, and the other using a **paralleling technique** with the mouth closed on a film-holding device. The coronoid process intrudes into the vestibular space on the film taken with the mouth open, making it difficult to get a clear image on film. However, on the second film, taken with the mouth closed, the coronoid process does not impinge on the space, demonstrating the benefit of a film-holding device, which eliminates exposure to radiation of the finger and a much more stabilized and accurate film.

The coronoid process may also cause some problems when you are trying to take maxillary impressions to fabricate study models. When the mouth is open wide, the coronoid process may tend to push on the posterior part of the impression tray and cause it to be displaced, making it difficult to obtain a good impression of the third molars and maxillary tuberosity regions. It may also impinge on the posterolateral portion of a patient's maxillary denture and cause possible dislodgment of the denture. It is necessary to remove as much bulk as possible from both the impression tray and denture in that area so this does not happen.

Alveolar Bone Loss

When teeth are lost, some loss occurs of the alveolar bone that formed the sockets for the teeth. If too much bone loss occurs, then there may not be enough room in the remaining bone to anchor a dental implant.

Mucosa

Study the texture of the inner surface of the lip. Pull the lower lip down, dry it with a tissue, and stretch it. Notice the small drops of fluid on the lip, indicating the openings of many small salivary glands. These of course are also found in many other areas of the oral cavity (see Chapter 25).

The mucosa of the lips, cheeks, and **retromolar pad** area (see Fig. 1.8), posterior to the mandibular molars, are also the most common sites of misplaced **sebaceous glands**, which are commonly referred to as **Fordyce granules**. These glands are normally associated with hair follicles, which are only found on skin. In about 60% to 80% of the population, some sebaceous glands may be located on mucosa in areas of the oral cavity. They appear as yellowish granular structures embedded in the mucosa. These may be of some concern to patients, but with verification of their true identity, the patients should be reassured that they are harmless and are only a cosmetic situation. Look for these harmless glands in your own mouth.

Buccal Alveolar Bone

Another condition found on the buccal **cortical plate** of the mandible and maxillae in a large portion of the population are small bony growths called **exostoses**. They are generally seen more often on the mandible than on the maxilla. They are normally of no consequence unless they become tender from brushing in the area.

Oral Cavity Proper

When the mouth is open, you can see the oral cavity proper. First examine the roof of the mouth and study the hard and soft palates.

Hard Palate

The **hard** palate is the boney roof of the mouth (see Fig. 1.5). See Chapter 26 for the extent and makeup of the hard palate. In the anterior portion of the hard palate are transverse ridges of epithelial and connective tissue known as **rugae**. During speech and mastication, the tongue contacts these rugae. They are covered with keratinized epithelium and are often burned by hot foods, which can cause an ulcerated area of mucosa lingual to the maxillary incisor.

Also within the hard palate is a singular bulge of tissue at the midline immediately posterior to the central incisors known as the **incisive papilla**. Beneath this papilla is the **incisive foramen**, which carries the nasopalatine nerves and blood vessels to the mucous membrane lingual to the maxillary incisor teeth (Fig. 1.4). This is a point of injection for anesthetizing the anterior palate area between the canines. At the posterolateral part of the hard palate, lingual to the second and third maxillary molars, are two openings in the bone on each side: (1) the greater palatine foramina (Fig. 1.5), through which the nerves and blood vessels serving the soft tissue lingual to the molars and premolars enter to the hard palate, and (2) the lesser palatine foramen, which carries nerves and blood vessels to the soft palate.

The tissue beneath the palatal epithelium varies from region to region in the palate. In the midline of the hard palate the connective tissue is rather thin, and the palate feels hard and bony. In the anterolateral part of the hard palate the connective tissue contains fat cells and is thicker than at the midline. In the posterolateral portion the fat cells are still present, but numerous minor salivary glands secrete mucus. The soft palate also contains these mucus-secreting minor salivary glands, which serve to keep the epithelium moist.

The shape and size of the hard palate vary from individual to individual. It may be wide or narrow; have a high, arching curvature or vault; or be quite flat in its contours.

The junction of the hard and soft palates forms a double curving line, and the **posterior nasal spine** of the palatine bone is the primary landmark at the midline (review Figs. 1.4 and 1.5). Although you cannot see this posterior nasal spine, you can palpate it. Additionally, two small depressions are located on each side of the spine and are known as **fovea palatinae (see Fig.1.8)**, which marks the spine as a landmark in the construction of an upper denture. This demarcates the imaginary line of where the hard palate ends and the soft palate begins.

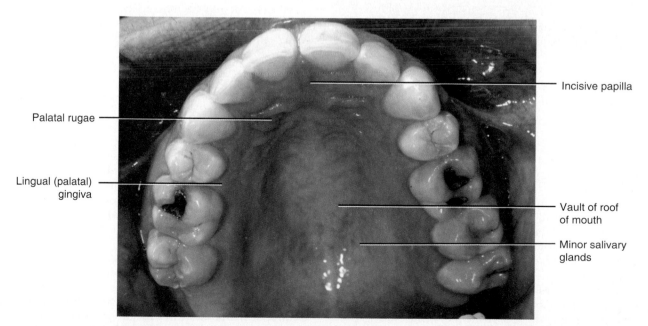

Palatal rugae

Lingual (palatal) gingiva

Incisive papilla

Vault of roof of mouth

Minor salivary glands

• **Figure 1.4** View of palate. The incisive papilla and rugae. (From Liebgott B. *The Anatomical Basis of Dentistry.* 3rd ed. St. Louis: Mosby; 2011.)

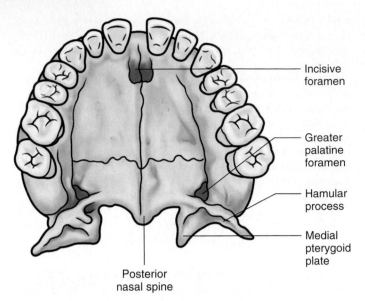

• **Figure 1.5** Hard palate. Notice how the posterior area curves toward the posterior nasal spine, indicating the end of the hard palate. Laterally, notice the hamular process of the medial pterygoid plate.

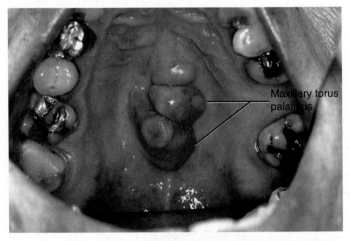

• **Figure 1.6** Typical torus palatinus. Notice the slightly constricted area in which it attaches to the hard palate. (From Regezi JA, Sciubba JJ, Jordan RCK. *Oral Pathology: Clinical Pathologic Correlations.* 6th ed. St. Louis: Saunders; 2012.)

Soft Palate

The **soft palate** is the moveable soft tissue area posterior to and contiguous with the hard palate. It helps close off the nasal cavity from the oral cavity during swallowing. Most of the posterior portion of the soft palate is actually part of the oral pharynx. The soft palate stretches back from the hard palate and in its most posterior portion at the midline is a downward projecting muscle known as the **uvula**. In a relaxed state, the soft palate has a slightly arching form from one side to the other. However, in speech and swallowing, the soft palate moves into various positions and closes off the oral pharynx from the nasal pharynx. This is accomplished by the *levator veli palatini* muscle, which pulls the soft palate up and back until it contacts the posterior throat *(pharyngeal)* wall.

In Chapter 18 the cleft lip and palate are discussed. Both are drastic medicodental problems and are generally treated by a team of dental and medical professionals. Another variation of cleft palate is the **short palate**. The soft palate may look normal, but it does not contact the posterior pharyngeal wall when it is elevated during swallowing or speech, producing a nasal or cleft speech sound. A dental appliance or speech therapy can correct this problem with gratifying results.

Lateral Borders

The lateral borders of the oral cavity proper are bounded primarily by the teeth and associated mucosa. In the posterolateral part of the oral cavity the boundary is the palatine tonsil and its associated **pillars**. The more prominent fold behind the tonsil, extending from the soft palate downward into the lateral pharyngeal wall, is referred to as the **posterior pillar** or **palatopharyngeal arch** or **fold**. Immediately in front of the palatine tonsil is the **anterior pillar** or **palatoglossal arch** or **fold**. The palatopharyngeal and palatoglossal muscles, respectively (Fig. 1.7), form these folds.

Posterior Borders

Just distal to the mandibular second molar in Fig. 1.8 is a small elevation of tissue known as the *retromolar pad.* This dense pad of tissue is immediately posterior to the last tooth in the mandible and covers the retromandibular triangle. This is usually a second or third molar, but in a child the last molar could be a first molar. The posterior extent of the oral cavity is the space between the left and right tonsils and is known as the **fauces**. The word fauces literally means a slit or opening between two places. In this case the fauces is the opening between the oral cavity and the throat. Looking into the oral cavity, you can see the tongue and soft palate. If you depress the tongue with a tongue depressor blade and ask the patient to say "ahhh," the soft palate will rise, enabling examination beyond the oral cavity into the oral pharynx. The posterior pharyngeal wall can be an indicator of the health status of the patient.

Tongue and Floor of Mouth

Tongue

Chapter 24 contains descriptions of structures on the tongue such as filiform, fungiform, vallate or circumvallate papillae, and the roughened lateral surface of the tongue opposite the vallate papillae, which represents rudimentary foliate papillae. These foliate papillae should be carefully examined in a routine oral examination because it is a difficult area to see and might hide early signs of oral cancer. There may also be enlargements of lymphoid tissue at the base of the tongue, which are referred to collectively as the **lingual tonsils**.

If the patient elevates the tongue, the underside or ventral surface of the tongue shows many blood vessels close to the surface. Extending from an area near the tip of the tongue down to the floor of the mouth is a fold of tissue known as the **lingual frenum** or **frenulum**. If this frenum is attached close to the tip of the tongue and is rather short, the tongue will have limited movement.

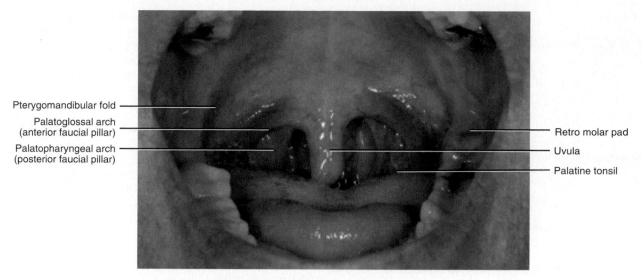

Pterygomandibular fold

Palatoglossal arch
(anterior faucial pillar)

Palatopharyngeal arch
(posterior faucial pillar)

Retro molar pad

Uvula

Palatine tonsil

• **Figure 1.7** Various posterior palatal structures.

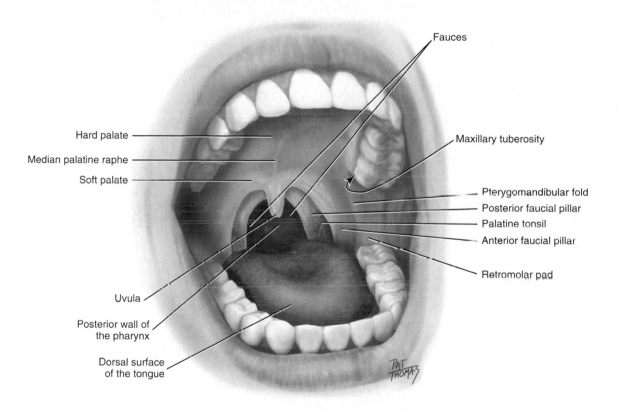

Fauces

Hard palate

Median palatine raphe

Soft palate

Maxillary tuberosity

Pterygomandibular fold

Posterior faucial pillar

Palatine tonsil

Anterior faucial pillar

Retromolar pad

Uvula

Posterior wall of
the pharynx

Dorsal surface
of the tongue

• **Figure 1.8** Note the retromolar pad behind mandibular third molar. The fovea palatinae are located at the junction of the hard and soft palate.

Floor of Mouth

At the base of the lingual frenum is a small elevation on each side known as the **sublingual caruncle**. This is the opening for the ducts of two of the major salivary glands, the submandibular and sublingual glands. Extending from the sublingual caruncle back along the floor of the mouth on either side is a fold of tissue called the **sublingual fold**. A number of small openings of the multiple ducts of the sublingual salivary gland can be found along the anterior and middle parts of this fold. This fold of tissue also marks the paths of a number of structures as they run forward in the floor of the mouth (Fig. 1.9).

Clinical Considerations

Bony swellings on the lingual surface of the mandible at the canine area often occur. These are similar in nature to the palatal tori and are called **mandibular tori** (Fig. 1.10). They may present a problem in radiology because correct image placement may be difficult and sometimes painful for the patient. If the patient requires a lower denture, it is usually necessary to remove the mandibular tori to eliminate undercuts or improper contours that would make denture construction and fit difficult. The same condition can present problems when you are trying to take impressions to fabricate study models. The flange of the tray may strike the area and cause irritation and may also make it difficult to correctly seat the impression tray.

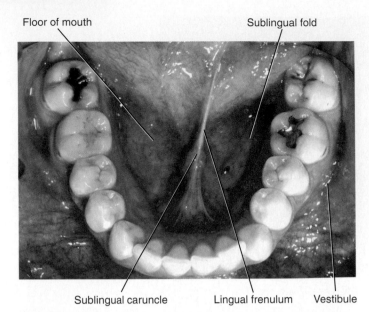

• **Figure 1.9** Sublingual region demonstrating the lingual frenum, attached to the lingual of the tongue. (From Liebgott B. *The Anatomical Basis of Dentistry.* 3rd ed. St. Louis; Mosby; 2011.)

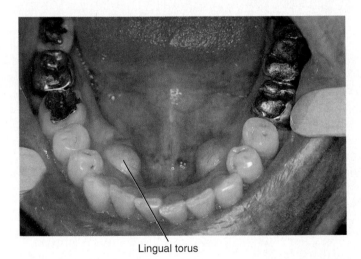

• **Figure 1.10** Another sublingual view demonstrating bony mandibular tori. (From Regezi JA, Scuibba JJ, Jordan RCK. *Oral Pathology: Clinical Pathologic Correlations.* 6th ed. St. Louis: Saunders; 2012.)

The floor of the mouth is supported by the paired mylohyoid muscles, which form a sling from the mylohyoid line on one side of the medial surface of the mandible to the same line on the other side. Contraction of these muscles raises the tongue and floor of the mouth (see Chapter 28). If you look in a mirror while raising your tongue as high as possible, you will see the movement and get an idea of where the mylohyoid muscle is attached to the mandible. This area of attachment is important in denture construction and determines how far into the floor of the mouth the denture flange should extend on the lingual side. If it extends below the mylohyoid line, the denture may be dislodged during elevation of the tongue, or it may irritate the lingual mucosa in that area.

The oral tissue beneath the tongue in the floor of the mouth is one of the thinnest in the oral cavity and therefore quite sensitive to trauma. Note that any of the oral tissues may be traumatized, but some are more susceptible than others. Some of the common injuries seen in a dental practice may relate to hot foods and liquids. Potato chips or bone in foods may cause cutting injuries to various areas of the oral cavity, especially the gingiva. *Be aware that these tissues may be easily injured.*

Other Clinical Manifestations of the Oral Cavity

Although many other chapters in this book refer to the oral cavity, it is important to stress that all readers should be aware of the need for a solid background in the normal anatomy of the oral cavity. It is the responsibility of all who view the intraoral anatomy of the patient to be aware of what the normal anatomy of the oral cavity looks like, regardless of whether you are a dental assistant, laboratory technologist, dental hygienist, or dentist. Legally, the dentist bears the primary responsibility for much of the diagnosis and treatment of the patient, but every member of the team should look carefully for anything that appears abnormal. Because significant differences within the oral cavity exist, it is beneficial for students to examine as many other students in their class as possible. This provides proper perspective on anatomic variation within the general population.

Clinical Considerations

We often think about the effects of oral diseases on other parts of the body, and we consider the spread of dental infections, oral cancers, and so forth. However, we should never lose sight of the fact that problems in other parts of the body may show up early or late in the disease state in the oral cavity. Early stages of measles show up as spots in the oral cavity. Many times, AIDS may be suspected because of oral lesions relating to Kaposi's sarcoma, which is a disease that may be found in association with AIDS. Many types of cancer from other parts of the body may spread to the oral cavity. A young child may be brought to the office because of bleeding gums. The child may have good oral hygiene, and the tissues may not appear notably abnormal, and yet the gums, or gingiva, bleed readily on brushing. One should seriously consider having blood tests run because bleeding gingival tissues in a mouth with good oral hygiene are a possible early sign of leukemia. A reddened, painful tongue may be a sign of vitamin deficiencies, and oral lesions may occur that can be associated with a number of other diseases.

This chapter is not meant to be comprehensive; rather, it is meant to reinforce the fact that all members of the dental team have the responsibility to be observant as they work within the oral cavity. Our patients deserve the very best care and concern that we can provide, and a good, solid knowledge of the normal anatomy of the oral cavity enables any member of the team to spot something abnormal and have the dentist examine it carefully.

Brain Buster

- Perform an oral inspection of your own oral cavity following proper hand hygiene. What did you find?
- The glossary section of a textbook provides definitions of important terms in a book. Please look up the following key terms in the glossary section of this text (at the end of this textbook): **frenum, gingiva, buccal, diastema, pharyngeal.**
- The index section of a textbook indicates what topics can be found in a textbook. Please look up the following pictures using the index of this book, which is located toward the end of this textbook: **uvula, philtrum, retromolar pad, maxillary tori.**

Review Questions

1. What are tori and exostoses? What clinical complications might they cause?
2. Define the boundaries of the vestibule.
3. Are muscles contained in the frenum attachments of the lips?
4. Why is the alveolar mucosa redder than the gingiva?
5. What are the divisions of the palate? What are the transverse ridges in the anterior palate?
6. Where and what is the posterior nasal spine?
7. Which muscle supports the floor of the mouth?
8. What and where is the sublingual caruncle?
9. What makes up the anterior and posterior pillars? What lies between them?
10. What are the fauces?
11. What are the two parts of the oral cavity? What are the boundaries of each part?
12. Why is knowledge of normal anatomy of the oral cavity so important for all members of the dental team?
13. Name three generalized disease states that can be detected by the presence of oral signs or oral lesions.
14. What are Fordyce granules? Describe the appearance of Fordyce granules.

Unit I Test

1. Small, localized growths of bone on the buccal cortical plate are known as
   a. torus mandibularis
   b. exostoses
   c. torus palatinus
   d. torus buccalis
   e. none of the above
2. What are Fordyce granules?
   a. abnormal minor salivary glands
   b. excessive numbers of salivary glands
   c. misplaced sebaceous glands
   d. abnormal hair follicles
   e. intraoral acne pustules/oral pimples
3. What is the location of the fovea palatinae?
   a. in the posterior lateral palate over the opening of the greater palatine foramen
   b. in the anterior palate over the incisive foramen
   c. on either side of the posterior nasal spine
   d. between the anterior and posterior tonsillar pillars
   e. none of the above
4. The space between the left and right palatine tonsils is known as
   a. anterior pillars
   b. posterior pillars
   c. palatoglossal folds
   d. fauces
   e. uvula
5. If denture flanges are overextended, which of the following muscles may cause displacement of the mandibular denture?
   a. styloglossus
   b. hyoglossus
   c. mylohyoid
   d. all of the above
   e. none of the above
6. When the tongue comes forward, which of the following may inhibit its movement?
   a. mandibular condyle
   b. labial frenum
   c. torus mandibularis
   d. lingual frenum
   e. none of the above
7. Which of the following structures is often the cause of a diastema?
   a. maxillary lingual frenum
   b. mandibular lingual frenum
   c. maxillary labial frenum
   d. mandibular labial frenum
   e. all of the above
8. Rugae are located on which landmark in the oral cavity?
   a. hard palate
   b. soft palate
   c. vestibule
   d. tonsillar pillars
9. Which term is commonly called "tongue tied" and refers to a short lingual frenum, limiting tongue movement?
   a. sublingual caruncle
   b. lingual flange
   c. ankyloglossia
   d. fovea lingual
10. The oral cavity is divided into which two parts?
    a. anterior vestibule and posterior vestibule
    b. vestibule and fauces
    c. oral cavity anterior and oral cavity posterior
    d. oral cavity proper and vestibule
    e. fauces and oral cavity proper

Unit I Suggested Readings

Berkovitz BK, Holland GR, Moxham BJ. *Head and Neck Anatomy: A Clinical Reference*. 1st ed. Fall River, Maine: Isis Med; 2001.

Berkovitz BK, et al. *Color Atlas and Textbook of Oral Anatomy, Histology, and Embryology*. 2nd ed. London: Mosby; 2009.

Berkovitz S. *The Cleft Palate Story*. Carol Stream, IL: Quintessence; 2021.

Bevelander G. *Outline of Histology*. 8th ed. St. Louis: Mosby; 1979.

Bhaskar SN. *Orban's Oral Histology and Embryology*. 11th ed. St. Louis: Mosby; 1991.

Carlson BM. *Human Embryology and Developmental Biology*. 6th ed. St. Louis: Mosby; 2019.

Chiego D. *Essentials of Oral Histology and Embryology*. 5th ed. A Clinical Approach. St. Louis: Elsevier; 2018.

Fehrenbach M. *Illustrated Anatomy of the Head and Neck*. 6th ed. St. Louis: Elsevier; 2021.

Larsen WJ. *Essentials of Human Embryology*. 3rd ed. Philadelphia: Harcourt Health Sciences; 2001.

Melfi R. *Permar's Oral Embryo Logy and Microscopic Anatomy: A Textbook for Students in Dental Hygiene*. Philadelphia: Lippincott, Williams & Wilkins; 2000.

Moss-Salentijn L, Hendricks-Klyvert M. *Dental and Oral Tissues: An Introduction*. 3rd ed. Baltimore: Williams & Wilkins; 1990.

Nanci A. *Ten Cate's Oral Histology, Development, Structure and Function*. 9th ed. St. Louis: Elsevier; 2013.

Sadler TW. *Medical Embryology*. 14th ed. Philadelphia: Lippincott, Williams & Wilkins; 2018.

Dental Anatomy

2

The Tooth: Functions and Terms

OBJECTIVES

- To identify the different functions of the teeth
- To identify the different tissues that compose the teeth
- To differentiate between clinical and anatomic crowns and roots
- To define single, bifurcated, and trifurcated roots
- To understand the significance of the crown/root ratio
- To recognize how the functions of teeth determine their shape and size
- To understand the individual functions and therefore the individual differences that exist among incisors, canines, premolars, and molars
- To name and identify the location of the various tooth surfaces
- To name and identify the line angles of the teeth
- To name and identify the point angles of the teeth
- To define the terminology used in naming the landmarks of the teeth

Function of Teeth

Teeth are important in many functions of the body. They are essential for protecting the oral cavity, in acquiring and chewing food, and in aiding the digestive system in breaking down food. The teeth form a hard physical barrier that protects the oral cavity. This shield not only affords protection to the oral structures, but the teeth themselves are formidable weapons. One group of mammals belonging to the order *Carnivora* demonstrates this particularly well. Lions and tigers are members of this order and have well-developed canines that they use as weapons to defend themselves and to attack and kill their prey. The teeth also function in communication. They are necessary for proper speech, phonetics, and even whistling. In many cultures their appearance can be a very attactive feature. In dental anatomy the teeth are studied individually and collectively, including their functions, anchorages, and relationships to one another. Our study, therefore, begins with a discussion of the individual tooth.

Crown and Root

Each tooth has a **crown** and **root** portion. The crown is covered with **enamel,** and the root portion is covered with **cementum.** The crown and root are joined at the **cementoenamel junction (CEJ).** The line that demarcates the crown and root is called the **cervical line,** which is a line that is formed by the junction of the cementum of the root and the enamel of the crown (Fig. 2.1).

The crown portion of the tooth erupts through the **bone** and **gingival tissue.** After eruption it will never again be covered with **gingiva.** Only the cervical third of the crown in healthy young adults is partly covered by this tissue. The tooth continues to erupt from the bone and gingiva until the entire crown is exposed (Fig. 2.2).

A clinical difference is evident between the amount of crown that could be erupted and the actual amount that is visible in the mouth. The **anatomic crown** is the entire crown of the tooth that is covered by enamel, regardless of whether it is erupted. The **clinical crown** is only that part seen above the gingiva. Any part of the unerupted crown is not a part of the clinical crown of the tooth; therefore if the entire anatomic crown does not erupt, the part that is visible is considered the clinical crown, and the unerupted portion is part of the **clinical root** (Fig. 2.3). **Eruption** of a tooth is thus the moving of that tooth through its surrounding tissues so that the clinical crown gradually appears longer.

The tooth has **coronal, cervical, and apical** areas. The coronal portion (crown area) is the part of the tooth that is most incisal or occlusal. The point of a cusp or the incisal edge would be the very most coronal part of a tooth. The cervical area is the area that forms the junction of the crown and the root. The cervical line marks this junction, and that part of the tooth located in this area would be called the **cervix** of the tooth (Fig. 2.4). The apical area ends at the terminal end of the root and is called the **apex.** It is here at the apex of the root that the **apical foramen** of the root canal is located. This apical foramen is the opening into the root canal and is where the blood vessels, nerves, and lymphatic tissues enter the tooth.

The root is held in its position relative to the other teeth in the **dental arch** by being firmly anchored in the bony process of the jaw. The portion of the jaw that supports the teeth is called the **alveolar process.** The bony socket in which the tooth fits is called the **alveolus** (Fig. 2.5). Teeth in the upper part of the jaw are called **maxillary** teeth because they are anchored in the **maxilla.** In the lower jaw they are called **mandibular** teeth because they are anchored in the bone called the **mandible.**

The tooth may have a **single root** (see Fig. 2.1) or **multiple roots** with **bifurcation** or **trifurcation**—that is, division of the root portion into two or three segments (Figs. 2.6 and 2.7). Each root has one **apex** or terminal end. The area between multirooted teeth is called the **furcal region,** and in a healthy bone–tooth relationship it would be filled with bone (see Fig. 2.4). In an unhealthy situation the gingiva and possibly the bone would be missing, and this space would be open and exposed.

Root-to-Crown Ratio

The root anchors the tooth in the bone. The longer and wider the root is, the more it offers resistance to displacement of the tooth.

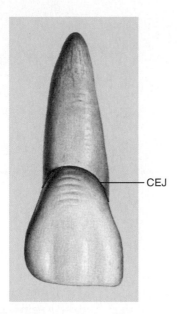

• **Figure 2.1** Maxillary right central incisor. The crown and root are separated by the cementoenamel junction (CEJ). (Modified from Zeisz RC, Nuckolls J. *Dental Anatomy.* St. Louis: Mosby; 1949.)

A tooth with a wider root offers more surface area for periodontal ligaments to attach the tooth to the bone. Both length and surface area play a part in resisting displacement.

It is also true that the longer the tooth root is the more surface area for periodontal attachment. If one root is longer than another (both teeth having the same crown length), the longer root offers more resistance to displacement of the tooth because the longer the root is the more force is necessary to cause movement. This is called the lever principle, which explains the greater proportional force required to displace a small incremental increase in length. It is related purely to length and not surface area. The fulcrum is the bone attached to the tooth, and the lever is that part of the clinical crown exposed above the bone. The longer the clinical crown is the greater the lever and the easier it is to displace the tooth (Fig. 2.8).

This ratio has clinical significance in restorative dentistry in which the length of a clinical crown might make it necessary to change supporting teeth because of an unfavorable root-to-crown ratio (Fig. 2.9). The ratio could also be expressed inversely as a crown to root ratio. The higher the crown-to-root ratio the larger the crown compared with the root and the lower the root-to-crown ratio.

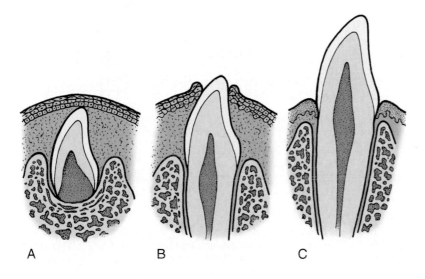

A   B   C

• **Figure 2.2** **(A)** Unerupted tooth. **(B)** Beginning eruption. **(C)** Young adult in which the eruption is almost completed.

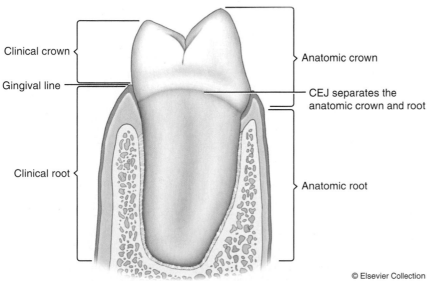

Clinical crown

Gingival line

Clinical root

Anatomic crown

CEJ separates the anatomic crown and root

Anatomic root

© Elsevier Collection

• **Figure 2.3** Longitudinal section of a tooth. The clinical crown and root can change, but the anatomic crown and root always remain the same for any one tooth. *CEJ,* cementoenamel junction.

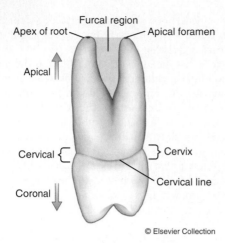

• **Figure 2.4** The closer the location to the apex of the tooth root the more apical is the location. Conversely, the closer the location to the tip of the crown cusp the more coronal it is. The area between the bifurcated roots is called the furcal region. The cervix of the tooth is located in the cervical area.

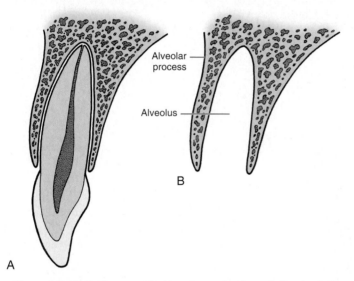

• **Figure 2.5** (A) Tooth surrounded by a bony alveolus. (B) Alveolus is the tooth socket in the alveolar process. This is an upper tooth, so it is an alveolus of the maxillary bone.

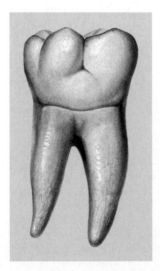

• **Figure 2.6** Bifurcated root: one mesial and one distal. (Modified from Zeisz RC, Nuckolls J. *Dental Anatomy*. St. Louis: Mosby; 1949.)

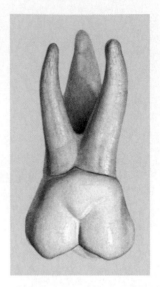

• **Figure 2.7** Trifurcated root: one mesiobuccal, one distobuccal, and one lingual. (Modified from Zeisz RC, Nuckolls J. *Dental Anatomy*. St. Louis: Mosby; 1949.)

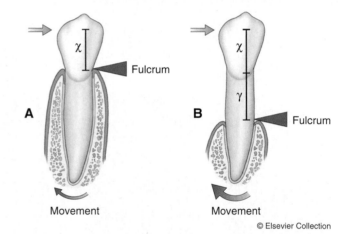

• **Figure 2.8** The force exerted on these two identical teeth is the same. The clinical crowns are different: (A) has a shorter clinical crown than (B). Because the clinical crown acts as a lever and the bone as a fulcrum the tooth with the longer lever magnifies the effects of the force; thus, (B) is affected more. The fact that there is less bone attached to (B) makes it easier to move than (A).

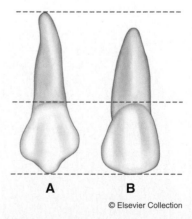

• **Figure 2.9** Tooth (A) has a larger *root-to-crown* ratio than (B). The crowns are nearly equal in length, but the root of (A) is much longer than (B). Another way to say the same thing is (A) has a lesser *crown-to-root ratio*.

Tooth Tissues

The four tooth tissues are enamel, **dentin**, cementum, and **dental pulp** (Fig. 2.10). The first three are **hard tissues,** and the pulp is **soft tissue.**

Enamel

Enamel forms the outer surface of the anatomic crown. It is thickest over the tip of the crown and becomes thinner until it ends at the cervical line. The color of enamel varies with its thickness and mineralization. The thicker the enamel is the whiter it appears. The thinner the enamel is the more it varies, from grayish white at the crown cusps' edges to white in the middle of the tooth to yellow-white at the cervical line where the thin enamel covering is translucent enough to show the yellow tint of the dentin underneath. The more mineralized the enamel the more it lends itself to translucency. These two factors, the mineralization and thickness of enamel, coupled with skin pigmentation, determine the color of the enamel. Older individuals and people with darker skin coloration often display brownish or grayish tones of coloration. Individuals with red or auburn-colored hair often exhibit a slight reddish or brown-red coloration.

Our teeth get darker as we get older. As we age the dentin in our teeth gets darker as the pulp recedes and is replaced by secondary dentin. Years of wear causes our enamel and cementum

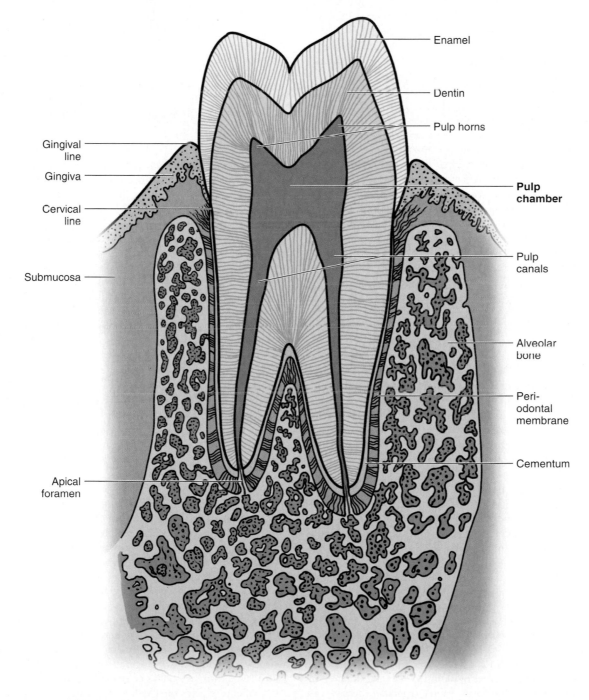

• **Figure 2.10** A pulp cavity is composed of pulp chambers, pulp horns, and root canals. This tooth has two bifurcated roots: one buccal and one lingual. Each root has its own root canal.

to become thinner, allowing the dentin to show through. Stains accumulate on the surface of our teeth with age.

Enamel is the most densely mineralized and hardest tissue in the human body. The chemical composition of enamel is 96% inorganic and 4% organic matter and water. This dense mineralization gives enamel the ability to be more resistant to the wear that the crown of a tooth is subjected to. The hard enamel does not wear very readily; rather, it wears down, grinds up, and crushes almost anything to which it is subjected, including nuts; seeds; ice cubes; and even particles of bone, grit, sand, and leather.

Our ancestors wore the enamel off the occlusal of their teeth because their diet consisted of hard uncooked nuts, fruits, and grains. In addition, their food was unprocessed so that pieces of rock, sand, dirt, and grit were embedded in it. Their lifestyle required chewing leather or bone to fabricate clothing. Often the life expectancy of our ancestors was directly related to whether they still possessed functional teeth. Those who were fortunate enough to have adequate enamel (durable and wear-resistant) were able to live longer and produce more offspring.

Present-day humans rarely wear the enamel off of their teeth. Enamel is not only resistant to wear, but it is very durable and rather resistant to bacteria, mild acids, and tooth decay. The densely packed enamel is smooth, which gives the crown of the tooth a self-cleaning ability, making it difficult for food particles, bacteria, sticky carbohydrate material, and other debris to adhere to the surface of the tooth crown. This self-cleaning ability of enamel and its extreme hardness and resistance to wear make it a nearly perfect outer covering for the crown. Enamel is the hardest and most resilient body tissue and is able to withstand extreme temperatures. The only natural material harder than enamel is a diamond. Still, enamel can be eroded away with severe abrasion and can be broken or chipped under pressure. Even today there is no dental restorative material that possesses the unique qualities of enamel.

Dentin

Dentin forms the main portion or body of the tooth; it comprises the greatest bulk of the tooth because it forms the largest portion of the crown and root. Dentin is wrapped in an envelope of enamel, which covers the crown, and an envelope of cementum, which covers the root.

Dentin is a hard, dense, calcified tissue. It is softer than enamel but harder than cementum or bone. It is yellow in color and elastic in nature. Its chemical composition is 70% inorganic and 30% organic matter and water. Unlike enamel, dentin is capable of adding to itself. When it does this, the new dentin is called **secondary dentin or tertiary dentin.**

Secondary dentin is formed throughout the pulp chamber after the tooth erupts. In time, secondary dentin could completely fill the pulp chamber. When it does completely obliterate the pulp cavity with dentin the tooth becomes nonvital because no nerve or vascular tissue remains inside the tooth. This process does not occur until the individual is well into old age. Secondary dentin grows very slowly and seems to be initiated by regular attrition and wear, which is a normal process of aging.

Tertiary dentin, often called **reparative dentin,** is the dentin that is laid down in response to caries or trauma (Fig. 2.11). It is not clear whether these same odontoblasts or modified odontoblasts form tertiary dentin. Tertiary dentin can take several forms, and each is probably formed by different types of modified cells and initiated by specific types of stimuli. One form, called reparative dentin, can quickly form in response to injuries such as deep decay, fracture, or

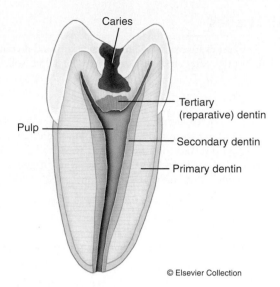

© Elsevier Collection

• **Figure 2.11** Longitudinal section. New dentin is laid down during the entire life of the tooth. Secondary dentin is formed as a normal process of aging. Reparative dentin is formed more quickly in response to major trauma.

when the tooth is subjected to bacterial invasion. Another form, called sclerotic dentin, forms less rapidly and is seen in elderly patients with slow-growing root caries. It can appear as a translucent form of dentin. It is less elastic, very hard, and also occurs under slow-failing restorations.

Tertiary dentin can be initiated by many different traumas, including the following: cracked teeth, occlusal trauma, leaky restorations, exposure into the pulp cavity, deep caries, slowly developing caries, deep restorations, attrition, abrasion, erosion, and any other traumas causing damage to the odontoblastic cell layer. The odontoblastic tissues are the cells within the pulp chamber that form the dentin initially and later in response to the previously listed traumas.

Cementum

Cementum is a bonelike substance that covers the root, although the root is not covered with a perfect layer of cementum. Voids expose small patches of dentin. The main function of cementum is to provide a medium for the attachment of the tooth to the alveolar bone. It is not as dense or as hard as enamel or dentin but is denser than bone, to which it bears a physiologic resemblance. The chemical composition of cementum is 45% to 50% inorganic and 50% to 55% organic, making it a less durable tissue than dentin or enamel. Cementum is quite thin at the cervical line but increases slightly in thickness at the apex of the root. The union of cementum and dentin is called the **dentinocemental junction.**

The two types of cementum are **cellular** and **acellular** (Fig. 2.12). Acellular cementum can cover most of the anatomic root. Cellular cementum is confined to the apical third of the root and can reproduce itself, compensating for the attrition (wear) that occurs on the crown of the tooth and other microtraumas. Cellular cementum derives its name from the fact that the very cells that lie down and form the cementum eventually become entrapped within newly formed cementum. The cells that produce cementum are called **cementoblasts.**

Cementum gives the tooth a mechanism of anchorage that protects and supports the tooth, yet it is self-adjusting and independent

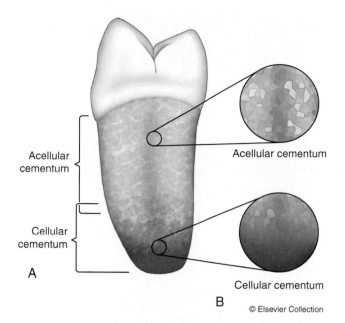

A

Acellular cementum

Cellular cementum

Acellular cementum

Cellular cementum

B
© Elsevier Collection

• **Figure 2.12 (A)** The coronal two-thirds of the root are covered by acellular cementum. The apical third of the root is covered by cellular cementum. At this area the two meet and overlap, and one becomes thinner as the other phases in. **(B)** Cellular cementum covers the root in a meshlike layer of cementum with bare spots of dentin exposed in small areas. The cellular cementum is much thicker, has no bare spots, and is laid down in layers parallel to the root surface.

of the tooth's main nourishment system. The nutrition for cementum is derived from the outside of the tooth through blood vessels that come directly from the bone.

Acellular cementum's primary function is to be part of the attachment system of the tooth. Acellular cementum has Sharpey's fibers embedded in it to anchor the tooth in bone. One end of the Sharpey's fiber is embedded in acellular cementum and the other in bone. Bare spots denuded of cementum can be found in the coronal two-thirds of the root. Although cementum nearly covers the root surface completely, it has a meshlike opening exposing the underlying dentin.

Cellular cementum does not have Sharpey's fibers or bare spots. It is so dense that it has the same cementoblasts that form the cellular cementum that can be trapped inside of it. This is because cellular cementum forms very quickly in response to microtraumas, such as when one tooth chronically hits before the rest of the teeth. It is laid down in layers parallel to the root surface, and new layers are added one on the other. Cellular cementum covers the apical third of the root with the thickest part of the cellular cementum at the apex of the root. Cellular and acellular cementum overlap each other where they meet in the apical third of the root. As the acellular cementum begins to thin out, the cellular cementum phases in and becomes thicker. Cellular cementum does not appear to have an attachment function; instead, it is more of a cushioning function.

Clinical Considerations

When the tooth lays down new layers of cellular cementum in response to trauma, there is a period of new calcification. The newly forming calcified area appears darker on an x-ray image and resembles an infection. If the tooth is sensitive because of this trauma and the x-ray image looks like an infection, then a misdiagnosis could easily occur, and the wrong treatment applied.

Pulp

Dental pulp is the nourishing, sensory, and dentin-reparative system of the tooth. It is composed of blood vessels, lymph vessels, connective tissue, nerve tissue, and special dentin-formation cells called **odontoblasts.**

The pulp is housed in the center of the tooth, with dentin surrounding the pulp tissue. The walls of the **pulp cavity** are lined with odontoblasts, the chief function of which is to lay down primary, secondary, and tertiary dentin. The odontoblasts lay down primary dentin when the tooth is first formed. After the tooth has erupted and is in occlusion, odontoblasts begin to form secondary dentin. Later the tooth lays down tertiary dentin in response to specific types of trauma.

In all instances, the blood vessels of the pulp bring in the nourishment necessary to activate and support the formation of dentin. In addition, the blood vessels also supply the white blood cells necessary to fight bacterial invasion within the pulp. The lymph tissue filters the fluids within the tooth, and the nerve tissue responds to pain and does not differentiate the cause. The nerves in the tooth cannot respond to cold or heat, only pain. Pressure can be felt but that is a response elicited from the periodontal ligament outside the tooth and not the pulp tissue inside the tooth.

Anatomically the pulp is divided into two areas: the **pulp chamber** and the **pulp canals** or **root canals.** The pulp chamber is housed within the coronal portion of the tooth, and the pulp canals are located within the roots of the tooth. Together the pulp chamber and pulp canals are referred to as the pulp cavity; thus the pulp cavity runs the entire length of the interior of the tooth from the tip of the pulp chamber (the **pulp horns**) to the apical foramen at the apex of the root canal (see Fig. 2.10).

Clinical Considerations

In the case of a patient with a possible infection at the end of the root, the treatment is dependent knowing if the tooth is alive. If the tooth is nonvital (dead) a root canal or extraction would be indicated. If the tooth is sensitive to pressure, is mobile, and shows a dark area (radiolucency) on the radiograph it could be an infection caused by a dying tooth, or it could be an alive tooth with newly formed cellular cementum and the tooth might be sensitive and loose because of occlusal trauma. The dental provider would perform vitality tests to determine whether the tooth is alive. These tests sometimes rely on ice or heat touching the tooth and causing a pain response in a vital (alive) tooth. The tooth cannot differentiate between hot or cold, but it can elicit a pain response if the ice or heat causes discomfort. If the patient feels pain the dental practitioner knows the tooth is alive.

Types of Teeth

The functions of teeth vary, depending on their individual shape and size and their location in the jaws. The three basic food-processing functions of the teeth are cutting, holding, and grinding.

Incisors

The **incisors** are designed to cut (incisor means "that which makes an incision, or cut"), and the biting edge is called an *incisal edge* (Fig. 2.13). The tongue side, or lingual surface, is shaped like a *shovel* to aid in guiding the food into the mouth (Fig. 2.14). When we bite into something we are actually using the incisal edges of our incisors as scissors to shear off a piece of food. In this example these edges are used as cutting tools. All teeth can also be used as holding or grasping tools and as tearing tools to some

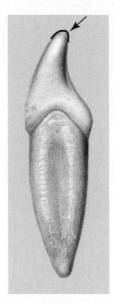

• **Figure 2.13** Mandibular central incisor. Notice the incisal edge *(arrow),* which incises or cuts food. (Modified from Zeiss RC, Nuckolls J. *Dental Anatomy.* St. Louis: Mosby; 1949.)

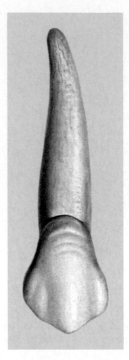

• **Figure 2.15** Maxillary canine. The bulk of the canine root affords resistance to displacement. (Modified from Zeisz RC, Nuckolls J. *Dental Anatomy.* St. Louis: Mosby; 1949.)

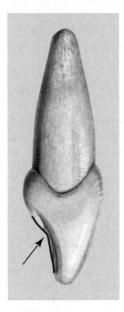

• **Figure 2.14** Shoveled-out lingual aspect of a maxillary right central incisor *(arrow).* (Modified from Zeisz RC, Nuckolls J. *Dental Anatomy.* St. Louis: Mosby; 1949.)

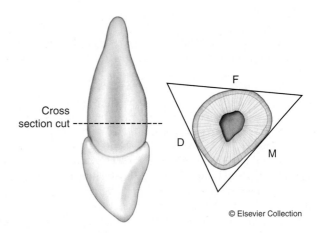

© Elsevier Collection

• **Figure 2.16** Cross-section of maxillary right canine. The triangular shape of the maxillary canine root affords resistance to forces that would dislodge it.

extent, but the primary function of incisors is to cut through something. In humans there are eight incisors: four maxillary and four mandibular with two on each side.

Canines

The **canines** are designed to function as holding or grasping teeth. When we look at canines they resemble spearheads, which are used primarily to pierce and grasp. The importance of these teeth can be seen in dogs, for example, whose genus, *Canis,* is named for these teeth. The dog uses the canines as a weapon to pierce and hold its prey.

In humans the canines also function to protect the jaw joint during side jaw movements (see Chapters 6 and 13). The canines

are often the only teeth touching when you move your jaw sideways. This affords a level of protection to both the teeth and the jaws. The greater length and thickness of the canines allows for lateral stress-bearing support during side-to-side jaw excursions. The canines are the longest teeth in human dentition. They are also some of the best-anchored and most stable teeth because they have the longest roots of any teeth (Fig. 2.15); therefore maxillary canines have the highest root-to-crown ratio of any teeth. Canine roots are shaped triangularly in cross-section. This triangular root shape makes it possible for a canine to hold its place in the corner of the mouth. This shape resists anterior, posterior, and lateral forces of displacement as well as forces that would rotate or turn the tooth within its bony socket (Fig. 2.16). There are two maxillary and two mandibular canines, one on each side.

Premolars

Premolars are a cross between canines and molars and are not as long as canines. They usually have at least two **cusps** rather than one large incisal edge. Like canines, they aid in holding food, but they function to help grind rather than incise food. Their pointed buccal cusps hold the food while the lingual cusps grind it, making their function similar to that of the molars.

Premolars are sometimes referred to as **bicuspids.** The term *bicuspid* is not accurate, however, because it implies only two cusps and some premolars have three. Therefore the term *premolar* is preferred (Fig. 2.17). There are four maxillary and four mandibular **premolars** with two on each side.

Molars

Molars are much larger than premolars and usually have four or more cusps. Each molar resembles two premolars fused together as one. Also, molars are located more posteriorly than the premolars. The function of the 12 molars is to chew or grind up food. The maxillary molars interlock with the mandibular molars and form a crushing mechanism. They do not incise food, and, like premolars, they do not have incisal edges; instead, they have cusps, which are designed to interlock together. This intertwining of the upper and lower molars allows for a grinding and crushing of food. There can be three, four, or five cusps on the occlusal surface of each molar, depending on its location and the occurrence of normal variations (Fig. 2.18). Maxillary and mandibular molars differ greatly from each other in shape, size, number of cusps, and number of roots. There are three maxillary and three mandibular molars on each side.

The incisors and canines are called **anterior** teeth because they occupy the anterior, or front, of the dental arch. Premolars and molars occupy the back portion of the arch and are called **posterior** teeth.

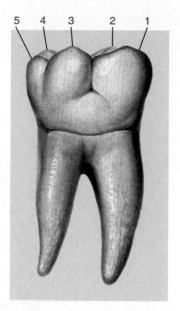

• **Figure 2.18** Mandibular first molar. This lower molar has five cusps. (Modified from Zeisz RC, Nuckolls J. *Dental Anatomy.* St. Louis: Mosby; 1949.)

Surfaces of Teeth

If one dentist wants to communicate a specific location on a specific tooth to another dentist, a staff member, or an insurance company, both parties must use and understand the same dental terminology. In this way they can convey the proper concepts in an oral or written form, and each party knows what the exact location is on the tooth they are discussing. Just as a map is divided into north, south, east, and west, the crowns of teeth are divided into **surfaces,** which are named according to the direction in which they face in a perfect dentition. Anterior teeth have four surfaces and a ridge, whereas posterior teeth have five surfaces (Fig. 2.19), including the four sides and the top of a tooth. The side surfaces can also be used to identify locations on the tooth root.

If the surface of a tooth faces the tongue, it is called the **lingual surface.** If the surface faces the cheek or lip, it is called the **facial surface,** also known as the **labial** (lip) **surface** if it is an anterior tooth or the **buccal** (cheek) **surface** if it is a posterior tooth (see Fig. 2.19). The surface of a tooth that faces the neighboring tooth's surface in the same arch (next to each other) is called a **proximal surface,** and each tooth has two proximal surfaces, mesial and distal. The **mesial proximal surface** of a tooth is closest to the **midline** of the face, and the **distal proximal surface** faces away from the midline. The fifth surface of the posterior teeth is called the **occlusal surface,** or biting surface of the tooth. It is also called the **occluding** or chewing surface. The occlusal surfaces of the mandibular posterior teeth hit against the occlusal surfaces of the maxillary teeth when the jaw closes (Figs. 2.19 and 2.20).

There are differing viewpoints as to whether the anterior teeth have a fifth surface. They have a biting edge called an *incisal ridge,* and some authors contend that this **incisal ridge** is an incisal surface. Therefore any reference to the incisal surface is referring to the incisal ridge of an anterior tooth. After studying the following sections on line and point angles, it will make more sense to consider the anterior teeth as having five surfaces (Fig. 2.21).

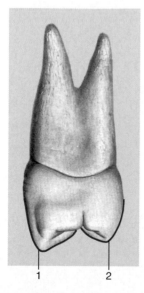

• **Figure 2.17** Maxillary first premolar with two cusps. (Modified from Zeisz RC, Nuckolls J. *Dental Anatomy.* St. Louis: Mosby; 1949.)

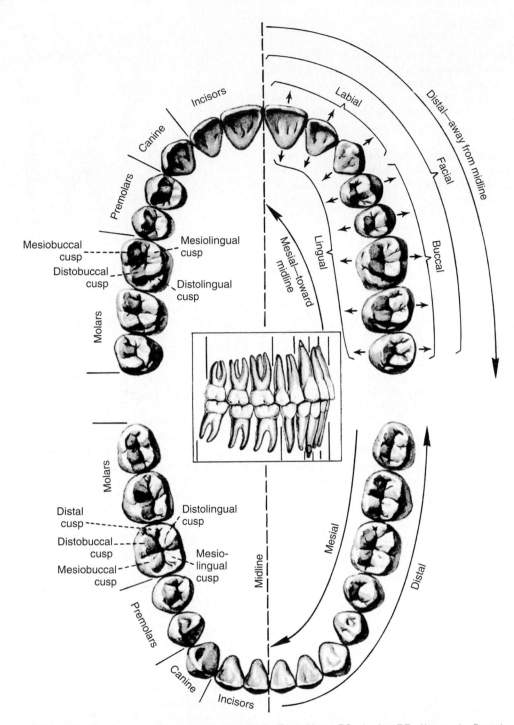

• **Figure 2.19** Permanent arch (terms of orientation). (From Kraus BS, Jordon RE, Abrams L. *Dental Anatomy and Occlusion*. Baltimore: Williams & Wilkins; 1969.)

Division of Surfaces

For the purpose of facilitating the location of various areas within a specific surface of a tooth, the surface is divided into thirds. The lingual surface of a tooth is divided into a **mesial, middle,** and **distal third.** The facial surfaces are divided in the same manner (Fig. 2.22). The proximal surfaces of a tooth are divided into a **facial,** middle, and **lingual third.** Each third is named for the surface to which it is closest, except for the **middle third.**

The teeth can be divided into divisions perpendicular to these surfaces so that any of the proximal, facial, or lingual surfaces can be further divided into an **incisal,** middle, and **cervical third.** On posterior teeth the **incisal third** is called the **occlusal third.**

Line Angles

A **line angle** separates two surfaces of a tooth by forming the junction of the two surfaces (Figs. 2.23 and 2.24). For instance,

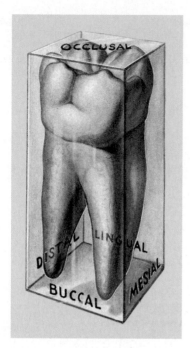

• **Figure 2.20** Surfaces of a mandibular right first molar. (Modified from Zeisz RC, Nuckolls J. *Dental Anatomy.* St. Louis: Mosby; 1949.)

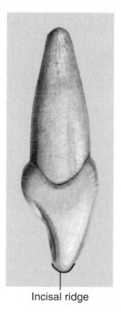

Incisal ridge

• **Figure 2.21** Incisal ridge of the central incisor. Even though the incisal ridge is small, it is treated independently. (Modified from Zeisz RC, Nuckolls J. *Dental Anatomy.* St. Louis: Mosby; 1949.)

the junction of the buccal surface and the occlusal surface of a tooth is a line angle. Because the line angles are named according to the surfaces they join, the line angle that separates the buccal and the occlusal surfaces is called the *buccoocclusal line angle*. Line angles are named by their proximal name (mesial or distal) first and their incisal or occlusal last. The various combinations are listed in the following tables.

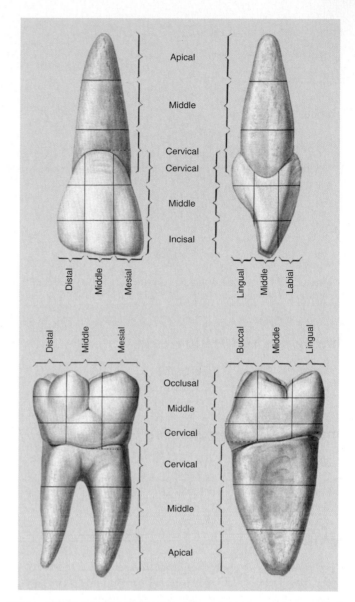

• **Figure 2.22** A maxillary right permanent central incisor and a mandibular right permanent first molar. (Modified from Zeisz RC, Nuckolls J. *Dental Anatomy.* St. Louis: Mosby; 1949.)

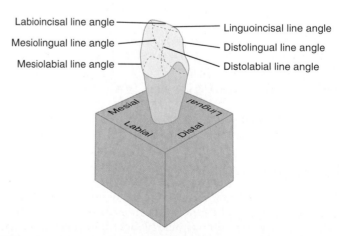

Labioincisal line angle — Linguoincisal line angle
Mesiolingual line angle — Distolingual line angle
Mesiolabial line angle — Distolabial line angle

• **Figure 2.23** Line angles for anterior teeth. (From Nelson SJ, Ash M. *Wheeler's Dental Anatomy.* 9th ed. St. Louis: Saunders; 2010.)

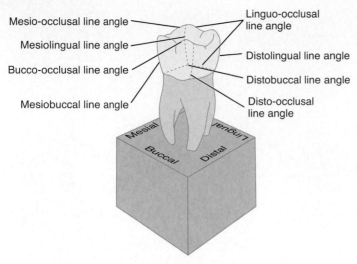

• **Figure 2.24** Line angles for posterior teeth. (From Nelson SJ, Ash M. *Wheeler's Dental Anatomy.* 9th ed. St. Louis; Saunders, 2010.)

Line Angles for Anterior Teeth

Distolabial	Mesiolingual
Mesiolabial	Linguoincisal
Distolingual	Labioincisal

Line Angles for Posterior Teeth

Distobuccal	Distoocclusal
Mesiobuccal	Mesioocclusal
Distolingual	Buccoocclusal
Mesiolingual	Linguoocclusal

Point Angles

A **point angle** is the point at which three surfaces meet. For instance, the point at which the mesial, labial, and incisal surfaces join is called the *mesiolabioincisal point angle* (Figs. 2.25 and 2.26). The point angles are named in this order: first the proximal (mesial or distal), then the facial (labial or buccal) or lingual, and then the incisal or occlusal.

Point Angles for Anterior Teeth

Mesiolabioincisal	Distolabioincisal
Mesiolinguoincisal	Distolinguoincisal

Point Angles for Posterior Teeth

Mesiobuccoocclusal	Distobuccoocclusal
Mesiolinguoocclusal	Distolinguoocclusal

Landmarks

The student must know basic landmarks to be able to study individual teeth. When the crowns are formed, they develop from four or more growth centers called **lobes.** These lobes grow and eventually fuse, but a line remains on the erupted tooth where fusion of the lobes took place. These shallow grooves or lines that

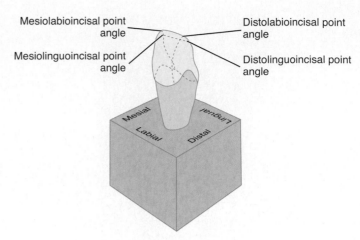

• **Figure 2.25** Point angles for anterior teeth. (From Nelson SJ, Ash M. *Wheeler's Dental Anatomy.* 9th ed. St. Louis: Saunders; 2010.)

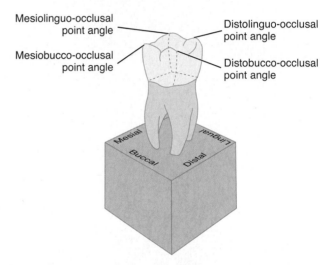

• **Figure 2.26** Point angles for posterior teeth. (From Nelson SJ, Ash M. *Wheeler's Dental Anatomy.* 9th ed. St. Louis: Saunders; 2010.)

separate primary parts of the crown or root are called **developmental grooves** (Fig. 2.27).

Incisors, canines, and most premolars are developed from three facial lobes and one lingual lobe. Second molars are developed from four lobes, two facial and two lingual. Most first molars are developed from five lobes; the maxillary has two facial and three lingual lobes, and the mandibular has two lingual and three facial lobes. Viewpoints vary as to whether the fifth cusp or cusp of Carabelli of the maxillary molars is a true cusp. If this fifth cusp is well pronounced and developed then many believe it is a true cusp and is formed from its own separate lobe. This is the case for many maxillary first molars when there may be five cusps from five lobes (Fig. 2.28). Maxillary second and (less frequently) third molars may have a small tubercle but not a true fifth cusp. In the latter cases the cusp of Carabelli (if present) is a tubercle not a cusp. In rare instances maxillary third molars may only have three cusps although most have four, whereas many have five and a very few have six or more cusps. Most second premolars have three cusps but some will have four. In Fig. 2.27 the lines separating the lobes represent developmental grooves, and the lobes are numbered. These variations will be studied in later sections of this book.

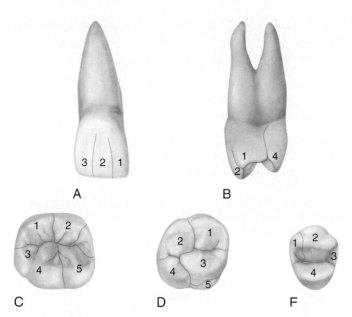

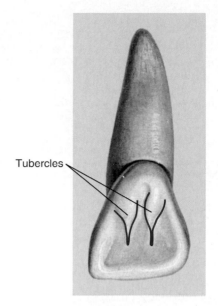

• **Figure 2.27** Lobes of teeth. **(A)** Maxillary central incisor. **(B)** Maxillary first premolar. **(C)** Mandibular first molar. **(D)** Maxillary first molar. **(E)** Maxillary premolar. Lines separating the lobes are developmental grooves. (From Nelson SJ, Ash M. *Wheeler's Dental Anatomy.* 9th ed. St. Louis: Saunders; 2010.)

• **Figure 2.29** Maxillary central incisor, lingual view. Tubercles of an anterior tooth extend from the cingulum onto the lingual fossa. (Modified from Zeisz RC, Nuckolls J. *Dental Anatomy.* St. Louis: Mosby; 1949.)

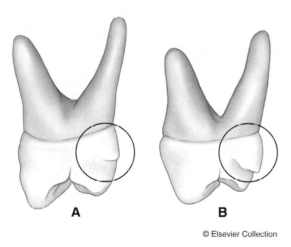

© Elsevier Collection

• **Figure 2.28** **(A)** Shows a maxillary right first molar with a small fifth cusp. In reality it is not a cusp but a tubercle. **(B)** Shows a more developed cusp of Carabelli, which may have been formed from its own lobe.

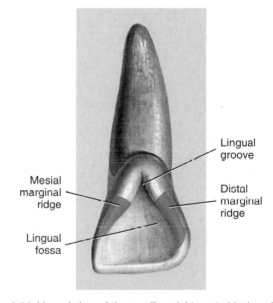

• **Figure 2.30** Lingual view of the maxillary right central incisor. (Modified from Zeisz RC, Nuckolls J. *Dental Anatomy.* St. Louis: Mosby; 1949.)

A **tubercle** is a small elevation of enamel on some portion of the crown of the tooth. It does not always occur on the lingual surface of a tooth but can occur on an area such as the labial or occlusal surface (Fig. 2.29).

The **fossa** of a tooth is a depression or concavity, which is an area on the tooth that is indented, or concave. Fossae are named for their location; for instance, a lingual fossa is on the lingual surface of a tooth (Fig. 2.30). On the anterior teeth a lingual fossa is between the **marginal ridges** and incisal to the **cingulum**. On canines, two lingual fossae are evident; on premolars, triangular fossae are on the occlusal surfaces, mesial or distal to the marginal ridges, and between cusps along the central developmental groove.

When a pinpoint hole is evident within the fossa or anywhere on the tooth, this depression is called a **pit.** Pits usually occur along the developmental grooves or in the fossae (Fig. 2.31). Pits are named for their location on a tooth; a lingual pit occurs on the lingual surface of a tooth, a buccal pit occurs on the buccal surface of a tooth, and an occlusal pit on the occlusal surface.

A **cusp** is a mound on the crown portion of the tooth that makes up a major division of its occlusal or incisal surface. Cusps are found on premolars, molars, and canines. They are not, however, found on incisors. The difference between a tubercle, which is a smaller elevation on a tooth, and a cusp is that a cusp makes up a major or divisional part of the occlusal or incisal surface, and a tubercle does not.

A **ridge** is an elevated portion of a tooth that runs in a line (Fig. 2.32). Ridges are named for their location, such as the

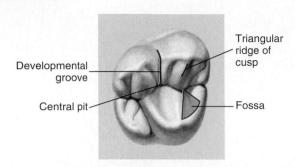

• Figure 2.31 Maxillary right second molar. (Modified from Zeisz RC, Nickels J. *Dental Anatomy.* St. Louis: Mosby; 1942.)

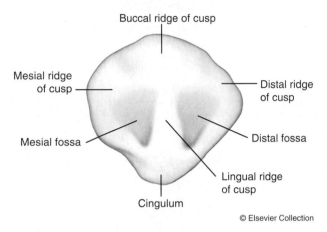

© Elsevier Collection

• Figure 2.32 Mandibular right canine, occlusal view. Four ridges form every cusp. The lower canine also has two fossae, one on each side of the lingual ridge of the cusp.

linguocervical ridge or the distal and mesial marginal ridges. All cusps have four ridges: buccal (or labial), lingual, mesial, and distal.

Marginal ridges are the rounded borders of enamel that form the mesial and distal shoulders of the occlusal surfaces of the posterior teeth and the mesial and distal shoulders of the lingual surface of the anterior teeth (Fig. 2.33).

A **concavity** is a carved-out section or area, like a cave or empty bowl; fossae and pits are concavities. The opposite of concavity is **convexity,** or a bulging out. The ridges of a tooth, a tubercle, and a cusp tip are convex (Fig. 2.34).

Anterior Teeth

Anterior teeth show two developmental grooves on their labial surfaces. These two grooves separate the three lobes that form the labial surface (see Fig. 2.27A). The fourth developmental lobe of anterior teeth occurs on the lingual surface of the crown (Fig. 2.35). This fourth lobe is the cingulum, and it makes up the bulk of the cervical third of the lingual surface of an anterior tooth. The developmental line that separates this fourth lobe from the labial lobes is called the **lingual groove** (see Fig. 2.35). A lingual developmental groove may not always be a single groove; rather, it may be several grooves interrupted by a tubercle (see Fig. 2.32).

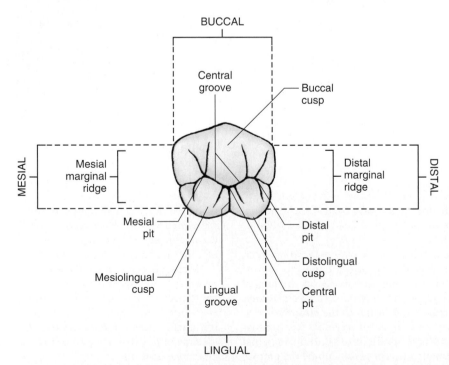

• Figure 2.33 Occlusal surface of a mandibular right second premolar (three-cusp variety). (Modified from Zeisz RC, Nickels J. *Dental Anatomy.* St. Louis: Mosby; 1942.)

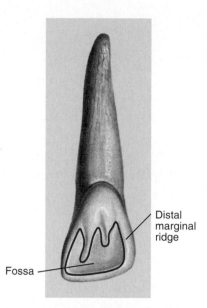

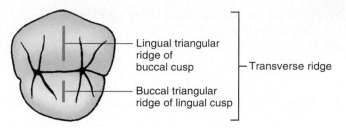

• **Figure 2.36** Occlusal view of maxillary right first premolar. (Modified from Zeisz RC, Nuckolls J. *Dental Anatomy.* St. Louis: Mosby; 1949.)

• **Figure 2.34** Fossa and ridges of a tooth. The fossa is a concavity or depression, and the ridge is a convexity or bulge. (Modified from Zeisz RC, Nuckolls J. *Dental Anatomy.* St. Louis: Mosby; 1949.)

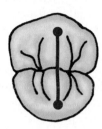

• **Figure 2.37** Maxillary right first premolar. The transverse ridge is formed by the lingual ridge of the buccal cusp and the buccal ridge of the lingual cusp.

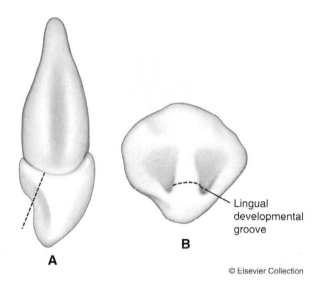

© Elsevier Collection

• **Figure 2.35** **(A)** Maxillary right canine distal view. The dotted line separates the lingual lobe from the facial lobe. **(B)** Occlusal view. The lingual developmental groove separates the facial lobes from the lingual lobe.

Posterior Teeth

The most obvious landmarks on the posterior teeth are the cusps. The number varies according to the tooth; these were discussed earlier under the individual teeth.

The cusps are formed by four ridges. The most obvious of which are the triangular ridges (Fig. 2.36). **Triangular ridges** are the main ridges on each cusp that run from the tip of the cusp to the central part of the occlusal surface. Thus the triangular ridge of the mesiobuccal cusp is the lingual ridge of the cusp that runs to the center of the occlusal surface, whereas the triangular ridge of the mesiolingual cusp is the buccal ridge that runs from the tip of the cusp to the center of the occlusal surface (see Fig. 2.27). A **transverse ridge** is the union of two triangular ridges, a buccal and a lingual, which cross the occlusal surface of a posterior tooth (Fig. 2.37).

Review Questions

1. What line separates the enamel from the cementum of the tooth?
2. How could a portion of the anatomic crown be a part of the clinical root?
3. How many roots are present in a trifurcated and in a bifurcated tooth?
4. Are maxillary teeth upper or lower jaw teeth?
5. Which tooth tissue composes the bulk of the tooth?
6. Which tooth tissue is the hardest?
7. Which tooth tissue is the softest?
8. Which tooth tissues have their own nourishment system?
9. Which tooth tissue is most like bone?
10. What is the main nourishment system of the tooth?
11. Name the different parts of the pulp cavity.
12. Is the pulp horn a part of the pulp chamber or the pulp canal?
13. What does the pulp tissue comprise?
14. The longer the root is, compared with the crown of a tooth, the more resistant a tooth has to displacement. How does a longer root affect a tooth's resistance to displacement?
15. What is the difference between the alveolus and the alveolar process?
16. Which is seen in the mouth first, the clinical or anatomic crown?
17. What is the percentage of inorganic material in enamel? In dentin? In cementum?
18. Enamel is harder than dentin, and dentin is harder than cementum. How does this correlate to the percentages of inorganic versus organic materials present in these tissues?

19. What are the basic functions of the teeth? What determines each tooth's functions?
20. What are the longest teeth in human dentition? Why are they considered the longest? How do the maxillary and mandibular compare?
21. Why is the term *bicuspid* inaccurate compared with *premolar*?
22. What is the function of the molars, and how do the cusps perform this function?
23. How many premolars and how many molars are there in permanent dentition?
24. How many surfaces are on a posterior tooth? Name them.
25. Which proximal surface is farther away from the midline, and which is closest to the midline?
26. If the anterior teeth do not have a fifth surface, what do they have that replaces the fifth surface?
27. What is a line angle? Name the six line angles for the anterior teeth and the eight for the posterior teeth.
28. What is a point angle?
29. The developmental grooves separate the lobes of a tooth. How many lobes does an anterior tooth have?
30. What separates the cingulum on an anterior tooth from the labial lobes?
31. What is the small elevation of enamel on some portion of the crown of a tooth?
32. What is the small pinpoint depression that occurs along a developmental groove?
33. Explain the difference between a tubercle and a cusp.
34. Which of the following are considered convex or concave?
    a. empty swimming pool
    b. empty soup bowl
    c. cave
    d. ridge of a mountain
    e. cusp tip
    f. valley between two hills
    g. a marginal ridge
    h. lingual fossa of an anterior tooth
35. Explain the difference between a developmental groove and a pit.
36. Identify the unlabeled surfaces of the mandibular right first molar that are missing in Fig. 2.38.
37. How many lobes or growth centers does it take to form the tooth in Fig. 2.39?
38. Identify the two triangular ridges in Fig. 2.40.
39. The developmental, elevated, rounded mound of the crown that forms a major division of the occlusal surface is a
    a. lobe
    b. tubercle
    c. cusp
    d. ridge

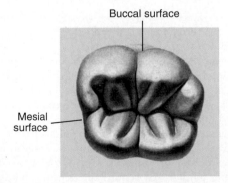

Buccal surface

Mesial surface

• **Figure 2.38** (Modified from Zeisz RC, Nuckolls J. *Dental Anatomy.* St. Louis: Mosby; 1949.)

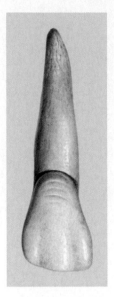

• **Figure 2.39** (Modified from Zeisz RC, Nuckolls J. *Dental Anatomy.* St. Louis: Mosby; 1949.)

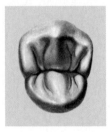

• **Figure 2.40** (Modified from Zeisz RC, Nuckolls J. *Dental Anatomy.* St. Louis: Mosby; 1949.)

40. A developmental elevated projection on the lingual surface of a newly erupted incisor is a
    a. ridge
    b. tubercle
    c. cusp
    d. cingulum
41. If a maxillary central incisor has an almost transparent incisal edge and a maxillary lateral incisor has a very white line covering its incisal edge, which incisor is more mineralized at its incisal edge?
    a. the central
    b. the lateral
    c. not enough evidence to determine
    d. the white spot is a sign of a more mineralized and healthier incisal edge area.
42. What type of specialized cells form dentin?
43. Which type of cementum is part of the system that anchors the tooth to the bone?
44. Name the two types of cementum.
45. What types of dentin form in response to deep tooth decay? Refer to the sections in Chapter 20 concerning enamel composition, dentin composition, formation of regular dentin, and formation of secondary dentin, and the section in Chapter 21 concerning cementum formation. These discussions contain much more detailed information about the material covered.

3

Fundamental and Preventative Curvatures
Proximal Alignment of the Teeth and Protection of the Periodontium

OBJECTIVES

- To identify the successful characteristics of tooth shape and alignment in protecting the periodontium
- To understand that the teeth are shaped to align next to each other to preserve the dentition
- To identify the proximal contact areas
- To identify contact points

2. Size and location of interproximal spaces formed by the proximal contact surfaces
3. Location and effectiveness of the embrasures or spillways
4. Facial and lingual **contours** on the labial, buccal, and lingual surfaces of crowns
5. Amount of curvature of the cementoenamel junction (CEJ) on the mesial and distal surfaces of the various teeth
6. Self-cleaning qualities of the tooth, smoothness of the enamel, and overall shape of the tooth to meet its function
7. Occlusal and incisal curvatures and contours

Evolution of Fundamental and Preventative Curvatures and Proximal Alignment of the Teeth

Over millions of years of evolution, the teeth have gradually developed a specific shape, with fundamental curvatures at certain areas on each tooth representing successful adaptation toward the maintenance of the teeth within the dental arch. In other words, the curvatures aid the teeth in preventing disease, damage, bacterial invasion, and calculus buildup; dispersing excessive occlusal trauma and biting forces; and protecting the gingiva and **periodontium.** The periodontium comprises the supporting structures surrounding the teeth. If these tissues are damaged, then the vascularity, interdental papillary tissue, gingiva, and finally the bone between and surrounding the teeth will be jeopardized, decreasing the life expectancy of the tooth within the dental arch.

Throughout evolution, the curvatures, by preserving the teeth, also increased the life expectancy and productivity of the possessor. As the life expectancy of the animal or person increased, so did the number of potential offspring. Thus through the process of evolution and through successful traits outnumbering, outlasting, and outproducing the less successful traits, the teeth of modern humans possess certain successful characteristics of shape and **alignment** (their position in the jaw). Some of these successful adaptations and characteristics are as follows:

1. Specific location and size of proximal (mesial or distal) contact areas of various teeth

Proximal Contact Areas

The **proximal** (mesial or distal) **contact areas** of the teeth are the areas on the surfaces of the teeth in which the proximal surfaces touch one another. The contact area between two teeth prevents food from packing between them. In a healthy mouth, the contact surface formed is small enough to prevent a buildup of excessive amounts of bacteria, food, and proximal debris but large enough to be an effective barrier to prevent food from packing between the teeth. This affords protection to the underlying gingiva tissue between teeth. Finally, because the teeth do slightly touch, they offer support and anchorage to one another and resistance to displacement from traumatic forces.

Finally, we must remember that two adjacent teeth share the same interproximal bone. The same bone that supports the distal root portion of the first tooth also supports the mesial root portion of the second tooth. If something happens to cause the loss of this bone, it affects both teeth. Sometimes a periodontally involved tooth is removed to protect a neighboring tooth. By removing the tooth with the most bone loss, the periodontium of the adjacent tooth has a chance to heal.

The proximal contact areas are located on the mesial and distal surfaces of each tooth at the widest portion and the greatest curvature. The **distal contact area** of one tooth touches the **mesial contact area** of the tooth posterior to it. For example, the distal contact area of the mandibular first premolar touches its posterior neighbor, the mandibular second premolar.

Fig. 3.1 shows the contact areas of two premolars. The contact area on the distal surface of the first premolar is called the *distal*

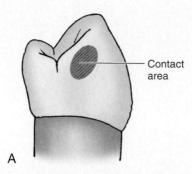
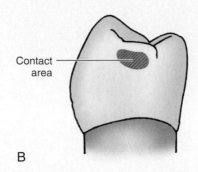

• **Figure 3.1** This is where the distal contact area (shaded) of the mandibular first premolar **(A)** touches the mesial contact area (shaded) of the second premolar **(B)**. (Modified from Zeisz RC, Nuckolls J. *Dental Anatomy.* St. Louis: Mosby; 1949.)

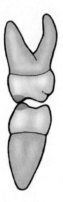
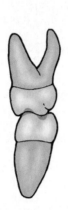
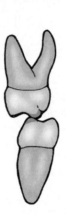

• **Figure 3.2** Contact points of a maxillary molar occluding with a mandibular molar in three different positions. A contact area is where two teeth in the same arch touch; a contact point is where a tooth in one arch touches a tooth in the opposite arch. (From Nelson SJ, Ash M. *Wheeler's Dental Anatomy.* 9th ed. St. Louis: Saunders; 2010.)

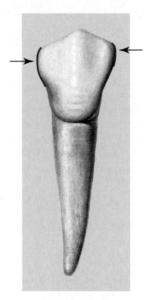

• **Figure 3.3** Buccal view of a lower first premolar with contact areas *(arrows)*. (Modified from Zeisz RC, Nuckolls J. *Dental Anatomy.* St. Louis: Mosby; 1949.)

contact area. What would the contact area on the mesial surface of the second premolar be called? The contact area is not just a point but rather a flattened portion of the tooth where it actually touches the tooth next to it in the same dental arch.

A **contact point** differs from a contact area. A contact point is where the occlusal cusp of one tooth touches the occlusal portion of another tooth in the opposing arch (Fig. 3.2). The contact point of a maxillary tooth hits (occludes and makes contact with) the occlusal surface of a mandibular tooth.

Looking at a buccal view of a tooth (Fig. 3.3), notice that the contact area occurs at the portion of the tooth that has the greatest curvature. In other words, the distal contact area occurs at the part of the distal portion of the tooth that bulges or curves out the most.

Even from an occlusal view (see Fig 3.8), it is apparent that, although the proximal contacts do not take up the entire surface, at least a considerable portion of the proximal surface does touch the adjacent tooth.

Interproximal Spaces

Interproximal spaces are triangular-shaped spaces between the teeth formed by the gingiva on one side and the proximal surfaces and their contact area on the other side (Fig. 3.4). The contact area forms the apex of the triangle, the proximal surfaces form the

sides, and the gingiva makes up the base. These spaces are normally filled with gingival tissue called **papillary gingiva** or **interdental papilla.** By its presence, the interdental papilla keeps food from collecting cervically to the contact areas between the teeth. The normal **interdental space** (space between teeth) provides a place for a bulk of bone, thus affording better anchorage and support. This space is wider cervically than occlusally to provide more access for the vascular support to nourish the interdental bone and papillary tissue. This also affords a stronger bony base.

The interdental space could be very large if a tooth is missing or if a diastema is present (Fig. 3.5) A **diastema** is the space between teeth in the same dental arch; it can be a tiny space that just barely traps food or a large space like in Fig. 3.5.

When gingival recession occurs between the teeth, the interdental papilla and bone no longer fill the entire interdental space; a void exists cervically to the contact area. This void is called a **cervical embrasure.** The more interdental papilla missing, the larger the interproximal space or cervical embrasure. When the papillary tissue recedes, the gingiva goes away as well as the supporting bone, periodontal ligaments, connective tissue, and vascular tissues. Cervical embrasures, also called **gingival**

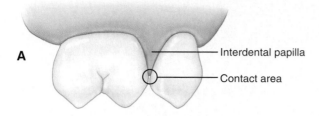

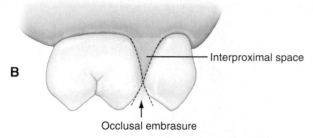

• **Figure 3.4** Buccal view of interdental papilla. Healthy papillary gingiva exhibits very small interproximal spaces.

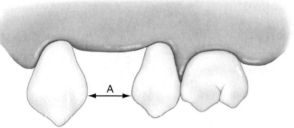

• **Figure 3.5** Buccal view maxillary left permanent arch. Interdental space represented by arrow *(A)* is the space between teeth. In this case the space is as large as a tooth. The space is being held for a yet-to-erupt first premolar.

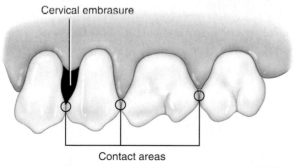

• **Figure 3.6** Buccal view maxillary left permanent arch. Cervical embrasure, also called gingival embrasure, occupies the interproximal space.

embrasures, occur often as pathologic consequences from periodontal or orthodontic causes, and these embrasures offer a place in which bacteria, calculus, and food debris can accumulate (Fig. 3.6). An open contact exists if two adjacent teeth do not touch tightly at their contact areas. This open space between the contact areas

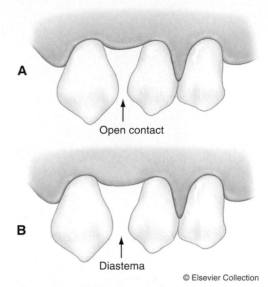

• **Figure 3.7** Buccal view maxillary left permanent arch. **(A)** An open contact can catch food and harbor bacteria, which can cause dental caries and periodontal disease. **(B)** A very large open contact area is called a diastema. If it is open enough it could allow food to be washed away rather than be trapped between contact areas.

traps food debris. Bacteria feed off this debris, multiply, and attach the gingiva leading to periodontal disease. They also attach the tooth surfaces and cause dental caries (tooth decay).

If the open contact is very wide it is called a diastema (Fig. 3.7). A large diastema could be big enough so that food does not get trapped and can be washed away. A small open contact is therefore more likely to cause dental disease (periodontal and caries) than a large diastema.

Embrasures

Embrasures are the spaces between the teeth that are occlusal to the contact areas (Fig. 3.8). They allow for the passage of food around the teeth so that food is not forced into the contact area between the teeth. Embrasures act as sluiceways or spillways and allow food to escape between teeth. By doing this they help dissipate the pressures brought to bear on the teeth from eating. These embrasures are named for their location in relation to the contact area. For instance, the space buccal to the contact area is the **buccal embrasure;** the **lingual embrasure** is lingual to the contact area (Fig. 3.9). The names of the embrasures are **facial** (buccal or labial), lingual, incisal, or **occlusal** (Fig. 3.10). Gingival embrasures are also

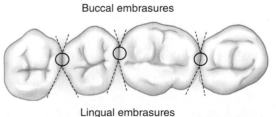

• **Figure 3.8** Occlusal view. Contact areas are circled. Embrasures flare out from each side of the contact areas.

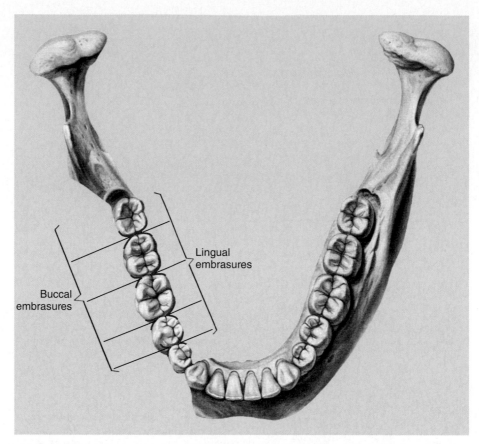

• **Figure 3.9** An occlusal view of proximal contact areas and embrasures. The width of the contact areas is not just a small point but an area of contact. Notice the position of the contact area with respect to the buccolingual dimensions of the tooth. (Modified from Zeisz RC, Nuckolls J. *Dental Anatomy*. St. Louis: Mosby; 1949.)

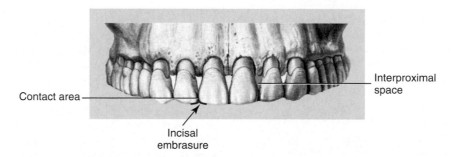

• **Figure 3.10** Incisal embrasure *(arrow)*. The area cervical to the contact area is a gingival embrasure, also called an *interproximal space (triangle)*. (Modified from Zeisz RC, Nuckolls J. *Dental Anatomy*. St. Louis: Mosby; 1949.)

evident, but only if the interproximal space is not occupied by any gingiva or bone. The gingival embrasure is gingival to the contact area and not usually present in a healthy mouth; it is the same as the cervical embrasure and interproximal space already discussed.

The embrasures have the following purposes:

1. They allow food to be shunted away from contact areas, which keeps food from being packed between the teeth.
2. They dissipate and reduce the forces of occlusal trauma brought to bear on the teeth, again by shunting food away from contact areas.
3. They are self-cleaning because of the rounded smooth surfaces that form the embrasures, allowing food to be swished away by saliva; ingested liquids; the cleaning action of other foods; and the friction of the tongue, cheeks, and lips.
4. They permit a slight amount of stimulation to the gingiva by frictional massage of food while protecting the gingiva from undue trauma. A poorly contoured embrasure leads to gingival irritation and breakdown.

Location of the Contact Areas, Interproximal Spaces, and Embrasures

Facial View

The contact areas of the anterior teeth are located closer to the incisal surfaces of the teeth. The posterior teeth have their contact areas nearer to the middle third of the teeth. The more posterior the tooth, the more cervical the location of its contact area. The one exception is the distal contact area of the maxillary canine, the location of which is in the center of the middle third of the tooth. This is more cervical than that of the first and second premolars, where the contact areas are just cervical to the junction of the occlusal and middle thirds of the tooth.

The more posterior teeth also have wider embrasures than the more anterior teeth, at least when compared with the occlusocervical dimensions of the tooth. The interproximal spaces of posterior teeth become shorter occlusocervically. Although the contact areas are at the same location, the teeth are shorter.

Occlusal View

The location of the contact areas and embrasures, as seen from the occlusal surface, shows that the contact areas of the anterior teeth are located in the center between the labial and lingual surfaces of the tooth. The posterior teeth have contact areas slightly buccal to the center of the teeth. Buccolingually the lingual embrasures are wider than the facial embrasures because from their contact point outward, teeth are narrower on the lingual side than on the facial side (see Fig. 3.8).

Facial and Lingual Contours

Facial and **lingual contours** of the teeth also afford the correct amount of frictional massage to the gingiva by directing food off the teeth and against the gingiva at a proper angle (Fig. 3.11) (see the section Periodontium later in this chapter). Too much deflection of the food would leave some gingiva without the right amount of stimulation, whereas too little deflection would allow some food to be forced into the gingival crevice, the space that separates the tooth from the gingiva. Food packed into this crevice could cause gingival inflammation, periodontal disease, or tissue recession.

The correct degree of facial or lingual curvature allows for the proper deflection of food so that the right amount of tissue stimulation occurs, and the gingival crevices are protected. In addition to these effects, the contour on the lingual surface should allow the tongue to rest against the tooth to promote efficient cleaning. Likewise, the facial height of contour allows for maximum cleaning of the lips and cheeks.

This contour varies in degree from tooth to tooth, but generally the location of the buccal height of contour of anterior and

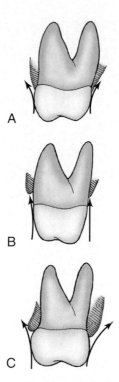

• **Figure 3.11** The angle at which normal contour (**A**), undercontour (**B**), and food (**C**) is deflected from a tooth surface is determined by the buccal and lingual contours.

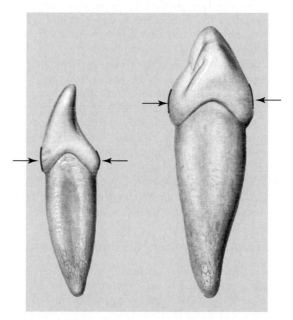

• **Figure 3.12** Labial and lingual heights of curvature of mandibular and maxillary incisors and canines are located within the cervical thirds of teeth. Facial and lingual crests of curvature *(arrows)*. Notice the curvature of the cervical lines (cementoenamel junction). (Modified from Zeisz RC, Nuckolls J. *Dental Anatomy.* St. Louis: Mosby; 1949.)

posterior teeth is always the same—at the cervical third of the tooth. The lingual height of contour of anterior teeth is at the cervical third of the tooth, but the **lingual crest of curvature** of posterior teeth is at or near the middle third (Figs. 3.12 and 3.13). The *crest of curvature* refers to the widest part of the crown of the tooth; it is the same as the height of contour.

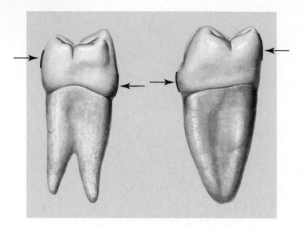

• **Figure 3.13** The buccal height of curvature is at the cervical third, and the lingual height of curvature is at the middle third on the maxillary and mandibular premolars and molars. Buccal and lingual crests of curvature *(arrows)*. Notice the curvatures of the cervical lines (cementoenamel junction). (Modified from Zeisz RC, Nuckolls J. *Dental Anatomy.* St. Louis: Mosby; 1949.)

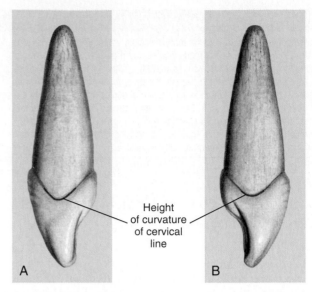

• **Figure 3.14** The mesial curvature of the cementoenamel junction is greater than the distal curvature. **(A)** Mesial view. **(B)** Distal view. (Modified from Zeisz RC, Nuckolls J. *Dental Anatomy.* St. Louis: Mosby; 1949.)

In young people, most curvatures, buccal and lingual, lie beneath the gingiva. As the teeth erupt, the curvature becomes more clinically apparent. In the normal adult whose tooth eruption has been completed, the **gingival crest** is cervical to the buccal and labial contours of all maxillary teeth and the lingual contour of anterior teeth. The **free gingiva** of the **cervical crest** covers the cervical enamel of the tooth. The normal amount of curvature found on most facial contours is approximately 0.5 mm and is somewhat less lingual on the anterior teeth.

On the lingual side of posterior teeth the crest of the gingiva is considerably more cervical than the lingual contour of the tooth. This is true because the height of contour on the lingual side of posterior teeth is located on the middle third of the crown. The amount of curvature on the lingual side of maxillary posterior teeth averages approximately 0.5 mm, and on the mandibular posterior teeth, it averages approximately 1 mm (see Figs. 3.12 and 3.13). The height of contour is the same as the crest of curvature and refers to the *buccal* or *lingual width* of a tooth. The *contact areas* refer to the mesial or distal crests of curvature of the tooth where it contacts adjacent teeth (see Fig. 3.3).

Curvature of the Cementoenamel Junction

As defined earlier, the cementoenamel junction (CEJ) is the junction where the enamel meets the cementum. This CEJ line curves as it goes around the tooth. It curves toward the incisal or occlusal on the mesial and distal of a tooth (Fig. 3.14). The CEJ is also called the *cervical line.*

The curvature of the cervical lines, or CEJ, on the mesial and distal surfaces of the teeth depends on the height of the contact area above the crown **cervix** and on the diameter of the crown labiolingually or buccolingually. The crowns of the anterior teeth show greater curvature of the cervical line than do the posterior teeth. The anterior teeth are narrower labiolingually, and to afford more anchorage and bony support, nature may have allowed interdental bone between the teeth to protrude more incisally. The posterior teeth, which are wider buccolingually, have more bone support and do not need this raised portion of bone between the teeth. Because of their cervicoincisal length, the anterior teeth

need this added portion of bone for anchorage. The tooth crown is shaped on the mesial and distal surfaces to accommodate this needed bone. The enamel does not go so far gingivally on the mesial and distal surfaces as it could; instead, the cementum rises in an incisal direction in the middle of the tooth. This affords more cementum on which the bone can attach itself. The periodontal attachment follows the cervical line and connects the gingiva and the cementum. The periodontal ligament attaches the cementum to the bone.

The maxillary anterior teeth show the greatest amount of curvature of the cervical line. The more anterior the tooth the greater the curvature. On the other hand, the mesial curvature of a tooth is greater than the distal curvature of the same tooth. The mandibular anterior teeth show less curvature than do their maxillary counterparts—generally less than 1 mm variation in cervical curvatures.

The posterior teeth in both arches show little variation. The mesial curvature of all posterior teeth usually averages about 1 mm, and the distal curvature is generally nonexistent or at least very slight at less than 0.5 mm. As a general rule, the curvature of the CEJ is usually about 1 mm less on the distal surface of the tooth than on the mesial surface. If a maxillary incisor has a 3.5 mm mesial curvature of the CEJ, the distal curvature may be 2.5 mm. Fig. 3.14 shows a very slight increase in the height of the cervical line on the mesial compared with the distal. In almost all teeth, the mesial curvature of the CEJ is greater than the distal curvature. Look again at Fig. 3.13 and compare the curvatures of the cervical lines to Fig. 3.14. Note how much greater the curvature is in anterior teeth as compared to posterior teeth.

Self-Cleaning Qualities of the Teeth

To a large extent the teeth are self-cleaning because the crowns of the teeth are covered by a very smooth enamel. As mentioned previously, the smoothness of this enamel helps food and sticky substances slip off the crown of the tooth and allows the tooth to remain relatively free of bacteria, lessening decay and periodontal disease.

The shape of the crown also aids greatly in the prevention of periodontal disease by stimulating and cleaning the gingival tissue. It does this by deflecting the food onto the gingival tissue at a specific and proper angle. For instance, the shape of the incisors is like a shovel, and, accordingly, the incisor cuts its way through food and forces it toward the lingual surface onto the gingiva. In the case of the maxillary teeth, the food is directed toward the gingiva and onto the palate. Thus the shape of the incisor directs food off the incisor and onto the gingiva.

The shape of the teeth also reflect their functions and self-cleaning ability. The canine is a piercing tool. Like a spear, it pierces through food. Because it is wedge shaped, it forces the food off the pointed canine cusp onto the cingulum and the gingiva. The premolars are shaped in such a way that food is deflected onto the occlusal surface of the premolar, where it is ground up by the cusps of the teeth in the opposing arch.

When food is introduced into the mouth, it is aided by the tongue and cheek in pushing the previously pulverized food back onto the surface of the molars. This process continues from molar to molar until the food reaches the back of the mouth and is swallowed. If deep pits and **fissures** on the occlusal surface of the tooth are evident, some of the food debris remains after eating. It would seem that deep pits, fissures, or holes in the enamel of the teeth would make cleaning difficult. Yet these pits and fissures do provide a method of dissipating the extreme occlusal forces that result from the interdigitation of the cusps in the process of grinding up food. These little pits and fissures act as spillways on the occlusal surfaces of the teeth. Should these pits and fissures be too deep, nature has devised a way to eliminate them.

Primitive people, by eating natural raw foods, wore down some of the enamel of their teeth in the process of chewing, which resulted in the gradual obliteration of the pits and fissures. The wearing down of these pits and fissures could only be accomplished by a coarse fibrous diet. For tens of thousands of years, humans chose to eat foods that were semiraw or uncooked. In this form, the food presented a certain amount of roughage because it was hard and coarse and helped wear down the enamel, but the modern approach has found a way to avoid all of this. Our diet of soft, overcooked, tacky, and sticky foods has resulted in an inability to wear down enamel; additionally, the stickiness of the food allows it to adhere to the tooth surface even when pits and fissures are not present.

> ## Clinical Considerations
>
> Although our diet may leave a lot to be desired, our ingenuity does not. Modern dentistry has found many more painless ways to obliterate the pits and fissures of teeth than through the abrasive action of eating. A pit can be polished out, making a tiny uncleanable hole into a small, more cleanable fossa. This process is called an *odontectomy* or *odontoplasty*. A pit can also be filled in and covered with a sealant or bonding procedure. Pit and fissure sealants, bondings, and composite materials are all painlessly and easily applied. They fill in the pits, fissures, and other voids to make smooth, easy-to-clean tooth surfaces, preventing bacterial buildup and dental disease. Great care must be taken in restoring teeth to allow the right amount of sluiceways and still keep the teeth self-cleansable.

Periodontium

The periodontium is the supporting tissue adjacent to the teeth. It consists of the free gingiva, attached gingiva, and **alveolar mucosa,** as well as the cementum, periodontal ligament, and bone.

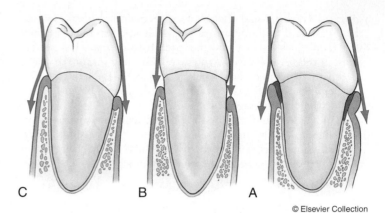

© Elsevier Collection

• **Figure 3.15** **(A)** Normal curvatures as found on a maxillary molar. Arrows show the path of food as it is deflected over the curvatures onto the gingiva. **(B)** A molar with little curvature and underdeveloped contours. The gingiva is likely to be stripped or pushed apically because of lack of protection and consequent overstimulation. **(C)** A molar with excess curvature. The gingiva is protected too much and experiences a lack of proper stimulation. Food and bacteria may lodge under these curvatures, promoting pathologic disturbance. (From Nelson SJ, Ash M. *Wheeler's Dental Anatomy.* 9th ed. St. Louis: Saunders; 2010.)

These tissues are essential for the support and anchorage of the teeth. The curvatures and contact areas of the teeth must be shaped in such a way that they not only protect these tissues from excessive trauma but also keep them free of bacteria and offer frictional massage and stimulation.

The buccal and lingual contours of a tooth are shaped so that food is deflected off the tooth and onto the gingival tissue. The angle at which the food is deflected is specific (Fig. 3.15). The mechanical friction of the food must not place extreme pressure on the free gingiva because this part of the gingival apparatus cannot tolerate extreme trauma.

If the curvature is too extreme, the food is deflected in such a way that the gingival tissue is not stimulated and cleaned by the frictional action of the food that deflects off it. In this situation, bacteria cannot be removed from the free gingival collar around the tooth and could then begin to destroy the gingival tissue. The tissue would become edematous, puffy, and inflamed and bleed easily, eventually leading to the periodontal breakdown of the supporting structures.

> ## Clinical Considerations
>
> When placing restorations or fillings, dental practitioners must be careful not to overcontour or undercontour the restoration. However, although both overcontouring and undercontouring of the buccal and lingual surfaces of teeth can cause periodontal disease, it is usually safer to undercontour a restoration than to overcontour it. Undercontoured surfaces can occur through the normal aging process during which more and more root shows as an individual gets older.

The contact areas are equally essential to the health and maintenance of the periodontal tissue in the interproximal spaces. If **open contacts** are present, then the teeth do not touch each other at their contact areas, and food is allowed to pack between the teeth and remain there. The bacteria captured on and in the

gingival crevice could then cause a periodontal breakdown of these tissues. If the contact area is so wide open, as in a diastema, that food can be forced into the interproximal space but not remain in this area because of the extremely large size of the space, then pathology can be prevented (see Fig. 3.7). The space must be large enough to ensure that bacteria and debris will be flushed out by the frictional massage of the food.

If the deflection of the food is at an extreme angle, a **recession** of the tissues away from the crown of the teeth could result. When gingival tissue recedes from the tooth, the root of the tooth becomes exposed. It is possible to have so much tissue stimulation or an improper angle of food deflection that the gum tissue recedes from the tooth.

Clinical Considerations

The radiograph shows an open contact between the maxillary molars. Open contacts allow food to be entrapped between the contact areas. This allows bacteria to build up, multiply, and attach to the gingiva and the tooth surfaces. This causes inflammation and eventual infection and results in the loss of papillary gingiva and bone. It also allows for the formation of tooth decay on the tooth surface. The overhanging restorations harbor food debris and bacteria as well. These two conditions make oral hygiene extremely difficult.

Review Questions

1. What normally fills the interproximal spaces between teeth? If this is missing, what is the void called?
2. Name the embrasures and explain their function. Which embrasure is not always present and why?
3. Which teeth have the greater curvature of the cementoenamel junction, anterior or posterior? Mesial or distal?
4. What term is synonymous with the cementoenamel junction?
5. Explain how the diet a person chooses affects gingival and tooth health.
6. What happens if a tooth is restored so that it is overcontoured?
7. What happens if two adjacent teeth have open contact areas?
8. What is the difference between a contact area and a contact point?
9. Which of the following spaces in Fig. 3.16 present the greatest potential for food impaction, periodontal disease, and caries?
   a. interproximal space mesial to the maxillary first molar
   b. interproximal space distal to the maxillary first molar
   c. edentulous space mesial to the mandibular first molar

10. Complete the blanks with the correct answer choices provided. Answers may be used more than once. The buccal height of contour of the anterior teeth is the _____ and that of the posterior teeth is the _____. The lingual height of contour of the anterior teeth is the _____ and that of the posterior teeth is the _____.
    a. cervical third of the crown
    b. near the middle of the crown
11. The buccal crest of curvature is _____ the buccal height of the contour.
    a. less than
    b. the same as
    c. lower than
    d. higher than
12. What is the normal amount of crest of curvature?
    a. 1 mm
    b. 0.5 mm
    c. less than 0.5 mm on the lingual of incisors
    d. at the cervical third except for mandibular posterior teeth
    e. b, c, and d
13. While examining this patient, you notice an open contact between the two mandibular premolars. What are your concerns? See Fig. 3.17.

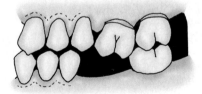

• **Figure 3.16**

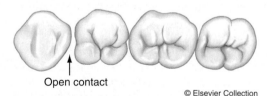

Open contact

© Elsevier Collection

• **Figure 3.17**

4

Dentition

OBJECTIVES

- To understand the difference between primary dentition, secondary dentition, and mixed dentition
- To understand the arrangement of the teeth into dentitions, arches, and quadrants
- To name and code any individual tooth
- To code teeth using the Universal system, the Palmer notation system, and the Federation Dentaire Internationale system
- To identify a tooth when given a code from one of the three systems

Arrangement of Teeth

The general arrangement of teeth is referred to as **dentition. Primary dentition** refers to the 20 **deciduous** teeth, often called *baby teeth.* **Secondary dentition** refers to the 32 permanent teeth (Figs. 4.1 and 4.2).

Dentition is divided into upper and lower arches. The teeth anchored within the upper jaw belong to the **maxillary arch.** The mandible is the bone that supports the lower arch of teeth, hence, the name **mandibular arch.**

The mandibular and maxillary arches each compose one-half of the dentition. In the permanent dentition of 32 teeth, each arch comprises 16 teeth. How many teeth are in an arch of the primary dentition? How many teeth compose the total primary dentition? Each arch is further divided into a right and a left half, making four **quadrants,** two in each arch. In the Palmer notation system, the quadrants are determined by the intersection of a vertical and a horizontal line. The maxillary quadrants are represented by numbers or letters above the horizontal line, and the mandibular quadrants are indicated below the line. The technical term for the dividing line between the right and left sides of the body is the **midsagittal plane.** In dentistry this is called the **midline,** or **median line,** of the face. The right and left quadrants are separated by this vertical line, which represents the midline of the skull when facing the patient. Thus each quadrant consists of one-fourth of the dentition and has a mirror image on the other side of the arch and an opposing quadrant in the opposite arch.

Note that a permanent dentition quadrant has eight teeth: central and lateral incisor; canine; first and second premolar; and a first, second, and third molar. A deciduous (primary) quadrant has five teeth: two incisors, canine, and first and second molars. No deciduous premolars are evident.

The permanent teeth that replace or succeed the deciduous teeth are called **succedaneous** teeth. The permanent molars are called **nonsuccedaneous** teeth. They do not have predecessors,

and they do not succeed or replace deciduous teeth. The permanent premolars replace the deciduous molars. How many teeth in the secondary dentition are nonsuccedaneous? How many are in each arch? How many are in each quadrant?

A **mixed dentition** refers to one that comprises some permanent teeth and some deciduous teeth. After a child's permanent teeth begin to erupt, several years of mixed dentition follow. Not all the deciduous teeth are replaced at one time. Some adults may also have mixed dentition; this occurs when a deciduous tooth is retained even though the remainder of the teeth are permanent. If any combination of primary and secondary teeth are in the same dentition, then a mixed dentition is present.

If an adult has one retained primary tooth, with the rest being secondary teeth, what type of dentition does that person have? What would have to happen for that person to have a permanent dentition?

Naming and Coding Teeth

When identifying a specific tooth, list the dentition, arch, quadrant, and tooth name in that order (e.g., permanent [dentition], mandibular [arch], right [quadrant], central incisor [tooth]). Therefore *permanent mandibular right central incisor* is the correct wording over *right mandibular permanent central incisor.*

Each dental team should be familiar with the various systems of naming and coding teeth. Although each office may use only one system, the staff should be familiar with all systems so that communication among dental offices is possible. Therefore the most popular systems are discussed here.

Universal System

The **Universal system** uses the Arabic numerals 1 through 32 for permanent teeth and the letters A through T for the primary teeth. The number **1** is assigned to the most posterior molar on the upper right, the permanent maxillary right third molar. The highest number is given to the permanent mandibular right third molar (Fig. 4.3). Likewise, the letter A is given to the primary maxillary right second molar, and the letter T to the primary mandibular right second molar (Fig. 4.4).

What symbol would represent each of the following?
1. Secondary mandibular left first molar
2. Secondary maxillary right first premolar
3. Primary maxillary right first molar
4. Primary mandibular left central incisor
5. Permanent maxillary left first premolar
6. Deciduous mandibular right canine

What tooth is represented by each of the following symbols of the Universal system?

Answer: 19, 5, B, O, 31, A, and I

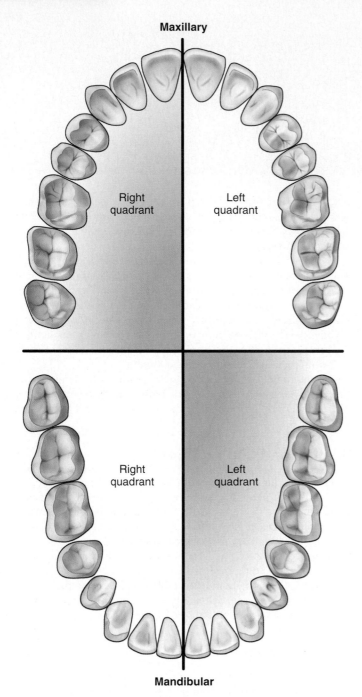

Maxillary

Right quadrant

Left quadrant

Right quadrant

Left quadrant

Mandibular

• **Figure 4.1** Permanent teeth or secondary dentition. Horizontal and vertical lines divide arches into quadrants.

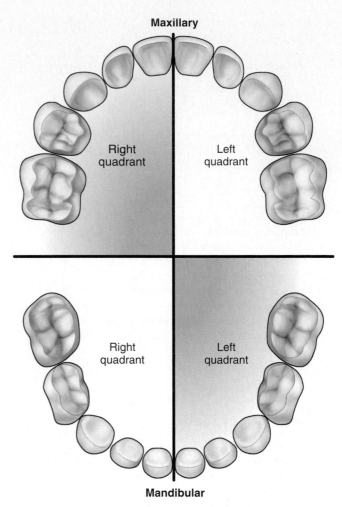

Maxillary

Right quadrant

Left quadrant

Right quadrant

Left quadrant

Mandibular

• **Figure 4.2** Deciduous teeth or primary dentition.

Palmer Notation System

In the **Palmer notation system** each of the four quadrants is given its own prefix symbol or quadrant bracket. For example, if the tooth is a maxillary tooth, the number or letter should be placed above the line of the bracket, indicating an upper tooth. Conversely, a mandibular tooth symbol should be placed below the line, indicating a lower tooth. Numbers or letters representing teeth from the right quadrant should be placed in a bracket with a line to their immediate right as the practitioner views it. This line indicates the midline or the midsagittal plane (see the diagram that follows). This system is a shorthand diagram of the teeth as if the practitioner was viewing the patient's teeth from the outside. The teeth in the right quadrant would have the midline bracket to the right of the numbers or letters. View the bracket as if you were looking at a patient. The teeth in the right quadrant would then have the midline bracket to their right.

The number or letter assigned to each tooth depends on its position relative to the midline. For example, the central incisors, the teeth closest to the midline, have the lowest number—that is, the number 1 for permanent teeth and the letter A for deciduous teeth.

Study the diagram that follows and note that 32 individual numbers, four of each number ranging from 1 to 8, are shown. In the Palmer notation system, the lowest number is closest to the midline. For example, all central incisors, maxillary and mandibular, right or left, are given the number 1. All lateral incisors are given the number 2, all canines are given the number 3, and the number 8 is assigned to the third molars. The farther the teeth are from the midline, the higher is the number assigned to the tooth. The number 6 is assigned to the first molars because it is the sixth tooth from the midline.

Each tooth is further identified as being maxillary or mandibular by its position above or below the horizontal maxillary-mandibular dividing line. In the diagram, notice that the number 1 appears at the four locations closest to the midline. Number 1 in all instances refers to a *central incisor*. By studying the midline bracket, whether the tooth belongs to a right or left quadrant can be identified. If the bracket is to the left of the letter or number,

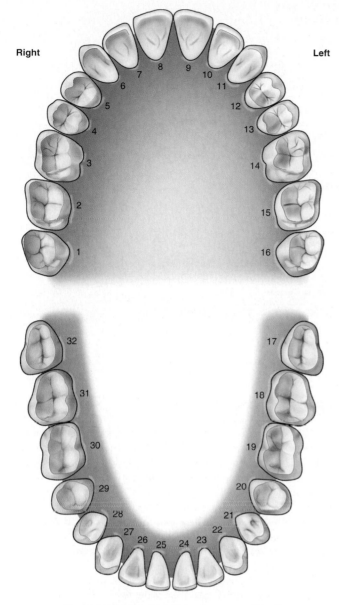

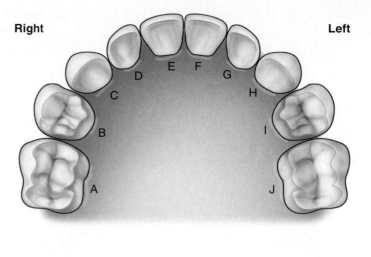

• **Figure 4.3** Universal system of permanent teeth.

• **Figure 4.4** Universal system of deciduous teeth.

then the tooth belongs to the left quadrant. The teeth are placed in relation to the midline as if the practitioner was looking at the patient and not from within the patient's mouth.

Study the following symbols:

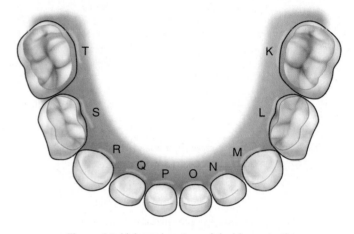

What can be determined from this diagram?
1. Three of the symbols (1, 2, and 4) are maxillary teeth because they are above the horizontal line.
2. One of the teeth (3) is a mandibular tooth. Why?
3. Numbers 1, 2, and 4 are in the maxillary left quadrant because the vertical line is to the immediate left of these numbers. This would also be the relationship of the vertical line to the teeth if one were looking *at* the patient.

4. Number 3 refers to a tooth in the mandibular right quadrant. Why?
5. Because number 1 refers to a central incisor, number 2 to a lateral incisor, and number 4 to the first premolar, these numbers refer to the maxillary left central and lateral incisors and the first premolar.
6. Because number 3 refers to a canine, number 3 in this diagram refers to the mandibular right canine.

If only one tooth was represented, such as the secondary maxillary left lateral incisor, the following symbol would be used:

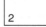

All that has been done here is that some of the horizontal and vertical lines have been eliminated. The original symbol would have looked like this:

Thus far secondary (permanent) teeth have been used in the examples of the Palmer notation system. Remember that the numbers 1 through 8 are used for permanent teeth and capital letters A through E for primary teeth. Refer to the following diagram for primary teeth.

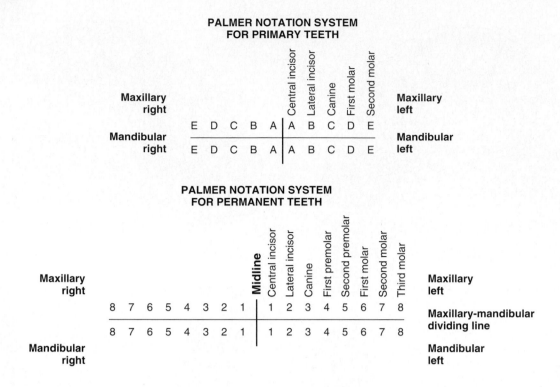

PALMER NOTATION SYSTEM FOR PRIMARY TEETH

PALMER NOTATION SYSTEM FOR PERMANENT TEETH

Which tooth is represented in each of the following?

E ⌐

D ⌐

What is the symbol for the primary mandibular right first molar? Refer to the diagram at bottom of page showing Palmer notation system.

Federation Dentaire Internationale System

In the **Federation Dentaire Internationale (FDI) system** each tooth, deciduous or permanent, is given a two-digit number. No letters or duplicate numbers are used. It is similar to the Palmer notation system in that the second digit indicates the position of the tooth relative to the midline. The first digit indicates the quadrant and whether the tooth is permanent or deciduous. Fig. 4.5 shows that each tooth has its own specific two-digit number. The permanent maxillary right quadrant teeth are assigned numbers from 11 to 18, and the permanent maxillary left quadrant teeth are assigned numbers 21 through 28. The permanent mandibular teeth are numbered 31 to 38 in the left quadrant and 41 to 48 in the right. Each quadrant is symbolized by a specific first digit, and all teeth in that quadrant have the same first digit. The second digit depends on the position the tooth occupies relative to the midline. The lowest number is given to the tooth closest to the midline.

Likewise, the deciduous teeth have their own first-digit number identifying each specific quadrant. Again, the second digit denotes the position the tooth occupies relative to the midline. See Fig. 4.6 for quadrant numbers.

Dental Formula

The **dental formula** is an abbreviated method used to express the number and types of teeth in the maxillary and mandibular arches

of mammalian teeth. The number of teeth is written for *one side* of the mouth. This represents one maxillary and one mandibular quadrant. The total number of teeth is twice the dental formula, because it represents only *one side* of the mouth. Modern man's permanent dentition on one side only would be two incisors, one canine, two premolars, and three molars in each the maxillary and the mandibular quadrants for a total of 16 teeth per side, therefore, $16 \times 2 = 32$ permanent teeth.

The formula is written in a specific order (I, C, P, M) and always represents the same side: first incisors (I), second canines (C), third premolars (P), and finally molars viewed as if looking at the left side.

There are two dental formulas for modern man: one for permanent dentition and one for deciduous dentition. The dental formula for the permanent dentition of man is I-2/2 C-1/1 P-2/2 M-3/3. The number 2 before the slash mark (/) means two maxillary teeth, which in this case are incisors. The 2 after the slash mark (/) means two mandibular teeth. Therefore I-2/2 means two maxillary and two mandibular incisors, C-1/1 means one maxillary and one mandibular canine, P-2/2 means two maxillary and two mandibular premolars, and M-3/3 means three maxillary and three mandibular molars. If you add all the teeth it results in a sum of eight maxillary and eight mandibular teeth per quadrant. Because there are four quadrants $4 \times 8 = 32$ total permanent teeth. Remember there is a maxillary and a mandibular quadrant on each side.

The deciduous formula is I-2/2 C-1/1 M-2/2, which is sometimes written with a D in front of the tooth type. Then it would be DI-2/2 DC-1/1 DM-2/2. In the deciduous dentition there are 5 maxillary and 5 mandibular teeth per quadrant for a total of 20 deciduous teeth ($5 \times 4 = 20$).

Additional Fun Information

The dental formula is just a small piece of information about each mammal. It tells us the number of incisors, canines, premolars,

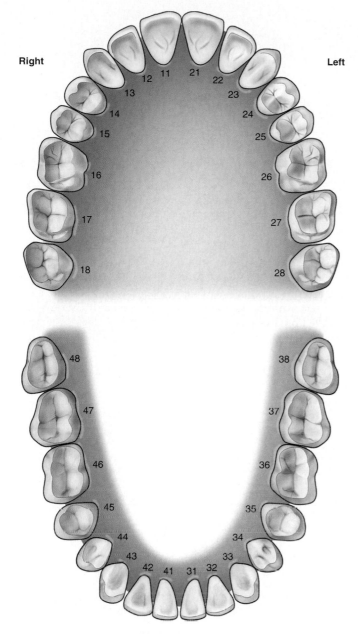

Right

Left

- **Figure 4.5** Federation Dentaire Internationale system of permanent teeth.

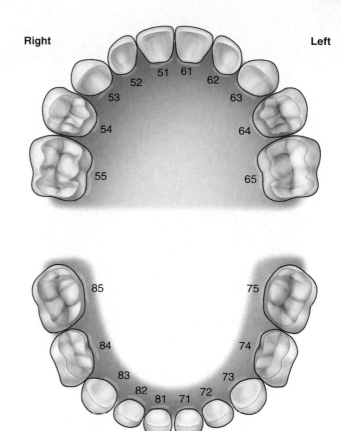

Right

Left

- **Figure 4.6** Federation Dentaire Internationale system of deciduous teeth.

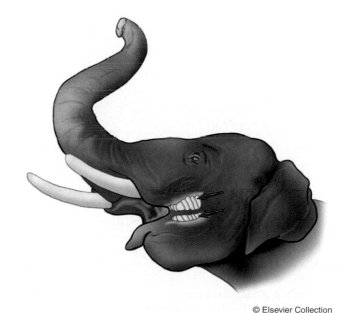

© Elsevier Collection

- **Figure 4.7** Elephants have marching molars. The new molars come in from the rear of the mouth and advance forward replacing the old molars. This is different from most mammals in which the teeth are replaced by teeth directly beneath them. Usually only one molar per quadrant is present at a time. The picture shows what looks like several teeth; it is really one molar with vertical striations. The occlusal shape differs between elephants, mammoths, and mastodons.

and molars and their location (upper or lower). It does not tell us the size, shape, or functional differences (Fig. 4.7).

For instance, the dental formula for elephants is I-1/0 C-0/0 P-3/3 M-3/3. It does not tell us that I-1/0 is one upper tusk on each side. The incisors in elephants are extraoral tusks, not intraoral incisors. It also does not tell us that the elephants have six rather than two sets of teeth. Elephants usually only have one molar at a time; as one molar is worn out another replaces it. The permanent molars are replaced three times. These molars are called *marching molars*, because the new molar marches in from the posterior to replace the worn out molar.

This formula does not tell us about the shape or function of the teeth. For instance, many carnivores have **carnassial** teeth—one molar and one premolar that together act like scissors. In carnivores such as wolves a modified fourth maxillary premolar

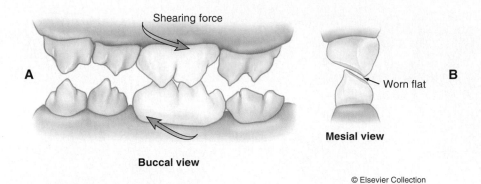

Shearing force

A

B

Worn flat

Mesial view

Buccal view

© Elsevier Collection

• **Figure 4.8** Carnassial teeth of a wolf. (A) Although carnassial teeth are molars and premolars, they are shearing teeth not grinding teeth. (B) The carnassial teeth work together as scissors and even sharpen themselves as they wear.

and the first mandibular molar act as a shearing tool to shear and cut tissue off bone. These modified teeth are also self-sharpening (Fig. 4.8).

Still this dental formula is of value when comparing mammals. It is worth noting that although the size, shape, and function of the teeth vary between species, the dental formula often is the same within the same genus. Within the same genus the interdental spaces and diastemae remain rather consistent. Primates are so consistent with the location of their diastemae that these spaces are called primate spaces.

Dental Formula for Several Species

Canines (wolves, dogs)	DI-3/3 DC-1/1 DP-3/3 DM-0/0 = 14 × 2 = 28 deciduous teeth I-3/3 C-1/1 P-4/4 M-2/3 = 21 × 2 = 42 permanent teeth
Cats	DI-3/3 DC-1/1 DP-3/2 DM-0/0 = 13 × 2 = 26 deciduous teeth I-3/3 C-1/1 P-3/2 M-1/1 = 15 × 2 = 30 permanent teeth
Cattle	DI-0/4 DC-0/0 DP-3/3 DM-0/0 = 10 × 2 = 20 deciduous teeth I-0/4 C-0/0 P-3/3 M-3/3 = 16 × 2 = 32 permanent teeth
Horse	DI-3/3 DC-0/0 DP-3/3 DM-0/0 = 12 × 2 = 24 deciduous teeth I-3/3 C-1/1 P-3 or 4/3 M-3/3 = 20 (or 21) × 2 = 40 (or 42) permanent teeth
Lion	I-3/3 C-1/1 P-3/2 M-1/1 = 15 × 2 = 30 permanent teeth
Opossum	I-5/4 C-1/1 P-3/3 M-4/4 = 25 × 2 = 50 permanent teeth
Elephant	I-1/0 C-0/0 DM-3/3 = 13 × 2 = 26 (24 temporary molars, 1 per quadrant at a time and 2 permanent tusks) I-1/0 C-0/0 P-0/0 M-3/3 = 13 × 2 = 26 (1 molar per quadrant at a time and 2 permanent tusks)

Review Questions

1. Name two types of human dentition and the number of teeth in each.
2. Name the different arches. How many teeth are present in a primary arch and how many in a secondary mandibular arch?
3. List the number of different quadrants.
4. Are any primary teeth succedaneous? If not, why not?
5. Name all the nonsuccedaneous permanent teeth.
6. Are secondary molars nonsuccedaneous?
7. What dentition is composed of both primary and secondary teeth?
8. How many dentitions are there?
9. Identify the following in the Universal system:
   a. numbers 3, 5, 19, 28, 32
   b. letters A, E, J, M, S
10. Give the correct Universal system symbol for the following:
    a. primary maxillary left central
    b. primary mandibular right first molar
    c. primary maxillary right canine
    d. permanent maxillary right second premolar
    e. permanent mandibular right central incisor

11. Identify the following by dentition, arch, and quadrant:
    a. $\underline{8}$
    b. $\underline{E}$
    c. $\underline{1}$
    d. $6\underline{|}$
12. Translate the previous four symbols of the Palmer system into symbols of the Universal system.
13. Give the Palmer, Universal, and FDI symbols for the permanent mandibular right first molar.
14. Identify the following symbols. Which systems are they derived from, and which teeth do they represent?
    a. 8
    b. $8\underline{|}$
    c. E
    d. $1\underline{|}$
    e. 11
    f. 18
15. How many permanent incisors do cats have?

5

Development, Form, and Eruption

OBJECTIVES

- To understand how the tooth germs develop within the crypts
- To understand how the growth centers or lobes fuse and form a tooth
- To understand that this fusion can take a variety of forms, which result in different types of teeth such as incisors, premolars, and molars
- To know how many lobes form each type of tooth and where the lobes are located
- To understand the eruption schedule of the deciduous and permanent teeth
- To understand general rules about the eruption of teeth
- To understand the phenomena of mesial drift, root resorption, and exfoliation
- To understand the implications of the terms *impacted teeth, congenitally missing teeth, attrition, occlusal plane,* and *curve of Spee*
- To understand the periods of primary, mixed, and permanent dentition

Developmental and Form

During the sixth week of fetal life (7 or 8 months before birth), tiny tooth buds, sometimes called **tooth germs,** begin to grow within the alveolar process of the fetus. Tooth germs are small clumps of cells that have the ability to form the tooth tissues (dentin, enamel, cementum, and pulp). Both the primary and secondary teeth develop from these tooth germs, which later are located within cavities of the alveolar process called **crypts.** The primary tooth germs give rise to their permanent tooth replacements (see Chapter 19).

The earliest evidence of tooth formation occurs during the sixth week of embryonic life, which is when the dental lamina begins to form (see Chapter 19).

At this time the dentin and enamel begin to form, followed later in development of the cementum. The type of dentin formed at this early stage is called *primary dentin,* and it occurs before root completion. Secondary dentin is continually formed within the tooth, presumably by the same odontoblasts that form regular dentin. This process continues throughout one's entire lifetime. Secondary dentin differs from tertiary dentin and specifically reparative dentin in that reparative dentin is laid down locally as protection for the pulp from irritation, caries, or trauma. The

tertiary dentins are laid down most probably by different types of odontoblasts that are different from those that form secondary dentin (see Chapters 2 and 20).

The primary teeth begin to calcify by about the fourth or fifth month of fetal life. The process of **calcification** is the hardening of the tooth tissues by the deposition of mineral salts within these tissues (Fig. 5.1). This process continues until about the third or fourth year after birth, when the deciduous roots become fully formed.

Soon after birth the permanent teeth begin to calcify and continue until about the 25th year, which is when the roots of the third molars become calcified. The last area of the tooth to become calcified is the apex of the root (see Chapter 21).

Developmental Lobes

Each tooth begins to develop from four or more growth centers. These centers grow out from the tooth germ and are known as **developmental lobes.** The lobes grow and develop within their bony crypt until they fuse. This fusion of the lobes is called **coalescence.** The junction that forms the union of these lobes is marked by lines on the tooth called **developmental grooves,** which can still be seen on the tooth after it has erupted (see Chapter 2).

The number of developmental lobes necessary for the formation of a tooth depends on the particular tooth and how many cusps it has; for instance, all the anterior teeth develop from four lobes—three labial and one lingual. The three labial lobes form the labial surface of each tooth. The **mamelons,** which are immediately evident after the eruption of an incisor tooth, show the division of the labial half of the incisor into three parts. Each of the three mamelons has its own rounded incisal ridge. These three labial developmental lobes are separated by two developmental grooves (Fig. 5.2), whereas the three labial lobes fuse to form the entire labial surface. The only evidence that three separate lobes existed is at the incisal ridge, in which the mamelons are distinct and separate, and on the labial surface of the tooth, in which developmental lines or grooves are evident. The three labial developmental lobes are called the *mesiofacial, centrofacial,* and *distofacial* lobes. The sole lingual lobe is appropriately called the *lingual lobe* and makes up the entire cingulum on the lingual surface of the incisor.

Mamelons are only present when the incisors first erupt. The mamelons soon wear off, forming a flat incisal edge that shows little or no evidence of developmental grooves (Fig. 5.3).

Clinical Considerations

When the incisors are well aligned, the mandibular incisors contact their maxillary antagonists. This causes the wearing off of the

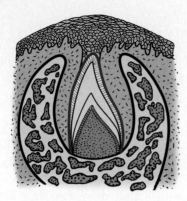

• **Figure 5.1** Beginning of tooth calcification. The small hole in the bone in which a tooth bud germ forms is called a crypt; it later becomes a tooth socket, which houses the root of the tooth.

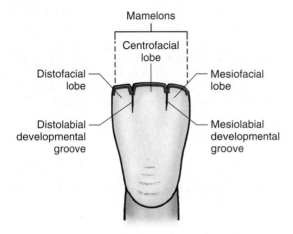

• **Figure 5.2** Incisal ridge of the three labial lobes is formed from mamelons. (Modified from Zeisz RC, Nuckolls J. *Dental Anatomy.* St. Louis: Mosby; 1949.)

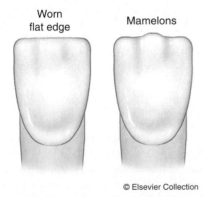

© Elsevier Collection

• **Figure 5.3** Incisors erupt with mamelons forming their incisal ridge. After the mamelons are worn off the incisal edges are flat and show no evidence of the once-rounded ridges.

mamelons of both the mandibular and the maxillary incisors. If an adolescent or adult presents with mamelons on his or her incisors, then the dental provider knows automatically that the incisors are malinged. In proper occlusion the incisor teeth wear off the mamelons within a year or two of the teeth touching. Some

situations in which this can cause an *open bite* (incisors not touching) include thumb-sucking, mouth breathing, tongue thrusting, speech problems, and swallowing and breathing difficulties.

Lobes and Cusps

Premolars

The maxillary premolars are like the anterior teeth because they have three facial lobes and one lingual lobe. However, unlike the anterior teeth, the three facial lobes of maxillary premolars form one high buccal cusp instead of an incisal ridge, and the single lingual cusp forms a large lingual *cusp* rather than a *cingulum* (Fig. 5.4). The names of the lobes are the same as those for the anterior teeth. Remember that the term "*facial*" replaces the terms "*labial*" in anterior teeth and "*buccal*" in posterior teeth (Fig. 5.5).

The mandibular first premolar has the same number and arrangement of lobes as the maxillary premolars; however, the lingual cusp of the mandibular first premolar is smaller than its maxillary counterpart (Fig. 5.6). These teeth are termed *bicuspids* because they have only two cusps, a buccal and a lingual. The mandibular second premolar varies; it may be a two-cusped or three-cusped form. Because not all these premolars have only two cusps, the term *premolar* is preferred.

There are two separate two-cusp varieties of the mandibular second premolar, a "U"-shaped and an "H"-shaped occlusal (Fig. 5.7A and C). They have exactly the same number and arrangement of lobes as the mandibular first premolar. The lingual cusps of these *bicuspids* are longer than that of the mandibular first premolar. The facial lobes and cusps of these two-cusp varieties

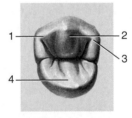

• **Figure 5.4** Four lobes of a maxillary right second premolar. *1,* Distobuccal lobe; *2,* centrobuccal lobe; *3,* mesiobuccal lobe; and *4,* lingual lobe. (Modified from Zeisz RC, Nuckolls J. *Dental Anatomy.* St. Louis: Mosby; 1949.)

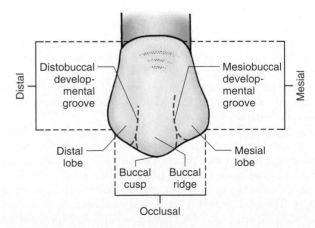

• **Figure 5.5** Buccal surface of a maxillary right second premolar. (Modified from Zeisz RC, Nuckolls J. *Dental Anatomy.* St. Louis: Mosby; 1949.)

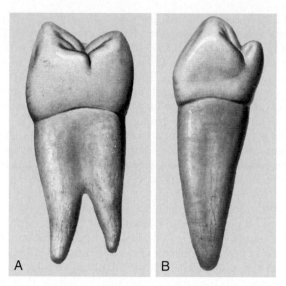

• **Figure 5.6** The maxillary first premolar **(A)** has a much larger lingual cusp than the mandibular first premolar **(B)**.

of the mandibular second premolar are exactly the same as on the first premolar, but the lingual lobes are quite different.

The third occlusal form of the mandibular second premolar is the three-cusp form or "Y" type. It differs from the two-cusp varieties because there are two lingual lobes (mesiolingual and distolingual) instead of a single lobe. This results in two separate lingual cusps, with the mesiolingual cusp usually larger than the distolingual cusp (see Fig. 5.7B, "Y" type). Unlike other premolars, this three-cusp form develops from five lobes (not four); each of the two lingual lobes is formed from its own lobe. The labial cusp is formed from three lobes.

A considerable difference is also apparent in the number and location of the developmental grooves, with an additional groove located between the two lingual cusps. This results in three separate occlusal forms for the mandibular second premolar consisting of a "U," "Y," or "H" shape. Further differences in anatomy are discussed in Chapter 14. These types are named by looking at the occlusal of the teeth. The developmental grooves form a U, Y, or H.

Molars

All molars have two facial and two lingual lobes, except the first molars, which usually have a fifth or minor lobe. For example, the maxillary first molar generally has five developing lobes: two major facial lobes (mesiobuccal and distobuccal); a mesiolingual lobe; one minor lobe (distolingual); and one **rudimentary lobe,** called the **lobe of Carabelli** or the **cusp of Carabelli**. Each of the four major and minor lobes develops into a cusp, which is named according to its lobe (e.g., the mesiobuccal lobe forms the mesiobuccal cusp). The lobe of Carabelli, which is located on the lingual surface of the mesiolingual cusp, develops into a tubercle (a small cusplike elevation).

The maxillary second molar often does not have a cusp of Carabelli; if it is present then it is much smaller in proportion to

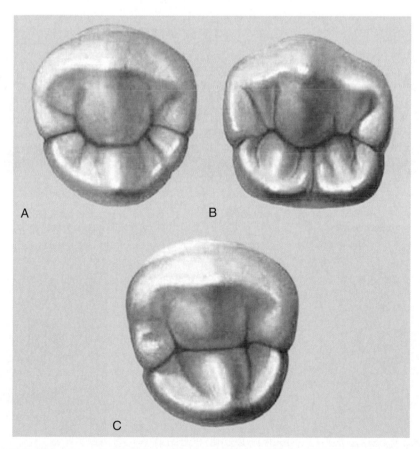

• **Figure 5.7** The three types of mandibular second premolar occlusals, C **(A)**, Y **(B)**, and H **(C)**, are named after the shape of their occlusal developmental grooves.

the other lobes. Second molars, maxillary and mandibular, are much smaller than first molars in all cusp proportions as a rule, and the distolingual cusp, which is a minor cusp, is often even smaller in proportion. The minor cusp becomes smaller as the tooth location becomes more posterior. Therefore it is not unusual for third molars to have only major cusps and no minor cusps. A maxillary third molar might have only three cusps, with little or no distolingual cusp. Additionally, the crown is usually smaller and the roots shorter than those of second or first molars (Figs. 5.8 and 5.9).

Special mention should be made about third molars in general. They are the most unpredictable of all the teeth. For instance, it is quite possible for mandibular third molars to be extremely well developed and better proportioned and larger than the first molars in the same mouth; however, they are more likely to be poorly formed and varying from three to eight cusps and to be deviated in form or missing entirely. Therefore any general rule that applies to the regression of minor cusps or the size of teeth must be limited by the extreme variability of third molars.

Eruption

The first teeth to emerge into the oral cavity are the deciduous or primary teeth. Calcification of these teeth begins around the fourth month of fetal life. By the end of the sixth month, all the deciduous teeth have begun to develop. Normally no teeth are visible in the mouth at birth. Occasionally infants are born with erupted incisor teeth, but these premature teeth are usually lost soon after birth and are not a part of the deciduous dentition.

The calcification process first forms the crown of the tooth, and root formation follows later. No two people are exactly alike in calcification, crown and root formation, or eruption schedules. During enamel and dentin development, minerals are deposited in the forming tooth germs. However, any fever, metabolic dysfunction, childhood or nutritional disease, or physical illness or trauma can alter the formation of the teeth and even stop their formation or mineralization completely.

Although human dentition varies somewhat in all people, certain approximations or averages are recognizable. The following is a list of deciduous teeth and approximate eruption times. Table 5.1 shows the approximate eruption dates for primary teeth. The mean number gives us an easier way to remember these dates.

The first general rule concerning eruption is that mandibular teeth usually precede the maxillary teeth of the same type; a mandibular central will usually erupt before a maxillary central. The second rule is that the teeth in both jaws erupt in pairs, one on the right and one on the left. The third rule is that *permanent teeth* usually erupt slightly earlier in girls than in boys. A slight difference between genders with respect to the eruption of *deciduous molars* may exist, but it is not apparent in the other deciduous teeth. Remember that these rules are not firm, and exceptions are numerous. The rules generalize, for instance, that the mandibular centrals may erupt only 60% of the time ahead of the maxillary centrals, which leaves the maxillary centrals to erupt first 40% of the time. At this point it is very helpful to refer to Fig. 5.10 as you review the following sections. Remember there is a great deal of variation in the eruption sequence, and notice how the previously mentioned rules seem to apply.

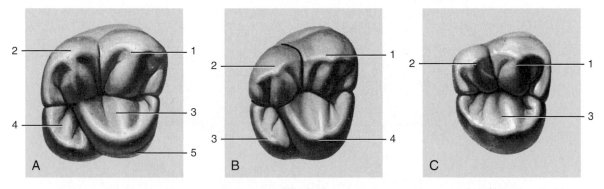

• **Figure 5.8** **(A)** Maxillary first molar with five lobes. **(B)** Maxillary second molar with four lobes. **(C)** Maxillary third molar with three lobes. (Modified from Zeisz RC, Nuckolls J. *Dental Anatomy*. St. Louis: Mosby; 1949.)

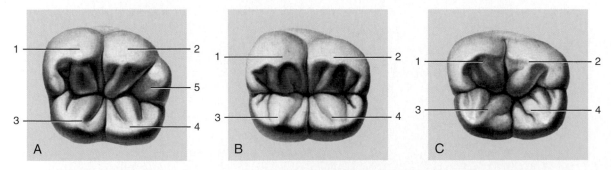

• **Figure 5.9** **(A)** Mandibular first molar with five cusps. **(B)** Mandibular second molar with four cusps. **(C)** Mandibular third molar. Each cusp is formed from one lobe. (Modified from Zeisz RC, Nuckolls J. *Dental Anatomy*. St. Louis: Mosby; 1949.)

TABLE 5.1	Eruption of Primary Teeth			
	Tooth	Universal System	Emergence of Teeth (Months)	
Upper	i1	E, F	10 (8–12)	
	i2	D, G	11 (9–13)	
	c	C, H	19 (16–22)	
	m1	B, I	16 (13–19)♂ (14–18)♀	
	m2	A, J	29 (25–33)	
Lower	i1	P, O	8 (6–10)	
	i2	Q, N	13 (10–16)	
	c	R, M	20 (17–23)	
	m1	S, L	16 (14–18)	
	m2	T, K	27 (23–31)♂ (24–30)♀	

i1, Central incisor; *i2,* lateral incisor; *c,* canine; *m1,* first molar; *m2,* second molar.
From Nelson SJ. *Wheeler's Dental Anatomy, Physiology, and Occlusion.* St. Louis: Elsevier Saunders; 2015.

The first teeth to appear in the mouth are usually the deciduous mandibular central incisors. They generally erupt at the age of approximately 6 to 8 months. Approximately 2 months later, the maxillary central incisors can be seen. The deciduous maxillary lateral incisors emerge around the end of the first year. They are followed by the mandibular laterals a month or two later. It is the exception when the maxillary teeth erupt earlier than the mandibular teeth.

Next to erupt, at approximately 16 months of age, are the mandibular first deciduous molars, closely followed by the maxillary first deciduous molars. They erupt before the canines. The deciduous canines erupt between 16 and 20 months of age, and they must fit in between the first molars and the laterals, both of which erupt earlier than the canines. Canines erupt into the corner of the mouth. As the canines erupt they bring their supporting bone with them, building up and developing the boney canine eminences at the corners of the dental arches (Fig. 5.11).

The second molars are the last deciduous teeth, usually erupting several months after a child's second birthday. The deciduous second molars are often called the *2-year molars,* and much of the cantankerous attitude of 2-year-olds is credited to the fact that the eruption of these large molars is painful.

All of the deciduous teeth are expected to have erupted by the time the child is 2½ years old. For the next 36 months, as the child continues to grow, the jaws also grow, which support the teeth. The erupted teeth, however, do not become any larger. Consequently, by age 5 it is normal to have spaces (diastemas) between the teeth, which are caused by the increased growth of the jaws. When the first permanent molars erupt in a mesial direction, this mesial movement of the teeth will close these spaces.

Unfortunately, many people do not realize the importance of the deciduous teeth. They believe that because these teeth will be lost in the process of making way for the permanent teeth, they are unimportant and are left to suffer dental neglect. Terms such as *baby teeth* or *milk teeth* lend credence to this fallacy and should be discouraged.

With premature loss of deciduous teeth, normal jaw growth and development may not take place. The deciduous teeth must remain intact to retain the proper spacing for the permanent teeth that will replace them. The deciduous dental arch must also help guide the first permanent molars into their normal positions. These molars act as the foundation for the rest of the permanent dentition. To a large extent the proper position and location of the other permanent teeth are dependent on the first permanent molars being in their proper position.

Permanent Dentition

The first permanent teeth to emerge into the oral cavity are usually the mandibular first molars, which are followed by the maxillary first molars several months later. They emerge immediately distal to the deciduous second molars. They are often called the *6-year molars* because they erupt at approximately 6 years of age. Much larger than the deciduous molars, they cannot emerge into the oral cavity until sufficient jaw growth has occurred to allow space for them.

Along with the eruption of the permanent molars comes the phenomenon of **mesial drift.** Mesial drift is the tendency of the permanent molars to have an eruptive force toward the midline. This means that the permanent molars not only erupt occlusally to meet their antagonists in the opposite arch, but they also have an eruptive force that causes them to move mesially. This force is strong enough to move the permanent molars into available space mesial to them. This phenomenon has two direct effects on the deciduous dentition: (1) the spaces between the deciduous teeth are closed as the first molar pushes the deciduous molars together, and (2) if a deciduous tooth is prematurely lost or if interproximal decay on the deciduous molar is not restored, then the permanent first molar moves mesially into the available space. Because little extra space is left to allow room for the eruption of premolars and canines, the infringement of the permanent molar into this space may keep a premolar or canine from properly erupting (Fig. 5.12).

Clinical Considerations

The deciduous molars are wider mesial distally than the permanent premolars that replace them.

They need this extra space to compensate for the time it takes for the permanent premolars to erupt. During this eruption time the permanent first molars begin to push anteriorly and start to move into this eruption space needed for the premolars. This *mesial drift* shortens the span between teeth, and if it were not for the fact that deciduous molars were longer (anterior to posterior) than the premolars, these premolars would be blocked from erupting.

After eruption of the mandibular first molars, the next permanent teeth to erupt are the central incisors, with the mandibular erupting at about 6 or 7 years of age and the maxillary erupting at about 7 or 8 years. The permanent incisors take over the position that the deciduous incisors held. This is made possible because the deciduous incisors are exfoliated. **Exfoliation** is the process by which the roots of a baby tooth are resorbed and dissolved until so little root remains that the baby tooth falls out. As the permanent tooth erupts, osteoclastic cells destroy the root of the deciduous tooth. This phenomenon is called **resorption.** The pressure brought to bear on the deciduous root by the eruption of the permanent tooth triggers the body to activate certain bone-destroying cells called **osteoclasts,** which destroy the roots of the deciduous teeth. As each deciduous root is destroyed, the tooth

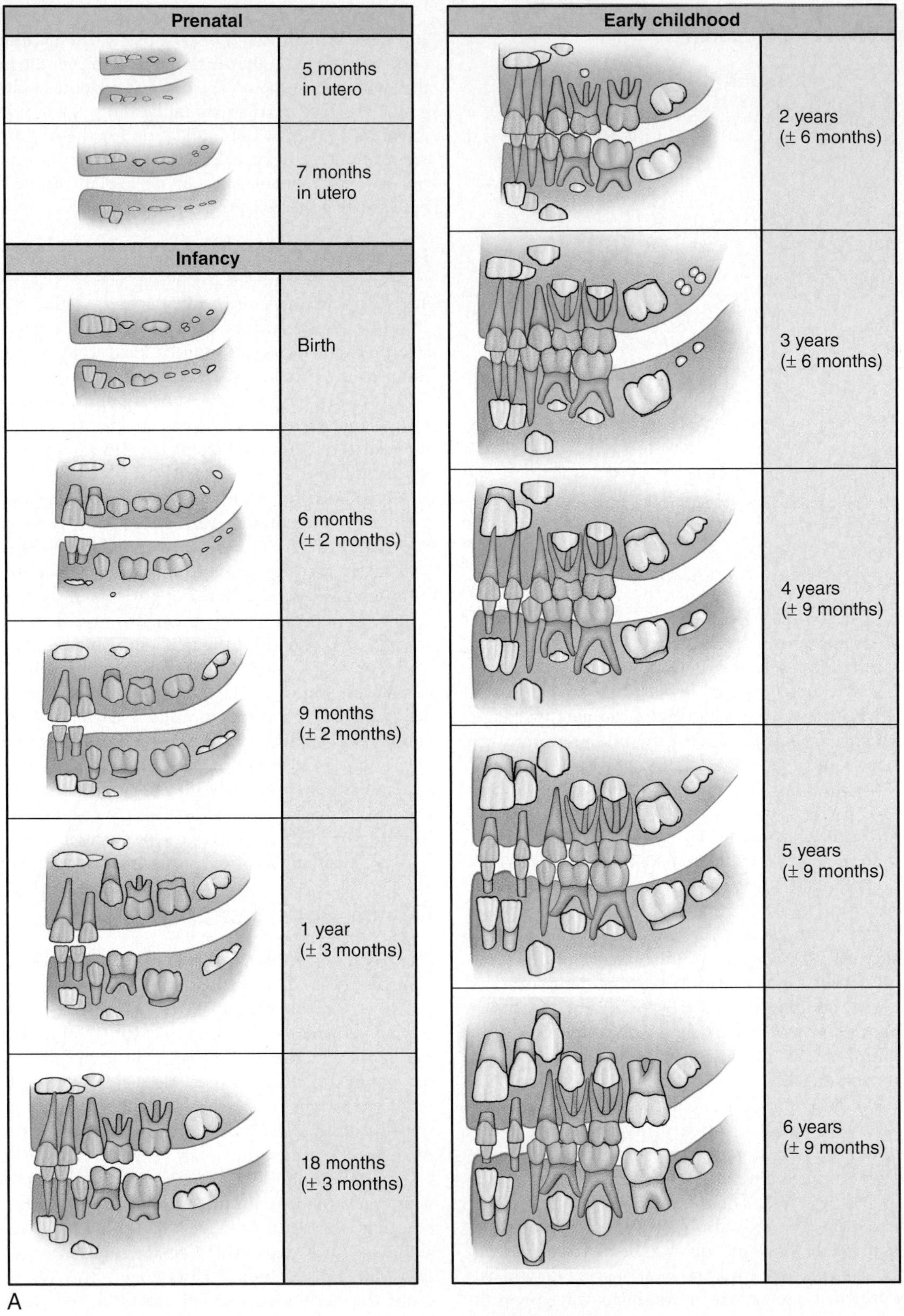

Prenatal	
	5 months in utero
	7 months in utero

Infancy	
	Birth
	6 months (± 2 months)
	9 months (± 2 months)
	1 year (± 3 months)
	18 months (± 3 months)

Early childhood	
	2 years (± 6 months)
	3 years (± 6 months)
	4 years (± 9 months)
	5 years (± 9 months)
	6 years (± 9 months)

A

• **Figure 5.10** Development of human dentition. **(A)** Deciduous dentition.

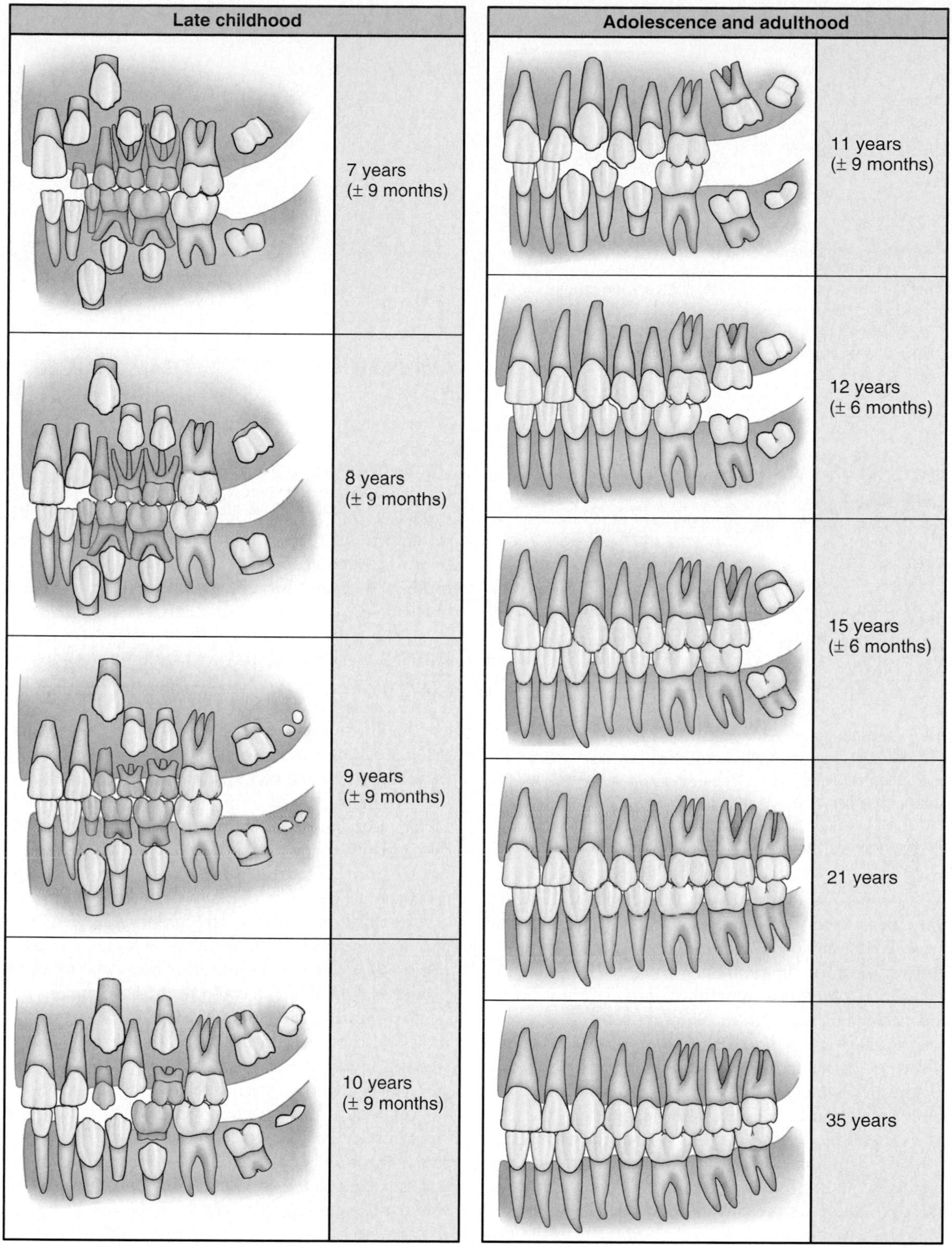

Late childhood	
	7 years (± 9 months)
	8 years (± 9 months)
	9 years (± 9 months)
	10 years (± 9 months)

Adolescence and adulthood	
	11 years (± 9 months)
	12 years (± 6 months)
	15 years (± 6 months)
	21 years
	35 years

B

C

• **Figure 5.10, cont'd** **(B)** Mixed dentition, late childhood. **(C)** Permanent dentition, adolescence and adulthood.

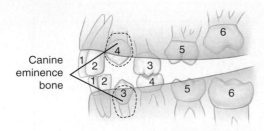

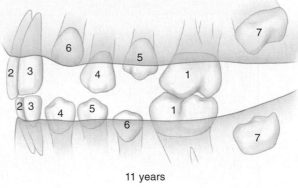

Canine
eminence
bone

18 months
Deciduous eruption sequence

• **Figure 5.11** Teeth in an 18-month-old. Note the canines erupt after the first deciduous molars. Their eruption develops the canine eminence of each dental arch. They bring bone with them as they erupt, which increases the labial amount of bone at the canine eminence.

© Elsevier Collection

• **Figure 5.13** Optimal eruption sequence of permanent teeth in each arch.

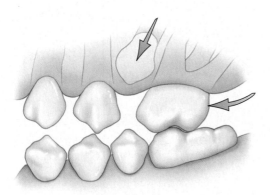

11 years

• **Figure 5.12** If a deciduous second molar is prematurely extracted and no space maintainer is placed, then the permanent first molar most likely will move into its vacated space. This closes the space needed for the second permanent premolar to erupt, thus preventing the eruption of this second premolar.

loses its anchorage, becomes loose, and finally exfoliates. During this process, the permanent tooth moves into the space that was occupied by the deciduous tooth.

It is not uncommon for the permanent incisors to erupt lingually to the deciduous incisors. Sometimes both central incisors, deciduous and permanent, are still in place, with the permanent central incisor located immediately lingual to the deciduous tooth. When the deciduous tooth is finally lost, pressure from the tongue forces the permanent tooth facially until it occupies its correct position in a balance between the lingual forces of the tongue and the facial forces of the lips. Remember the permanent tooth buds initially form lingually to their deciduous predecessors and move facially as the deciduous teeth are exfoliated.

The next teeth to erupt are the lateral incisors at 7 to 9 years of age. The developing incisors are in a position lingual to the deciduous roots. Like the central incisors, they can erupt lingual to their predecessors.

The incisors are followed by the mandibular canines, then the first premolar at 10 or 12 years. The maxillary canines do not erupt at this time. The mandibular canines are followed by the mandibular first premolars, but usually the maxillary first premolar erupts at about the same time or soon after.

The second premolars erupt at 10 to 12 years of age, with the maxillary premolars erupting slightly later than the mandibular premolars.

The maxillary canines then erupt at 11 or 12 years of age. It is very important that the deciduous teeth have maintained the proper amount of space for the canines to erupt. If the space is insufficient, the canine is forced to erupt facially toward the cheek or is unable to erupt at all. The latter situation occurs when the tooth is blocked out by the already erupted teeth and little room is available.

At about the same time (11 to 13 years of age), the mandibular second molars emerge, followed within months by their maxillary counterparts. The permanent second molars are often called *12-year molars* (Fig. 5.13).

The third molars do not appear in the oral cavity until age 17 or later. Much variation is seen in the eruption of third molars, especially when one considers that third molars are the teeth most likely to be **impacted.** Impacted teeth are those that do not completely erupt but remain embedded in bone or soft tissue. Mandibular third molars are most often affected because the mandible has to grow enough to accommodate them. The maxillary third molars are the next most likely teeth to be impacted.

The third molars, maxillary and mandibular, are also the most common teeth to be congenitally missing. A **congenitally missing** tooth is one that never forms because a tooth bud was never produced from which it could form. This can be a hereditary trait.

The eruptive forces do not cease after the eruption of the third molars. Eruption continues because of **attrition,** which is the wearing away of the tooth through contact of its functioning surfaces. Studies of ancient skulls show excessive wear not only on the occlusal of the teeth but also on their proximal surfaces. This wear accumulatively could have allowed more room for third molar eruption. This could be one reason why these skulls showed less impacted teeth. Another reason is that the diet of ancient man was grittier and harder to chew. This resulted in larger muscles of mastication, slightly wider jaw sizes, and wear between proximal surfaces of the teeth. A modern inherited trait is congenitally missing third molars. It is still rare to find all four third molars congenitally missing, but it is more and more common to find one or two missing.

As the teeth erupt and meet their antagonist in the opposite arch, they form what is known as the **occlusal plane.** Von Spee noted that the cusps and incisal ridges of the teeth tended to follow a curved line when the arches were observed from a point opposite the first molars. This line of occlusal surfaces is the occlusal plane. The curved alignment of the occlusal plane is named

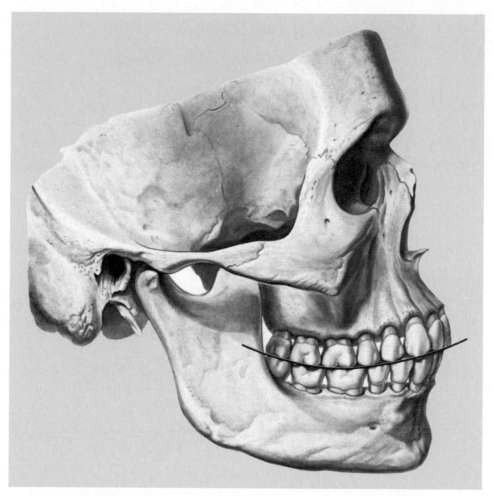

• **Figure 5.14** Occlusal plane (curve of Spee) rises to meet incisors and third molars. It dips down in the area of the first molars and second premolars. (Modified from Zeisz RC, Nuckolls J. *Dental Anatomy.* St. Louis: Mosby; 1949.)

after von Spee and is called the **curve of Spee** (Fig. 5.14). Not all occlusal planes follow a curve of Spee and some are flat. The flat occlusal plane is only possible if there is no crowding of the teeth within the arch. If crowding of the teeth exists, then the dental arch forms the curve of Spee. This curve allows for more occlusal space than a flat line.

The following is an approximate breakdown of permanent tooth eruption (Table 5.2).

Periods of Dentition

The period of **primary dentition** begins with the eruption of the first deciduous tooth. This tooth, a central incisor, usually erupts 7 months after birth, but some erupt as early as 6 months or as late as 9 months after birth. The period of primary dentition lasts as long as only deciduous teeth are present. When the first permanent molar erupts, the period of primary dentition ends.

At about 6 years of age the period of **mixed dentition** begins. This period exists while both primary and secondary teeth are simultaneously present and ends when the last deciduous tooth is exfoliated and only permanent teeth remain. Fig. 5.15 shows a radiographic x-ray taken of a child with a mixed dentition; notice the unerupted permanent teeth.

The period of permanent dentition begins when the last primary tooth is lost and ends when the last permanent tooth is lost. This period usually begins at about 12 years of age and, it is hoped, does not ever end. If all the permanent teeth are lost, no other period of dentition exists because no dentition is evident. Such a condition is termed **edentulous,** meaning *no teeth*.

Refer to Chapters 19 and 20 for a discussion of the formation of enamel, dentin, and pulp and to Chapter 16 for information concerning deciduous teeth.

Clinical Considerations

One of the functions of deciduous molars is to hold enough space into which the permanent premolars can erupt. If a deciduous tooth is prematurely lost, such as in the case of an extraction, that space is in jeopardy. One way to protect this space is for the dental provider to place a space retainer, which is a device that protects this space and prevents the permanent molar from moving into it. If a deciduous tooth is lost prematurely, it takes longer for the permanent tooth to erupt than if the deciduous tooth had not been lost. This is because it is harder for the osteoclasts to dissolve bone than a tooth root. Consequently the space retainer may need to be kept longer than the normal eruption period.

TABLE 5.2	**Chronology of Permanent Teeth**		
	Tooth	Universal System	Eruption (Years)
Upper	CI	8, 9	7–8
	LI	7, 10	8–9
	C	6, 11	11–12
	P1	5, 12	10–11
	P2	4, 13	10–12
	m1	3, 14	9–10
	m2	2, 15	12–13
	m3	1, 16	17–21
Lower	CI	24, 25	6–7
	LI	23, 26	7–8
	C	22, 27	9–10
	P1	21, 28	10–12
	P2	20, 29	11–12
	m1	19, 30	6–7
	m2	18, 31	11–13
	m3	17, 32	17–21

From Nelson SJ. *Wheeler's Dental Anatomy, Physiology, and Occlusion.* St. Louis: Elsevier Saunders; 2015.

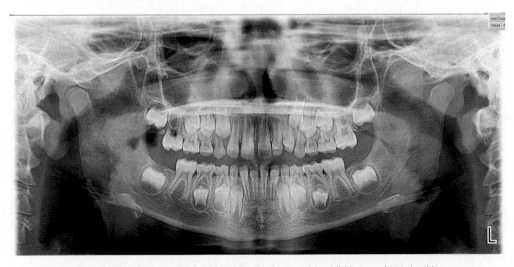

• **Figure 5.15** A panoramic radiograph of a 9-year-old exhibiting a mixed dentition.

Review Questions

1. Which hard tissue of the tooth forms last?
   a. enamel
   b. dentin
   c. cementum
2. What does the term *coalescence* mean?
3. What do developmental grooves or lines separate?
4. From what lobe does the cingulum of an anterior tooth form?
5. What is a rudimentary lobe of the maxillary first molar called?
6. Which teeth erupt first, the deciduous first molars or the canines?
7. Which of the following statements are usually true about eruption?
   a. Girls' teeth erupt earlier than boys' teeth.
   b. Maxillary teeth erupt before their mandibular counterparts.
   c. Teeth in both jaws do not erupt in pairs.
   d. The eruption sequence varies little from person to person.
8. Name the first permanent teeth to erupt in the oral cavity.
9. Of the following, which is the only acceptable dental term?
   a. bicuspid
   b. premolar
   c. milk teeth
   d. baby teeth
10. Explain all the various problems connected with premature loss of a deciduous molar.
11. With which teeth does the phenomenon of mesial drift occur, and what does it do?
12. Which teeth are the most likely to be congenitally missing?
   a. central incisors
   b. lateral incisors
   c. third molars
   d. canines
13. Name the structures now worn off that used to be present on the incisal ridge of Fig. 5.3.
14. How many lobes are present in the mandibular premolar in Fig. 5.7B? (HINT: It has three cusps.)
15. What are the periods of dentition for a 12-year-old boy? Give two possible reasons for each period of dentition.
16. When does the period of primary dentition end?
17. What deciduous teeth might an 11-year-old still have?
18. An orthodontist asks you to refer a patient back when the patient is out of mixed dentition. When would you send the patient to the orthodontist? What marks the end of the period of mixed dentition?
19. A new drug has been developed. It is a good drug with a bad side effect. The side effect is that this drug can discolor teeth if taken during the period of tooth development.
   a. What age of patient should avoid this drug to protect the permanent dentition?
   b. If this drug passes the placental barrier and affects the unborn fetus, then at what ages and what period of fetal development should it be avoided?

True or False

20. Only primary teeth begin to develop in utero (during fetal life).
21. If a child has spaces between the deciduous teeth at 5 years of age, these spaces will always remain, even after the permanent teeth have erupted.
22. Permanent teeth show no evidence of development until the sixth month after birth.
23. Deciduous teeth begin to calcify as early as the fourth month of fetal life.
24. Deciduous teeth become fully formed somewhere around 3.5 years after birth.
25. Permanent teeth continue to calcify until age 21 to 25.

6

Occlusion

OBJECTIVES

- To understand how the eruption schedule, growth, and ultimate alignment of the teeth are related
- To understand how muscle forces affect the alignment of the teeth
- To understand how the mesial step, flush terminal plane, and distal step affect occlusal classifications
- To understand the maxillary to mandibular vertical and horizontal alignment of teeth and which molars play a key part in this
- To define centric occlusion, centric relation, primate space, and leeway space
- To define overjet, overbite, crossbite, and open bite and to understand how they occur
- To identify the three occlusal classifications
- To understand the relationship that exists between the teeth during protrusive and lateral excursive movements

Position and Sequence of Eruption

Chapter 5 described eruption patterns of teeth. The eruption schedule helps permanent teeth emerge in their proper position. The loss of certain deciduous teeth at particular times allows the permanent teeth to move into key positions.

What about the deciduous teeth? What enables them to take their position for alignment? When examining the deciduous teeth, they not only appear in a certain position that is normal for each tooth but are also arranged in a row, which is referred to as *being in alignment.*

Normally, the eruption schedule helps the deciduous teeth take their proper position. For example, the central incisors come into position anterior to the lateral incisors because the centrals erupt before the laterals. Facial development and growth encourages the teeth to erupt properly. The anterior teeth are not covered by as much bone; therefore the tooth buds begin their formation earlier than those of the posterior teeth. The result is that most of the anterior teeth erupt before the posterior teeth. Some posterior teeth must actually wait until growth has occurred in the mandible because they are initially trapped under the **ramus of the mandible.** Thus the eruption pattern, facial development, and the sequence in which tooth buds begin forming all contribute to the eventual relationship of the teeth and jaws.

The development of **occlusion** begins with the eruption of the primary teeth (see Fig. 5.10A). Usually the first teeth to erupt are the central incisors, with the mandibular teeth erupting slightly

before the maxillary. The eruption of the lateral incisors, which occurs next, follows the same sequence.

At 16 months the primary molars erupt, which is an important event because the primary molars establish the vertical height of the primary occlusion. Primary molars also establish **intercuspation,** which is the mesial-distal and buccal-lingual relationships that determine how the maxillary teeth will touch, hit, and interlock with the mandibular teeth. The maxillary primary molars also help establish the anteroposterior (mesial-distal) relationship of the remaining deciduous teeth because their presence prompts the canines and second deciduous molars to erupt around them.

The primary dentition, which is usually complete by about 2.5 years of age, erupts in a more upright position than secondary teeth replacements. The average overjet of primary teeth is 3.0 mm, and the average overbite is 2.5 mm. The primary occlusion has one of three possible anteroposterior molar relationships called steps or planes. Most children have a **mesial step** between the distal surfaces of the second primary molars (Fig. 6.1A). The mandibular molars are situated more mesially than their maxillary counterparts, forming a mesial step. A smaller but still large group of children exhibits a **flush terminal plane,** with the distal surfaces of the deciduous second molars even with each other (Fig. 6.1B). A still smaller minority has a **distal step** (Fig. 6.1C). How would you describe a distal step compared with a mesial step or flush terminal plane? Also, note the large diastema or space in the mandibular arch between the canine and first molar (Fig. 6.1A–C).

As a child grows in height and weight, so too do the jaws. This growth of the mandible and maxilla results in horizontal and vertical growth of the dental arches. The teeth, however, remain the same size. Thus as the arches grow, spaces called **diastemae** (singular, **diastema**) form between the teeth. The largest spaces are often found mesial to the maxillary primary canines and distal to the mandibular canines. These spaces are called **primate spaces** and, although not always present, they are characteristic of all primates, including man (Fig. 6.2). As growth continues, diastemae also develop between the primary incisors.

Development of the Mesial Step

The permanent molars erupt and eventually touch the distal surfaces of the deciduous molars. As the permanent molars push up against the deciduous molars, they cause a chain reaction that pushes all the spaces between the teeth closed. A mesial step occurs in most individuals because as the permanent mandibular first molars erupt they push the primary molars mesially. This closes the primary space, allowing room for the permanent mandibular molars not only to erupt but to move mesially. The closing of the mandibular primary space allows for this extra room needed and results in the mandibular molars ending up in a more

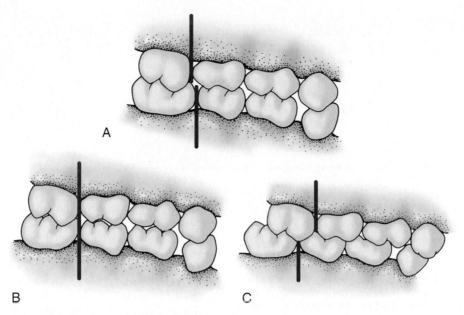

• **Figure 6.1** Relationships of the first permanent molars to each other determine the step or plane. **(A)** Mesial step; **(B)** flush terminal plane; **(C)** distal step.

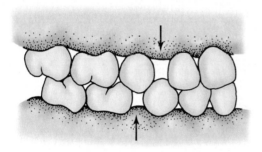

• **Figure 6.2** Primate spaces. These spaces occur in primary dentition. In the maxillary arch, they are anterior to the canines. In the mandibular arch, they are distal to the canines.

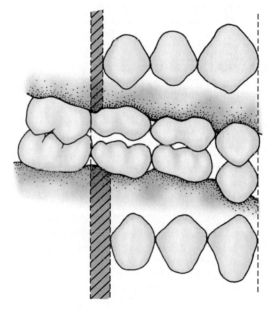

• **Figure 6.3** Leeway space is extra space that deciduous canines and molars occupy to help save room for their permanent successors. These permanent teeth take up less space. The difference between the space that deciduous teeth take up and that of their permanent replacements is called *leeway space*.

mesial position relative to their maxillary counterparts. The net result is the development of the mesial step.

A mesial step is further enhanced as the deciduous molars exfoliate and are replaced by the narrower permanent premolars. Extra space called **leeway space** is gained from this exchange of the second premolars. The earlier eruption cycle of the mandibular teeth allows them to capitalize on this exchange before the maxillary teeth, which further helps establish the mesial step (Fig. 6.3).

Finally, the mandible usually continues to grow later than the maxillae, allowing even further mesial mandibular advancement and usually ensuring a mesial step, thus forming a class I relationship. Too much further growth of the mandible could push the patient into an extreme mesial step, resulting in a class III relationship. A class II relationship could result if the mandible does not continue to grow or if the maxillae outgrow the mandible. It is possible for one type of relationship to occur on just one side while the other side maintains a class I relationship. Classes I, II, and III are covered later in this chapter, but it might help to see Figs. 6.19, 6.20, 6.21, and 6.22 to get a better understanding of what has just been covered.

A *deep bite* could result if the posterior teeth do not erupt enough, if the muscles of mastication are so hyperactive that they prevent the eruption of the posterior teeth, or for a variety of other reasons related to the jaw joint. A **deep bite** is the overclosing of the jaw to the extent that the occluding teeth do not erupt far enough. The vertical height is less than the normal bite (Fig. 6.4). The maxillary incisors will come further down, passing over more of the mandibular incisors, thus less of the length of the mandibular incisors can be seen when the teeth are closed together (occluding).

The development of the occlusion is further influenced by hereditary factors such as congenitally missing teeth, impacted teeth, or the size and shape of muscle and bone. Controllable factors that also affect occlusal development include the premature loss of deciduous teeth, decayed teeth that were not restored, and harmful habits.

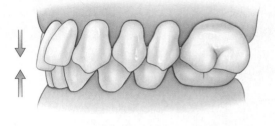
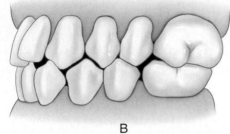

• **Figure 6.4** **(A)** Deep bite. The posterior teeth are not erupted vertically as much as in the slight posterior open bite **(B)**.

© Elsevier Collection

Clinical Considerations

Thumb-sucking and tongue thrusting are two such habits that if left uncorrected in the young child will leave the permanent incisors protruded. Once these incisors erupt, the forces exerted by the presence of a thumb or tongue habit push the incisors too far anteriorly. This not only causes the incisors to protrude but in some cases these forces are strong enough to move the alveolar ridge of the maxilla bone as well. As the anterior teeth are pushed forward they bring the surrounding bone with them. This makes it impossible to later move the teeth back because the entire alveolar ridge is so far forward that the only way to move the teeth back into proper alignment would require moving the teeth off their boney base. These habits must be stopped before the age of six and sometimes even five or younger in severe cases. Once the bone is moved it may be impossible to move it back, and the teeth can only go where the bone is. Bone does not always accompany the teeth if the guiding pressure is too great or if growth hormones are not present.

Horizontal Alignment

After the teeth erupt into the oral cavity, the tongue acts as a huge internal force that pushes the teeth toward the lips and cheeks. Conversely, resistance from the muscles that form the cheeks and lips is the controlling factor that prevents the teeth from moving too far facially. The balance or relative equilibrium between the tongue and the facial muscles allows the teeth to be brought into proper alignment and to be maintained in their proper positions once they have erupted.

Clinical Considerations

If this balance of forces is disturbed, a **malocclusion**, or an abnormal alignment of the teeth within the dental arches, can result. Abnormal forward thrusting of the tongue against the anterior teeth can cause such an imbalanced state (Fig. 6.5). Tongue thrusting causes the maxillary anterior teeth to **protrude** labially out of the mouth. This is especially true if an underdeveloped maxillary lip is evident along with the tongue thrust.

An opposite situation can also occur if the mandibular lip is overdeveloped; the **retrusion** of the mandibular anterior teeth

occurs. The patient is constantly tightening the lower lip against the mandibular anterior teeth (mentalis habit). These lip muscles are so strong that the mandibular teeth will be pushed back into the mouth by this overdeveloped lower lip (Fig. 6.6). If the mentalis habit involves placing the lower lip between the maxillary and mandibular incisors, the maxillary incisors will be pushed forward (protruded) while the mandibular incisors are pushed backward (retruded).

The lip, tongue, and cheek muscles and their relationship to one another are not the only factors that determine the alignment of the teeth. The intercuspation of the teeth helps prevent tooth deviations in a buccal or lingual direction. The maxillary posterior teeth have buccal and lingual cusps, and when the jaws are closed, the buccal cusps of the mandibular posterior teeth are interlocked

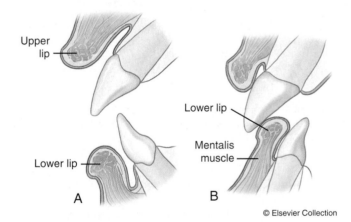

© Elsevier Collection

• **Figure 6.6** **(A)** Protrusion of maxillary incisors because of a lack of labial support from an upper lip that is too short. **(B)** Retrusion of lower incisors because of an overactive mentalis muscle habit. The habit of flexing the mentalis muscle forces the teeth to erupt in a lingual direction. If a lip habit is also involved, then the lip pushes up between maxillary and mandibular incisors and forces the upper teeth to protrude while retruding the lowers.

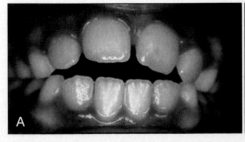
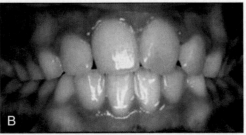

• **Figure 6.5** Open bite resulting from tongue thrusting. **(A)** Posterior teeth touch when jaws are closed, but space exists between anterior teeth. **(B)** During swallowing, the tongue closes space. (From Dean J. McDonald. *Avery's Dentistry for the Child and Adolescent*, Eleventh Edition. *Mosby*; 2021.)

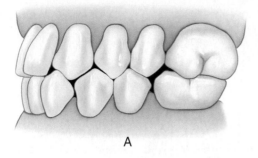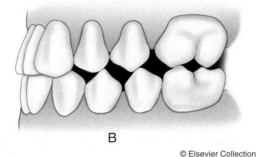

• **Figure 6.7** **(A)** The teeth interlock in maximum intercuspation. **(B)** The teeth are touching but not interlocking, and they are at an edge-to-edge bite.

between the buccal and lingual cusps of the maxillary teeth. This interlocking is similar to the interlocking of two gears. Fig. 6.7A–B shows how the interlocking of the cusps in Fig. 6.7A could help stability of the teeth as they occlude. This is not the case in Fig. 6.7B, in which the smooth tooth surfaces allow slippage because the cusps of the teeth do not interlock.

The alignment of previously erupted teeth in turn affects the alignment of successive teeth. Adequate space between teeth allows for complete and unhindered eruption of more teeth. If a tooth does not have room enough to erupt, it will deflect off the obstructing tooth and erupt out of alignment. It could also be blocked entirely by the obstruction and never erupt.

Other factors also influence the alignment of teeth. Mesial drift could account for the closure or loss of space necessary for tooth eruption. The size and shape of the jaws, the shape of the teeth, and the amount of lingual convergence of each tooth affect not only the alignment of the teeth but also the curvature of the dental arch and the spacing necessary for incoming teeth.

A slight *curve of Spee* can be seen in most normal occlusions (Fig. 6.8). This curve is higher in the anterior and posterior and dips downward in the middle. A flat plane of occlusion could also be considered a normal occlusion. If you look at the *curve of Spee* as seen in Fig. 6.8, you will notice that if the premolars were raised to the level of the molars and incisors it would require more total

arch space. In other words, if the teeth are slightly crowded and could not fit on a flat plane, they might be able to fit on a curved plane.

Clinical Considerations

A flat plane of occlusion is considered more stable and is one of the goals of orthodontics. However, if there is not enough room in the mouth to accommodate all the teeth in a flat plane, they sometimes could fit on a curved plane; the more room needed, the deeper the *curve of Spee*.

Vertical Alignment

Teeth are often thought to be vertically straight, but this is not true. They are not positioned straight up and down in the mouth. The mandibular posterior teeth tend to tip their crowns lingually and their roots laterally (Fig. 6.9). The maxillary posterior teeth tend to keep the crown straighter but with a slight buccal inclination and as a lingual inclination of the root (Fig. 6.10). From a lateral view, all the teeth (maxillary and mandibular and anterior and posterior) show a slight mesial inclination, with the possible exception of the maxillary third molar. Notice that the anterior teeth (Figs. 6.11 and 6.12) have a slight labial protrusion (a condition of being tipped forward), and from a frontal view, their crowns seem to incline laterally. In other words, the anterior teeth tip out to the side and toward the front (see Figs. 6.9 and 6.10).

Occlusion

Occlusion is the term used to describe the relationship of the mandibular and maxillary teeth when the teeth are closed together or during excursive movements when the teeth are touching. When the jaws are completely closed together, two possible relationships occur: (1) a relationship of the upper jaw to the lower jaw or (2) a relationship of the maxillary teeth to the mandibular teeth.

Centric Relation

Centric relation refers to the position of the mandible relative to the maxillae and is determined by the maximum contraction of the muscles of the jaw. *Centric relation* is defined as the relationship of the mandible to the maxillae in which healthy muscles and boney contours comfortably guide the mandible into its most posterior position as if there were no teeth to guide the mandible.

This relationship of the mandible to the maxillae occurs during strong muscle contractions such as swallowing. It is the most

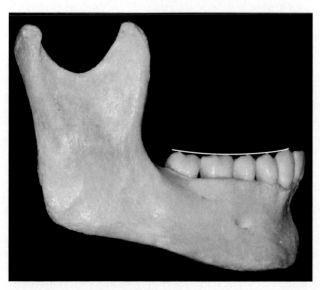

• **Figure 6.8** Curve of Spee.

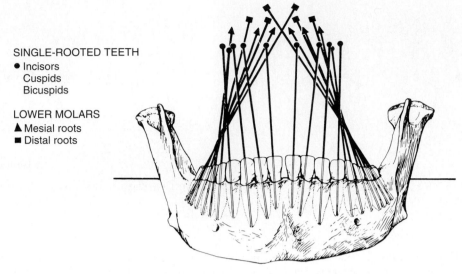

SINGLE-ROOTED TEETH
- ● Incisors
  Cuspids
  Bicuspids

LOWER MOLARS
- ▲ Mesial roots
- ■ Distal roots

• **Figure 6.9** Lines indicate the angle of inclination of teeth in relation to the mandible. (From Kraus BS, Jordon RE, Abrams L. *Dental Anatomy and Occlusion.* Baltimore: Williams & Wilkins; 1969.)

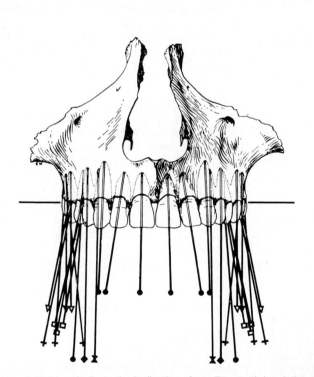

SINGLE-ROOTED TEETH
- ● Incisors
  Cuspids
  Upper second premolars

FIRST PREMOLAR
- ◆ Buccal roots
- ✗ Palatal roots

UPPER MOLARS
- ▽ Mesiobuccal roots
- ✚ Distobuccal roots
- ▫ Palatal roots

• **Figure 6.10** Lines indicate the inclination of maxillary teeth in relation to the maxillae. (From Kraus BS, Jordon RE, Abrams L. *Dental Anatomy and Occlusion.* Baltimore: Williams & Wilkins; 1969.)

stable and most posterior position that affords the strongest muscle contractions. It is a relationship of bone to bone brought about by allowing the muscles to contract in their most natural posture to their most comfortable and effective position. This posture does not have anything to do with the interdigitation of the teeth. Indeed, it may not be the position that allows the greatest intercuspation of the teeth. It is a bone-to-bone relationship guided by the temporomandibular joint.

To experience centric relation, tip your head as far back as possible and gently close your teeth together. Let your mandible go back as far as possible. You will notice this is different than your **habitual occlusion**. If you tip your head forward and close your

teeth together as you usually do, this is your centric occlusion. Is your mandible farther forward in your habitual centric occlusion or in your centric relation?

Centric Occlusion

Centric occlusion also refers to a position when the jaws are closed, but this position is determined by the way the teeth fit together. It is the jaw position that allows the greatest interdigitation of the teeth. It is related to tooth occlusion and not determined by muscle or TMJ. It is the habitual way that the teeth come together or the normal way people close their teeth together.

SINGLE-ROOTED TEETH
● Incisors
 Cuspids
 Upper second premolars

FIRST PREMOLAR
♦ Buccal roots
✗ Palatal roots

UPPER MOLARS
▽ Mesiobuccal roots
✚ Distobuccal roots
▢ Palatal roots

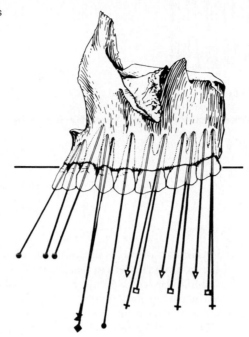

• **Figure 6.11** A lateral view of the inclination of maxillary teeth. (From Kraus BS, Jordon RE, Abrams L. *Dental Anatomy and Occlusion.* Baltimore: Williams & Wilkins; 1969.)

SINGLE-ROOTED TEETH
● Incisors
 Cuspids
 Bicuspids

LOWER MOLARS
▲ Mesial roots
■ Distal roots

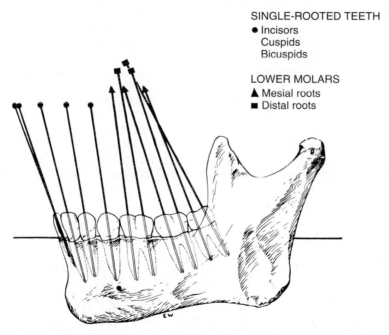

• **Figure 6.12** A lateral view of the inclination of mandibular teeth. (From Kraus BS, Jordon RE, Abrams L. *Dental Anatomy and Occlusion.* Baltimore: Williams & Wilkins; 1969.)

Centric occlusion is sometimes called **acquired centric occlusion, habitual occlusion, convenience occlusion,** or **intercuspal position.** This is the way your teeth fit together out of habit without planning or forethought. With the jaws closed, the occlusal surfaces of the maxillary teeth touch the occlusal surfaces of the mandibular teeth. The lingual cusps of the maxillary premolars and molars rest in the deepest parts of the occlusal sulci of the mandibular premolars and molars, and the buccal cusps of the mandibular premolars and molars rest in the deepest parts of the sulci of the maxillary premolars and molars (Figs. 6.13 and 6.14). It is a tooth-guided relationship and not a bone-guided or muscle-guided relationship.

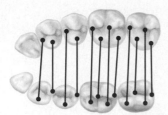

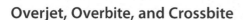

• **Figure 6.13** Centric occlusion. Contacting marginal ridge areas and occlusal cusp tips are indicated by circles. The buccal cusp tips of the mandibular teeth contact the maxillary marginal ridges and the central fossae of the maxillary molars. The lingual cusp tips of the maxillary teeth contact the marginal ridges and central fossae of the mandibular molars. (From Okeson JP. *Management of Temporomandibular Disorders and Occlusion.* 7th ed. St. Louis: Mosby; 2013.)

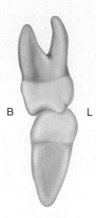

• **Figure 6.14** Mesial view of the left first molars. In centric occlusion, teeth interconnect to their greatest potential. (From Nelson SJ, Ash M. *Wheeler's Dental Anatomy.* 9th ed. St. Louis: Saunders; 2010.)

Overjet, Overbite, and Crossbite

When the jaws are closed in centric occlusion, the cusps of the maxillary teeth overlap the cusps of the mandibular teeth so that the maxillary teeth are facial to the mandibular teeth. Although the cusps of the maxillary teeth do not directly touch the cusps of the mandibular teeth on closure of the jaw, it is possible for the cusps to come into contact when the mandible slides from side to side. Notice that the maxillary cusps are located facial to the mandibular cusps.

The amount of facial horizontal overlap of the maxillary teeth is called an **overjet.** In Fig. 6.15, the maxillary incisors are facial to the mandibular incisors. Line A represents the amount of horizontal overlap, or overjet.

Fig. 6.16 shows that the maxillary incisors also vertically overlap the mandibular incisors. Line A indicates the amount of vertical overlap or **overbite.** Overbite is the extension of the incisal edges of the maxillary anterior teeth below the incisal edges of the mandibular anterior teeth in a vertical direction (Fig. 6.17).

If one or more teeth in the mandibular arch are located facial to their maxillary counterparts, a condition known as **crossbite** occurs. Fig. 6.18 illustrates a mandibular right first molar in crossbite. Notice that the buccal cusp of the mandibular molar is located facial to the buccal cusp of the maxillary molar. A crossbite condition can exist between any number of teeth. It can be caused by a loss of space in the deciduous arch such that a tooth could be blocked out of its normal position and moved into a more lingual position for a maxillary or more facially for a mandibular tooth. A crossbite of all the mandibular teeth can occur if a disease causes the patient's mandible but not the maxillae to continue growing. Such a condition is called **acromegaly.** In this disease, growth hormone causes the mandible to grow faster and wider than the maxilla. As a result, the mandibular teeth are eventually positioned in crossbite with the maxillary teeth. Because the mandible continues to grow for a longer period than the maxilla, this condition worsens with time.

An even more common cause of crossbite can occur if the maxillae bones do not grow in proportion to the mandible. When this happens, the maxillary teeth are bilaterally in crossbite or edge to edge with the mandibular teeth. In most of these situations the patient forces their teeth to one side to close completely together as in centric occlusion. The other side displays full crossbite of most or all the posterior teeth on that side. The midline of the anterior teeth is off, and the maxillary and mandibular midlines do not line up because the patient is forcing the mandible to one side to get a more functional bite.

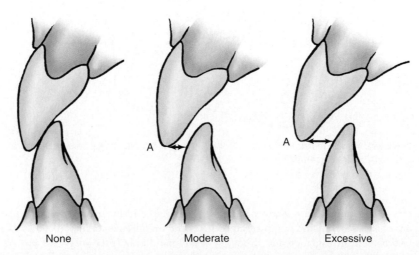

None   Moderate   Excessive

• **Figure 6.15** Moderate, slight, and extreme overjet. Line A indicates the difference in overjet; the amount of overbite is the same in all three examples. (Modified from Ross IF. *Occlusion: A Concept for the Clinician.* St. Louis: Mosby; 1970.)

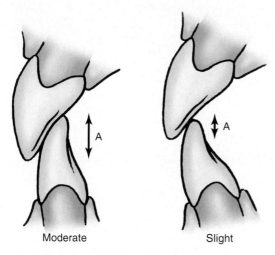

Moderate   Slight

• **Figure 6.16** Moderate and slight overbite. Line A indicates the difference in overbite; the amount of overjet is the same in both examples. (Modified from Ross IF. *Occlusion: A Concept for the Clinician.* St. Louis: Mosby; 1970.)

Open Bite

When the teeth are in centric occlusion, the maxillary and mandibular teeth should touch each other. The occlusal surfaces of the posterior teeth should touch, and the anterior teeth should touch in such a way that the incisal edges of the mandibular anterior teeth almost or just barely touch the lingual surfaces of the maxillary anterior teeth. If the anterior teeth do not touch but are widely separated when in centric occlusion, the condition known as **open bite** occurs. An open bite exists when the anterior teeth of the maxillary arch do not overlap the mandibular teeth in a vertical direction. Such a condition can be caused by either a thumb-sucking or a tongue-thrusting habit. In either situation a powerful force is exerted against the anterior teeth when the jaws close. In thumb-sucking, the patient's thumb or fingers rest between the maxillary and mandibular anterior teeth, preventing the teeth from touching each other. Thus a force is exerted that pushes the anterior teeth back into the bone and prevents them from erupting. The outcome is a wide separation of the anterior teeth when the jaws close (see Fig. 6.5).

A tongue-thrusting habit places the tongue between the anterior teeth every time the patient swallows. The act of swallowing requires the jaws to come together and the lips to close, which seals off air spaces and results in a negative pressure. If the patient has poor tongue placement or if open spaces exist between the front teeth, the following sequence occurs. First the patient places the tongue against these open spaces or against the anterior teeth. When the patient swallows, closing the jaws, the tongue pushes against the anterior teeth. The result is a protrusion of the maxillary anterior teeth, with the pressure preventing the teeth from erupting normally. In the normally developed swallowing pattern, this situation is prevented because the tongue is placed against the roof of the mouth, not against the teeth. When the tongue thrusts during jaw closure, it exerts pressure on the palate rather than on the teeth.

Occlusal Classification

The two basic classifications of occlusion are skeletal and dental. The first is based on the relationship of the bone of the maxilla to the bone of the mandible. This system, because it is related to the bones, is referred to as the skeletal classification. The second system is based on the relationship of the teeth of the mandible to the teeth of the maxilla. It is called the dental classification, because it is related to the teeth.

The skeletal classification is divided into the following three classes of relationship (Figs. 6.19–6.22):

Class I: The maxilla and mandible are in normal relationship to each other.

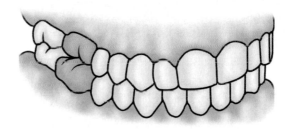

• **Figure 6.18** Posterior crossbite of right first molars, in blue. The mandibular first molars is buccal to the maxillary first molar.

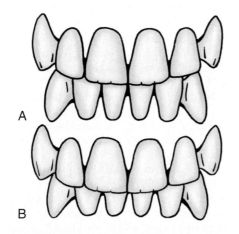

• **Figure 6.17** **(A)** Slight overbite. **(B)** Moderate overbite. **(C)** Excessive overbite. (Modified from Ross IF. *Occlusion: A Concept for the Clinician.* St. Louis: Mosby; 1970.)

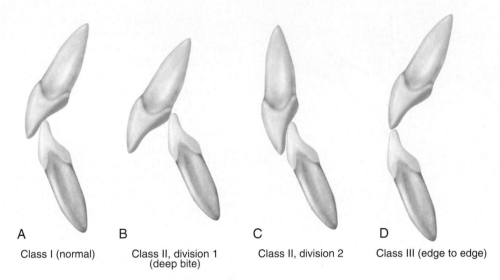

A	B	C	D
Class I (normal)	Class II, division 1 (deep bite)	Class II, division 2	Class III (edge to edge)

• **Figure 6.19** Types of malocclusion. **(A)** Class I. **(B)** Class II, division I, severe overjet, deep overbite. **(C)** Class II, division II, deep overbite, no overjet. **(D)** Class III, incisal edges of maxillary central even to or lingual to mandibular central incisal edges. (From Okeson JP. *Management of Temporomandibular Disorders and Occlusion.* 7th ed. St. Louis: Mosby; 2013.)

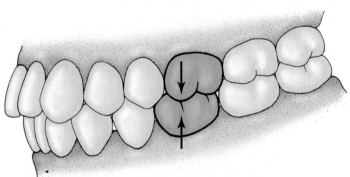

• **Figure 6.20** Class I occlusal relationship. *Vertical arrows* show the relationship of the mesiobuccal cusps of maxillary first molars in relation to the mesiobuccal groove of the lower first molars in all three classifications.

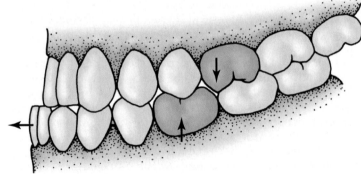

• **Figure 6.22** Class III occlusal relationship. *Arrow* indicates mandibular incisors are more anterior than maxillary.

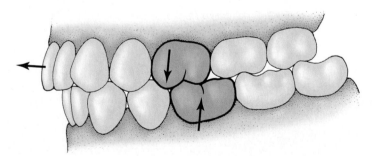

• **Figure 6.21** Class II, division I occlusal relationship. *Horizontal arrow* indicates maxillary incisors are more anterior than mandibular.

Class II: The mandible is retruded and thus retrognathic. It has a distal relationship with the maxilla.

Class III: The mandible is protruded and thus prognathic. It has a mesial relationship with the maxilla.

The dental classification is based on the relationship of the teeth. The canines or the first permanent molars are used in dental classifications. The first molars are easier to evaluate and their upper to lower relationship is the preferred way to determine the occlusal relationship.

E. H. Angle's classification system is the most popular dental classification system in use today. His system is based primarily on the relationship of the permanent first molars to each other and, to a lesser degree, on the relationship of the permanent canines to each other. In centric occlusion, three relationships exist among the first molars. In the normal relationship the maxillary first molar is slightly posterior to the mandibular first molar. The mesiobuccal cusp of the maxillary first molar is directly in line with the buccal groove of the mandibular first molar. Such a relationship is called a **class I occlusal relationship,** or a **neutroclusion** (see Figs. 6.19A and 6.20).

A **class II occlusal relationship,** or a **distoclusion,** exists when the maxillary first molar is even with or anterior to the mandibular first molar. In this relationship the buccal groove of the mandibular first molar is posterior to the mesiobuccal cusp of the maxillary first molar (see Fig. 6.21). Could such a relationship be present if the maxillary teeth protruded or if the mandibular teeth retruded (see Fig. 6.19B and C)?

Class II contains two separate divisions. Class II, division I occurs when the permanent first molars are in class II and the permanent maxillary central incisors are in their normal, slightly protruded position (Fig. 6.23A; see Figs. 6.19B and 6.21).

Class II, division II occurs when the permanent first molars are in class II relationship and the permanent maxillary central incisors are retruded and inclined lingually (see Figs. 6.19C, 6.21, and 6.23B). The maxillary incisors slightly overlap the centrals with the centrals being slightly lingual to the laterals.

A class II, division II relationship often occurs when the following scenario is present:
1. Deep overbite
2. Crowded maxillary anteriors
3. Normal overjet
4. Excessive masseter muscle development

Any class II occlusion can result in a retrognathic positioning of the mandible. In this relationship the mandible is positioned much more posteriorly to the maxilla than normally. A class II relationship can result in a deep bite with excess overbite. This occurs because when the jaws close together, they over-close. The teeth do not touch as soon as in a class I or III because the incisors do not touch, and the posterior teeth may be intruded. The net result is that the upper and lower jaws come closer together because the teeth don't stop them as soon.

A **class III occlusal relationship**, or a **mesioclusion**, exists when the buccal groove of the mandibular first molar is more anterior than normal to the mesiobuccal cusp of the maxillary first molar (see Figs. 6.19D and 6.22). This relationship would be present if the maxillary teeth were retruded or if the mandibular teeth protruded. Most class III relationships are due to **prognathic** positioning of the lower jaw. In this condition the mandible is positioned forward to the maxilla. This usually occurs because the mandible continues to grow forward faster than the maxilla. Eventually the lower teeth and jaw are positioned in a more anterior relationship to the maxilla.

It is possible for both sides of the mandible to be in different classes. Although the molar-to-molar classification is the main method of identifying the dental classification, it is not the only method. The canines can be used in a dental classification system as follows:

Class I: The distal surface of the mandibular canine is within one premolar's width of the mesial surface of the maxillary canine.
Class II: The distal surface of the mandibular canine is distal to the mesial surface of the maxillary canine by a width of at least one premolar.

Class III: The distal surface of the mandibular canine is mesial to the mesial surface of a maxillary canine by at least a width of one premolar.

Another form of dental classification involves the incisor relationships (see Fig. 6.19) as follows:
Class I: The mandibular incisors occlude with or lie directly below the middle of the lingual surfaces of the maxillary incisors (see Fig. 6.19A).
Class II: The incisal margins of the mandibular incisors lie behind the middle part of the lingual surfaces of the maxillary incisors. Division I means that the maxillary centrals (and possibly laterals) are protruded labially (see Figs. 6.19B and 6.23A). Division II means that the maxillary centrals only have their incisal edges tipped more lingually and the maxillary centrals may be retruded lingually to the laterals (see Figs. 6.19C and 6.23B).
Class III: The incisal margins of the mandibular incisors lie in front of the middle of the lingual surface of the maxillary incisors (see Fig. 6.19D and Fig. 6.22). If the incisal edges are meeting in centric, and no overjet exists, then the mandibular incisors are too far forward.

In many class III relationships the mandibular teeth are actually anterior to the maxillary incisors when the jaws are in centric relationship.

Lateral Mandibular Glide (Lateral Excursion)

In lateral excursion the mandible moves toward the right or left side. The side to which the mandible moves is referred to as the working side, and the other side is referred to as the nonworking side when no teeth are contacting on this side. When working with artificial teeth, as in denture construction, this nonworking side is referred to as the balancing side. When making dentures, it is important to have both sides continue to contact and touch even during side movements. This keeps the denture balanced and avoids tipping. Natural teeth do not need to balance, and none of the teeth on the nonworking side are in contact.

A working side exists when the mandible is moved to one side, with buccal cusps of the maxillary and mandibular teeth directly above each other and the lingual cusps directly over each other on the same side to which the mandible moved. If you slide your lower jaw to the right, the working side is on the right (Fig. 6.24).

A nonworking side occurs on the opposite side from which the jaw moves toward. If you move the lower jaw to the right, a nonworking side would exist on the left side.

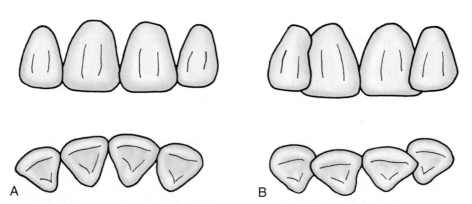

• **Figure 6.23** **(A)** Class II, division I: maxillary incisors are in good alignment. **(B)** Class II, division II: maxillary central incisors are retruded lingually behind the lateral incisors.

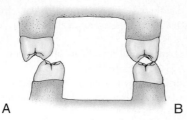

• **Figure 6.24** Lateral excursion. **(A)** Balancing side. **(B)** Working side.

In lateral mandibular glide (also called lateral excursion), usually only the canines are in contact as the jaw moves into its working side. If only the canines are touching, it is referred to as a **canine rise.** The mandibular canine opens the bite by gliding down the lingual surface of the maxillary canine. In lateral excursion, the last two teeth to touch, in an almost cusp tip–to–cusp tip arrangement, should be the canines. If the lateral glide is to the right, the last two teeth to touch should be the right canines.

It is common to sometimes have a slight premolar contact along with the canines in lateral excursion. When the premolars also occlude during lateral excursion, it is called **group function.** The canines should still be the dominant occluding teeth; the premolars only assist through part of the lateral slide.

In natural dentition the cusps on the nonworking side rarely touch at all. In fact, having balancing side interferences during lateral excursion can have detrimental effects on the temporomandibular jaw joint.

Protrusion

Protrusion is when the mandible moves forward from centric occlusion. In protrusion the only teeth that should touch are the anterior teeth. The mandibular anterior four incisors should glide across the maxillary four incisors as the mandible moves forward. No other teeth except possibly the canines may touch, and then only slightly. No posterior teeth should touch in a mandibular protrusive movement.

The anterior teeth in Fig. 6.22 resembles what a class I occlusion would look like in protrusive movement with the incisors touching as they guided the mandible in a forward position, but none of the posterior teeth would be touching as they are in class III centric relation.

Premature Contact

When the jaw closes, all the posterior teeth should come into contact at the same time. If one tooth hits ever so slightly more than the others, it becomes an interference and bears more force than the others, becoming a **premature contact area.** The anterior incisors may also hit but not harder than the posteriors. If the anteriors do hit in centric occlusion, it is called **anterior coupling.**

A premature contact causes the jaw to deflect before allowing the rest of the teeth to occlude. If the path of the lower jaw movement deflects from its true course, the temporomandibular jaw joint must be put into a stretched or abnormal position, which can cause the following results:

1. The temporomandibular joint undergoes abnormal stress, causing damage to the ligaments or to the muscles of the joint. Often the jaw joint affected is the one from the opposite side of the mouth that has the premature contact.

2. The closing muscles act to move the jaw in a direction that would avoid the teeth from hitting prematurely. In doing so they become tired, sore, and tender as one set of muscles is forced to be overexerted trying to prevent a premature contact. Eventually that set of muscles exhibits symptoms of discomfort from spasms, strains, and tears.

3. The tooth that is hitting prematurely becomes sensitive to percussion and is tender during chewing. It may become mobile, and x-ray examination may reveal a widening of the periodontal ligament.

4. The responsible tooth may become cracked or broken. Even under the normal stress of occlusion, when all the teeth are hitting at the same time, the occluding cusps undergo a contact pressure of 300 pounds per square inch. In premature contact the force could be enough to crack or break the tooth.

Fundamentals of Ideal Occlusion in Permanent Dentition

Ideal occlusion is the result of the maxillary bones and the mandibular bone in proper harmony with each other. The condyles of the mandible are in their most favorable location within the glenoid fossae. At the same time the muscles of the face and jaws must be in balance with each other and with the previously mentioned bones. Finally, the occlusion of the teeth and how they interlock is most stable when all the previously mentioned bones, muscles, and joints are synchronized to be in balance and harmony with one another. Is ideal occlusion a matter of luck, wishful thinking, or a dream? No, it actually happens. The function of the bones, muscles, and joints helps guide the teeth in a harmony of forces that results in a balanced occlusion.

The most ideal occlusion is a class I occlusion. The class I occlusion is also the most common occlusion. The class I molar relationship exists when the mesiobuccal cusps of the maxillary first permanent molar fall within the groove between the mesiobuccal and middle buccal cusps of the mandibular first molar. A *class I canine relationship* exists when the distal surface of the mandibular canine is within one premolar's width of the mesial surface of the maxillary canine. The mandibular canine should then be positioned in the embrasure located between the maxillary canine and the maxillary lateral incisor (see Fig. 6.20).

In the ideal occlusion, the occlusal plane is almost flat with a slight *curve of Spee,* which deepens with age. The teeth have good, tight proximal contacts with no spaces in between. No rotated teeth are evident, and the upper and lower arches are symmetric and well formed. All of the crowns of the teeth are tipped slightly mesially, with the exception of the maxillary third molar. The maxillary third molar is almost straight up and down with a slight distal inclination. The labiolingually and buccolingually crown inclination is such that the incisors flair labially and the rest of the teeth flair lingually. Finally, the maxillary first molar is tipped mesially so that it touches the mandibular first and second molars. This is called a **stolarized molar,** and in the ideal occlusion the distal marginal ridge of the permanent maxillary first molar touches the mesial marginal ridge of the permanent mandibular second molar and the middle of the mandibular first molar (Fig. 6.25).

Because all humans are different, only a few experience ideal occlusion. However, it is easier to discover malocclusions when one is familiar with the ideal. It is also helpful to study the skeletons of our ancestors to discover how our occlusion developed. In the 1930s, P. R. Begg studied more than 800 Australian aboriginal skulls. He noted that although some class II and III malocclusions occurred,

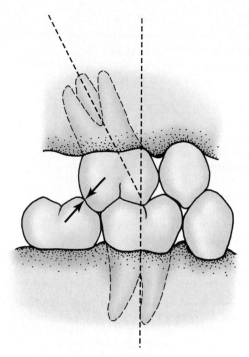

According to Begg: "Class II, division II and class III malocclusions are far more serious physical afflictions for [prehistoric] man than they are for civilized man. This is because of the harm that these two forms of malocclusion do to [prehistoric] man by interfering with his proper masticatory function and by producing severe dental disease." In prehistoric people the deep incisor overbite of class II, division II malocclusion interfered with lateral movement of the mandibular teeth and jaw.

This was a less effective form of mastication of food and required more effort and time. In addition, the incisors would undergo severe attrition faster because the maxillary incisors were inclined lingually, which caused the incisors to abscess when the pulps were exposed. The resulting bacterial infections could have adversely affected survival rates (Fig. 6.26). The extreme, early wear of the incisors in class III could have also resulted in lower survival rates for the same reason (Fig. 6.27).

According to Begg, the survival of our ancestors was affected by the class of dental occlusion they possessed. More class I occlusions were successfully passed on through genetics. This was the result of attrition rather than jaw placement, temporomandibular joint structure, or muscle-to-bone relationships.

• **Figure 6.25** Stolarized molars. The upper first molar is tipped forward so its distal marginal ridge touches the mesial marginal ridge of the lower second molar and the middle of the mandibular first molar. To do this the upper molar must have a mesial tip that allows its distal marginal ridge to come further occlusally than its mesial marginal ridge.

proportionately fewer were found in Australian aboriginal skulls than in modern humans. He also postulated that this occurred for two reasons: (1) far fewer malocclusions occurred because of overcrowding or excess tooth size, and (2) some of the more severe anomalies were so detrimental to Stone Age man that their incidence was kept relatively low by natural selection, which limited survival rates.

Begg noted that prehistoric people had extensive attrition of their teeth. He concluded that the diet of primitive aborigines was abrasive enough to wear down not only the occluding surfaces but also the interproximal surfaces of the teeth. An average of 1 mm of wear occurred on the proximal surfaces of each tooth, which accumulated to 7.5 mm/arch. Through mesial drift the posterior teeth took advantage of this wear and closed the arch length, and the extra space provided by interproximal wear allowed the third molars additional arch space to erupt.

Begg surmised that an adaptive mechanism seemed to allow the mandible to move anteriorly. As the incisors wore down, the mandible moved forward to maintain an edge-to-edge bite. This enabled the posterior teeth to occlude with the jaw in an anterior position with no overjet or overbite. The occlusal cusps were worn flat so the jaw could have full occlusion in class I or in protrusive movement.

This occlusal wear shortened the crown length, but the teeth erupted to compensate for the loss of vertical height. The supraeruptive forces of the teeth compensated for this occlusal wear just as mesial drift took advantage of the opportunity to close the spaces left from interproximal wear. The dentition of prehistoric people had extreme occlusal wear, which led to the shortening of the anatomic crowns and the preservation of the vertical bite through supraeruption.

The vast majority of prehistoric skulls studied by Begg had class I occlusions, with only 12% having class II, division I occlusions; 1% having class II, division II occlusions; and only 3% having class III occlusions.

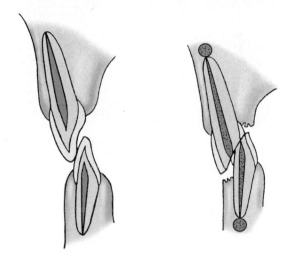

• **Figure 6.26** Incisal wear such as that seen in prehistoric human's attritional class II, division II malocclusion may cause exposure and death of the tooth pulp. (From Begg PR, Kesling PC. *Begg Orthodontic Theory and Technique.* Philadelphia: WB Saunders; 1977.)

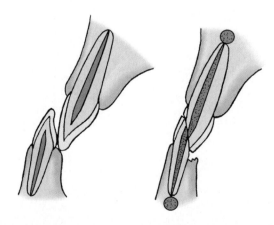

• **Figure 6.27** Incisal wear such as that seen in prehistoric human's attritional class III malocclusion may cause pulp exposure. (From Begg PR, Kesling PC. *Begg Orthodontic Theory and Technique.* Philadelphia: WB Saunders; 1977.)

Review Questions

1. What affects the alignment of the teeth?
2. Which muscle forces affect the alignment of the teeth?
3. What is the difference between the *curve of Spee* and a flat-planed occlusion?
4. Define the following terms:
    a. open bite
    b. overbite
    c. overjet
    d. centric occlusion
    e. crossbite
5. Which occlusal classification has the distal surface of the mandibular canine distal to the mesial surface of the maxillary canine by a width of at least one premolar?
6. Which occlusal classification is shown in Fig. 6.28?

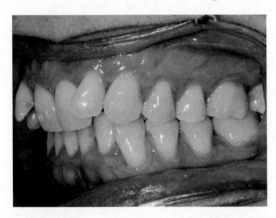

• **Figure 6.28** The molars and canines are in what classification? The incisors are in what division? (From Sergueef N. Ostéopathie orofaciale et temporomandibulaire. *Elsevier Massaon;* 2021.)

7. What is meant by mesial step?
8. If an occlusion with a mesial step proceeds without problems, which of the following most likely results?
    a. class I
    b. class II
    c. class III
    d. distal step
9. Which factors influence occlusion?
    a. heredity
    b. unrestored deciduous decayed molars
    c. impacted deciduous teeth
    d. congenitally missing teeth
    e. growth of the condyles
    f. eruption sequence of the teeth
    g. leeway space
    h. primate space
10. Outline the elements of the ideal occlusion.
11. Outline some of the differentiating features of the occlusion of primitive people.
12. What marks the beginning of the development of occlusion?
13. What determines the height of the primary occlusion?
14. Define or explain the term *intercuspation.*
15. Which molar relationship is more common in children: the flush terminal plane or the distal step?

7
Dental Anomalies

OBJECTIVES

- To define dental anomaly
- To discuss intrinsic factors
- To discuss extrinsic factors
- To discuss the difference between hereditary and congenital factors
- To define the various anomalies listed in this chapter

An **anomaly** is defined as something that is noticeably different or that deviates from the ordinary or normal. Dental anomalies are deviations of dental tissue origin and therefore are derived from the dental tissues: enamel, dentin, or cementum. Anomalies can be extreme variations or just slight deviations. They can be caused by a multitude of things or by just one small variation in the environment.

Some abnormalities result from **intrinsic** factors (those that originate from inside the body) such as heredity, metabolic dysfunction, or mutations; other causes are **extrinsic** (causes originating from outside the body) such as physical or chemical trauma, biologic agents, nutritional deficiencies, stress, habits, or environmental conditions. In many instances anomalies result from a combination of intrinsic and extrinsic factors.

If a condition occurs because of an individual's genetic makeup, the condition is termed **hereditary**. If the condition occurs at or before birth, it is termed **congenital**. A congenital condition is sometimes the result of heredity, and sometimes a hereditary condition does not become evident until years after birth. If a condition exhibits some evidence of an inherited tendency but such evidence is inconclusive, it is often referred to as a **familial tendency**. If a condition results during the formation and development of a dental structure, it is referred to as a *developmental anomaly*.

Classification of Dental Anomalies

Anomalies resulting in a variation in the size of teeth are called **macrodontia**, which is when teeth are larger than normal (Fig. 7.1), and **microdontia**, which is when teeth are smaller than normal (Fig. 7.2).

Anomalies resulting in a variation in the number of teeth are **hyperdontia** (multiple or extra teeth (Fig. 7.3) and **anodontia** (singular or multiple missing teeth; Fig. 7.4). Total anodontia exists if no teeth are present at all, and partial anodontia exists if less than the normal number of teeth are present. True anodontia is the congenital absence of teeth. It may involve the permanent dentition, the primary dentition, or both. If the primary teeth are

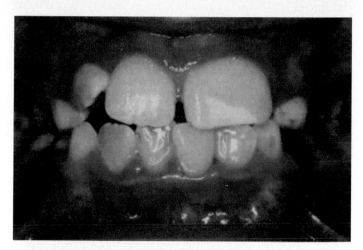

• **Figure 7.1** Macrodontia. The incisor teeth are too large for the size of the oral cavity. (From Berkovitz BKB, Holland GR, Moxham BJ. *Oral Anatomy, Histology and Embryology*. 4th ed. London: Mosby; 2009.)

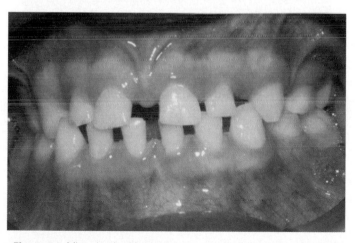

• **Figure 7.2** Microdontia. Note the large diastemae between the teeth, caused by the teeth being too small for the oral cavity. (From Neville BW, Damm DD, Allen C. *Oral and Maxillofacial Pathology*. 3rd ed. St. Louis: Saunders; 2009.)

congenitally missing, their permanent replacements will also be absent.

The most commonly missing permanent teeth are the third molars, and the maxillary thirds are absent more often than the mandibular ones. The next most likely teeth to be missing are the permanent maxillary lateral incisors. Between 1% and 2% of the population are missing at least one permanent maxillary

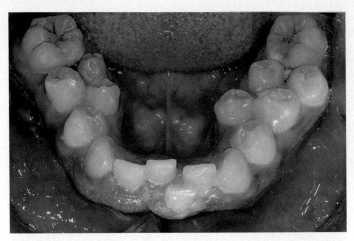

• **Figure 7.3** Hyperdontia or supernumerary teeth. There are extra teeth lingual to the regular dentition. (From Neville B., Damm D. Color *Atlas of Oral and Maxillofacial Diseases.* Elsevier; 2018.)

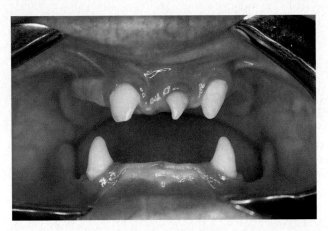

• **Figure 7.4** Anodontia. This particular case illustrates partial anodontia. There is a large number of missing teeth. (From Bird D. Robinson D. *Modern Dental Assisting*, 12e, Saunders; 2017.)

lateral incisor. The third most commonly missing tooth is the permanent mandibular second premolar. About 1% of the population is affected. The least likely permanent teeth to be missing are the canines.

Hyperdontia is not an uncommon anomaly. It has been reported that from 0.1% to 3.6% of individuals from various populations have too many teeth. These extra teeth are referred to as **supernumeraries**. Supernumerary teeth are most commonly located in the midline and molar regions of the maxillae, followed by the premolar region of the mandible, whereas other sites are only rarely involved. Maxillary supernumerary teeth outnumber mandibular nine to one.

Supernumerary teeth arising in the midline of the maxillae are termed **mesiodens** (Fig. 7.5) and are the most common supernumeraries. The maxillary distomolars are the next most common supernumerary teeth. These **distomolars** are also called *fourth molars* and are located distal to the maxillary third molars. Mandibular distomolars do occur but not nearly as often as in the maxilla. A supernumerary tooth situated buccally or lingually to a molar is called a **paramolar**; they are usually small and rudimentary. The next most likely location for supernumeraries is the premolar area of the mandible. Only 10% of all supernumeraries occur in the mandible.

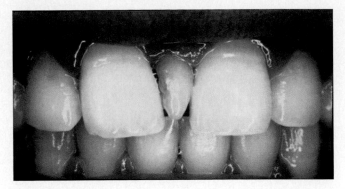

• **Figure 7.5** Mesiodens. Note the peg-shaped supernumerary tooth between maxillary incisors. (From Neville B., Damm D. *Oral and Maxillofacial pathology*, 4e. Saunders; 2015.)

If a supernumerary resembles a regular tooth, it is termed *supplemental*; if it is cone shaped, it is called **conical**; and if it is very small, it is called **tubercle**. Supernumerary teeth are much more common in the permanent than in the primary dentition.

Anomalies in Shape

Odontoma

An **odontoma** (Fig. 7.6) is a tumorous anomaly of calcified dental tissues. There are two types of odontoma: complex, which consists of a single mass of dentin, cementum, and enamel in a large blob or unspecified shape, and compound, which consists of several small masses that more or less resemble rudimentary teeth. Compound odontomas may sometimes resemble multiple mesiodens because they are similar to small, supplemental teeth, but they are even smaller.

Dens in Dente

Dens in dente (Fig. 7.7) is a developmental variation thought to occur when the outer surface of the tooth crown invaginates or

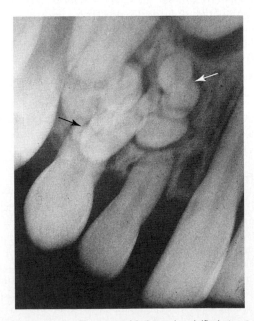

• **Figure 7.6** Odontoma. The two odd-shaped, calcified structures in the middle of the field are odontomas. (From Blue C. Darby's *Comprehensive Review of Dental Hygiene*, 9e. Mosby; 2021.)

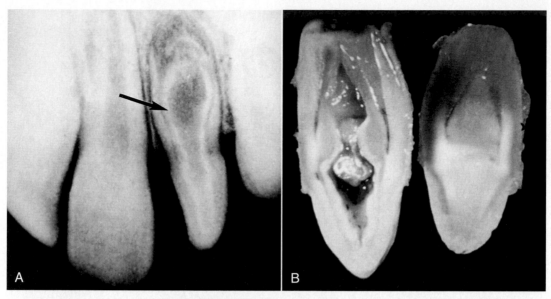

• **Figure 7.7 (A)** Radiograph of dens in dente. Enamel is growing within the tooth (tooth within a tooth) *(arrow)*. **(B)** A dens in dente has been extracted and sectioned in half, showing the enamel growing within the tooth.

turns itself inward before mineralization. The term *dens in dente* means "tooth within a tooth." An x-ray image of a dens in dente shows what appears to be a tooth actually within a tooth (see Fig. 7.7A). This invagination allows communication between the oral cavity and the inner enamel-lined cavity, which could be considered an extremely deep pit. Permanent maxillary lateral incisors are the teeth most often affected by dens in dente.

Dilaceration

A **dilacerated tooth** (Fig. 7.8) is a tooth that has a sharp bend or curve in the root or crown. It appears as though the tooth suddenly bent under pressure. The term **dilaceration** should only be used to describe teeth with very sharp bends.

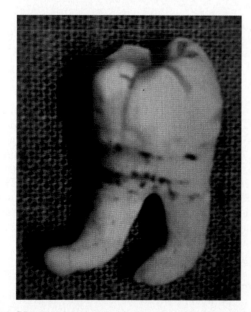

• **Figure 7.8** Dilacerated tooth with numerous bends in the root. This anomaly makes tooth extraction very difficult. (From Ongole R, BN P. *Textbook of oral medicine and oral diagnosis and oral radiology*, 2e. Elsevier India; 2012.)

Dwarfed Roots

A condition in which the roots of the teeth are extremely short compared with their crowns is called **dwarfed roots** (Fig. 7.9). Maxillary teeth with normal-size crowns and abnormally short roots are not uncommon. The condition of *dwarfed roots* can also occur in mandibular teeth as seen in Fig. 7.9.

Gemination

Gemination (Fig. 7.10) is an anomaly that arises when a tooth attempts to divide itself or partially twin itself by splitting its tooth germ; therefore, it is a developmental anomaly. Gemination could result in twin teeth. In most cases, however, geminated teeth are only partially split. Usually the geminated teeth have a single root and a common pulp canal. A tooth split into two crowns with one root would be termed a *bifid tooth* or *bifurcated crown*.

One form of gemination, called *twinning*, occurs when a single tooth germ splits, forming two nearly identical teeth but remaining fused as one, usually with a single root and a single pulp canal. This is more commonly seen in the anterior area and occurs more often in primary dentition than in permanent dentition.

Fusion

Fusion (Fig. 7.11) occurs when two adjacent tooth germs unite. The two teeth may be united along a part of or the entire length of the tooth. They may be joined by their crowns or their roots. The fusion of the teeth must be made at the dentin. If the teeth are only connected by their cementum, then it is not fusion but *concrescence* that has occurred. For fusion to exist, two teeth must be joined; therefore, one less tooth than the normal complement is present.

Concrescence

Concrescence (Fig. 7.12) is a type of fusion that occurs after the roots have formed. It is thought to occur sometimes as a result of

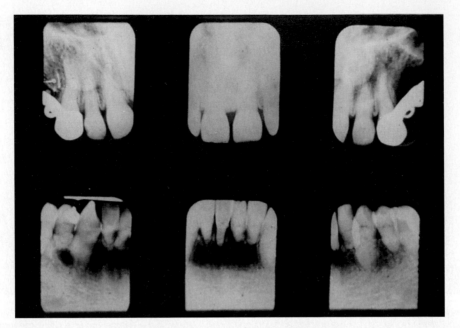

• **Figure 7.9** Dwarfed roots. The roots of the mandibular teeth of this patient have never fully developed.

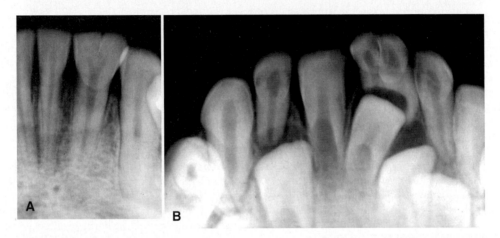

• **Figure 7.10** **(A)** Gemination. A groove is in the central incisor *(arrow)* in which two teeth have begun to develop. **(B)** Radiograph showing how two teeth have grown from one tooth. This anomaly is much more obvious than that illustrated in **(A)**. (Mallya S, Lam E. White and Pharoah's *Oral Radiology: Principles and Interpretation* 8th Edition. Mosby; 2018.)

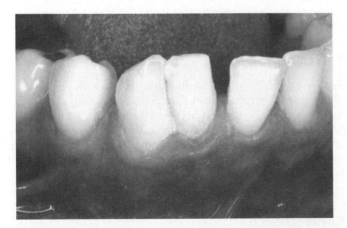

• **Figure 7.11** Fusion. The central and lateral incisors have fused in their development. They are fused at both the enamel and dentin. (From Babbush CA. *Mosby's Dental Dictionary.* 2nd ed. St. Louis: Mosby; 2008.)

trauma. It involves two approximating roots contacting and fusing by a deposition of cementum. If the teeth are connected by their dentin, then it is not concrescence but fusion that has occurred. Concrescence can occur before or after eruption. The condition of concrescence occurs when two adjacent teeth are fused together at their roots through cementum only. This is different from fusion because these teeth were originally separate and became joined after eruption. Concrescence is most often seen in the maxillary molar region.

Hypercementosis

Hypercementosis (Fig. 7.13) is the deposition of excessive amounts of secondary cementum. Although this usually occurs at the apex of the tooth, it may occur along the entire length of the root. Excessive cementum formation usually only forms around the apical third of a root and then only after a tooth has erupted.

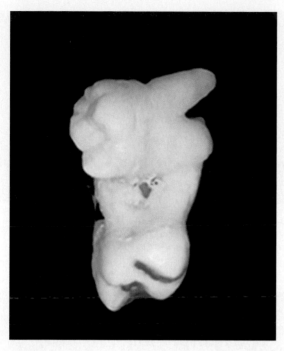

• **Figure 7.12** Concrescence. Two teeth grew separately but then fused at their cemental surfaces and were joined together. (From Babbush CA. *Mosby's Dental Dictionary.* 2nd ed. St. Louis: Mosby; 2008.)

It first appears on x-ray films as a radiolucent dark area that is sometimes mistaken for a periapical abscess. Later, this area appears opaque on x-ray film as it becomes more mineralized. This condition is not pathologic.

>*Cementoma*

Cementoma (Fig. 7.14) is a form of hypercementosis that is also associated with localized destruction of the bone.

Enamel Pearls

Enamel pearls (Fig. 7.15) are small masses of excess enamel on the surface of the teeth located apically to the cementoenamel junction. They are often found at the bifurcation or trifurcation area and are formed by a small, misplaced group of ameloblasts.

Hutchinson's Incisors

Hutchinson's incisors (Figs. 7.16 and 7.17) are notched incisors, sometimes called *screwdriver shaped,* that are formed as a result of prenatal syphilis. The notched incisors are characteristic of congenital syphilis, as are **mulberry molars** (Fig. 7.18), which are irregular-shaped molars with poorly formed cusps.

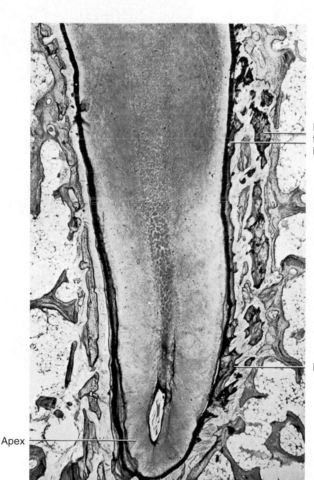

Remnants of fractured cementum
Hyperplastic cementum

Hyperplastic cementum

Apex

• **Figure 7.13** Hypercementosis. Note the localized area of hypercementosis, which may be referred to as *hyperplastic cementum.* (From Bhaskar SN. *Orban's Oral Histology and Embryology.* 10th ed. St. Louis: Mosby; 1986.)

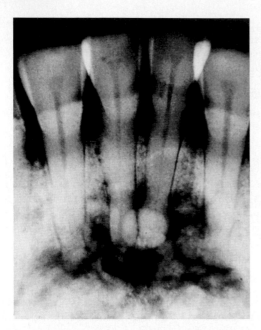

• **Figure 7.14** Cementoma. Note the thickened radiopaque area of cementum at the apexes of the central incisors, with localized bone destruction around them.

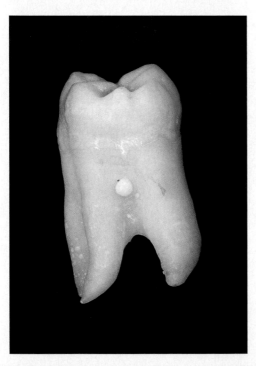

• **Figure 7.15** Enamel pearl. A small ball of enamel is in the bifurcation of this molar. It is always found in bifurcations or trifurcations of teeth. (From Regezi JA, Scuibba JJ, Jordan RCK. *Oral Pathology: Clinical Pathologic Correlations.* 6th ed. St. Louis: Saunders; 2012.)

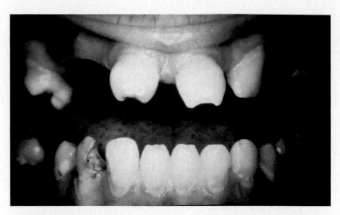

• **Figure 7.16** Hutchinson's incisors with the typical notching of the incisal edges of the incisors as a result of congenital syphilis. (From Neville B., Damm D. *Oral and Maxillofacial pathology*, 3e. Saunders; 2015.)

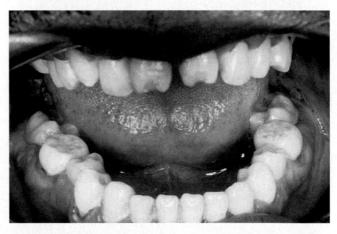

• **Figure 7.17** Notched Hutchinson's incisors and malformed molars.

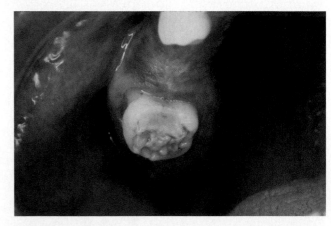

• **Figure 7.18** Mulberry molar with its poorly formed cusps.

Enamel Dysplasia

Enamel dysplasia includes two types of abnormal enamel development: **enamel hypoplasia** and **enamel hypocalcification**. Enamel hypoplasia, which is caused by any condition that inhibits enamel formation, may leave small pits or grooves at different levels in the crown (Fig. 7.19). They are formed by a local disturbance in the

enamel formation. Such situations can be caused by inflammation, fever, systemic disease, and even heredity. Enamel hypocalcification is caused by a condition that inhibits the calcification of enamel.

Enamel Fluorosis

One of the most common forms of enamel hypocalcification is **enamel fluorosis** (Fig. 7.20), a discoloration of enamel caused by

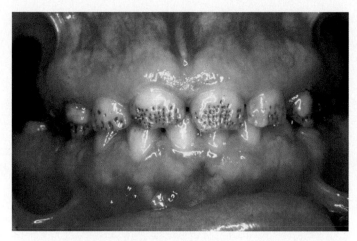

• **Figure 7.19** Enamel hypoplasia. Pitting occurs on the surfaces of the maxillary central and lateral incisors where the enamel is thin. (From Nelson SJ, Ash M. *Wheeler's Dental Anatomy.* Ed. 9. St. Louis: Saunders, 2010.)

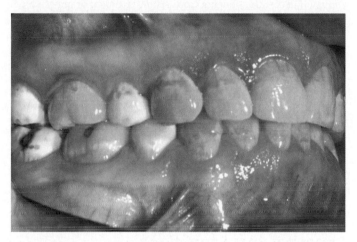

• **Figure 7.20** Enamel fluorosis discoloration of white, brown, and gray blotches on the surfaces of the teeth resulting from drinking natural well water with high fluoride content. (From Neville BW, Damm DD, Allen C. *Oral and Maxillofacial Pathology.* 3rd ed. St. Louis: Saunders; 2009.)

an excessive amount of fluoride in the tooth structure. This can occur naturally from well water with excess amounts of fluoride or accidentally by a child taking vitamins with fluoride, fluoride mouthwashes, or fluoride supplements either in excess or in combination with fluoridated water. The enamel discoloration can range from small, white flecks to large, opaque areas to brownish spots, sometimes with pits. In severe cases, large areas of the crown are a brownish color. These discolored areas are called **mottled enamel**. Fig. 5.7 shows at what age a developmental anomaly could occur to a maxillary permanent central incisor.

Amelogenesis Imperfecta

Amelogenesis imperfecta (Fig. 7.21) is another developmental anomaly related to hypocalcification, but it is hereditary rather than acquired. In the typical form of amelogenesis imperfecta, the enamel of the permanent and deciduous teeth is affected. Sometimes, however, only the permanent teeth are affected. The enamel, when present, is thin and stained various shades of yellow and brown and easily fractures away.

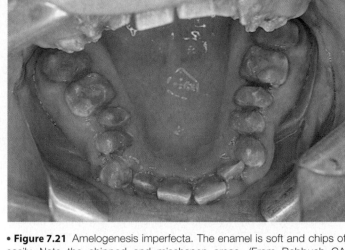

• **Figure 7.21** Amelogenesis imperfecta. The enamel is soft and chips off easily. Note the chipped and misshapen areas. (From Babbush CA. *Mosby's Dental Dictionary.* 2nd ed. St. Louis: Mosby; 2008.)

Turner's Tooth

Turner's tooth (Fig. 7.22) is a hypocalcification of a single tooth, usually a maxillary incisor. The condition occurs if a developing permanent tooth is affected by a local infection or trauma. Something, bacteria or trauma, disturbs the ameloblastic layer, which results in a hypoplasia of the enamel.

Dentinogenesis Imperfecta

Dentinogenesis imperfecta (Fig. 7.23) is a hereditary dentinal developmental abnormality. The dentin is colored gray, brown, or yellow, but the tooth exhibits an unusual translucent hue. The

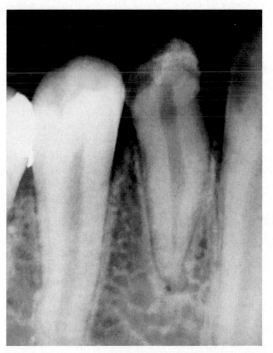

• **Figure 7.22** Turner's tooth. Note the lack of calcification of the crown of this tooth. The tooth was affected while the crown was forming but was not affected later when the root was forming.

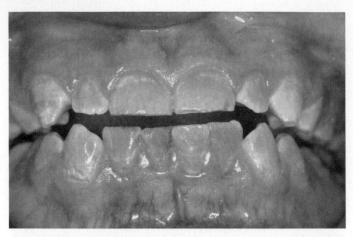

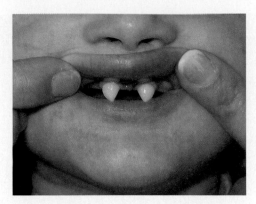

• **Figure 7.25**   Peg-shaped incisors.

• **Figure 7.23**   Dentinogenesis imperfecta with discoloration of the maxillary anterior teeth. Enamel often chips away because the poorly developed dentin beneath it does not support it. (From Neville BW, Damm DD, Allen C. *Oral and Maxillofacial Pathology.* 3rd ed. St. Louis: Saunders; 2009.)

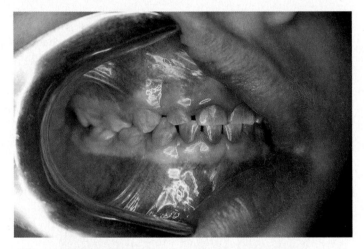

• **Figure 7.24**   Tetracycline staining. Note the discolored enamel of the teeth. This individual was taking tetracycline for an extended period, and most of the teeth were affected. (From Regezi JA, Scuibba JJ, Jordan RCK. *Oral Pathology: Clinical Pathologic Correlations.* 6th ed. St. Louis: Saunders; 2012.)

most striking feature of this condition is that the pulp chambers and root canals are completely filled with dentin. This total obliteration of the pulp tissue occurs because the dentinal tissue continues to form dentin until all of the root canal and pulp chambers are completely filled.

Tetracycline Staining

Another dentinal developmental condition is **tetracycline staining** (Fig. 7.24). This condition occurs when an expectant mother or a young child with tooth crowns that are still developing takes the antibiotic tetracycline. The teeth of the developing fetus or the young child discolor, ranging from yellow to brown or grayish blue.

Abnormal Crown Shapes

The maxillary third molars followed by the mandibular third molars are most likely to show variety and abnormalities in the size, number, and shape of the cusps. They can range from a single peg-shaped crown to a multicusped large or small variation of the first or second molar.

The most common malformed anterior tooth is the maxillary lateral incisor, which is **peg shaped** (Fig. 7.25) in more than 1% of the population. Mandibular second premolars vary from a two- to three-cusp form, with several variations of each. Accessory cusps or tubercles can occur on any tooth, but they are most commonly found on maxillary molars.

Abnormal Root Formation

The maxillary second premolars often have two bifurcated roots, although more often only one. The maxillary first premolars usually do have two roots, although in 40% of cases they have one. It is not uncommon for the mandibular second premolars or canines to have accessory roots, which is a second root that is sometimes bifurcated only at the apical third. In all the teeth mentioned previously, if two roots are present, then one will be buccal and one lingual.

Mandibular canines and premolars are the single-rooted teeth most likely to be affected by accessory roots. Third molars are the most likely multirooted teeth to possess accessory roots.

A severe bend or distortion in the tooth root and crown of more than 40 degrees is termed a *dilaceration,* most often seen in mandibular third molars. A sharp curvature or twist of a tooth root only is called **flexion**.

Review Questions

1. What is an anomaly?
2. Name some extrinsic and intrinsic factors that may cause anomalies.
3. What is the difference between hereditary and congenital factors?
4. What is the difference between hyperdontia and anodontia?
5. What is an odontoma?
6. What is the difference between gemination and fusion?
7. What is the cause of Hutchinson's incisors and mulberry molars?

8. What is the difference between amelogenesis imperfecta and dentinogenesis imperfecta?
9. How can tetracycline staining occur?
10. What is mottled enamel?
11. Which misplaced groups of tissue result in the presence of enamel pearls?
12. Which teeth are the most likely to be congenitally missing?
13. In which arch do supernumerary teeth occur with more frequency?
14. Of the following, which affect only the root of the tooth?
   a. flexion
   b. dilaceration
   c. dwarfed roots
   d. cementoma
   e. hypercementosis
   f. all but b
   g. all but a
15. An irregularly shaped mass of toothlike material (enamel cementum and dentin) was removed from the maxillary anterior area between a central incisor and a lateral incisor. The mass was 10 mm long and 8 mm wide (Fig. 7.26). This mass of tissue is likely a(n) _____?
   a. complex odontoma
   b. compound odontoma
   c. cementoma
   d. enamel pearl
16. A permanent maxillary right third molar was removed from an 18-year-old female. Three years later, this x-ray (Fig. 7.27) was taken. Name the anomaly seen in this x-ray.

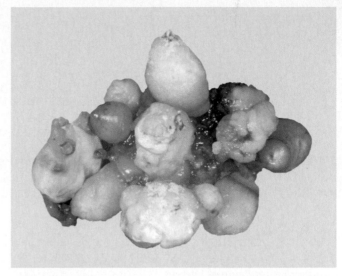

• **Figure 7.26** (Odell E, Cawson R. Cawsons *Essentials of oral pathology and oral medicine*, 8e. Churchill livingstone; 2008.)

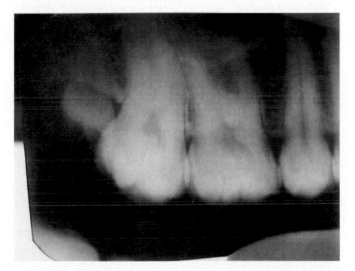

• **Figure 7.27** Note the very small molar distal to the maxillary second molar.

8

Supporting Structures
The Periodontium

OBJECTIVES

- To understand the relationships within the gingival unit, a supporting structure of the teeth
- To understand the terminology of the gingival unit and to identify its various parts
- To understand how the gingival unit functions
- To understand how the attachment apparatus is related to the gingival unit
- To understand the relationship of cementum, periodontal ligament, and alveolar bone
- To identify the components of the alveolar process
- To understand the clinical significance of the gingival sulcus
- To understand how the fibers of the periodontal ligament function in tooth movement and shock absorption

The periodontium consists of those tissues that support the teeth and is divided into a **gingival unit** and an **attachment unit** or **attachment apparatus**. The following is a list of the various parts of the periodontium.

Gingival Unit:	Attachment Unit:
Free gingiva	Cementum
Attached gingiva	Alveolar process
Alveolar mucosa	Periodontal ligament

Gingival Unit

The gingiva is made up of free and attached gingiva (Fig. 8.1). Composed of very dense mucosa called **masticatory mucosa**, it has a thick **epithelial** covering and **keratinized cells**. The underlying **mucosa** is composed of dense collagen fibers (Table 8.1). This type of masticatory mucosa is also found on the hard palate. Masticatory mucosa is well designed to withstand the trauma to which it is subjected while grinding food.

The rest of the mouth is lined with a different type of mucosa called **alveolar mucosa** (lining mucosa). Alveolar mucosa is found apical to the **mucogingival junction** and is continuous with the rest of the mucous membrane of the cheeks and lips and the floor of the mouth. It is thin and freely movable and tears or injures easily. The epithelium covering this lining mucosa is thin and nonkeratinized. Its mucosa is composed of loose connective tissue with some muscle fibers. In the strictest sense alveolar mucosa would not be considered part of the periodontium because it does not directly surround or support the teeth. In reality it is part of the gingival unit; therefore, it contributes to the well-being of the other gingival tissues that do directly support the teeth.

Free Gingiva (Marginal Gingiva)

Free gingiva is the gum tissue that extends from the gingival margin to the base of the gingival sulcus; it is also called **marginal gingiva**. The attached gingiva extends from the base of this sulcus to the **mucogingival junction**. Free gingiva is usually light pink in color and averages between 0.5 to 2 mm in depth (Fig. 8.2).

The free gingiva (marginal gingiva) mirrors the scalloped outline formed by following the cervical lines of the teeth. The free gingiva around a fully erupted tooth is located next to the enamel about 0.5 to 2 mm coronal to the cementoenamel junction (CEJ). It forms a collar, which is separated from the tooth by the gingival sulcus. This **gingival sulcus** is the space between the free gingiva and the tooth. The bottom of the sulcus is influenced by the curvature of the cervical line of the tooth. A healthy gingival sulcus is 3 mm or less in depth and does not bleed when probed or brushed. An inflamed gingival sulcus easily bleeds with gentle probing and can exceed 3 mm in depth. The deeper the sulcus depth, the more unhealthy the situation. Thus a periodontal probe measurement of 5 mm indicates more damage than a reading of 4 mm.

When a periodontal sulcus is probed, the probe is inserted until it meets resistance. No force can be used after that. It is possible to push the probe all the way through the attached gingiva, even past the root apex. A significant force is required to do this, but it is possible. Because of this no force is used when probing. When the probe meets any resistance the probing is stopped and the probe measurement is recorded. When the base of the pocket is reached, the tissue will blanch slightly to indicate to the clinician they have reached the attached gingiva. Any measurement >3 mm is significant.

The **gingival papilla** (interdental papilla) is the free gingiva located in the triangular interdental spaces. The apex in the anterior teeth is rather sharp, but it is blunter in the posterior teeth. The shape of gingival papilla is greatly affected by the location of the contact area of the adjacent teeth, the shape of the interproximal surfaces of the adjacent teeth, and the CEJ of the adjacent teeth. Inflammation of the gingival papilla is easily recognized because the area takes on a color that is more red than normal and exhibits a puffy appearance with some blunting of its apex.

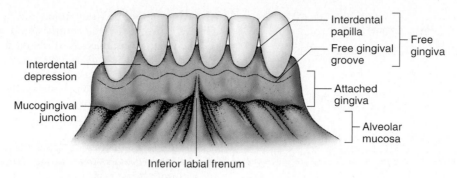

• **Figure 8.1** Anatomy of a normal gingival unit of a periodontium.

TABLE 8.1	Characteristics of Gingiva and Alveolar Mucosa	
Free (Marginal) Gingiva	**Attached Gingiva**	**Alveolar Mucosa**
Masticatory mucosa	Masticatory mucosa	Lining mucosa
Slight mobility	Tightly bound	Movable and elastic
Epithelium	Thick epithelial layer	Thinner epithelial layer
Slight keratinization	Keratinized	Nonkeratinized
No rete peg formation	Rete peg formation	No rete peg formation
Smooth	Stippled surface (like an orange peel)	Smooth
Light pink	Light red to dark pink	Pink to red
Collagenous fibers	Collagenous fibers	Collagenous fibers and some muscle fibers

Sometimes the color takes on a bluish-purple color instead of red, but healthy tissue is pink with some skin pigment exhibited in people of color. The marginal gingiva is so thin that discolored calculus and the metal of restorations can affect the color of the tissue, making it appear darker.

The inner portion of the gingival sulcus is lined with nonkeratinized epithelium, whereas the outer portion of the free gingiva is covered with keratinized epithelium. The attached gingiva begins at the base of the gingival sulcus. A gingival groove often occurs on the outside of the free gingiva and corresponds to the base of the sulcus. This groove is not always present, but it is considered to be a normal part of the anatomy when present; it is named the **free gingival groove**. The attached gingiva extends apically from the base of the sulcus and is attached to the bone and the cementum by a dense network of collagenous fibers (Fig. 8.3). Connective tissue fibers within the marginal and attached gingiva are called the **lamina propria**. The fibers of the lamina propria of the marginal gingiva intermingle with the lamina propria fibers of the attached gingiva and the **periodontal ligament (PDL)**. Circular fibers are confined to the free gingiva

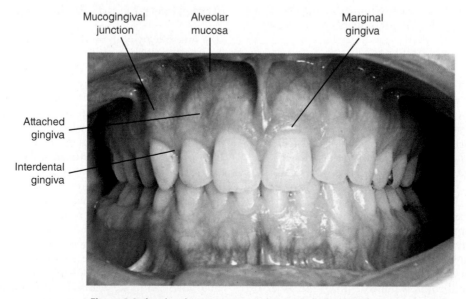

• **Figure 8.2** A color change occurs at the mucogingival junction.

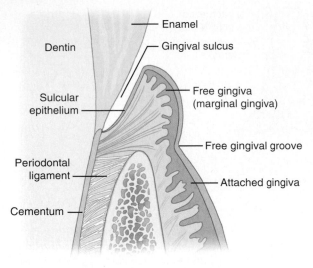

© Elsevier Collection

• **Figure 8.3** Sulcular epithelium is not keratinized, the free gingiva is slightly keratinized, and the attached gingiva is more keratinized. The more keratinized a tissue is, the less fragile it is.

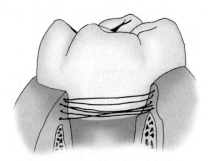

• **Figure 8.4** Circular fibers of the gingival unit encircle the tooth.

and encircle the tooth (Fig. 8.4). These circular bands of connective tissue fibers surround the teeth, tying them together They help keep the free gingiva firm. Gingival fibers do not embed in bone or cementum.

Attached Gingiva

Attached gingiva is not mobile like free gingiva because its **lamina propria** is attached to the bone underneath it. The lamina propria is the connective tissue region within the oral mucosa. This makes attached gingiva firm and immoveable. Attached gingiva is not as translucent as the marginal gingiva and exhibits a slight color variation from it. It is also more keratinized and less fragile.

The outside of the attached gingiva often displays a stippled texture, resembling the dimpled surface of an orange. Stippling becomes evident before the teeth erupt and becomes even more so in adult gingiva. The attached gingiva is highly keratinized and is covered by **stratified squamous epithelium** in which **rete peg formation** is evident. The dimpling effect is caused by the rete peg formation, which is simply the irregular binding of the epithelium to the bone by collagen fibers (Fig. 8.5). This causes depressions or dimples where the epithelium is pulled tight to the bone. The color of the gingiva varies from light to dark pink and may contain pigment, correlating to the skin pigmentation of the person.

The darker a person's skin color, the more likely it is that the gingiva is also darker and contains more **melanin**.

The gingiva is connected to the tooth by a meshwork of collagenous fibers. These fibers are formed by fibroblasts, which are the principal cells of connective tissue. Collagen fibers embedded in the cementum or alveolar bone are known as **Sharpey's fibers**; they extend from the cementum to the papillary area of the gingiva and to the attached gingiva. These fibers pass out from the cementum in small bundles.

The function of these gingival fibers is to keep the gingiva closely attached to the tooth surface. These fibers prevent the free gingiva from being peeled away from the tooth and keep the gingiva firmly attached. They also prevent the apical migration of the epithelial attachment and resist gingival recession.

Sharpey's fibers embed in bone or cementum, and they can extend not only tooth to bone, but also tooth to gingiva or even tooth to tooth.

The blood supply of the gingival tissue comes from the **supraperiosteal** vessels. These in turn originate from the lingual, mental, buccal, infraorbital, and palatine arteries.

Alveolar Mucosa

The **mucogingival junction** is where the moveable alveolar mucosa joins the attached gingiva. It is just apical to the attached gingiva. The alveolar mucosa joins the attached gingiva at the mucogingival junction and is continuous with the rest of the tissues of the **vestibule**. This tissue is thin and soft and rather loosely attached to the underlying bone. Alveolar mucosa is composed of lining mucosa, and its **submucosa** contains loose connective tissue, fat, and some muscle fibers. The epithelium is smooth, thin, and nonkeratinized. Alveolar mucosa covers the buccal surfaces of the mandibular and maxillary teeth, but covers only the lingual surfaces of the mandibular teeth because keratinized tissue from the hard palate attaches to the lingual surface of maxillary teeth. The gingiva is quite rich in capillary vascularity, and the alveolar mucosa is equally **vascular** but more red. Its deep color is attributed to numerous shallow blood vessels and thinner, more translucent nonkeratinized epithelium.

Attachment Unit: Periodontium

The attachment unit comprises the cementum, the periodontal ligament, and the alveolar process. Together these tissues form the attachment apparatus of the **periodontium**, and they are the supporting mechanism for the teeth. They attach the tooth to the alveolar bone. The periodontium is made of hard and soft tissue. Cementum is a hard, bonelike tissue covering the roots of the teeth. The PDL (periodontal ligament) is the soft connective tissue that surrounds the roots of the teeth and connects the teeth to alveolar bone. The **alveolar bone** is the thin covering of bone that surrounds the teeth. The function of the attachment apparatus is not only supportive but also nutritive, formative, and sensory. The supportive function is to maintain the support for the tooth in the bone and to prevent its movement. The nutritive and sensory functions are fulfilled by the blood vessels and nerves. The nerves act as indicators of pressure or pain around the tooth. The formative function is to replace cementum, PDL, and alveolar bone and is accomplished by specialized cells called **cementoblasts**, fibroblasts, and osteoblasts. In addition to accomplishing these functions, the PDL acts as a suspensory mechanism that keeps the root and bone from abrading each other. The PDL also acts as a

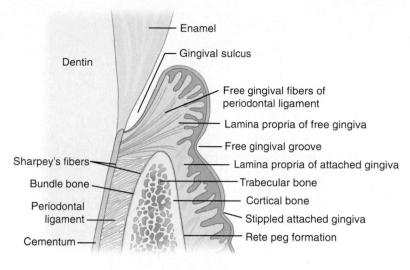

© Elsevier Collection

• **Figure 8.5** Fibers of the lamina propria of the free and attached gingiva intermingle with each other and the periodontal ligament. The rete peg formation holds the gingiva so tight it forms a dimple on the surface.

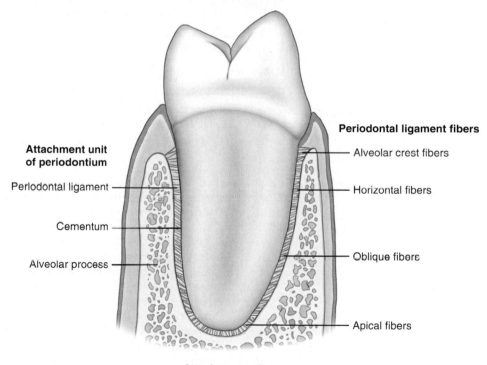

© Elsevier Collection

• **Figure 8.6** Fibers of the attachment unit form a hammock of tissue from the bone to the tooth.

hammock of live tissue whose fibers cushion the impact between tooth and bone when undergoing pressure. The fibers themselves become taut, thus dissipating the pressure and, at the same time, allowing the nerves associated with these fibers a way of measuring and equating the amount of pressure (Fig. 8.6).

Cementum

Cementum can be cellular or acellular. Both types are formed by cementoblasts, but in the cellular type, the cementoblasts become

embedded in the cementum. The acellular type is free of embedded cementoblasts and is clear and without structure.

Acellular cementum always covers the cervical third of the root and sometimes extends over almost all of the root, except the apical portion. Cellular cementum covers the apical portion of the root and sometimes may form over acellular cementum. Cellular cementum is like bone in character and in the way in which it grows and resorbs. Like bone, cementum grows by the **apposition** (addition) of new layers, one on top of another. Changes in function and pressure influence the growth activity of cementum.

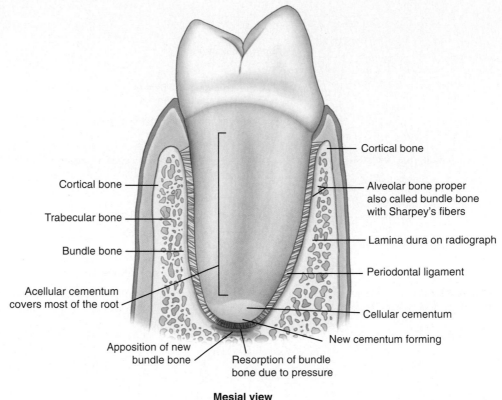

Cortical bone

Trabecular bone

Bundle bone

Acellular cementum
covers most of the root

Cortical bone

Alveolar bone proper
also called bundle bone
with Sharpey's fibers

Lamina dura on radiograph

Periodontal ligament

Cellular cementum

New cementum forming

Apposition of new
bundle bone

Resorption of bundle
bone due to pressure

Mesial view

© Elsevier Collection

• **Figure 8.7** As cellular cementum grows it puts pressure on the alveolar bone proper causing the bundle bone to resorb on the inside of the alveolus and add bone to the lamina dura on its trabecular side.

Both cellular and acellular cementum have collagen fibers embedded within them. These Sharpey's fibers are the embedded ends of connective tissue fibers of the PDL. Some are embedded in cementum, where some are embedded in bone (Fig. 8.7). See also Fig. 8.5 and note that Sharpey's fibers are the periodontal ligament fibers that are embedded in either bone or cementum.

Alveolar Bone

The type of bone that lines the sockets in which the roots of teeth are held is called **alveolar bone proper**. The socket in which the tooth rests is called an **alveolus**. These alveoli are a part of the **alveolar process** that surrounds and supports the teeth in the maxilla and mandible. Alveolar bone proper is thin and compact, with many small openings through which blood vessels, nerves, and lymphatic vessels pass. The alveolar bone that forms the inner bone of the alveolus is also called **bundle bone**. The term *bundle bone* applies when numerous layers of bone are added to the socket wall. Bundle bone forms the immediate attachment of the PDL with its Sharpey's fibers. When viewed radiographically, this attachment lining of bone around the tooth is called the **lamina dura** (Fig. 8.8).

The alveolar bone and cementum continually undergo change. Bone apposition and resorption are related to the functional demands placed on the bone. Compared with cementum, bone is an extremely active tissue. Very slow apposition of cementum occurs, whereas the alveolar bone undergoes changes readily. Under normal conditions bone is constantly in flux, undergoing tissue

growth (apposition) and resorption in a finely coordinated way. Bone may be laid down on one end and resorbed on the other. The extreme difference between bone and cementum in their ability to undergo remodeling poses a significant problem. The two tissues are tied together by the PDL, which must make adjustments for the variation in their abilities.

Bone, like cementum, consists of an **organic matrix** and **inorganic matter**. The organic matrix comprises collagen and intercellular substance, whereas the inorganic matter comprises **apatite crystals** of calcium, phosphate, and carbonates.

The alveolar process is composed of two types of bone: cortical and trabecular. The alveolar process is surrounded on the outside by a very dense **cortical bone**. **Trabecular bone** forms the inside of the alveolar process. The cortical bone is composed of dense compact bone and covers the buccal and lingual of the alveolar process. The **trabecular bone** is composed of a softer **cancellous bone (spongy bone)** and surrounds the alveolus. It fills the inside of the alveolar process with bone between the teeth, around the teeth, and in between the roots. It is a spongier bone with boney trabeculations running through it. A trabeculation is a crisscross of bone with holes running through it for blood vessels and nerves. It is less dense, softer, and looks like a sponge; therefore it is also called *spongy* bone.

The trabecular bone between the teeth is called **interdental bone**. The alveolar process between the teeth is called an **interdental septum**. The bone between teeth with multiple roots is called **interradicular bone** and forms the **interradicular septum**. It is found between the roots of multirooted teeth (Fig. 8.9).

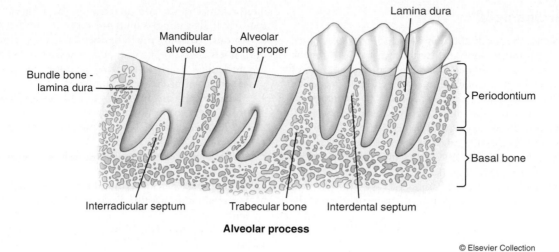

Alveolar process

© Elsevier Collection

• **Figure 8.8** Lamina dura is the outline of the bundle bone that shows up on a radiograph.

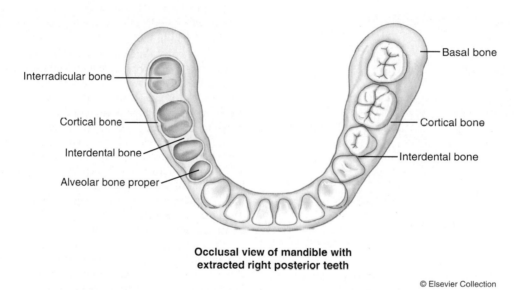

Occlusal view of mandible with
extracted right posterior teeth

© Elsevier Collection

• **Figure 8.9** Four posterior alveoli exposing the interradicular bone between the roots of the molars. The alveolar bone proper lines the inside of alveoli, and the cortical bone forms the outer lining. Interdental bone is the bone between the teeth. The basal bone forms that part of the maxilla or mandible that is not alveolar process. The alveolar process is the bone that surrounds and supports the teeth; it ends just apically to the roots of the teeth.

The bone forming the alveoli is dependent on the functional demands of the tooth. If a tooth undergoes long-standing loss of function, as when the antagonists in the opposite arch are lost, the alveolar bone undergoes changes. If the teeth are subjected to occlusal stress, the supporting bone will be composed of thicker and more numerous trabeculae. The lamina dura may become compressed. The bone itself may undergo resorption when continuous pressure is exerted on it and apposition when long-term tension is placed on it. Sharpey's fibers, embedded in the bone at one end and in the cementum at the other, are capable of expressing such tension. The architectural arrangement of the **trabeculae** is directly related to the demands of function. The bundle bone covering the trabecular bone undergoes these changes, and the trabecular bone follows its lead.

The bundle bone is very dense alveolar bone proper and, although it is formed from many layers, it does not have trabeculations. Instead it is continuous with trabecular bone and forms the inner covering of it; the outer covering of the trabecular bone is the cortical bone.

The denser cortical bone does not undergo apposition easily on its outside, but it can undergo reposition. Cortical bone does not expand after normal growth as easily as trabecular bone, making orthodontic treatment more challenging.

Basal bone is the main part of the maxilla and mandible and is different from alveolar process bone. Basal bone supports the alveolar process and is denser and formed of compact bone. Like cortical bone it does not respond easily to pressure or tension; however, basal bone does become weaker and less calcified in elderly patients. Both basal bone and alveolar process bone are covered with periosteum. Basal bone is not part of the periodontium because it does not surround and support the teeth.

Periodontal Ligament

The PDL surrounds the tooth and helps hold it in alveolar bone. It attaches the tooth to the bone and suspends it like a hammock in its boney socket. The ligament is actually a tiny meshwork of collagenous connective tissue fibers that runs from the bone to the tooth. These connective tissue fibers are Sharpey's fibers embedded in bone or cementum. For the sake of this discussion only, fibers that are embedded in alveolar bone and cementum will be considered PDL. The most occlusal connective tissue fibers attached to the tooth travel to the gingival tissues. They go from the tooth to the papilla of the free gingiva (Fig. 8.10). Other gingival connective tissue fibers pass into the free and attached gingiva. The next layer of fibers, the transseptal group, travels completely across the

interproximal space and attaches to the adjacent tooth. These transseptal fiber bundles bind one tooth to another (Fig. 8.11).

For our discussion the PDL fibers attach the tooth to the bone. PDL fibers align in specific groups based on the general direction in which they attach to the alveolar bone and cementum. They can be arranged in the following five groups:

1. **Alveolar crest group:** Fibers extending from the cervical area of the tooth to the alveolar crest
2. **Horizontal group:** Fibers running horizontally from the tooth to the alveolar bone
3. **Oblique group:** Fibers running obliquely from the cementum to the bone
4. **Apical group:** Fibers radiating apically from the tooth to the bone
5. **Interradicular group:** Periodontal fibers between roots of multirooted teeth

This arrangement of fibers provides a hammock of tissue bundles that support the tooth within the bone. They not only tie the tooth to the bone but also prevent it from being pushed into the bone. They also insulate the tooth and bone, minimizing the trauma of being pushed together. This shock absorption function is also helped by the roots of the teeth and by fluids within the spaces of the PDL. The shapes and sizes of the roots of the teeth help dissipate occlusal stresses in both a lateral and apical direction. In multirooted teeth, the forces can be distributed between the roots of the same tooth. Additionally, the fluids within the PDL act as a hydraulic pressure system on the walls of the alveolus.

Because the fibers are constantly subjected to a variety of pressures exerted on the tooth, the PDL is constantly undergoing functional change. The main portion of the PDL is composed of bundles of white collagenous connective tissue fibers. These fibers extend from and are embedded in the cementum of the tooth and alveolar bone and are bundled together like the many strands of a rope.

In addition to the collagen fibers, the PDL contains fibroblasts, one of the cellular elements of the PDL. Fibroblasts are found in alignment with the collagen fibers, arranged in groups. The PDL also contains small blood and lymph vessels and nerves. Loose connective tissue surrounds these vessels and nerves.

The tooth is actually suspended by this PDL in such a way that it is allowed some degree of movement within the bony cavity. For instance, if pressure is exerted on the mesial surface, the periodontal fibers on the distal surface are compressed and allow more space

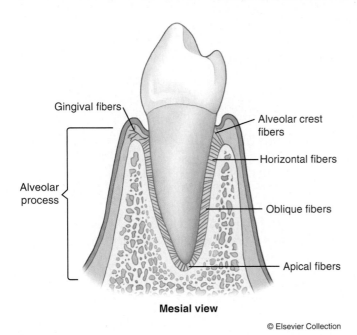

Mesial view

© Elsevier Collection

• **Figure 8.10** Periodontal fibers support the tooth in the alveolar process. They connect the bone to the tooth. The most occlusal fibers from the tooth go to the free gingiva.

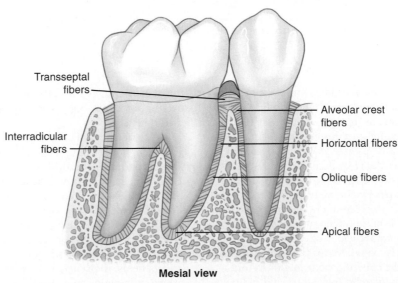

Mesial view

© Elsevier Collection

• **Figure 8.11** Transseptal fibers go from one tooth to another.

between the tooth and the bone. This ability of the PDL to expand allows the tooth to tip, rotate, or become compressed within the bony cavity. Even total bodily movement is possible because of the PDL, for example, the constant abrading of neighboring teeth, not only occlusally but also interproximally. This causes wear on the contact areas and occlusal surfaces. Two forces that are active within the mouth allow for movement of the tooth. The first is mesial drift, which allows the tooth to move forward within the oral cavity, thus closing the spaces lost from interproximal wear. The second is an active eruption force of the tooth, which causes the tooth to migrate occlusally until it occludes with an antagonist. Both forces can be activated fairly rapidly because of the PDL's ability to tense and compress and the bone's ability to change the shape and size of the socket. Finally, orthodontics would not be possible without the adaptability and versatility of the PDL and bundle bone.

Clinical Considerations

Several clinical situations should be discussed. The first of these concerns how a tooth can move within a bony alveolus. Such movement is accomplished by several mechanisms already discussed.

For a tooth to move through bone, a force of some type must be acting on it. This force causes pressure on the root, PDL, and bone. It compresses the PDL and the alveolar bone on one side of the root. If this force continues for a long enough time, a biomechanical system of osteoclastic cells (bone-destroying cells) is initiated. The osteoclasts destroy bone to make room for the compressed tissues. If the pressure is extreme and constant, the osteoclastic cells may even resorb portions of the root of the tooth.

On the other side of this same tooth root, the PDL is pulled taut. This results in a pulling force on the alveolar bone on that side of the socket. This constant tension causes an opposite biomechanical system. Osteoblastic cells (bone-forming cells) start laying down bone. These osteoblasts produce bone in response to tension, which aids in relieving the tension on the PDL. The net effect is that the tooth moves away from the force by remodeling bone. On one side, bone is destroyed; on the other side, bone is formed.

The following are some of the forces that exert pressure on the teeth:
1. *Active eruption:* Tooth eruption into the oral cavity and eruption to compensate for occlusal **abrasion**
2. *Mesial drift:* The mesial movement of molars to compensate for proximal abrasion
3. *Masticatory occlusal forces:* Tooth occlusion during chewing
4. *Orthodontic corrective forces:* Placing of pressure-causing appliances on the teeth to correct malocclusion by a dentist or an orthodontist
5. *Traumatic occlusal forces:* Teeth subjected to premature contact during occlusion

The first four of these forces can tip, rotate, or move the tooth because of the bone-remodeling system just mentioned. These forces must be relatively constant for the bone-remodeling mechanisms to be activated.

The last of these forces, occlusal trauma, is not a consistent, constant force. It is usually intermittent and, consequently, does not result in tooth movement as much as tooth mobility. Although some osteoclastic activity occurs, it may be the result of constant pressure from inflammation caused by trauma more than the external force of the occlusion. The tooth becomes loose and mobile because intermittent pressure causes the PDL space to widen. At the same time the immediate bone, *lamina dura,* becomes thicker. These actions occur around the entire tooth and are not aimed in any one direction. This does not cause the tooth to move, because the forces exerted on it are not constantly applied in one direction. The bone at the apex of the tooth may be resorbed as a result of constant inflammation, whereas this same inflammation may push the tooth occlusally causing tensions that result in the surrounding bone to thicken.

The important concept here is that a tooth cannot be moved with intermittent forces. To move a tooth, the forces must be consistent. However, even constant forces cannot be so great as to outpace the body's ability to manufacture bone.

Gingival Sulcus and Dentogingival Junction

Much of the dental providers' clinical concerns center around the gingival sulcus and the dentogingival junction in particular. Dental providers are concerned about maintaining the integrity of this tissue, preventing disease of the PDL, and protecting the health of the patient. When calculus (tartar), plaque (biofilm), food debris, or other materials are left in the gingival sulcus, an inflammatory process is initiated. Any bacterial or traumatic event could also trigger such a response.

The gingival sulcus is the space facing the sulcular gingiva. Ordinarily this space is the space between the tooth surface and the sulcular gingiva. In a healthy condition this space would be bordered by the tooth surface and marginal gingiva (free gingiva) and meet at the dentogingival junction (Fig. 8.12).

The sulcular gingiva is nonkeratinized squamous epithelium; it is smoother and more fragile than the more keratinized outer covering of the marginal gingiva. The dentogingival junction is where the tooth surface meets the gingival tissue. It is formed from both sulcular and junctional epithelium and is continuous with the PDL.

The junctional epithelium attaches to the tooth surface by an epithelial attachment. This attachment covers the tooth and stays attached to the tooth throughout its eruption. First it is attached to the enamel, and eventually to cementum, and then to dentin. This attachment covers the tooth throughout its eruption until the junctional epithelium ends up at the cervical portion of the tooth where it forms the PDL. The entire time a tooth is erupting the gingiva covers the tooth tightly, preventing bacteria from embedding below the gingival tissues.

The dentogingival junction is composed of cells that are less densely packed than the marginal gingiva. It is here that fluids seep from the lamina dura and into the gingival sulcus. It is also here that bacteria can invade the body.

Clinical Considerations

Pericoronitis is inflammation around the gum tissue surrounding a tooth. It is a frequent cause of infection in partially erupted mandibular third molars. It is caused because food debris becomes trapped between the gingiva and the unerupted tooth. Bacteria living off this food debris attacks the sulcular gingival tissues. These tissues are smooth, thin, and nonkeratinized; they are fragile and can be more easily invaded by bacteria. Once the bacteria is in the gingival tissue it spreads through the bloodstream to where it can attack other parts of the rest of the body. Before the invention of antibiotics, pericoronitis was often fatal. If untreated it could lead to a blocked airway, infection of the bloodstream, or infection of the heart lining.

Chronic inflammation in the area of the dentogingival junction can result in recession of the gingiva, periodontal pockets, gingivitis, and bone loss. Calculus harboring bacteria, biofilm, and other foreign materials must not be allowed to build up in this area. The very process of removing these irritants can result in a bacterial invasion of the bloodstream. Special precautions are used when performing dental prophylaxis on patients with certain types of heart valve damage, heart murmurs, and bleeding disorders, or who have moveable knee or hip prosthesis.

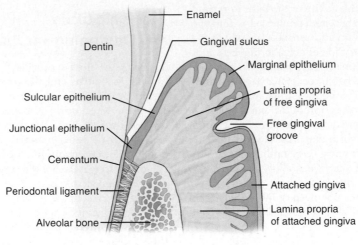

© Elsevier Collection

• **Figure 8.12** The dentogingival junction is formed by the tooth on one side, the sulcular epithelium is on the other side, and the junctional epithelium is in the middle. This is where the tooth attaches to the gingiva.

Review Questions

1. Which of the following are true of attached gingiva?
   a. The tissue is soft and movable.
   b. The epithelial layer is thick and keratinized.
   c. The tissue can have a stippled texture.
   d. The tissue is fixed and firmly attached to the bone and cementum.
2. Which is most true of cementum?
   a. Sharpey's fibers are embedded in it.
   b. It is always smooth.
   c. Acellular cementum covers the apical end of the tooth.
   d. It is resorbed as easily as bone.
3. Which is true of Sharpey's fibers?
   a. They can embed in bone only.
   b. They can embed in cementum only.
   c. They can embed in either bone or cementum.
   d. The same fiber can embed in bone at one end and in cementum at the other.
4. When the tooth is subjected to occlusal stress, it relieves this stress by which of the following mechanisms?
   a. The periodontal ligament tenses.
   b. The fluids in the periodontal ligament absorb some force.
   c. The walls of the alveolus spread the force out and divide it over a wider area.
5. Define the following by researching the index and glossary:
   a. rete peg formation
   b. stratified squamous epithelium
6. Which statements are true about fibers labeled A–C in Fig. 8.13?
   a. They are called *Sharpey's fibers*.
   b. They attach only the free gingiva to the cementum.
   c. They are called *transseptal fibers*.
   d. They are embedded in the cementum.
7. Draw and label the periodontal ligament fibers in Fig. 8.14 (a mandibular first molar).

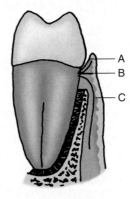

• **Figure 8.13** Mesial view of a permanent mandibular left first molar.

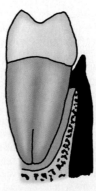

• **Figure 8.14** Mesial view of a permanent mandibular left first molar.

8. Which tissues are not keratinized?
   a. the sulcular epithelium of free gingiva
   b. alveolar mucosa
   c. attached gingiva
   d. the outer layer of free gingiva
   e. both a and b

True or False

9. The free gingiva extends from the gingival margins to the base of the gingival sulcus.

10. The attached gingiva extends from the gingival sulcus to the interdental space.

11. The gingival sulcus is the space between the tooth and the mucogingival fold.

12. The gingival papilla is located in the interdental space.

13. The alveolar bone when seen on the x-ray is called *lamina dura*.

9
Clinical Considerations

OBJECTIVES

- To understand how clinical experience is related to the theory and lecture portion of dental anatomy
- To understand how preventive clinical situations are related to tooth form and supportive dental structures
- To understand how occlusal trauma and the natural shape and contour of the teeth can contribute to dental disease
- To understand how the placement of a restoration can contribute to disease of the supporting tissues
- To evaluate the reliability of dental pain as a diagnostic aid
- To understand how tooth migration can affect the success of treatment or necessitate different treatment

When studying clinical considerations of an existing dental condition, there are two possible scenarios. The circumstances are preventive in nature, enhancing the ability of the oral tissues to protect themselves, or they are potentially pathologic. Recognizing the difference is important. Sometimes the best treatment is no treatment, and at other times the wrong treatment can make a bad situation even worse. Therefore a study of preventive clinical situations is important.

Preventive Clinical Considerations

Preventive clinical considerations include tooth form, shape, and arrangement that aid in the prevention of dental problems such as decay, occlusal trauma, and periodontal disease.

Decay and Periodontal Disease

The teeth are encased in a hard, smooth outer covering (enamel) that offers protection from the accumulation of bacteria and debris (plaque). The smoothness of the enamel makes the adherence of plaque more difficult. This self-cleaning ability of the enamel, therefore, helps resist decay, because decay is caused by acids produced by bacteria that etch away the tooth surface. If the bacteria cannot accumulate and adhere to the tooth surface, then decay cannot occur. Likewise, some prevention of periodontal disease is attributable to the very smoothness of this enamel because bacteria that destroy gum and bone tissue are also prevented from accumulating on the tooth.

However, not all periodontal disease is initially caused by bacteria. If the tooth has rough pits, grooves, or fissures, then these areas allow debris to accumulate and provide a breeding ground

for bacteria. The same is true if the tooth has rough margins on its restorations or if the tooth interproximally has an **overhanging restoration**—that is, a restoration that does not stay within the confines of the tooth form but protrudes into the gingival tissue (Fig. 9.1). Bacteria can adhere around the margins of the excess material and lead to disease within the gingival and tooth tissues. Restoration of any tooth must follow the normal anatomy of that tooth. A restoration must be polished smooth so that the tooth can resume normal function and the jaw its normal anatomy. Dental personnel provide a valuable service in preventive dentistry by polishing dental restorations. It is much more comfortable for patients to undergo the polishing of their restorations than a replacement

Likewise, tooth sealants can be placed in the grooves and pits on the occlusal surface of the molars and premolars. This is to prevent decay from forming in these hard-to-clean areas.

Rough surfaces on the roots of teeth and extra projections of cementum and calculus can also lead to decay, as in Fig. 9.1, as well as to the breakdown of periodontal tissues. Fig. 9.2 shows calculus spurs attached to the roots of the teeth. One can immediately see how these roughened areas would allow calculus, debris, and bacteria to build up in these areas.

It therefore becomes extremely important for dental professionals not only to remove calculus and stain from the roots of the teeth but also to smooth any rough areas on the root that may be formed from irregularities in the cementum or developmental defects. Regular root scaling can prevent disease by destroying any plaque-trapping areas that could harbor bacteria but may not be enough. A procedure called **root planing** will most likely be required as well. The dental professional must always remember how thin the envelope of cementum is that wraps around the root. A painful situation occurs when bare dentin is exposed, because the cementum is stripped away from part of the root of a tooth.

These interproximal areas are hard to clean. When the bone is healthy and no periodontal pockets exist, dental floss or water picks may be enough to clean these areas. In Fig. 9.3 we see a set of problems first caused by the early loss of a first molar but made worse when the second molar did not completely move into the first molar's position. A diastema developed, causing a food trap that eventually resulted in a deep periodontal pocket. If this area was kept clean, the pocket probably would not have formed. When calculus was left to build up as we see in the x-ray, then the bacteria built up on the root, causing the interproximal bone to become irritated, infected, and eventually lost. To correct this requires treatments such as scaling, root planning, and possibly surgery. Even after treatment the maintenance to prevent future pathology will require interproximal brushes in addition to flossing, water picks, and tooth brushing to get beneath the gum line of the pocket area and keep calculus and bacteria from building up on the roots. Even after successful treatment the patient will

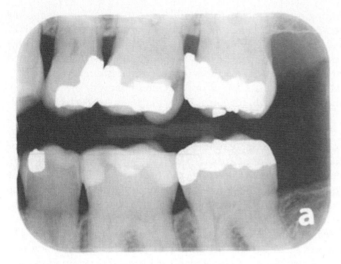

• **Figure 9.1** Overhang on the mesial of the second molar makes it a difficult area to clean. The adjacent first molar has large caries on its distal surface.

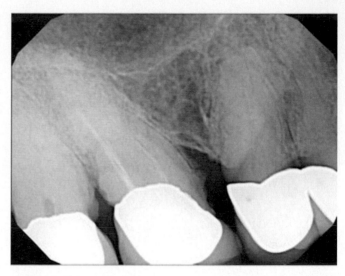

• **Figure 9.3** The second molar is shown here in the location where the first molar usually is. Note the bone loss on its mesial surface. There are also heavy calculus deposits on its root surface.

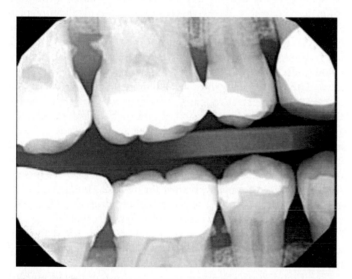

• **Figure 9.2** There are heavy calculus deposits between the maxillary molars and between the mandibular first molar and second premolar with accompanying bone loss.

forever be seen on a more frequent recall in order to detect beginning pathology as soon as possible. Remember the bone loss will not be regained, so it will be much harder for the patient to clean the area and prevent further problems. Future problems are not only harder to prevent, but should they occur the damage will begin at the level of the last periodontal pocket.

Trauma

The hardness of enamel helps prevent occlusal wear or attrition, but this same hardness allows the full impact of trauma to be transferred from tooth to bone. If a tooth prematurely contacts another, only the two teeth will bear the initial brunt of forces when the jaws are closed. A more ideal situation is to have all the teeth hit equally on closure of the jaw, without any teeth hitting prematurely. This allows for the forces exerted to be dissipated

over all the teeth. Should one tooth hit with a greater force than the rest of the teeth, it will be traumatized by this excess force. Such a situation is known as **occlusal trauma** and results in disease of the periodontal tissue, cracking of the enamel of the tooth, and possible fracture of the tooth.

Occlusal trauma can also occur during eating. It is necessary to have spillways between the teeth to allow for the dissipation of forces. This dissipation of occlusal forces occurs because the spillways allow the food to escape from between the teeth.

Contours of Teeth

The contours of the teeth, facially and lingually, determine the angle at which food is deflected from the teeth and onto the gingiva. If the buccal or lingual contours are underdeveloped (under contoured), food and debris are pushed into the gingival crevice. If the buccal and lingual contours are overdeveloped (over contoured), the food and debris pass off the tooth and onto the gingiva at a poor angle. This results in gingival inflammation because the gum tissue is denied proper frictional massage (see Fig. 3.11).

An excess of contour, such as more than 1 mm of lingual contour on mandibular molars, creates an oral hygiene problem. If the tooth contour presents extreme undercuts, the natural cleaning action of the tongue and friction of the food and cheeks become ineffective. Special oral hygiene devices and instructions must be given to the patient.

Therapeutic Considerations

Maintaining Form in Restorations

Because it is very important in the restoration of teeth to reconstruct a tooth in its anatomic form, knowing the anatomic shape of each individual tooth is also important. Contact areas and buccal and lingual contours should also be learned. For instance, an overhanging restoration or an open interproximal contact is undesirable in restoring a tooth in the interproximal area. Measures should be taken to keep the filling material from impinging on the tissue.

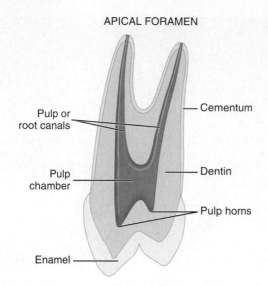

APICAL FORAMEN

Pulp or root canals

Cementum

Pulp chamber

Dentin

Pulp horns

Enamel

• **Figure 9.4** Pulp tissue of a tooth is encased by hard dentin. The only pathway for blood's vital support is through the apical foramen. (From Nelson SJ, Ash M. *Wheeler's Dental Anatomy.* 9th ed. Saunders; 2010.)

Deep pits and fissures that occur naturally should not be recreated in the teeth to be restored. The deep pits and grooves only become plaque traps. The buccal and lingual contours, however, should be restored in the best possible manner so that the gingiva is carefully protected.

The pulp tissue of the tooth should also be protected during a tooth restoration. Any trauma to the pulp tissue of a tooth creates serious complications. For example, if one were to hit his or her finger with a hammer, an inflammatory process would ensue. The finger would immediately be in pain, and blood would soon rush to the injured area. The finger would swell, and heat from the increased vascularity would be felt. The same factors exist for inflammation within the pulp cavity. If trauma occurs, the pulpal tissues become inflamed, which is caused by an increase in the blood flow to that area. Unlike the finger, however, pulpal tissue cannot swell because it is encased in hard tooth structures. The pulp cavity walls are formed from dentin (Fig. 9.4), which makes it virtually impossible for the pulpal tissue to expand. As the pressure from the increased vascularity builds up within the pulp cavity walls, the veins within the pulp tissue begin to close. Because arteries have thicker walls than veins and because they are less affected by pressure, they maintain the blood supply; however, the veins, with thinner walls, collapse. Because the only opening into the pulp cavity is the small **apical foramen** at the root apex, very little internal pressure closes this opening. As soon as the apical foramen is obstructed, blood flow is stopped and the tooth literally chokes itself off from fresh oxygenated blood. The result is that the tooth's pulpal tissues die of lack of oxygen. Once the tooth is dead it cannot fight off bacteria inside the pulp cavity. If bacteria get into this space, an infection could result. Such an infection could cause the loss of the tooth and could attack other parts of the body as well.

Maintaining Proper Bite in Restorations

The dentist and auxiliary should check a patient's bite after a restoration is in place by having the patient bite on articulating (ink) paper. This is done to ensure that no part of the restoration is

hitting prematurely, which would result in occlusal trauma to the tooth and possible fracture of the restoration or even the tooth itself. Even if the tooth hits with just slightly more contact than the rest of the teeth, the result is extreme trauma. First, the tooth, by hitting prematurely, becomes sore because it is carrying more than its share of the burden of occlusal stress. Second, the soreness of the tooth leads to inflammation of the periodontal and other supporting tissues. Third, with inflammation, edema occurs; pressure and swelling within the tissues push the tooth out of its bony socket to relieve some of these stresses. Fourth, the tooth now extends farther from the bony socket than it did before it was inflamed and hits the opposing teeth sooner and harder. Thus the tooth undergoes even more severe occlusal trauma, resulting in more inflammation, swelling, and pain. The tooth is forced to extend even farther from the bony socket to relieve this new pressure from the inflammation and edema. If untreated, the cycle could be irreversible. Therefore the dentist must make sure that any new dental restorations fit properly according to the patient's bite.

Pain

When diagnosing dental pain, note that nerve centers within the tooth are not the only nerve centers capable of eliciting pain around the tooth. If a tooth is severely damaged such that the nerve of the tooth has degenerated or even been obliterated, the tooth could still cause pain. Even an endodontically treated tooth, whose pulp cavity has been completely **debrided** of all traces of nerve tissue and filled with root canal filling material, can respond to pain if the tooth is touched. This happens because the nerve tissues in the periodontal ligament and surrounding bone tissue are still alive. If trauma or infection from any source such as periapical involvement or periodontal abscess is present, then the nerves in the supporting structures around the tooth will respond to the pain. The nerve within the pulp cavity can give only a response to pain, whereas nerves within the periodontal tissue can give either a pain response or a pressure response. A patient who reports feeling pain from within a tooth may be experiencing pain from the periodontal tissues or surrounding bone. A careful clinical examination is therefore necessary, because false and referred pains are common.

A common form of pain occurs when the gum recedes and the root of the tooth is exposed. The cementum leaves bare areas of dentin uncovered, and the dentin elicits pain whenever air, sweets, hot, or cold come into contact with it. Dentin can become nature's warning system of gum disease.

Tooth Migration

If a tooth is fractured so that it no longer hits its antagonist in the opposite arch, within 24 hours the tooth would begin to erupt to meet this antagonist. This is called **tooth migration**. The same thing would happen if a dentist cut a tooth for a crown preparation and the occlusal surface were cut away; the tooth would no longer hit its antagonist and would erupt to try to meet the antagonist. If an impression had been taken of the tooth preparation at that time so that the crown could be made, then when the crown was ready 2 weeks later, the tooth would have moved. The crown then might not fit. To avoid this problem, a well-placed temporary restoration is made to fit the crown preparation. This temporary restoration must replace the interproximal areas (to prevent mesial drift) and restore the cut preparation to a functional occlusion to prevent the tooth from erupting to meet its antagonist.

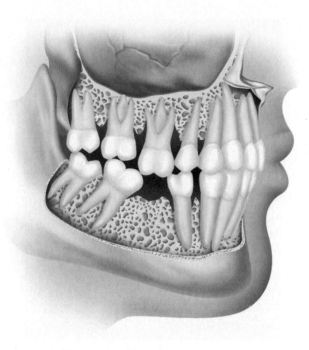

• **Figure 9.5** Dental tissues collapse because of a failure to replace the missing mandibular first molar.

If a tooth were removed and not replaced, the tooth in the opposite arch might **supraerupt** (erupt past the occlusal plane in an attempt to meet its antagonist), which would destroy the effectiveness of the contact areas between this tooth and its neighboring teeth. With the contact areas changed, food impaction could occur. In the opposite arch, mesial drift would begin to cause any teeth immediately posterior to the extraction site to move in a mesial direction. This would usually cause the posterior teeth also to become mesially tipped. Fig. 9.5 shows what happened to the interproximal spaces and contact areas when a tooth was removed and not replaced.

Interrelation of the Dental Structures

Notice the relocation of the mesial and distal contact areas of the maxillary first molar. This causes food impaction between the maxillary teeth interproximally. Plaque adheres to these poor contact areas, which results in decay. Food debris and plaque also cause gingival irritation and periodontal breakdown. Finally, premature occlusal contact occurs in centric occlusion because the distal area of the maxillary first molar prematurely hits the mesial area of the mandibular second molar. When the mandible goes into protrusive movement, the distal area of the maxillary first molar hits the mesial area of the mandibular second molar. (In protrusive movement only the anterior teeth should occlude; the posterior teeth disengage.)

This occlusal trauma results in mobility of the affected teeth and finally migration and tipping of these teeth. The mandibular second premolar migrates and tips distally and results in an open contact between the mandibular premolars. This open contact can cause a periodontal pocket with loss of the lamina dura and formation of intraosseous periodontal pockets.

The teeth are not the only structures traumatized. The temporomandibular joint (TMJ) and especially the lateral and medial pterygoid muscles experience trauma caused by premature occlusal contacts. The pterygoid muscles, which are smaller muscles, can go into spasm if they repeatedly have to move the jaw to avoid a traumatic premature contact.

The combination of occlusal trauma and mesial drift causes the mandibular second molar to move mesially and tip gingivally. This in turn causes a poor contact area between the distal mandibular second molar and the mandibular third molar, which results in a periodontal pocket between these two molars. This malpositioned contact area allows the bacteria to build up initial dental decay of the interproximal surfaces of these two molars. The mesial drift of the mandibular third molar causes the second molar to move into the decay area on the second molars, destroying the occlusal contact between the two molars.

All of this helps illustrate the importance of good preventive dentistry and the interrelationships that exist within the oral cavity. All of the dental structures interrelate in a biomechanical system. Each mechanism protects and supports the others in some way. The breakdown of any one of these systems destroys the circle of mutual protection. If the contour of teeth is destroyed, sooner or later the gingiva and bone tissue are destroyed. If the occlusal relationship is destroyed, damage to the bone, teeth, gums, and TMJ occurs. Even the muscles responsible for movement of the jaw become traumatized and spasmodic. When an occlusal prematurity exists, the patient subconsciously tries to avoid this occlusal discrepancy. To do this, the patient overexerts the lateral pterygoid muscle. This muscle becomes overworked trying to move the jaw to avoid the premature contact. This is only one example among numerous possibilities.

Study Fig. 9.6 and notice the position of the mandibular molars. They have tipped mesially, and the maxillary second premolar has supraerupted into the space vacated by the missing mandibular left first molar. Indeed the bite is totally collapsing; no occlusal plane is evident. In fact numerous teeth are broken, infection is rampant, bone loss is everywhere, and the roots of many teeth are trapped in the gingiva. This patient was fearful of going to the dentist. Instead of correcting the problem the patient persisted in pain until serious infections affected his total health.

Sometimes there are too many teeth, as seen in Fig. 9.7. Which tooth is not supposed to be there? There are two deciduous maxillary left canines. Correction of this involves removing the two canines and orthodontic treatment.

If teeth are congenitally missing, then orthodontics, a space maintainer, and eventually an implant might be required (Fig. 9.8). This congenitally missing maxillary lateral was replaced with an implant. Implants can also be used to replace extracted teeth (Fig. 9.9).

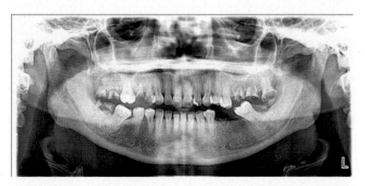

• **Figure 9.6** Movement of teeth because of the collapse of the bite due to caries. Numerous root tips remain in the gingiva. Apical infections are apparent.

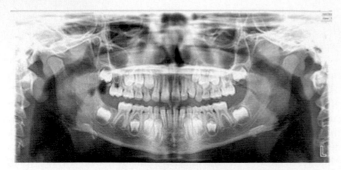

• **Figure 9.7** Which tooth is the supernumerary tooth?

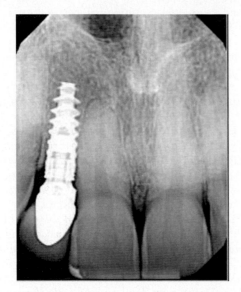

• **Figure 9.8** Congenitally missing maxillary lateral incisor replaced with an implant.

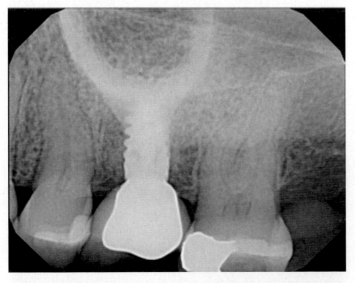

• **Figure 9.9** Maxillary molar replaced with an implant.

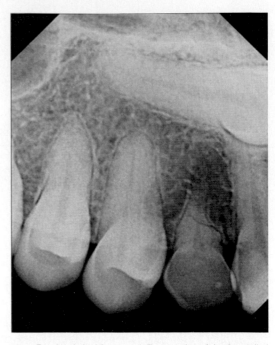

• **Figure 9.10** Retained deciduous maxillary canine. A horizontally impacted permanent canine is immediately above it.

Implants can also be used to replace retained deciduous teeth. If a deciduous tooth is not replaced by its permanent successor, it might stay in the mouth for 20 or more years. In most cases it will become loose with time. For some reason the body eventually starts to resorb the root, and the tooth becomes loose and eventually falls out. Dentists try to anticipate this and remove the retained deciduous tooth while there is still enough bone left to support the implant. Fig. 9.10 shows a retained deciduous canine. Note the horizontally impacted permanent canine above it. It will never replace the deciduous canine without serious intervention. Sometimes it is possible to orthodontically pull the canine into position. In other cases the deciduous tooth is removed and replaced with an implant. It is not always necessary to remove the impacted permanent canine. Sometimes it is just left in place if it does not continue to move within the roof of the mouth. However, it is also possible for an impacted tooth to form an invasive cyst. For this reason the impacted teeth are often removed.

The best dentistry is preventive dentistry. Preventive dentistry maintains the oral structures in their most mutually protective harmony. It intercepts disease at the earliest possible time so that the most natural, self-protective, functional, and preventive balances can be restored and maintained by these tissues. The clinical considerations are endless, but here it is intended that the student of dental anatomy merely have an example of how to apply the basic principles of dental anatomy to the clinical experience. Never cease to be alert and observant. Your reward will be the comfort of patients, pride in your work, and the progress of the dental profession.

Review Questions

1. If a dentist restores a tooth in such a way that it is the first tooth to touch its antagonist when the patient closes his or her mouth, which of the following clinical problems could result?
   a. inflammation of the nerve of the tooth
   b. occlusal trauma
   c. tooth mobility
   d. tooth migration
   e. pain
   f. nerve involvement
   g. fracture of the restoration or the tooth
   h. inflammation of the supporting structures of the tooth
   i. any of the above
2. If a dentist cuts a crown preparation but does not place a temporary restoration properly, which of the following could occur? Identify all that apply.
   a. gingival inflammation of the supporting structures because of bacterial buildup around the margins of the temporary restoration
   b. occlusal trauma to the tooth and temporary restoration
   c. tooth migration to avoid occlusal trauma
   d. supraeruption of the tooth to meet its antagonist
   e. pain caused by trauma, inflammation, or bacterial involvement
   f. sensitivity to hot or cold fluids
   g. tipping or mesial drifting of the tooth
3. What could happen to the nerve of a tooth if the tooth became inflamed because of occlusal traumatization?
4. Name three of the possible pathologic situations present in Fig. 9.11.
5. An overhanging restoration is evident on an x-ray but does not show any bone loss radiographically. An explorer is used to examine the gingival area next to the overhang in the patient's mouth. What findings would be considered healthy?
   a. the presence of a 4-mm pocket
   b. the depth of the gingival sulcus exceeding 3 mm
   c. the presence of pus and blood on probing the area
   d. no bleeding on probing the sulcus a depth of 2.5 mm (pink and firm papillary gingiva)
6. What can be done to prevent dental disease (caries and periodontal disease)?
   a. polishing restorations
   b. sealants
   c. smoothing off or replacing overhanging restorations
   d. grinding down teeth that are hitting prematurely
   e. all of the above

7. Which of the following elicits a pain response in an area of gum recession?
   a. cold
   b. sweets
   c. air
   d. heat
   e. all of these
   f. none of these
8. A healthy gingival sulcus rarely exceeds
   a. 3 mm
   b. 3.5 mm
   c. 4 mm
   d. 2.5 mm

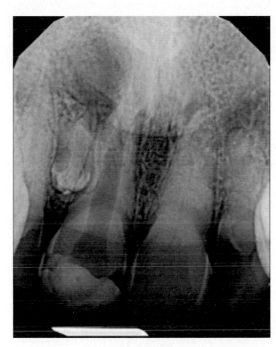

• Figure 9.11

10
Tooth Identification

OBJECTIVES

- To understand how to use landmarks to identify the incisors
- To understand how to use landmarks to identify the canines
- To understand how to use landmarks to identify the premolars
- To understand how to use landmarks to identify the molars
- The permanent teeth only will be studied here. The deciduous teeth will be discussed in Chapter 16.

It is rare to find a full set of teeth in which every tooth meets all the anatomic criteria of what a perfect tooth should be because too much variation occurs among individual teeth. When studying tooth identification, it is important to remember that extreme amounts of variation are possible. The individual tooth to be identified may meet most of the criteria of a maxillary central incisor, may be missing certain criteria for a maxillary central incisor, and may even meet some of the criteria of a maxillary canine or lateral incisor, yet it may still be a maxillary central incisor. Only after compiling all the characteristics of the tooth in question and categorizing these characteristics can the individual tooth be identified—and then only *after* it becomes apparent that the tooth meets more characteristics of one type of tooth than another (Fig. 10.1).

The following is a description of general characteristics of each of the teeth by their respective groupings: incisors, canines, premolars, and molars.[1] In identifying teeth, it is necessary to be able to differentiate among the left and right teeth in any particular group as well as if they are primary or secondary teeth. The proper name for each tooth is stated: **dentition** (permanent or deciduous), **dental arch** (maxillary or mandibular), **quadrant** (right or left), and **tooth name** (incisor, canine, premolar, or molar). An example is permanent maxillary left second premolar or deciduous mandibular left molar (review Chapter 4).

General Rules of Tooth Identification

1. The curvature of the cementoenamel junction (CEJ) is usually about 1 mm less on the distal surface of the tooth than on the mesial.
2. Tooth roots do not always curve; however, if they do curve, they usually curve distally, especially at the apex of the root. It is not uncommon, however, for the root to curve mesially.

---

1 Generally

3. The distal incisal edges of anterior teeth are more rounded than the mesial incisal edges.
4. Mandibular anterior teeth tend to wear on their labial incisal edges, whereas maxillary teeth wear on their lingual incisal edges. Unless a person has a class III occlusion, then the maxillary teeth are facial to the mandibular teeth.
5. Permanent molars are generally smaller in height and have fewer cusps the more posteriorly they are positioned. For example, the permanent first molar usually has five cusps and is larger than a second or third molar. A mandibular first molar has a distal cusp on its facial surface, and a maxillary first molar has a cusp of Carabelli. The second and third molars are less likely to have these cusps; however, when they do, cusps are less well developed and are more like tubercles than cusps.
6. Permanent molars tend to have more **secondary** and **tertiary anatomy** the more posterior they are positioned. **Secondary anatomy** consists of extra grooves and pits in addition to the main primary developmental anatomy. These grooves and pits are shallower than the primary anatomy and are more likely to be found on second and third molars. **Tertiary anatomy** refers

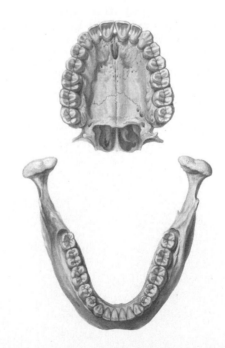

• **Figure 10.1** Occlusal view of the maxillary and mandibular permanent teeth. The permanent teeth are displayed in their proper position and alignment within their supporting bones. (Modified from Zeisz RC, Nuckolls J. *Dental Anatomy*. St. Louis: Mosby; 1949.)

to the extremely shallow and even more numerous grooves, pits, and lines that third molars often have, giving them a more wrinkled appearance than first or second molars.

7. The roots of molars tend to be shorter and closer together the more posterior the molars are positioned, and the roots are often fused into one. First molars have the widest and longest roots of all molars.

8. The more posterior the molars are positioned, the more variation of the anatomy is evident. Third molars are more wrinkled and unpredictable in shape than second or first molars; they could have six cusps or one single conical cusp. They are also more likely to be congenitally missing than other molars.

Incisors

1. Incisal two-thirds appear flattened on labial and lingual sides (Fig. 10.2).
2. Incisal "biting" edge, not a cusp.

Maxillary

1. Crown is wider mesiodistally than faciolingually (see Fig. 10.2; Fig. 10.3).
2. Crown is convex on labial and concave on lingual (Figs. 10.4 and 10.5).
3. Root has a triangular cross section, being broader on the facial side.
4. The incised edge is worn more on the lingual than the labial, so it slants lingually (see Fig. 10.5).

Central Incisor

1. Greater crown-to-root ratio than the lateral incisor (crown length divided by root length). The crown is larger; root is about the same or smaller (Figs. 10.5 and 10.6).
2. Mesioincisal angle is relatively sharp (90-degree angle), with contact area in incisal third.
3. Broad, smooth lingual fossa with well-developed cingulum (see Fig. 10.4).

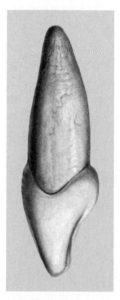

• **Figure 10.2** Maxillary right central incisor, mesial view. (Modified from Zeisz RC, Nuckolls J. *Dental Anatomy*. St. Louis: Mosby; 1949.)

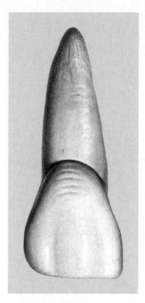

• **Figure 10.3** Maxillary right central incisor, labial view. (Modified from Zeisz RC, Nuckolls J. *Dental Anatomy*. St. Louis: Mosby; 1949.)

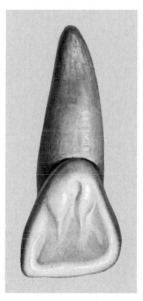

• **Figure 10.4** Maxillary right central incisor, lingual view. (Modified from Zeisz RC, Nuckolls J. *Dental Anatomy*. St. Louis: Mosby; 1949.)

Lateral Incisor

1. Lesser crown-to-root ratio than central incisors (crown smaller, root usually longer than central incisors).
2. Mesioincisal angle more rounded than central, with contact area at junction of middle and incisal thirds.
3. Small cingulum, often with a lingual pit.
4. Root longer and more slender than the central incisor (compare Fig. 10.7 with Fig. 10.8).

Right Versus Left

1. Mesioincisal angles are squarer than distoincisal angles (Fig. 10.9).
2. Crest of cervical line more often displaced toward distal from labial or lingual view.

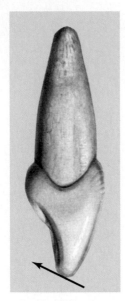

• **Figure 10.5** Maxillary right central incisor, distal view. The incised edge slants lingually as it is worn down. The *arrow* points in the direction of wear. (Modified from Zeisz RC, Nuckolls J. *Dental Anatomy.* St. Louis: Mosby; 1949.)

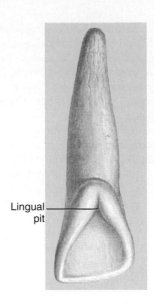

• **Figure 10.7** Maxillary right lateral incisor, lingual view displaying location of lingual pit. (Modified from Zeisz RC, Nuckolls J. *Dental Anatomy.* St. Louis: Mosby; 1949.)

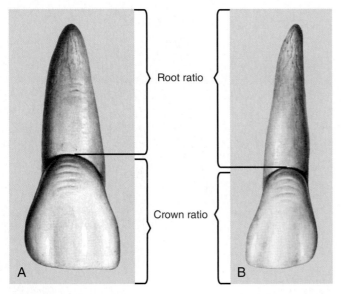

• **Figure 10.6** Maxillary right central incisor, labial view. Central crown is wider and longer but the root shorter than a lateral. (Modified from Zeisz RC, Nuckolls J. *Dental Anatomy.* St. Louis: Mosby; 1949.)

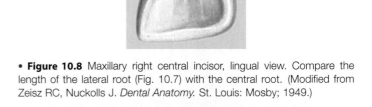

• **Figure 10.8** Maxillary right central incisor, lingual view. Compare the length of the lateral root (Fig. 10.7) with the central root. (Modified from Zeisz RC, Nuckolls J. *Dental Anatomy.* St. Louis: Mosby; 1949.)

3. Mesiocervical line curves more incisally than distocervical line (Fig. 10.10).

Mandibular

1. Smaller than maxillary central or lateral incisor (Figs. 10.11 and 10.12).
2. Crown wider faciolingually than mesiodistally.
3. Root with oval cross section.
4. Incisal edge wears on labial surface (Fig. 10.13); incisal edge is worn more on labial than lingual, so it slants from incisor edge toward labial.

Central Incisor

1. Incisal view: incisal edge perpendicular to faciolingual axis of tooth.
2. Mesial and distal lobes appear identical (Fig. 10.14).
3. Most difficult tooth in mouth to differentiate right from left—almost identical.

Right Versus Left

1. Cervical line curves more incisally on mesial than on distal surface.
2. Height of curvature of cervical line on mesial greater than on distal surface.

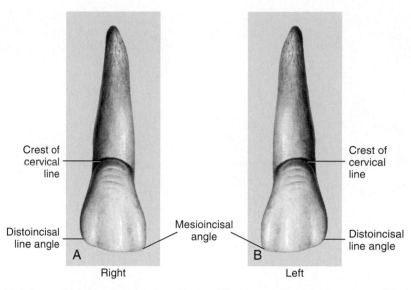

• **Figure 10.9** Comparing a maxillary right lateral incisor (**A**) with a maxillary left lateral incisor (**B**). (Modified from Zeisz RC, Nuckolls J. *Dental Anatomy*. St. Louis: Mosby; 1949.)

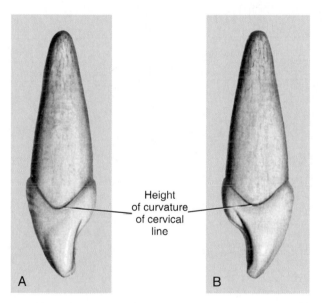

• **Figure 10.10** (**A**) Maxillary right lateral incisor, mesial view. (**B**) Maxillary right lateral incisor, distal view. (Modified from Zeisz RC, Nuckolls J. *Dental Anatomy*. St. Louis: Mosby; 1949.)

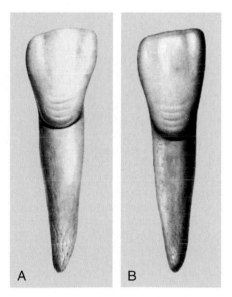

• **Figure 10.11** Maxillary left lateral incisor (**A**) is shown inverted for comparison with mandibular right lateral incisor (**B**). (Modified from Zeisz RC, Nuckolls J. *Dental Anatomy*. St. Louis: Mosby; 1949.)

3. Root tip may have slight distal curve.
4. Incisal edge worn wider on distal surface.

Lateral Incisor

1. Incisal view: distoincisal edge angled toward lingual side.
2. Distal lobe appears larger than mesial lobe (Fig. 10.15).
3. Larger than mandibular central and often confused with it or maxillary lateral incisor.

Right Versus Left

1. Cervical line curves more incisally on mesial than on distal surface.
2. Incisal view: distal half of incisal edge rotated toward lingual side.

3. Incisal edge worn wider and longer on distal surface (see Fig. 10.15).

Canines

1. Single conical cusp with well-developed mesiofacial lobe.
2. Lingual cusp ridge from cusp tip to lingual fossa (Fig. 10.16; see Fig. 10.20).

Maxillary

1. Lingual surface has well-developed marginal ridges, cingulum, and fossa (see Fig. 10.16).

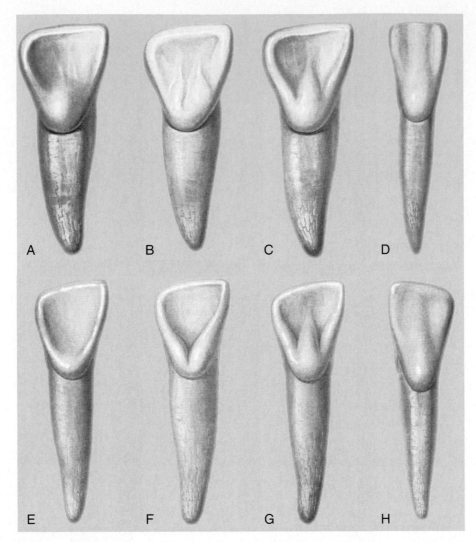

• **Figure 10.12 (A–C)** Maxillary right central incisors. **(D)** Mandibular right central incisor. **(E–G)** Maxillary lateral incisors. **(H)** Mandibular right lateral incisor. All are lingual views. Compare the smooth lingual surface of the mandibular incisors with the maxillary incisors. (Modified from Zeisz RC, Nuckolls J. *Dental Anatomy.* St. Louis: Mosby; 1949.)

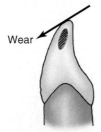

• **Figure 10.13** Mandibular right lateral incisor, mesial view.

• **Figure 10.14** Mandibular right central incisor, incisal view. (Modified from Zeisz RC, Nuckolls J. *Dental Anatomy.* St. Louis: Mosby; 1949.)

• **Figure 10.15** Mandibular right lateral incisor, incisal view. (Modified from Zeisz RC, Nuckolls J. *Dental Anatomy.* St. Louis: Mosby; 1949.)

2. Larger and bulkier crown than incisors and lower canines; more distal convexity (Fig. 10.17).
3. Cusp tip directly midcenter over root.

Right Versus Left

1. Cervical line curves more incisally on mesial than on distal surface (Figs. 10.18 and 10.19).
2. Incisal view: distofacial lobe elongated or pulled out.
3. Facial view: distal surface rounded and contact area located more cervically.

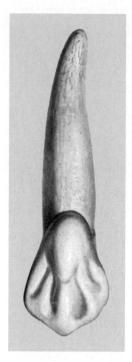

• **Figure 10.16** Maxillary right canine, lingual view. (Modified from Zeisz RC, Nuckolls J. *Dental Anatomy.* St. Louis: Mosby; 1949.)

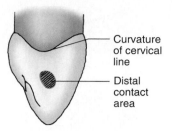

• **Figure 10.18** Maxillary right canine, distal view. (Modified from Zeisz RC, Nuckolls J. *Dental Anatomy.* St. Louis: Mosby; 1949.)

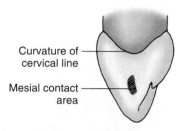

• **Figure 10.19** Maxillary right canine, mesial view. (Modified from Zeisz RC, Nuckolls J. *Dental Anatomy.* St. Louis: Mosby; 1949.)

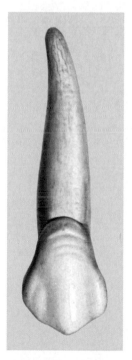

• **Figure 10.17** Maxillary right canine, labial view. (Modified from Zeisz RC, Nuckolls J. *Dental Anatomy.* St. Louis: Mosby; 1949.)

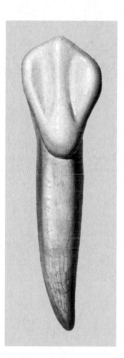

• **Figure 10.20** Mandibular right canine, lingual view. (Modified from Zeisz RC, Nuckolls J. *Dental Anatomy.* St. Louis: Mosby; 1949.)

Mandibular

1. Lingual surface almost smooth with poorly developed ridges, cingulum, and fossa (Fig. 10.20).
2. Narrower mesiodistal width than maxillary.
3. More wear on facial (labial) surface (Fig. 10.21) compared with maxillary canine.

Premolars

At least two cusps, one a single facial cusp, with one or two lingual cusps.

Maxillary

1. Two major cusps, one buccal and one lingual, approximately equal in size.
2. Distinctly wider faciolingually than mesiodistally.

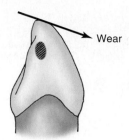

• **Figure 10.21** Mandibular right canine, mesial view. (Modified from Zeisz RC, Nuckolls J. *Dental Anatomy.* St. Louis: Mosby; 1949.)

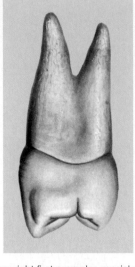

• **Figure 10.23** Maxillary right first premolar, mesial view. Notice the mesial depression above the contact area. (Modified from Zeisz RC, Nuckolls J. *Dental Anatomy.* St. Louis: Mosby; 1949.)

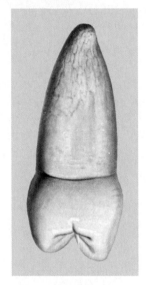

• **Figure 10.22** Maxillary right second premolar, distal view. (Modified from Zeisz RC, Nuckolls J. *Dental Anatomy.* St. Louis: Mosby; 1949.)

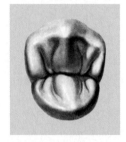

• **Figure 10.24** Maxillary right first premolar, occlusal view. (Modified from Zeisz RC, Nuckolls J. *Dental Anatomy.* St. Louis: Mosby; 1949.)

3. Proximal view: facial and lingual cusps nearly same height and both located over root trunk (Fig. 10.22).

First Premolar

1. Facial cusp slightly longer than lingual cusp (Fig. 10.23).
2. Often has two roots, buccal and lingual.
3. Occlusal surface has well-developed central groove, with little supplemental grooving.
4. Mesial surface has depression above contact area starting below cervical line and usually extending onto root.

Right Versus Left

1. Mesial marginal groove.
2. Cervical line on mesial surface curves more occlusally than on distal surface.
3. Occlusal view: mesiofacial cusp ridge forms 90-degree angle with mesial marginal ridge; distofacial cusp ridge forms rounded angle with distal marginal ridge (Fig. 10.24).

Second Premolar

1. Facial and lingual cusps are nearly same height (Fig. 10.25).
2. Usually single rooted, but often bifurcated.

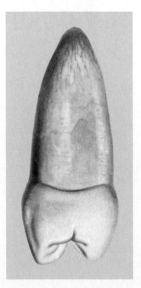

• **Figure 10.25** Maxillary right second premolar, mesial view. (Modified from Zeisz RC, Nuckolls J. *Dental Anatomy.* St. Louis: Mosby; 1949.)

3. Short central groove, with frequent and numerous supplemental grooves.
4. No depression on mesial or distal crown surfaces.

Right Versus Left

Lingual cusp displaced slightly toward mesial side (Fig. 10.26).

Mandibular

1. Prominent facial cusp with one or two much smaller lingual cusps.
2. Nearly equal faciolingual and mesiodistal widths.
3. Proximal view: facial cusp much larger; facial cusp tip at or near midaxis of root; lingual cusp(s) extend lingually past lingual border of root (Fig. 10.27).

First Premolar

1. Proximal view: occlusal surface tilted strongly toward lingual side (Fig. 10.28).
2. Occlusal view: oval outline with strong transverse ridge and no central pit (Fig. 10.29).

Right Versus Left

1. Cervical line on mesial surface curves more occlusally than on distal surface.

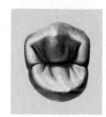

• **Figure 10.26** Maxillary right second premolar, occlusal view. The lingual cusp tip is more distal than on the first premolar. (Modified from Zeisz RC, Nuckolls J. *Dental Anatomy.* St. Louis: Mosby; 1949.)

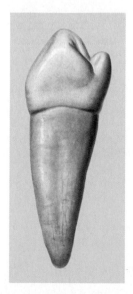

• **Figure 10.27** Mandibular right first premolar, mesial view. (Modified from Zeisz RC, Nuckolls J. *Dental Anatomy.* St. Louis: Mosby; 1949.)

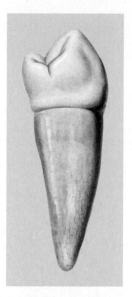

• **Figure 10.28** Mandibular right first premolar, proximal view. (Modified from Zeisz RC, Nuckolls J. *Dental Anatomy.* St. Louis: Mosby; 1949.)

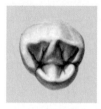

• **Figure 10.29** Mandibular right first premolar, occlusal view. (Modified from Zeisz RC, Nuckolls J. *Dental Anatomy.* St. Louis: Mosby; 1949.)

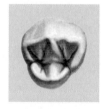

• **Figure 10.30** Mandibular left first premolar, occlusal view. (Modified from Zeisz RC, Nuckolls J. *Dental Anatomy.* St. Louis: Mosby; 1949.)

2. Often a depression or groove where mesial marginal ridge joins lingual cusp ridge (Fig. 10.30).
3. Distal marginal ridge more prominent.

Second Premolar

1. Occlusal view: pentagonal outline, with a central pit and no transverse ridge (Fig. 10.31).
2. Proximal view: occlusal surface less lingually tilted (Fig. 10.32).
3. May have two lingual cusps.

Right Versus Left

Proximal view: more of occlusal surface visible from distal than from mesial because of distal inclination of crown-to-root axis.

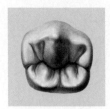

• **Figure 10.31** Mandibular right second premolar, occlusal view. (Modified from Zeisz RC, Nuckolls J. *Dental Anatomy.* St. Louis: Mosby; 1949.)

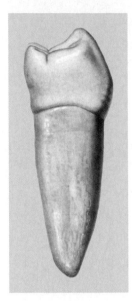

• **Figure 10.32** Mandibular right second premolar, distal view. (Modified from Zeisz RC, Nuckolls J. *Dental Anatomy.* St. Louis: Mosby; 1949.)

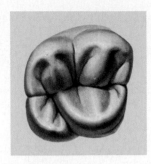

• **Figure 10.33** Maxillary right first molar, occlusal view. (Modified from Zeisz RC, Nuckolls J. *Dental Anatomy.* St. Louis: Mosby; 1949.)

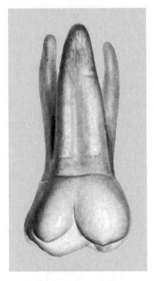

• **Figure 10.34** Maxillary right first molar, lingual view. (Modified from Zeisz RC, Nuckolls J. *Dental Anatomy.* St. Louis: Mosby; 1949.)

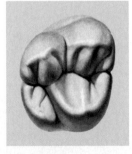

• **Figure 10.35** Maxillary right second molar, occlusal view. (Modified from Zeisz RC, Nuckolls J. *Dental Anatomy.* St. Louis: Mosby; 1949.)

Molars

Three to five cusps, with at least two facial cusps.

Maxillary

1. Crowns wider faciolingually than mesiodistally.
2. Three roots: two on facial and one on lingual side.

First Molar

1. Occlusal view: strong **oblique ridge** less likely to be crossed by a groove (Fig. 10.33).
2. Three roots widely separated.
3. Often has a fifth cusp (cusp of Carabelli) on mesiolingual cusp (Fig. 10.34).

Right Versus Left

Mesiolingual cusp always much larger than distolingual cusp.

Second Molar

1. Occlusal view: smaller oblique ridge usually interrupted by a groove (Fig. 10.35).
2. Roots closer together (Fig. 10.36).
3. No fifth cusp or much smaller tubercle rather than cusp.
4. Distolingual cusp smaller than on first molar.

Right Versus Left

Mesiolingual cusp always much larger than distolingual cusp.

Third Molar

1. Distolingual cusp progressively smaller or missing entirely (Fig. 10.37).
2. Roots either fused or very close together and much shorter.
3. No oblique ridge (Fig. 10.38).

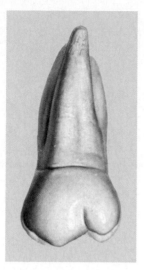

• **Figure 10.36** Maxillary right second molar, lingual view. Note no cusp of Carabelli. (Modified from Zeisz RC, Nuckolls J. *Dental Anatomy.* St. Louis: Mosby; 1949.)

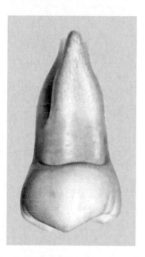

• **Figure 10.37** Maxillary right third molar, lingual view. (Modified from Zeisz RC, Nuckolls J. *Dental Anatomy.* St. Louis: Mosby; 1949.)

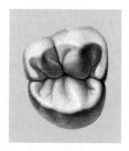

• **Figure 10.38** Maxillary right third molar, occlusal view. (Modified from Zeisz RC, Nuckolls J. *Dental Anatomy.* St. Louis: Mosby; 1949.)

4. Roots shorter than first or second molars.
5. No cusp of Carabelli usually, but third molars vary considerably.
6. Occlusal anatomy quite varied.

Right Versus Left

1. Distofacial cusp much shorter than other molars.
2. Roots curved distally.

Mandibular

1. Crowns wider mesiodistally than faciolingually.
2. Two roots: one mesial and one distal.
3. Mesial root larger, wider, and longer than distal root.

First Molar

1. Three facial cusps and two facial grooves (Fig. 10.39).
2. Bifurcated roots widely separated and relatively vertical.

Right Versus Left

Distal cusp is smallest facial cusp (Fig. 10.40).

Second Molar

1. Only two facial cusps and one facial groove (Fig. 10.41).
2. Occlusal groove well defined but travels straight mesial to distal and forms a cross (+) with facial and lingual grooves (Fig. 10.42).
3. Roots are bifurcated and close together.

Right Versus Left

Buccal height of contour in cervical third; lingual height of contour in middle third (Fig. 10.43).

Third Molar

1. Secondary and tertiary anatomy (Fig. 10.44).
2. Short roots, often fused and frequently curved distally.

Right Versus Left

Crown tapers distally; wider faciolingually on mesial than on distal surface (also true of mandibular first and second molars).

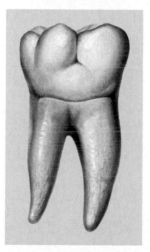

• **Figure 10.39** Mandibular right first molar, buccal view. (Modified from Zeisz RC, Nuckolls J. *Dental Anatomy.* St. Louis: Mosby; 1949.)

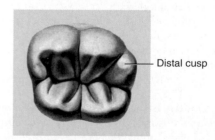

Distal cusp

• **Figure 10.40** Mandibular right first molar, occlusal view. (Modified from Zeisz RC, Nuckolls J. *Dental Anatomy.* St. Louis: Mosby; 1949.)

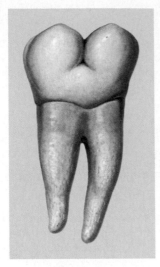

• **Figure 10.41** Mandibular right second molar, buccal view. Note the lack of distal cusp. (Modified from Zeisz RC, Nuckolls J. *Dental Anatomy.* St. Louis: Mosby; 1949.)

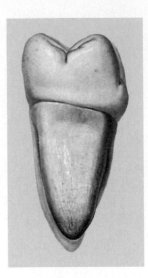

• **Figure 10.43** Mandibular right second molar, distal view. (Modified from Zeisz RC, Nuckolls J. *Dental Anatomy.* St. Louis: Mosby; 1949.)

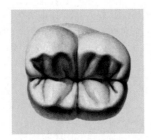

• **Figure 10.42** Mandibular right second molar, occlusal view. (Modified from Zeisz RC, Nuckolls J. *Dental Anatomy.* St. Louis: Mosby; 1949.)

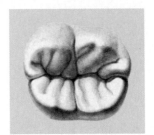

• **Figure 10.44** Mandibular right third molar, occlusal view. Note this third molar has a tiny distal cusp. Second molars can also sometimes have a distal cusp. The mandibular first molar will have the larger, more developed distal cusp. (Modified from Zeisz RC, Nuckolls J. *Dental Anatomy.* St. Louis: Mosby; 1949.)

Review Questions

1. Which anterior incisors are much wider mesiodistally than faciolingually?
2. Which incisors have the greater crown-to-root ratio? Centrals or laterals?
3. Which incisors are nearly identical?
4. In general, does the cervical line curve more incisally on the mesial or the distal surface?
5. Which has more developed lingual marginal ridges, the maxillary or mandible?
6. On incisors, which incisal line angle is more rounded, mesial or distal?
7. Which incisor has its incisal edge worn on the labial side, maxillary or mandibular?
8. Which mandibular incisor is longer?
9. Which canine has more distal convexity?
10. On a maxillary incisor, is the labial surface of the crown convex or concave?
11. On canines, which surface is least convex, mesial or distal?
12. Which premolars are most likely to have two roots?
13. Which premolar is most likely to have three cusps?
14. Which premolar is most likely to have a well-defined mesial marginal groove?
15. Which molars are most likely to have five cusps?

16. Name the smallest of the five cusps of a mandibular first molar.
17. The fifth cusp of a maxillary first molar is located on what other cusp?
18. Are the roots closer together on a first or second molar?
19. Are the roots longer on a first or second molar?
20. Which molar is most likely to have three buccal cusps?
21. If two teeth look identical, such as two mandibular incisors, the one that shows greater curvature of the CEJ is more likely which of the following:
    a. central
    b. lateral
    c. neither
22. If the root of the tooth described in question 21 has a curve of the root at its apex, this curve more likely points in which of the following ways?
    a. mesially
    b. distally
    c. neither
23. If this same tooth from question #21 has a rounded incisal ridge on the same side toward which the root curves, this rounded edge is more likely to be which of the following?
    a. mesial incisal ridge
    b. distal incisal ridge

11

Root Morphology

OBJECTIVES

- To understand the functions of the roots of teeth
- To understand how the shape of the root affects the support of the tooth
- To understand how orthodontic tooth movement is possible
- To understand how root shape protects the health and hygiene of periodontal tissue
- To understand the anatomic differences between root canals

Functions of Roots

The roots of teeth have several general functions. First, the roots afford a sensory system to warn of threats to teeth. Second, the roots house the nourishment system of teeth and afford external and internal reparative methods to respond to pathology, pressure, or trauma. Third, the roots offer a system of support or anchorage for the teeth.

Sensory Functions

The inner part of tooth roots is composed of **dental pulpal** tissue. This tissue not only nourishes the tooth but also contains nerves that can elicit a pain response. In fact, once the pulpal nerves are stimulated, the only response they can emit is a pain response.

Pulpal nerves can be stimulated in a variety of ways. The most common way is for the dentinal tubules to carry a stimulus from the root surface through the dentinal tubules to the nerve tissue lining the root canal. If that stimulus is dehydration, caused by air or chemicals, the response is pain. Root decay, root resorption, or abrasion can allow the tubules to be opened, and air, sweets, or other chemicals, such as bleaching agents, can cause the tubules to become dehydrated. Rubbing the root surface with an instrument, friction, or abrasion can also elicit a pain response.

The dentin that surrounds the pulpal tissue of the root is itself covered by an imperfect layer of cementum. This patchwork of cementum has bare areas where dentin is exposed. If the tooth root is exposed because of periodontal disease, recession, trauma, or any form of pathology, these exposed spots of dentin can stimulate the pulpal nerves through their tubules (Fig. 11.1).

The roots are a warning system that indicates external or internal trauma. If the pulpal tissue inside the root canal becomes inflamed, then hot or cold stimulation can cause pain. If the nerve is alive but severely inflamed, a cold stimulus, such as cold water, can cause a painful response. The longer the response takes to subside, the more damaged the pulpal tissue is. If gases are present within the pulpal tissue, such as when the pulp is infected or necrotic, these gases can be expanded with a heated stimulus, such as hot coffee, tea, food, or water. Once affected by heat, the gases expand, but the root canal that houses these gases remains the same size. These expanded gases put pressure on any nerve tissue that remains vital. The expanded gases then force themselves out the root apex into the surrounding bone and periodontal ligament. This, in turn, causes a serious pain response that lingers, sometimes with extreme intensity and duration.

Pressure and temperature responses are not elicited by the pulpal tissue. Instead the nerve tissue within bone, gums, and the periodontal ligament elicits these responses. The root canal tissue does not have nerves that can stimulate sensations of temperature or pressure. The root canals can only respond to pain.

Reparative and Nourishment Functions

The pulp canals house the nourishment system of the tooth. It is here within the root canal that arteries, veins, and lymph tissue nourish the tooth from the inside. These vessels enter and exit through an orifice in the apex of the root called the **apical foramen**. They allow nutrients and oxygen to circulate throughout the pulp chamber. They also provide a system to remove harmful products and carbon dioxide from the tooth. This is the way that the nerves and odontoblasts within the tooth are nourished and replenished.

If the flow of these vessels is restricted over a long time or totally constricted for as little as several minutes, then the nerves and other tissues inside the pulp chamber could die of anoxia (lack of oxygen).

Inside the tooth the odontoblasts allow secondary and reparative dentin to be formed in response to trauma (see Chapter 20). This process is not restricted to the root but is applicable to the entire pulp chamber.

The apical third of the root at or near its apex can continue to form cementum on the outside of the root. If this process is extreme, it is called *hypercementosis,* and it forms a cementoma at the apex of the root (see the sections on Dental Anomalies in Chapter 7 and Root Formation in Chapter 21). A cementoma is usually associated with bone destruction and/or trauma. This cementum is different from the cementum that lines the rest of the root. First, it can continue to grow and add on to itself. Second, in this process of adding on to itself, cells that form cementum are trapped within it. This cementum is called *cellular cementum* (see Fig. 11.1).

Support Functions

The shape and length of the roots have a direct effect on how much anchorage and support they can afford. The longer and

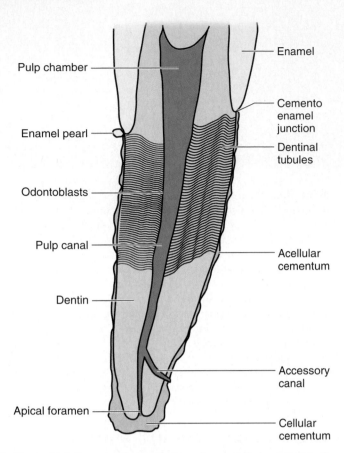

- **Figure 11.1** Cross-sectional drawing of a mandibular lateral incisor. Note how the dentinal tubules communicate with the pulp canal. In this way, external stimuli can initiate pain responses and even odontoblastic activity within the pulp chamber. The pulp chamber *(red-colored area)* houses nerves, arteries, veins, lymph tissue, and odontoblasts.

Labels for Figure 11.1: Pulp chamber, Enamel pearl, Odontoblasts, Pulp canal, Dentin, Apical foramen, Enamel, Cemento enamel junction, Dentinal tubules, Acellular cementum, Accessory canal, Cellular cementum

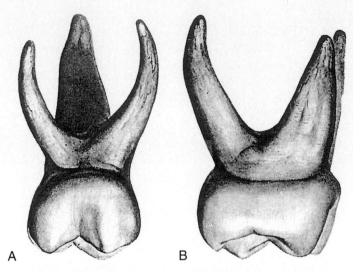

- **Figure 11.2** The roots of a deciduous maxillary right second molar are flared wide apart. These roots not only afford anchorage for the tooth but also offer protection to the developing permanent premolar tooth bud, nestled between these roots. **(A)** Buccal view. **(B)** Distal view.

Tooth Movement

Teeth are not embedded into bone but rather they are supported between the root and bone by a hammock of periodontal fibers. These fibers attach to the cementum of the root on one end and to alveolar bone on the other. This hammock of living tissue is called the *periodontal ligament (PDL).* It is composed of collagenous fibers of connective tissue and is capable of being tensed or compressed.

The PDL fills the thin area of space that exists between the tooth and bone. Pressure exerted on the tooth compresses the PDL fibers on one side and tenses them on the other. If you push on a tooth with an instrument, you can see the tooth move ever so slightly. This small movement is called *mobility.* A slight amount of mobility is healthy and normal.

When the external force is strong enough to exert pressure on bone, it triggers a resorption process within alveolar bone. This causes certain white blood cells (WBCs), or osteoclasts, to dissolve bone in the area of the pressure. When enough bone is resorbed, the pressure ceases, the PDL regains its normal width, and the tooth moves away from the external force and into this newly remodeled area.

On the opposite side of the tooth, the PDL is tensed to accommodate the tooth's movement. This tension is exerted on bone. Osteoblastic bone-forming cells respond to the tension by forming new bone (Fig. 11.3).

In this way, responding to pressure and tension, the bone is remodeled. The net result is that the tooth moves away from the external force into a new location.

Orthodontics is accomplished by exerting force onto a tooth. This sustained force causes the tooth to move gradually into the desired new location. Only a slight amount of movement is possible during a specific amount of time. Many orthodontic cases require 2 years or more to complete.

For orthodontics to succeed, the tooth must be held fixed in its new location long enough for the collagenous fibers of the PDL to remodel. While in this *retention* phase, the PDL fibers that were lengthened from tension must have sufficient time to

wider the root, the more support the tooth receives. The longer the root, the more firmly the root is embedded into bone. The greater the surface area of the root, the more the periodontal fibers can attach the root to bone and the better the root can resist displacement from the forces exerted on it. A tooth with multiple roots has its periodontal ligaments more disbursed in different directions compared with a single-rooted tooth. This allows resistance to displacement from a greater variety of forces. Likewise, concavities and grooves in the root also allow for more surface area and for the periodontal ligament to attach at different angles.

A root with a triangular cross section offers more resistance to lateral displacement than a round cross-sectional root. Curved roots afford resistance to occlusal, apical, and distal forces. Multiple directions of periodontal fibers in the furcation areas between the roots give the tooth direct resistance to occlusal displacement.

The width, shape, length, curvature, number of roots, concavities, and direction of the periodontal fibers all affect the amount and direction of resistance a tooth can offer to withstand the forces exerted on it (Fig. 11.2).

The direction of the root tip can even offer resistance to movement. Most single-rooted teeth have their root tips pointed distally. This distal slant offers slightly more resistance to movement compared with a straight vertical upright shape.

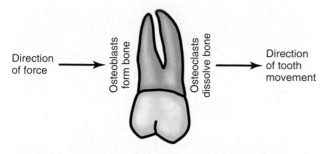

• **Figure 11.3** The tooth moves into the space where osteoclasts have dissolved bone. Osteoblasts fill bone in the space vacated by the tooth.

relax and relieve this tension. Otherwise the residual tension in these fibers causes the tooth to move back and *relapse.*

If the pressure is too extreme, both bone and the root can be resorbed. The same cells that resorb bone can also resorb the root. However, the root does require a greater pressure to be resorbed compared with bone.

Even without external forces, a tooth still moves. If all of the occlusal forces are removed from a tooth and it has no occlusal antagonist, the tooth continues to erupt. A tooth moves mesially if it does not have another tooth mesial to it; this is called *mesial drift* (see Chapter 5). The shape of the roots and the residual tension within the PDL may play some part in causing these phenomena.

Periodontal and Hygiene Considerations

The grooves and depressions on the roots make these areas harder to clean and thus more susceptible to periodontal disease. Canines and premolars have longitudinal grooves and depressions, but these areas seem much easier to clean compared with the mesial roots of molars. Molars are not only farther back in the mouth and harder to reach, but the molar roots are wider buccolingually, and it is harder to gain access to the middle of the root areas. Mandibular canines have deeper longitudinal grooves on their distal roots than on their mesial roots. Remember they often also have two root canals. Any of the teeth that may have two root canals within the same root often have deep longitudinal grooves. In fact, these grooves may be so deep that they actually divide the root into two roots. The maxillary premolars are the most likely teeth to do this. The mandibular canines sometimes bifurcate in the apical area. Mandibular lateral incisors and the mesial roots of molars usually do not bifurcate but often have deep longitudinal grooves and two root canals within the same root.

Some of the greatest periodontal problems result from furcation involvement. A furcation is the point where the roots of multirooted teeth are separated. Maxillary premolars and occasionally mandibular canines may have a bifurcation where buccal and lingual roots divide. Because these roots do not divide until near the apical third of the root, furcations are seldom noticed.

Maxillary molars have a longer root trunk compared with mandibular molars. Three separate roots emerge from this longer root trunk, with three separate furcations, resulting in a trifurcated root. The three different furcation areas for maxillary molars are between the two buccal roots, between distobuccal and lingual roots, and between mesiobuccal and lingual roots. Furcations are hard to keep clean and usually result in severe periodontal problems (Fig. 11.4A).

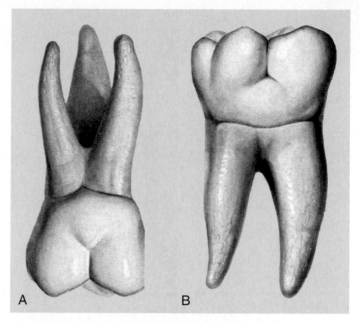

• **Figure 11.4** **(A)** A maxillary first molar has a trifurcation at the point of junction where the three roots join the root trunk. **(B)** A mandibular first molar has a bifurcation where its two roots join its root trunk. (Modified from Zeisz RC, Nuckolls J. *Dental Anatomy.* St. Louis, MO: Mosby; 1949.)

Mandibular molars have a bifurcation at the junction of their mesial and distal roots. Because their root trunks are shorter than those of maxillary teeth, these bifurcated areas are closer to the cementoenamel junction (CEJ). The buccal bifurcation is more likely to be seen clinically because the lingual root trunk is longer than the buccal root trunk, and thus the lingual furcation is further from the CEJ (see Fig. 11.4B and Fig. 15.20 A–B).

The outer surfaces of roots are much rougher than the smooth enamel covering of crowns. This makes hygiene more difficult because it is harder to clean plaque, tartar, and other debris from the root surface. Occasionally the root may be even rougher and harder to clean than usual because of excess or uneven deposits of cementum. Sometimes enamel pearls, which are small elevations of enamel on the root surface, also make hygiene more difficult. If enamel pearls develop, they usually are found in furcation areas.

It is important to remember where the grooves are on each tooth you scale. When one scales the root of a tooth, she or he must keep in mind where the grooves are on that particular tooth.

It is in these grooves that periodontal problems are the hardest to prevent. The grooves are harder for the patient to keep clean and more difficult for the dental professional to clean, treat, and maintain. It is for that reason we study how the roots may vary, where their furcations and grooves are, what is normal and unusual, the probable location of grooves and furcations, and how to find effective ways for our patients to clean and maintain these areas according to their own specific abilities.

Root Canals

Anterior teeth usually have one large root canal per tooth. Most incisors have a large root canal that is the continuation of the pulp chamber. The one anterior tooth that sometimes has two canals is the mandibular canine. If it has two canals, one is buccal and the other lingual. They are usually separated by a deep longitudinal groove, which is more obvious on the distal canal (Fig. 11.5).

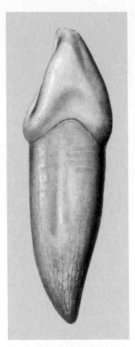

• **Figure 11.5** A mandibular right canine distal view. A deep groove may separate the root into buccal and lingual portions. The mandibular canine usually has only one root canal. Often, however, this tooth may have two root canals. When this happens, one root canal is in the buccal portion of the root and the other in the lingual portion. (Modified from Zeisz RC, Nuckolls J. *Dental Anatomy.* St. Louis, MO: Mosby; 1949.)

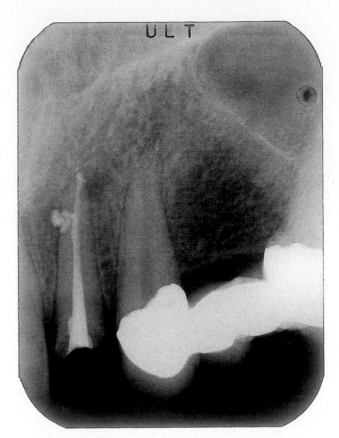

• **Figure 11.6** X-ray of a maxillary left lateral incisor. Note the accessory canal exiting mesial to the main root canal foramen at the apex of the root. The main canal exits at the apex of the root.

Nerves and blood vessels enter and leave the root through the root apex. Often more than one opening in the apex is evident. Usually one is the main apical foramen for the root canal, and the others are **accessory root canals** (Fig. 11.6).

It is possible for a tooth to have several possible orifices into the root canal. Fig. 11.7 shows only one apical foramen. Although Fig. 11.7B shows two root canals, they join together to form one canal with one apical foramen. Fig. 11.7C–D show two apical openings. In the case of Fig. 11.7C two separate root canals exit the same root through two separate openings. Fig. 11.7D shows one single root canal that divides at the apical end of the tooth, but it becomes two separate but smaller apical openings. If the **orifices** are lateral rather than apical, they are referred to as *accessory canals*. A root can have several accessory canals, as depicted in Fig. 11.7E. All anterior teeth, upper and lower, usually have one canal. Mandibular laterals and canines occasionally have two canals or at least two canals that merge into one apical opening (see Fig. 11.5).

Whenever a root has two apical openings, they are each smaller than a singular apical foramen. If a tooth has two root canals in the same root, they are each smaller than if that root had only one root canal. The maxillary first molar has three roots, and each root has at least one canal. The mesiobuccal root often has two canals, each of which is smaller than the canals in the other two roots.

Mandibular premolars usually have one canal. Maxillary premolars often have two canals. The maxillary first premolar is more likely to have two canals and even two roots compared with the maxillary second premolar. When two canals are evident, one is buccal and the other lingual; it is the same for a two-rooted tooth.

One canal is located in the buccal root and one is located in the lingual root (Fig. 11.8).

Mandibular molars usually have two root canals, one mesial and the other distal. The mesial canal is usually wider and bigger than the distal canal. The mandibular first molar is the most likely tooth to have two canals in its mesial root. When this occurs, the mesial root has a buccal canal and a lingual canal, both of which are considerably smaller than the distal canal in the same tooth (Fig. 11.9).

Second molars rarely have three root canals; usually they only have a mesial canal and a distal canal (see Fig. 11.9). Mandibular third molars can have one, two, three, or more root canals. Because third molar roots are usually curved, their root canals are very unpredictable.

Maxillary molars usually have three root canals—mesiobuccal, distobuccal, and lingual—one for each root. The first molar is the most likely tooth to have four root canals. When this happens, two root canals occur in one root, the mesiobuccal root.

If third molars are allowed to develop with more room in the mandible, the roots are longer and straighter, and the molars are bigger in general. This is often observed when the second molars are missing before age 14 years. After age 14 years, tooth tissues become calcified. The roots continue to grow until age 18 or 19 years. When the roots are straighter and longer, the root canals within these roots are as well.

Review and compare illustrations of the pulp cavities in Figs. 11.10 to 11.22.

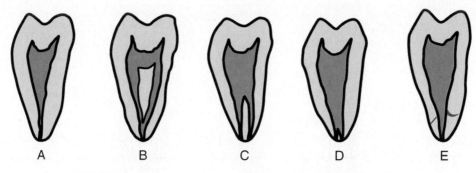

• **Figure 11.7** Variations of root canals, canal orifices, and apical foramen within the root.

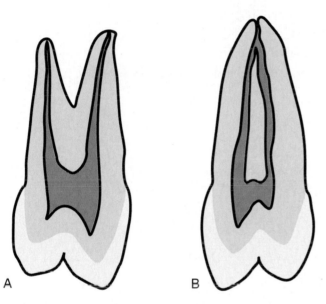

• **Figure 11.8** (A) A maxillary left premolar with two roots and two canals. (B) A maxillary right premolar with one root and two canals.

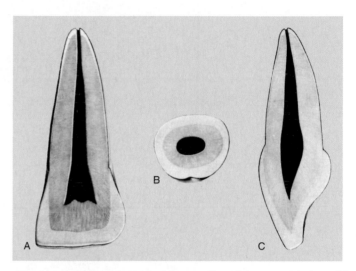

• **Figure 11.10** The pulp cavity of a maxillary right central incisor. **(A)** Distomesial section, lingual view. **(B)** Cross section, incisal view. (C) Linguolabial section, mesial view. (Modified from Zeisz RC, Nuckolls J. *Dental Anatomy.* St. Louis, MO: Mosby; 1949.)

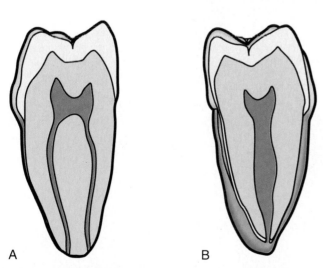

• **Figure 11.9** Mandibular right first molar. **(A)** Linguobuccal section, mesial view. **(B)** Linguobuccal section, distal view. (From Zeisz RC, Nuckolls J. *Dental Anatomy*. St. Louis, MO: Mosby; 1949.)

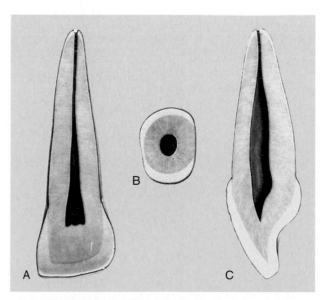

• **Figure 11.11** The pulp cavity of a maxillary right lateral incisor. **(A)** Distomesial section, lingual view. **(B)** Cross section, incisal view. **(C)** Linguolabial section, mesial view. (Modified from Zeisz RC, Nuckolls J. *Dental Anatomy.* St. Louis, MO: Mosby; 1949.)

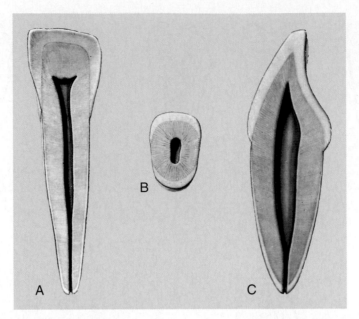

• **Figure 11.12** The pulp cavity of a mandibular right lateral incisor. The pulp cavity of a mandibular central is nearly identical to the lateral but smaller. **(A)** Mesiodistal section, lingual view. **(B)** Cross section, incisal view. **(C)** Labiolingual section, mesial view. (Modified from Zeisz RC, Nuckolls J. *Dental Anatomy.* St. Louis, MO: Mosby; 1949.)

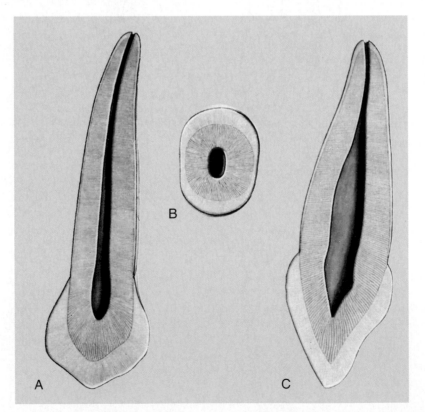

• **Figure 11.13** The pulp cavity of a maxillary right canine. **(A)** Distomesial section, lingual view. **(B)** Cross section, incisal view. **(C)** Linguolabial section, mesial view. (Modified from Zeisz RC, Nuckolls J. *Dental Anatomy.* St. Louis, MO: Mosby; 1949.)

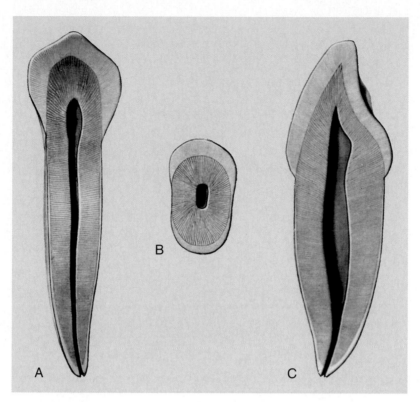

• **Figure 11.14** The pulp cavity of a mandibular right canine. **(A)** Mesiodistal section, lingual view. **(B)** Cross section, incisal view. **(C)** Labiolingual section, mesial view. (Modified from Zeisz RC, Nuckolls J. *Dental Anatomy.* St. Louis, MO: Mosby; 1949.)

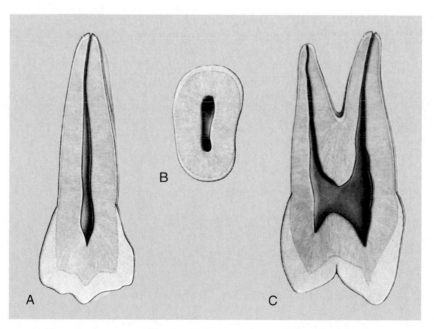

• **Figure 11.15** The pulp cavity of a maxillary right first premolar. **(A)** Mesiodistal section, buccal view. **(B)** Cross section, occlusal view. **(C)** Buccolingual section, distal view. (Modified from Zeisz RC, Nuckolls J. *Dental Anatomy.* St. Louis, MO: Mosby; 1949.)

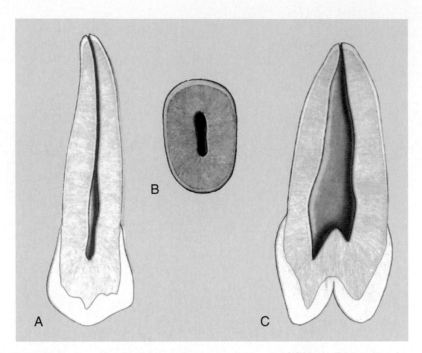

• **Figure 11.16** The pulp cavity of a right maxillary second premolar. **(A)** Mesiodistal section, buccal view. **(B)** Cross section, occlusal view. **(C)** Linguobuccal section, mesial view. (Modified from Zeisz RC, Nuckolls J. *Dental Anatomy.* St. Louis, MO: Mosby; 1949.)

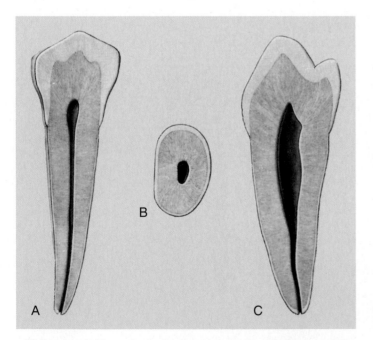

• **Figure 11.17** The pulp cavity of a mandibular right first premolar. **(A)** Mesiodistal section, buccal view. **(B)** Cross section, occlusal view. **(C)** Buccolingual section, mesial view. (Modified from Zeisz RC, Nuckolls J. *Dental Anatomy.* St. Louis, MO: Mosby; 1949.)

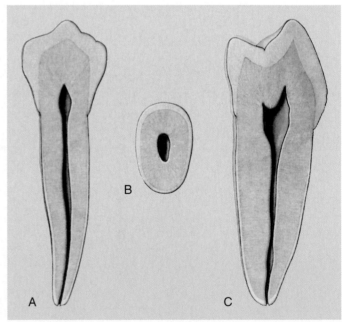

• **Figure 11.18** The pulp cavity of a mandibular right second premolar. **(A)** Mesiodistal section, buccal view. **(B)** Cross section, occlusal view. **(C)** Buccolingual section, mesial view. (Modified from Zeisz RC, Nuckolls J. *Dental Anatomy.* St. Louis, MO: Mosby; 1949.)

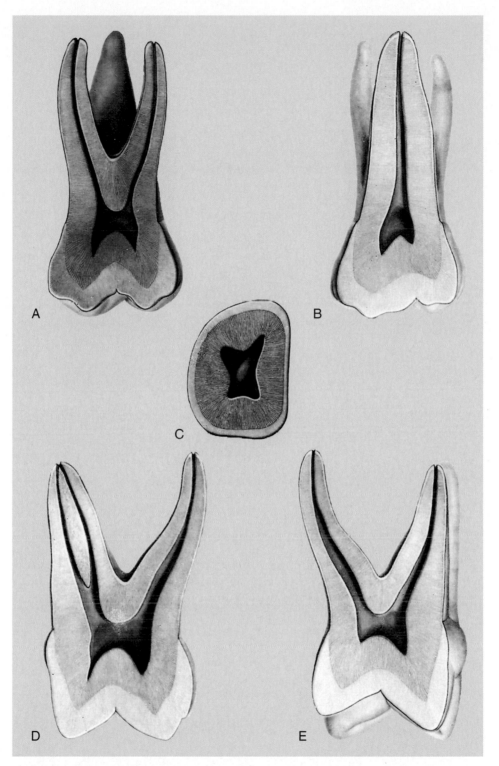

• **Figure 11.19** The pulp cavity of a maxillary right first molar. **(A)** Mesiodistal section, buccal view. **(B)** Distomesial section, lingual view. **(C)** Cross section, occlusal view. **(D)** Linguobuccal section, mesial view. **(E)** Buccolingual section, distal view. Note that the mesiobuccal root has two root canals within one root. (Modified from Zeisz RC, Nuckolls J. *Dental Anatomy*. St. Louis, MO: Mosby; 1949.)

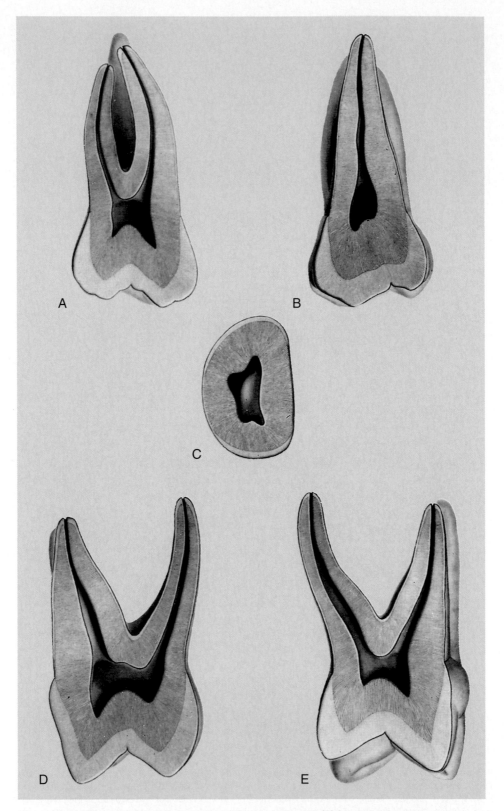

• **Figure 11.20** The pulp cavity of a maxillary right second molar. **(A)** Mesiodistal section, buccal view. **(B)** Distomesial section, lingual view. **(C)** Cross section, occlusal view. **(D)** Linguobuccal section, mesial view. **(E)** Buccolingual section, distal view. Note that the mesiobuccal root has two root canals within one root. (Modified from Zeisz RC, Nuckolls J. *Dental Anatomy.* St. Louis, MO: Mosby; 1949.)

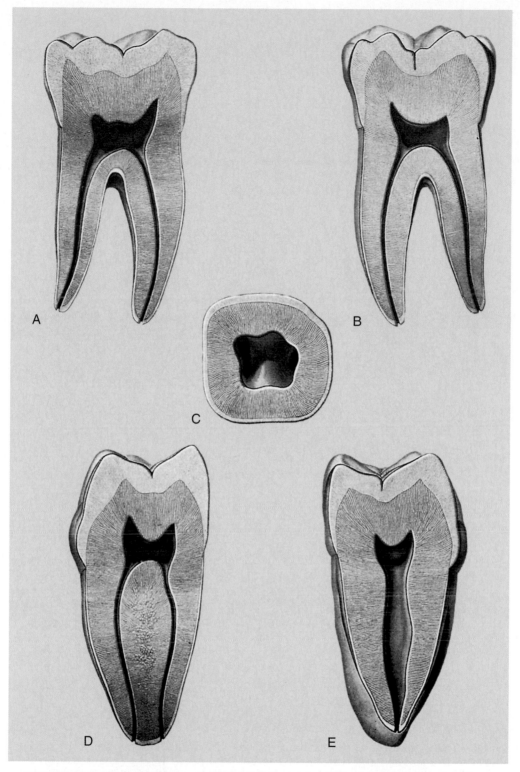

• **Figure 11.21** The pulp cavity of a mandibular right first molar. **(A)** Mesiodistal section, buccal view. **(B)** Distomesial section, lingual view. **(C)** Cross section, occlusal view. **(D)** Linguobuccal section, mesial view. Usually the mesial root has two canals. **(E)** Buccolingual section, distal view. (Modified from Zeisz RC, Nuckolls J. *Dental Anatomy.* St. Louis, MO: Mosby; 1949.)

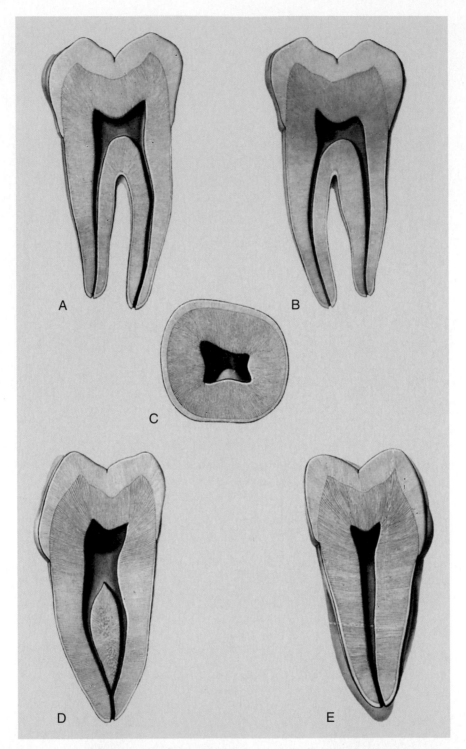

• **Figure 11.22** The pulp cavity of a mandibular right second molar. **(A)** Distomesial section, buccal view. **(B)** Mesiodistal section, lingual view. **(C)** Cross section, occlusal view. **(D)** Buccolingual section, mesial view. **(E)** Linguobuccal section, distal view. Note: Sometimes the mesial root of the second molar will have two canals, although more often it will only have one. (Modified from Zeisz RC, Nuckolls J. *Dental Anatomy.* St. Louis, MO: Mosby; 1949.)

Review Questions

1. A healthy nerve inside the pulp chamber
   a. elicits a quicker response to cold stimulation compared with an inflamed nerve
   b. elicits the strongest pain response to cold stimulation
   c. elicits a quick but proportionate response to cold stimulation
   d. has no response to cold stimulation
2. Sweets can initiate a pain response in a tooth because of their high caloric content.
   a. Statement is true; reason is true.
   b. Statement is false; reason is false.
   c. Statement is true; reason is false.
   d. Statement is false; reason is true.
3. The greater the surface area of the root, the more the periodontal fibers can attach the root to bone and the better the root can resist displacement.
   a. Statement is true; reason is true.
   b. Statement is false; reason is false.
   c. Statement is true; reason is false.
   d. Statement is false; reason is true.
4. Orthodontics are possible because
   a. the force that initiates bone resorption is less than the force that initiates root resorption
   b. osteoclasts and osteoblasts remodel bone
   c. the periodontal ligament is capable of tensing and compressing
   d. all of the above
5. A slight amount of tooth mobility
   a. is healthy and desirable
   b. is a sign of pathology
   c. is a sign of trauma
   d. both b and c
6. When a molar has a trifurcation, how many possible apical foramen openings can there be?
   a. two
   b. three
   c. four
   d. three or four
7. A root can have more than one accessory canal. It is through these accessory canals that the main artery and the nerve of the pulp chamber enter and exit.
   a. Statement is true; reason is true.
   b. Statement is false; reason is false.
   c. Statement is true; reason is false.
   d. Statement is false; reason is true.

8. Deep longitude grooves on the roots of teeth such as maxillary premolars and mandibular canines
   a. make dental hygiene more difficult for the patient
   b. create a place for calculus formation
   c. afford a place for periodontal ligaments to attach to the bone in different directions
   d. actually help teeth resist forces of displacement
   e. may indicate that two root canals are within the same root because the deeper the groove, the more the tooth structure separates the canals
   f. all of the above
   g. a and b only
   h. c and e only
9. The root of a tooth can be more difficult to clean if which of the following are present?
   a. uneven or rough cementum
   b. enamel pearls
   c. furcation areas
   d. accessory canals
   e. apical foramen
   f. a, b, and c
   g. d and e
   h. all of the above
10. Accessory canals can
    a. be smaller than the main root canal at the apical foramen
    b. never have the orifice on the side of the root rather than at the apex
    c. never be multiple within the same root (more than one on the same root)
    d. only be confined to the apical third of the root
    e. all of the above
11. The root tips of most single-rooted teeth
    a. tip usually to the mesial
    b. tip usually to the distal
    c. do not tip, lean, slant, or point; they are vertically straight
    d. a and b

12

Incisors

- To identify the particular anatomic features of incisors
- To compare maxillary central incisors with maxillary lateral incisors
- To compare maxillary incisors with their mandibular counterparts
- To identify an extracted incisor
- To recognize the normal and deviated anatomic forms of incisors

The eight permanent incisors are four maxillary (upper) incisors and four mandibular (lower) incisors. Maxillary incisors consist of two central and two lateral incisors, as do the four mandibular incisors (Fig. 12.1). The eight incisors, four maxillary and four mandibular, together with the four canines form the *anterior* teeth of the mouth. All permanent anterior teeth are *succedaneous* and replace primary teeth.

The most prominent teeth in the mouth are maxillary incisors. The maxillary central incisors are larger than lateral incisors, but these teeth complement each other in form and function. Central incisors erupt in the seventh or eighth year and lateral incisors 1 year or more later.

Incisors are shovel shaped, with sharp incisor edges and wider cervical areas. They function as cutting shears that incise or cut through tissue. Their shape helps shovel the cut food particles back toward the inside of the mouth. Incisors are wider mesiodistally than labiolingually. Their **height of contour**, or **crest of curvature**, is in the cervical third of their crowns both on the labial and the lingual aspects. The **curvature of their cervical lines** (cementoenamel junctions [CEJs]) is greater on their mesial aspect than on the distal aspect. Of all the permanent teeth, both maxillary and mandibular, the maxillary central incisor has the greatest curvature of its cervical line. The greatest curvature of the cervical line is on the mesial surface of maxillary central incisors. In general, the mesial surface of all permanent teeth has a greater curvature of their cervical lines compared with their distal surface; however, exceptions do exist.

Clinical Considerations

Anterior teeth first erupt with rounded ridges, called *mamelons,* which are worn off to form flat incisal edges. These edges are further worn in the direction that teeth slide over each other (Fig. 12.2; see Fig. 12.22). This wear results in maxillary incisors being inclined lingually, whereas mandibular incisors are inclined labially.

Incisors are prone to trauma because of their anterior position in the mouth. They are frequently fractured and occasionally completely avulsed. When a tooth is avulsed, the entire tooth root and crown are completely displaced from the alveolar socket.

Maxillary Permanent Incisors

Central Incisors

Evidence of calcification: 3 months
Eruption: 7 to 8 years
Root completed: 10 to 11 years

A maxillary central incisor (Fig. 12.3) is the widest mesiodistally of any of the anterior teeth. Its labial appearance is less rounded than that of a maxillary lateral incisor or canine. The crown usually looks symmetric and normally formed, having a nearly straight incisal edge, a mesial side with a straight outline, and the distal side that is more curved. The mesioincisal angle forms a right angle, and the distoincisal angle is much more rounded.

Please refer to Table 12.1 for measurements of all permanent teeth. Please also refer to flashcards at the back of the book. You will need to refer to this information for comparison reasons between not only incisors but all permanent teeth in subsequent chapters.

Maxillary central incisors usually develop normally. Two anomalies that sometimes occur are a short root or an unusually long crown. A third is gemination, where the tooth shows evidence of attempting to divide itself. (Please refer to Table 12.1 for measurements of incisor and all permanent teeth.)

Clinical Considerations

If a pregnant woman has syphilis caused by the spirochete *Treponema pallidum,* her fetus could also become infected. Congenital syphilis occurs if the spirochete transmits across the placental barrier and infects the fetus. This child could be affected with enamel hypoplasia of molars and incisors. Incisors appear screw shaped, with the incisal area of the tooth narrower than the cervical area and with notches in the incisal edges. This is referred to as *Hutchinson's incisors.* See Chapter 7 for more information and pictures.

Labial Aspect (see Figs. 12.3 and 12.10A)

The labial surface of the crown of the maxillary central incisor is slightly convex, bulging out from the cervical portion of the crown. The enamel surface is very smooth. When the tooth first erupts, mamelons can be seen on the incisal ridge (see Fig. 5.3). These mamelons are rounded portions of the incisal ridge of newly erupted teeth. Each mamelon forms the incisal ridge portion of one of the labial primary lobes. Developmental lines on the labial face divide the surface into three parts, each developmental line separating a primary lobe. In Fig. 12.4, follow the developmental lines to see how they separate the three facial lobes, and you can see the outline of the mamelons with their incisor portion worn off.

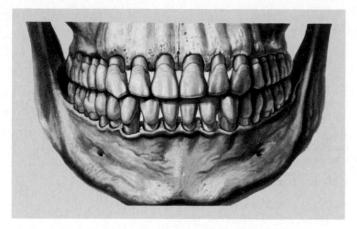

• **Figure 12.1** Anterior view of the lower portion of an adult skull. (Modified from Zeisz RC, Nuckolls J. *Dental Anatomy*. St. Louis: Mosby; 1949.)

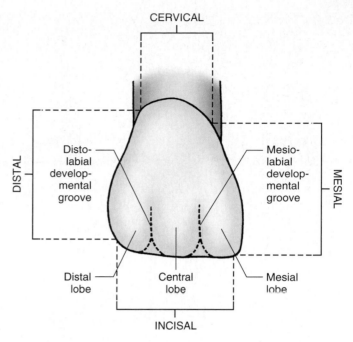

• **Figure 12.4** The arrow points in the direction of wear toward the lingual. The lingual side of the incisal edge is worn as a result of attrition.

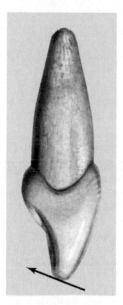

• **Figure 12.2** Maxillary right central incisor. (Modified from Zeisz RC, Nuckolls J. *Dental Anatomy*. St. Louis: Mosby; 1040.)

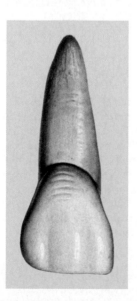

• **Figure 12.3** Labial surface of a maxillary right central incisor. (Modified from Zeisz RC, Nuckolls J. *Dental Anatomy*. St. Louis: Mosby; 1949.)

From this facial view, the distal outline of the crown is more rounded or convex than the mesial outline. The distal contact area is higher toward the cervical line compared with the mesial contact area. From this facial view, the cervical line crests slightly distal to the center of the tooth.

The incisal outline is usually straight across the incisal ridge after the tooth has been in function long enough to wear down the mamelons. When an incisor first erupts, the incisal portion of the crown is rounded, and the mamelons are quite distinct. This ridge portion is then called the *incisal ridge*. However, normal use eventually wears down the rounded ridge into a flat edge, and therefore the term *incisal edge* is more appropriate than *ridge*. Note the incised edge wears on the facial because of where it occludes with the mandibular incisors (see Fig. 12.2).

The root of a central incisor from the labial aspect is cone shaped and has a blunt apex in most instances. The root is usually 2 to 3 mm longer than the crown, although the root-to-crown ratio varies considerably.

Lingual Aspect (Figs. 12.5 and 12.6; see also Fig. 12.10B)

The lingual outline of a maxillary central incisor is the reverse of that found on the labial aspect. The labial surface of the crown is smooth, whereas the lingual surface is bordered by rounded convexities and a concavity. The outline of the cervical line is similar, but immediately below the cervical line is usually a smooth convexity called the *cingulum*. Sometimes there are two or more *lingual ridges* running from the cingulum and sometimes there is a *cingulum with* a *fossa* instead (see Fig. 12.5).

A *lingual fossa* is present on either side of the cingulum. Marginal and incisal ridges, which are rounded convexities, border the lingual fossa. Usually there are developmental grooves extending from the cingulum into the lingual fossa. Fig. 12.6 shows how diverse the lingual anatomy of the maxillary central incisors can be. Five examples have been provided in the figure.

The crown and root taper lingually; the lingual portion of the root is narrower than the labial portion.

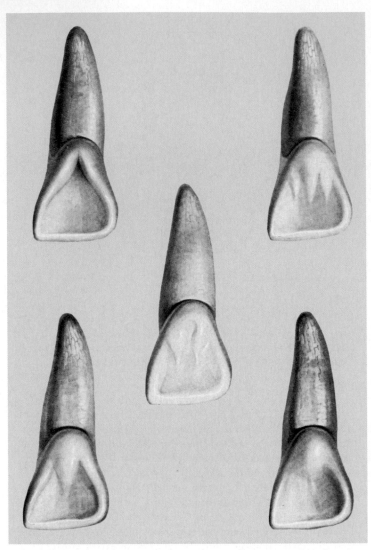

• **Figure 12.5** Lingual views of five permanent right central incisors. (Modified from Zeisz RC, Nuckolls J: *Dental Anatomy.* St. Louis: Mosby; 1949.)

curvature is greater. For example, if mesial curvature is 2.5 mm, the distal might be 1.5 mm.

Incisal Aspect (Fig. 12.9; see also Fig. 12.10C)

The incisal ridge tends to slope lingually as a result of the lower incisors coming more frequently into contact with the lingual edge than with the facial edge of the maxillary incisor. From an incisal view, the crown has a triangular shape, with its apex on the lingual surface. (See Fig. 12.10 for all of the views of a maxillary right central incisor.)

Lateral Incisors

Evidence of calcification: 1 year
Eruption: 8 to 9 years
Root completed: 11 years

Maxillary lateral incisors complement central incisors in function, and they resemble each other in form. Lateral incisors are small in all dimensions except root length. The features—curvatures, concavities, and convexities—of lateral incisors are more prominent and show more distinction and contrast compared with those of central incisors. These teeth differ from central incisors in that their individual development varies considerably. Maxillary lateral incisors vary in form more than any other teeth in the mouth except the third molars. If the variation is too great, it is considered a developmental anomaly.

Clinical Consideration

Of all anterior teeth, maxillary lateral incisors are the most likely to be malformed. A common situation is to find maxillary lateral incisors that have a nondescript, pointed form; such teeth are called *peg-shaped lateral incisors.* In some individuals, lateral incisors are missing entirely. *Maxillary lateral incisors are more likely to be congenitally missing than any other teeth except the third molars.* Some maxillary lateral incisors show twisted roots or distorted crowns. One type of malformed maxillary lateral incisor displays a large, pointed tubercle as part of the cingulum; some have deep developmental grooves that extend down the root lingually with a deep fold in the cingulum. One developmental anomaly is *dens in dente,* in which the tooth has a deep fold in the enamel organ into the dental papilla. The outer surface literally folds inward, hence the term "tooth within a tooth." See Chapter 7 for pictures and more information.

Mesial Aspect (Fig. 12.7; see also Fig. 12.10D)

The crown of a maxillary central incisor is triangular, with the base of the triangle at the cervix and the apex at the incisal ridge. The incisal ridge of the crown is centered over the middle of the root. This alignment is characteristic of maxillary central and lateral incisors.

The labial outline of the crown is slightly convex from the incisal edge to the cervical line. The height of contour (crest of curvature) is about one-third of the way down from the cervical line. *The cervical curvature (curvature of the cervical line) is greater on the mesial surface of maxillary central incisors than on any surface of any other teeth in the mouth.*

Distal Aspect (Fig. 12.8; see also Fig. 12.10E)

Little difference is evident between the distal and mesial outlines of maxillary central incisors. The cervical line indicating the CEJ is less curved on the distal surface than on the mesial surface. It is generally true that if a difference exists in the curvatures of the mesial and distal cervical lines of the same tooth, the mesial

Labial Aspect

Although the labial aspect (Fig. 12.11A) of a maxillary lateral incisor may appear to resemble that of a central incisor, it usually has more curvature, with a rounded incisal ridge and rounded angles mesially and distally. The distal outline is always more rounded, and the height of the contour is more cervical compared with the mesial outline.

The labial surface of the crown is more convex than that of a central incisor, and as a rule, the root length is greater in proportion to the crown length than that of a central incisor. The root is often about 1.5 times the length of the crown.

Lingual Aspect

The lingual view (see Fig. 12.11B; Fig. 12.12) of a lateral incisor shows more contrast compared with the same view of a central incisor. Both teeth display different types of lingual anatomy (see Figs. 12.5 and 12.12). However, the anatomy of the lateral incisor

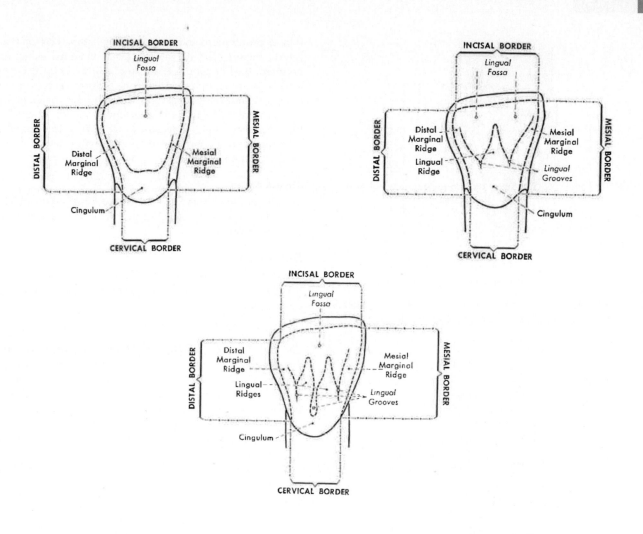

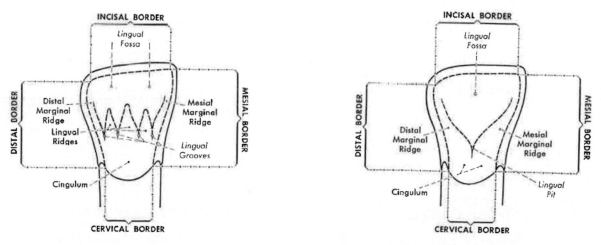

• **Figure 12.6** Maxillary right permanent central incisor—five lingual views. (Modified from Zeisz RC, Nuckolls J. *Dental Anatomy*. St. Louis: Mosby; 1949.)

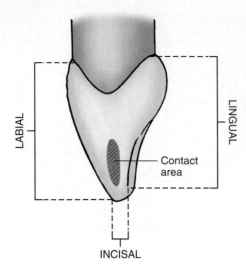

• **Figure 12.7** Mesial surface of a maxillary right central incisor. (Modified from Zeisz RC, Nuckolls J. *Dental Anatomy*. St. Louis: Mosby; 1949.)

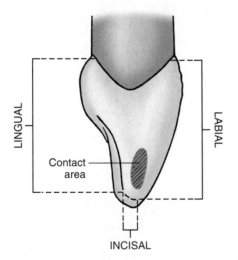

• **Figure 12.8** Distal surface of a maxillary right central incisor. (Modified from Zeisz RC, Nuckolls J. *Dental Anatomy*. St. Louis: Mosby; 1949.)

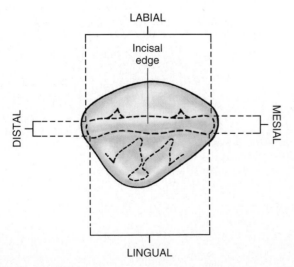

• **Figure 12.9** Incisal edge of a maxillary right central incisor. (Modified from Zeisz RC, Nuckolls J. *Dental Anatomy*. St. Louis: Mosby; 1949.)

is more pronounced and more rounded compared with that of the central incisor. The mesial and distal marginal ridges are pronounced, the lingual ridges are more convex, and the cingulum is usually prominent, with a tendency to form deep developmental grooves within the lingual fossa where it joins the cingulum. The linguoincisal ridge is better developed, and the lingual fossa is more concave and circumscribed than that of the central incisor. A lingual pit is more frequently present on the lateral incisor than on the central incisor.

Mesial Aspect

The mesial aspect (see Fig. 12.11D) of a maxillary lateral incisor is similar to that of a small central incisor, except that the root appears longer.

Distal Aspect

The distal aspect (see Fig. 12.11E) of the maxillary lateral incisor is the same as the mesial aspect, except for less curvature of the cervical line.

Incisal Aspect

The incisal aspect (see Fig. 12.11C) of these teeth sometimes resembles that of central incisors or a small canine. However, the cingulum and the incisal ridge may be large; the labiolingual dimension may be greater than usual in comparison with the mesiodistal dimension. If these variations are present, these teeth show a strong resemblance to the canines.

All maxillary lateral incisors exhibit more convexity labially and lingually from the incisal aspect compared with maxillary central incisors.

Root

The maxillary central incisor usually has a straight, thick, cylindrically shaped root. The maxillary lateral incisor has a narrower root mesiodistally; the root is as long as that of the central incisor but appears thinner. The apical portion of the lateral incisor's root often curves distally and ends in a sharp apex rather than in a blunt, straight apex as in the central incisor.

Clinical Consideration

The space between the permanent maxillary central incisors causes several potential problems. A common location for extra teeth, called **supernumerary teeth**, is between these two maxillary central incisors. Supernumerary teeth between maxillary central incisors are called *mesiodens*. Odontomas also favor this site. Odontomas are composed of tooth tissues—dentin, enamel, and cementum—but they are not shaped like a tooth. They are toothlike masses that did not properly form into teeth (see Chapter 7).

Sometimes the space between central incisors is just that—a space. A *diastema* between central incisors is also quite common. Large spaces between maxillary central incisors may form if the attachment for the *maxillary frenum* is too low and prevents the central incisors from moving into this space. In this case, the frenum resists the movement of the central incisors and prevents them from moving together (Fig. 12.13).

Pulp Cavity

The pulp cavity varies in size with the age of the tooth. When the tooth first erupts, the pulp cavity is very large, and the root is incompletely formed, so the canal becomes funnel shaped in the region of the apical foramen. As the tooth develops completely,

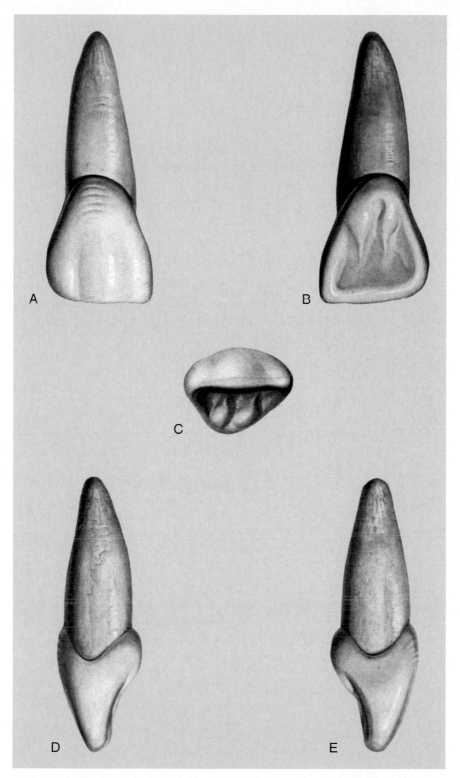

• **Figure 12.10** A maxillary right central incisor. **(A)** Labial view. **(B)** Lingual view. **(C)** Incisal view. **(D)** Mesial view. **(E)** Distal view. (Modified from Zeisz RC, Nuckolls J. *Dental Anatomy*. St. Louis: Mosby; 1949.)

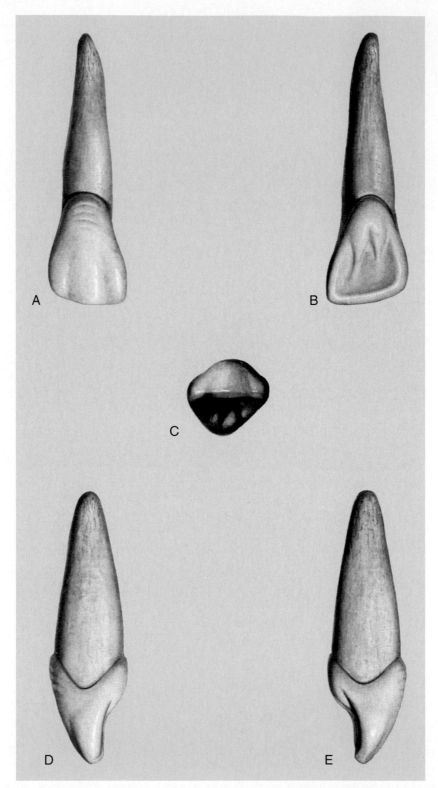

• **Figure 12.11** A maxillary right lateral incisor. **(A)** Labial view. **(B)** Lingual view. **(C)** Incisal view. **(D)** Mesial view. **(E)** Distal view. (Modified from Zeisz RC, Nuckolls J. *Dental Anatomy*. St. Louis: Mosby; 1949.)

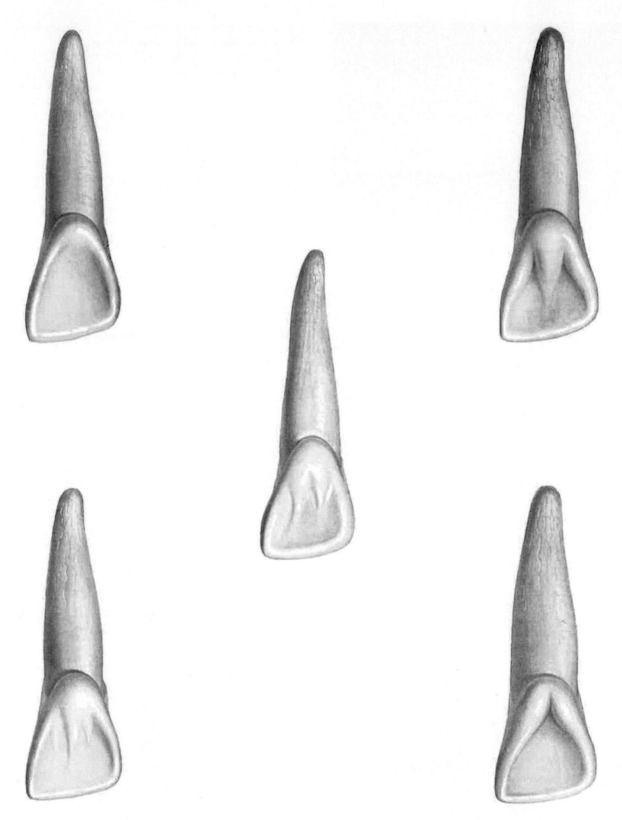

• **Figure 12.12** Lingual views of five permanent right lateral incisors. (Modified from Zeisz RC, Nuckolls J. *Dental Anatomy*. St. Louis: Mosby; 1949.)

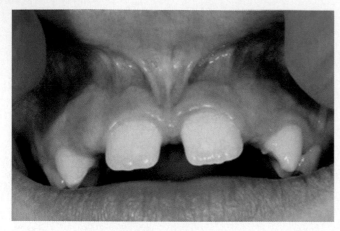

• **Figure 12.13** A large diastema is created because the frenum is so wide and attaches so low that its presence prevents the central incisors from coming together.

the entire pulp cavity to the apex of the root becomes smaller, and dentin becomes thicker in both the crown and the root. The apical foramen is then very small. This process continues throughout the life of the tooth. In very old individuals, it is not unusual to find calcification of the entire pulp cavity and solid dentin filling the entire root canal. This variation in the size of the pulp cavity with aging is common to all of the permanent teeth.

The pulp cavity of the maxillary central incisor (Fig. 12.14) mirrors the configuration of the tooth. Only one root canal is evident, which is rather large. The pulp chamber lies in the coronal portion of the tooth and presents three sharp elongations: mesial,

distal, and central pulp horns. The central pulp horn is usually shorter and more rounded than the other two.

The pulp cavity of the maxillary lateral incisor is quite simple, comprising only a pulp chamber and a single pulp canal. The chamber is similar to that of the maxillary central incisor but usually does not have three sharp pulp horns. More often, the pulp chamber ends incisally as one rounded form or two less sharp pulp horns: mesial and distal pulp horns (Fig. 12.15).

Pertinent Data

Maxillary Central Incisors

	Right	Left
Universal code	8	9
International code	11	21
Palmer notation:	1⌋	⌊1

Number of roots: 1
Number of pulp horns: 3
Number of developmental lobes: 4

Location of Proximal Contact Areas
Mesial: incisal third
Distal: junction of incisal and middle thirds

Height of Contour
Facial: cervical third, 0.5 mm
Lingual: cervical third, 0.5 mm

Identifying Characteristics
These incisors are the largest and most prominent incisors. The distoincisal angle is more rounded than the mesioincisal angle.

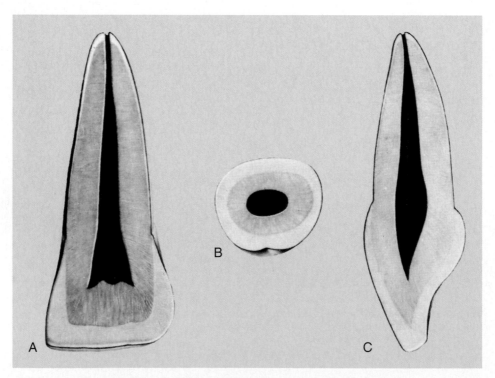

• **Figure 12.14** The pulp cavity of a maxillary right central incisor. **(A)** Distomesial section, lingual view. **(B)** Cross section, incisal view. **(C)** Linguolabial section, mesial view. (Modified from Zeisz RC, Nuckolls J. *Dental Anatomy*. St. Louis: Mosby; 1949.)

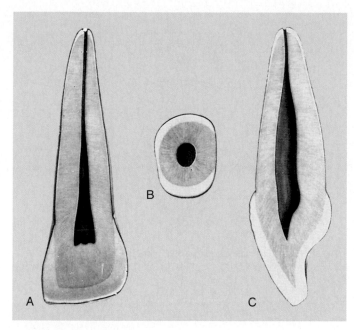

• **Figure 12.15** The pulp cavity of a maxillary right lateral incisor. **(A)** Distomesial section, lingual view. **(B)** Cross section, incisal view. **(C)** Linguolabial section, mesial view. (Modified from Zeisz RC, Nuckolls J. *Dental Anatomy*. St. Louis: Mosby; 1949.)

The lingual surface has a prominent cingulum, broad lingual fossa, and distinct marginal ridges. The pulp cavity is one large single chamber and root canal.

Maxillary Lateral Incisors

	Right	Left
Universal code	7	10
International code	12	22

Palmer notation: 1⌋ ⌊1
Number of roots: 1
Number of pulp horns: 1 to 3
Number of developmental lobes: 4

Location of Proximal Contact Areas
Mesial: junction of incisal and middle thirds
Distal: middle third

Height of Contour
Facial: cervical third, 0.5 mm
Lingual: cervical third, 0.5 mm

Identifying Characteristics
The lingual anatomic features are similar to those of the central incisors but are more highly developed and have more prominent marginal ridges and deeper lingual fossae. Lateral incisors are more likely to have a lingual pit compared with central incisors. The cingulum may be smaller or even almost absent. The labial surface resembles that of a central incisor but is more convex. The crown-to-root ratio is less than that of a central incisor because the crown is usually smaller, whereas the root is almost as long. In all other ways, lateral incisors appear as smaller, more rounded versions of central incisors.

Mandibular Incisors

Central Incisors

Evidence of calcification: 3 months
Eruption: 6 to 7 years
Root completed: 9 years

The *smallest teeth* in the mouth are mandibular central incisors. How does this differ from maxillary teeth? Which are larger—maxillary central incisors or lateral incisors? A mandibular central incisor occludes only with one opposing tooth, a maxillary central incisor (see Fig. 12.1).

Similar to other anterior teeth, a mandibular central incisor is derived from four lobes—three labial and one lingual. When mandibular incisors erupt, mamelons can be seen on the incisal ridges.

Of all teeth, mandibular central incisors are the *most difficult to identify as right or left.* They are bilaterally symmetric and difficult to differentiate. The following features are not always obvious, but if present, they may support a good guess:
1. The distoincisal angle is just slightly greater than the mesioincisal angle.
2. The distofacial line angle is more rounded than the mesiofacial line angle (Fig. 12.16).
3. The cervical line crests slightly toward the distal side (Fig. 12.17).
4. A straight line drawn between the endpoints of the distofacial line angle (*y*) compared with a straight line drawn between the endpoints of the mesiofacial line angle (*x*) is shorter (Fig. 12.18).

Labial Aspect
The labial aspect (Figs. 12.19; see Fig. 12.24A) exhibits a very smooth facial surface. The gingivoincisal outline is almost straight up and down. The height of contour is at the incisal third on both the mesial and distal surfaces.

Lingual Aspect
The lingual view (Fig. 12.20; see Fig.12.24B) presents a cingulum much smaller than that of maxillary anterior incisors. No

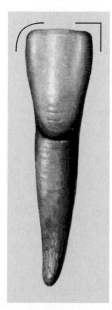

• **Figure 12.16** The distofacial line angle of a mandibular right central incisor is more convex than the mesiofacial line angle. (Modified from Zeisz RC, Nuckolls J. *Dental Anatomy*. St. Louis: Mosby; 1949.)

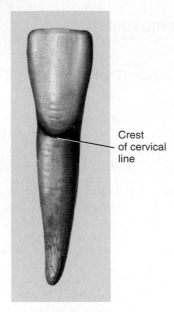

Crest of cervical line

• **Figure 12.17** The cervical line of a mandibular right central incisor has its crest slightly toward the distal surface. (Modified from Zeisz RC, Nuckolls J. *Dental Anatomy*. St. Louis: Mosby; 1949.)

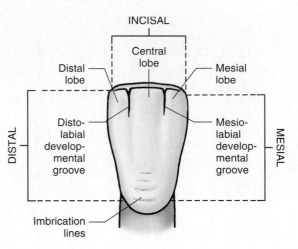

INCISAL

Central lobe

Distal lobe — Mesial lobe

DISTAL

Disto-labial develop-mental groove — Mesio-labial develop-mental groove

MESIAL

Imbrication lines

• **Figure 12.19** The labial surface of a mandibular right central incisor. (Modified from Zeisz RC, Nuckolls J. *Dental Anatomy*. St. Louis: Mosby; 1949.)

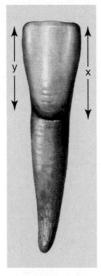

y   x

• **Figure 12.18** Line *x* is longer than line *y*. (Modified from Zeisz RC, Nuckolls J. *Dental Anatomy*. St. Louis: Mosby; 1949.)

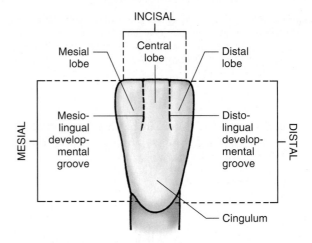

INCISAL

Mesial lobe — Central lobe — Distal lobe

MESIAL

Mesio-lingual develop-mental groove — Disto-lingual develop-mental groove

DISTAL

Cingulum

• **Figure 12.20** The lingual surface of a mandibular right central incisor. Note that no pits or tubercles are present. (Modified from Zeisz RC, Nuckolls J. *Dental Anatomy*. St. Louis: Mosby; 1949.)

tubercle extensions or lingual pits are evident, and the fossa is very shallow.

Mesial and Distal Aspects

The proximal views (Fig. 12.21; and see Figs. 12.24D, E) reveal that the incisal edge tends toward the lingual half of the tooth and slants labially from this edge. The incised edge shows wear toward the facial aspect. How do maxillary central incisors wear out? When the upper teeth touch the lower teeth, mandibular incisors touch the lingual surface of maxillary incisors. Therefore maxillary incisors wear down the lingual part of their incisal ridges, and the mandibular incisors wear down the labial portion of their incisal ridges. Fig. 12.22 shows the direction of wear toward the labial.

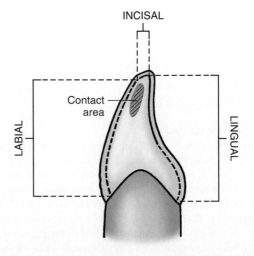

INCISAL

Contact area

LABIAL

LINGUAL

• **Figure 12.21** The mesial surface of a mandibular right central incisor. (Modified from Zeisz RC, Nuckolls J. *Dental Anatomy*. St. Louis: Mosby; 1949.)

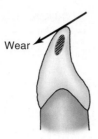

• **Figure 12.22** The arrow shows the direction of wear.

Compare Fig. 12.22 to Fig. 12.4 to see how the maxillary and mandibular incisors vary in the way they wear their incised edges. This is very useful in tooth identification.

The height of the contour at the cervical third is about 0.5 mm on the labial and lingual surfaces. Is the cervical curvature greater mesially or distally? A difference is not always evident between the amount of cervical curvature on the mesial and distal sides, but if a difference exists, the mesial side shows more curvature.

Incisal Aspect

The incisal view (see Figs. 12.24C and Fig. 12.23) shows wear on the incisal ridge. Note that incisal wear occurs toward the facial aspect. In what way do maxillary central incisors wear out? When the upper teeth touch the lower teeth, the lower incisors touch the lingual surface of the upper incisors. Therefore the upper incisors wear down the lingual part of their incisal ridges, and the lower incisors wear down the labial portion of their incisal ridges. In Fig. 12.24C (from this view), it would be impossible to determine if it were right or left central.

Lateral Incisors

Evidence of calcification: 4 months
Eruption: 7 to 8 years
Root completed: 10 years

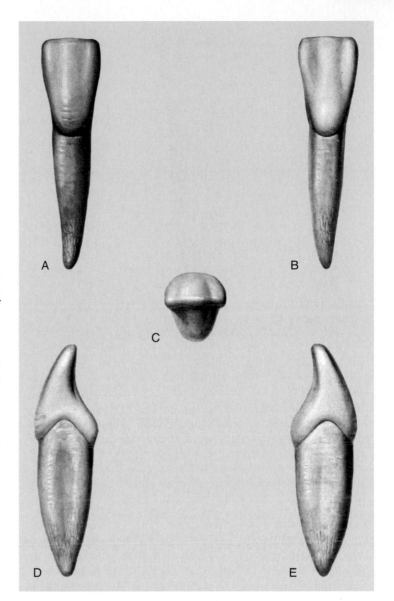

• **Figure 12.24** A mandibular right central incisor. **(A)** Labial view. **(B)** Lingual view. **(C)** Incisal view. **(D)** Mesial view. **(E)** Distal view. (Modified from Zeisz RC, Nuckolls J. *Dental Anatomy*. St. Louis: Mosby; 1949.)

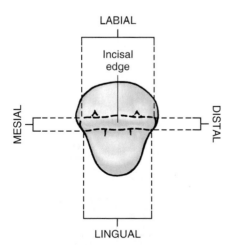

• **Figure 12.23** The incisal surface of a mandibular right central incisor. The permanent mandibular central is the most symmetric tooth in the mouth. It is very hard to tell a right central incisor from a left central incisor if from the same mouth. (Modified from Zeisz RC, Nuckolls J. *Dental Anatomy*. St. Louis: Mosby; 1949.)

Mandibular lateral incisors appear to have nearly the same form as mandibular central incisors. Indeed, it is very difficult to tell them apart. In general, the following principles help differentiate between mandibular lateral and central incisors in the same mouth. Mandibular lateral incisors are bigger, wider, and longer than mandibular central incisors; they are wider mesiodistally and longer gingivoincisally. *This situation is different from that of maxillary incisors.* Lateral incisors are wider because their distal developmental lobe is larger than the distal lobe of mandibular central incisors. Lateral incisors have more prominent anatomic features on the lingual aspect compared with central incisors. In mandibular teeth, the difference is not as extreme as in maxillary teeth; however, lateral incisors are still slightly more convex and concave than their counterparts, the central incisors, in the same mouth.

Lateral incisors have greater facial curvature compared with central incisors. The endpoints of the mesiofacial line angle are farther apart than those of the distofacial line angle (Fig. 12.25).

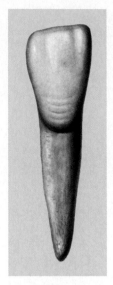

• **Figure 12.25** The distal lobe of a mandibular right lateral incisor is larger than the distal lobe of a mandibular right central incisor (facial view). (Modified from Zeisz RC, Nuckolls J. *Dental Anatomy*. St. Louis: Mosby; 1949.)

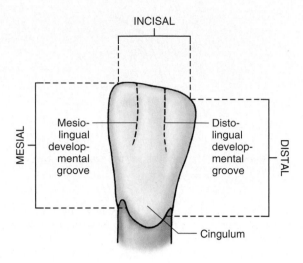

• **Figure 12.27** The lingual surface of a mandibular right lateral incisor. (Modified from Zeisz RC, Nuckolls J. *Dental Anatomy*. St. Louis: Mosby; 1949.)

Labial Aspect

The labial view (Fig. 12.26; and see 12.30A) shows a more rounded appearance mesially and distally. The developmental grooves on the labial surface are all deeper on lateral incisors compared with those on central incisors. The height of contour at the contact areas is at the incisal third on the mesial and distal aspects. The distal contact area is slightly more gingival than the mesial. *This is generally true of all teeth.*

Lingual Aspect

Compared with the lingual view of central incisors, the lingual view of lateral incisors (Fig. 12.27; and see 12.30B) shows more prominent features. The ridges are more developed, the fossa appears, and enamel tubercles often extend into the fossa. A lingual

pit is still rare in lateral incisors but is present more often compared with central incisors.

Much more deviation occurs in the form of a lateral incisor. All features are usually more prominent, if present.

Mesial and Distal Aspects

The proximal views (Fig. 12.28; and see 12.30D, E) reveal that the height of contour on the labial and lingual surfaces is highest at the gingival third of the crown. Note that a lateral incisor is thicker than a central incisor at the linguoincisal ridge.

A mandibular lateral incisor is wider labiolingually than a mandibular central in the same mouth. Once again the cervical curvature is greater on the mesial side than on the distal side.

Incisal Aspect

The incisal view (Fig. 12.29; and see Fig. 12.30C) depicts a rounded general appearance of lateral incisors, and the developmental grooves appear deeper.

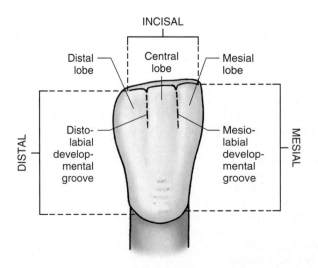

• **Figure 12.26** The labial surface of a mandibular right lateral incisor. (Modified from Zeisz RC, Nuckolls J. *Dental Anatomy*. St. Louis: Mosby; 1949.)

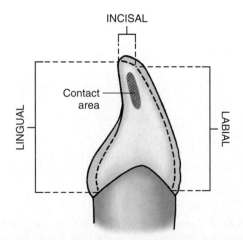

• **Figure 12.28** The distal surface of a mandibular right lateral incisor. (Modified from Zeisz RC, Nuckolls J. *Dental Anatomy*. St. Louis: Mosby; 1949.)

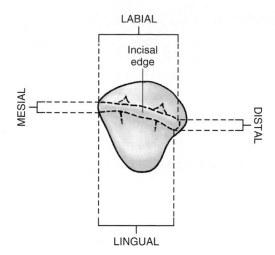

LABIAL

Incisal
edge

MESIAL

DISTAL

LINGUAL

• **Figure 12.29** The incisal surface of a mandibular right lateral incisor. (Modified from Zeisz RC, Nuckolls J. *Dental Anatomy*. St. Louis: Mosby; 1949.)

Lateral incisors appear to be rotated on their root axes because the distal developmental lobes of mandibular lateral incisors are larger and located more lingually compared with the mesial lobes. The reason for this extra bulk and lingual location is that lateral incisors have to curve distally to fit into the mandibular arch. Remember that the mandibular arch is more curved than the maxillary arch because it has to fit inside the maxillary arch.

Root

The root of a mandibular incisor is usually straight. The root of the lateral incisor is slightly wider, thicker, and longer than that of the central incisor. The apex of the lateral incisor's root may point labially or distally. Proximal grooves are commonly found on the root surface, giving the appearance of a double root (Fig. 12.30).

Pulp Cavity

The pulp cavities of mandibular central and lateral incisors are simple. They usually have three pulp horns and a single root canal.

The root canals of all four mandibular incisors are similar to their maxillary counterparts. They are straight and narrow and present very little variation. The mandibular lateral pulp canal is larger and may show more variation than the central pulp canal. It is rare for either of them to have two root canals (Fig. 12.31).

Pertinent Data

Mandibular Central Incisors

	Right	Left
Universal code	25	24
International code	41	31
Palmer notation:	1⌋	⌊1

Number of roots: 1
Number of pulp horns: 3
Number of developmental lobes: 4

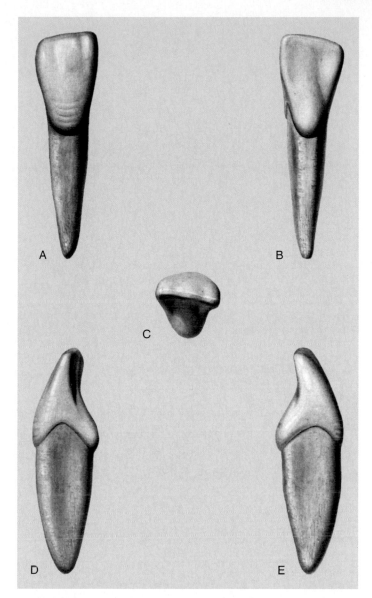

A

B

C

D

E

• **Figure 12.30** A mandibular right lateral incisor. **(A)** Labial view. **(B)** Lingual view. **(C)** Incisal view. **(D)** Mesial view. **(E)** Distal view. (Modified from Zeisz RC, Nuckolls J. *Dental Anatomy*. St. Louis: Mosby; 1949.)

Location of Proximal Contact Areas
Mesial: incisal third
Distal: incisal third

Height of Contour
Facial: cervical third, less than 0.5 mm
Lingual: cervical third, less than 0.5 mm

Identifying Characteristics
The distoincisal and mesioincisal angles are nearly identical. The lingual surface is shallow, with no prominent features. The crown is wider faciolingually than mesiodistally. The root is oval shaped in cross section. The incisal edge shows wear on the facioincisal edge. From a proximal view, the incisal edge appears to be tilted toward the lingual side.

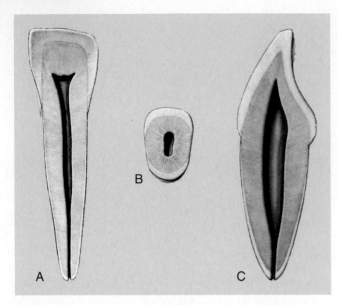

• **Figure 12.31** The pulp cavity of a mandibular right lateral incisor. The pulp cavity of a mandibular central incisor is nearly identical to the lateral incisor but smaller. **(A)** Mesiodistal section, lingual view. **(B)** Cross section, incisal view. **(C)** Labiolingual section, mesial view. (Modified from Zeisz RC, Nuckolls J. *Dental Anatomy*. St. Louis: Mosby; 1949.)

Mandibular Lateral Incisors

	Right	Left
Universal code	26	23
International code	42	32
Palmer notation:	2⌐	⌐2

Number of roots: 1
Number of pulp horns: 3
Number of developmental lobes: 4

Location of Proximal Contact Areas
Mesial: incisal third
Distal: incisal third

Height of Contour
Facial: cervical third, less than 0.5 mm
Lingual: cervical third, less than 0.5 mm

Identifying Characteristics
The crown is similar to that of mandibular central incisors. The distal lobe is more highly developed than the mesial lobe. The distal incisal ridge angles toward the lingual aspect as if rotating on the root axis. The crown and the root are slightly larger than those of central incisors.

TABLE 12.1   Average Permanent Teeth Dimensions as Recorded by Russell C. Wheeler

	Length of Crown	Length of Root	Mesiodistal Diameter of Crown*	Mesiodistal Diameter at Cervix	Labio- or Buccolingual Diameter	Labio- or Buccolingual Diameter at Cervix	Curvature of Cervical Line (Mesial)	Curvature of Cervical Line (Distal)
Maxillary Teeth								
Central incisor	10.5	13.0	8.5	7.0	7.0	6.0	3.5	2.5
Lateral incisor	9.0	13.0	6.5	5.0	6.0	5.0	3.0	2.0
Canine	10.0	17.0	7.5	5.5	8.0	7.0	2.5	1.5
First premolar	8.5	14.0	7.0	5.0	9.0	8.0	1.0	0.0
Second premolar	8.5	14.0	7.0	5.0	9.0	8.0	1.0	0.0
First molar	7.5	B 12 L 13	10.0	8.0	11.0	10.0	1.0	0.0
Second molar	7.0	B 11 L 12	9.0	7.0	11.0	10.0	1.0	0.0
Third molar	6.5	11.0	8.5	6.5	10.0	9.5	1.0	0.0
Mandibular Teeth								
Central incisor	9.0†	12.5	5.0	3.5	6.0	5.3	3.0	2.0
Lateral incisor	9.5†	14.0	5.5	4.0	6.5	5.8	3.0	2.0
Canine	11.0	16.0	7.0	5.5	7.5	7.0	2.5	1.0
First premolar	8.5	14.0	7.0	5.0	7.5	6.5	1.0	0.0
Second premolar	8.0	14.5	7.0	5.0	8.0	7.0	1.0	0.0
First molar	7.5	14.0	11.0	9.0	10.5	9.0	1.0	0.0
Second molar	7.0	13.0	10.5	8.0	10.0	9.0	1.0	0.0
Third molar	7.0	11.0	10.0	7.5	9.5	9.0	1.0	0.0

*The sum of the mesiodistal diameters, both right and left, which give the arch length, is 128 mm for maxillary teeth and 126 mm for mandibular teeth.
†Lingual measurement is approximately 0.5 mm longer.
Wheeler RC. *A Textbook of Dental Anatomy and Physiology*. 4th ed. Philadelphia: WB Saunders; 1965.

Review Questions

1. A permanent maxillary central incisor, compared with a maxillary lateral incisor in a proximal view, is
   a. thicker at the incisal edge
   b. identical at the incisal edge
   c. thinner at the incisal edge
   d. similar but smaller overall

2. Which of the following is *not* characteristic of the maxillary central incisors?
   a. distolabial line angle is shorter than the mesiolabial line angle
   b. rounded distoincisal angle
   c. mesial line angle that is nearly straight
   d. rounded mesioincisal line angle

3. With normal wear, the incisal edge of the maxillary incisors (choose all that apply)
   a. slopes toward the facial side
   b. flattens
   c. slopes toward the lingual side
   d. becomes more rounded

4. The mesiofacial line angle of the maxillary central incisors differs from the distofacial in that it is
   a. less rounded
   b. longer
   c. sharper
   d. all of the above

5. In contrast to maxillary lateral incisors, maxillary central incisors usually have how many pulp horns?
   a. 1 or 2
   b. 2 or 3
   c. 3
   d. 4

6. Which of the following anatomic features of the mandibular incisors provide evidence of the four developmental lobes of these teeth?
   a. mamelons and faint developmental lines at eruption
   b. lingual pit, marginal ridges, and incisal edge
   c. mamelons, faint developmental lines at eruption, and cingulum
   d. incisal edge and lingual concavity

7. The proximal contact area on the distal surface of a mandibular lateral incisor is located
   a. slightly more gingival than mesial
   b. slightly more incisor than the mesial
   c. slightly more mesial than distal
   d. slightly more apical than distal

8. The structure of mandibular lateral incisors, compared with mandibular central incisors, is
   a. identical but larger
   b. almost identical but smaller
   c. almost identical but larger
   d. the same

9. The mesiodistal crown width of maxillary lateral incisors, compared with maxillary central incisors, is
   a. greater
   b. smaller
   c. about equal
   d. sometimes smaller but more often greater

10. The distofacial line angle of maxillary lateral incisors, compared with maxillary central incisors, is
    a. the same
    b. more rounded
    c. less rounded
    d. very straight

11. Which is the more acute incisal angle on the maxillary central incisors?
    a. distal
    b. mesial

12. In contrast to a mandibular incisor, a maxillary incisor can be identified by which of these (choose all that apply)?
    a. its rotated incisal edge
    b. central location of its cingulum
    c. prominent longitudinal grooves on the root
    d. prominent lingual features of the crown

13. Where does the height of contour of the facial and lingual surfaces of the anterior teeth occur?
    a. mesial third
    b. incisal third
    c. middle third
    d. cervical third

14. Which anterior teeth have the most prominent and widest crowns (mesiodistally) in the permanent dentition?
    a. maxillary lateral incisors
    b. mandibular lateral incisors
    c. mandibular central incisors
    d. maxillary central incisors

15. A more prominent cingulum is found on which tooth?
    a. maxillary central
    b. mandibular central
    c. mandibular lateral
    d. maxillary lateral

16. The curvature of the cementoenamel junction (CEJ) of the maxillary central incisor is
    a. higher on the mesial aspect than any other tooth distally or mesially
    b. higher on the distal aspect than on the mesial aspect
    c. highest toward the mesial aspect on the facial surface
    d. the same as the cervical line and crests more toward the mesial aspect on the facial surface

17. Which incisor is more likely to be congenitally missing?
    a. maxillary central
    b. mandibular central
    c. mandibular lateral
    d. maxillary lateral

18. Which incisor can have fewer than three pulp horns?
    a. maxillary central
    b. mandibular central
    c. mandibular lateral
    d. maxillary lateral

19. Which incisor occludes with only one tooth?
    a. maxillary central
    b. mandibular central
    c. mandibular lateral
    d. maxillary lateral

20. Which incisor is the smallest in the crown and the root?
    a. maxillary central
    b. mandibular central
    c. mandibular lateral
    d. maxillary lateral

13

Canines

OBJECTIVES

- To understand the function of a canine in relation to its shape
- To understand the calcification and root completion schedules in relation to the eruption dates of canines
- To recognize the resemblance of canines to other anterior teeth
- To understand how canines are different from other anterior teeth
- To recognize how canines are similar to some premolar teeth
- To recognize and identify the anatomic structure and landmarks of the canine
- To compare maxillary and mandibular canines and identify each

Maxillary and Mandibular Permanent Canines

The four permanent maxillary and mandibular canines, one on each side of each jaw, are the longest teeth in the mouth. Located at the corners of the mouth, they are well anchored in bone by their extremely long roots. Their location requires extra anchorage, which is furnished by the length and the shape of their roots and a special projection of bone called the **canine eminence.** The term *canine* brings to mind the fanglike teeth of dogs, which are members of the animal family *Canidae.*

In function, canines act as holding and tearing tools and assist both incisors and premolars. In addition, their "V" shape at the corner of the mouth allows for dissipation of pressures that can force premolars to protrude out of the mouth or incisors farther into the mouth. The self-cleaning qualities of canines; their smooth, pointed shape; the thickness of their crowns; and their strong anchorage make them the most stable teeth in the mouth.

Maxillary Canines

Evidence of calcification: 4 months
Enamel completed: 6 to 7 years
Eruption: 11 to 12 years
Root completed: 13 to 15 years

A maxillary canine (Fig. 13.1) resembles an incisor in its composition of four developmental lobes—three facial and one lingual. The three facial lobes resemble the facial lobes of incisors except that the middle facial lobe extends farther incisally when the tooth is viewed from the labial or lingual aspect. This middle lobe extension results in

the formation of a single cusp. The cusp tip is formed by the junction of four ridges. One of the ridges extends along the middle lobe of the tooth on its most facial part; another extends along the lingual part. The other two ridges run from the mesioincisal and distoincisal corners. All four ridges converge to form the cusp tip.

The lingual lobe of a canine is much larger and thicker than the lingual lobe of an incisor, which results in the canine being much wider labiolingually compared with a maxillary incisor. The cingulum of a maxillary canine also shows greater development in that it is larger and bulkier than the cingulum on any other anterior teeth.

Labial Aspect (Fig. 13.2; see Fig. 13.1A)

The crown and root of a maxillary canine are narrower mesiodistally compared with those of a maxillary central incisor. The cervicoincisal length of the crown is much larger on a maxillary canine than on any other anterior tooth except the maxillary central incisor and the mandibular canine. Although these teeth usually have longer crowns compared with a maxillary canine, the roots of the maxillary canines are longer, making them the longest teeth in the mouth. Mesially, the outline of the crown is straighter than on the distal with a slight convexity at the contact area. The center of the mesial contact area is approximately at the junction of the middle and incisal thirds of the crown.

Distally, the outline of the crown is rounded in appearance because the distal contact area is usually at the center of the middle third of the crown. This position makes the distal convexity appear larger and more uniform. How does this differ from the location of the mesial contact area? Which contact area is located more incisally—mesial or distal? Like all anterior teeth the distal contact area is more cervical than the mesial.

The labial surface of the crown is smooth. The developmental lines are two shallow depressions dividing the three labial lobes. The middle lobe is much larger and has greater development than the other lobes, resulting in a ridge on the labial surface of the crown. This ridge ends incisally at the cusp tip, which is centered in the middle of the tooth (from the facial view).

The cervical line crests slightly mesial to the center of the tooth.

The root of a maxillary canine is slender in comparison with the crown and is conical in shape with a blunt root apex. It is not unusual for the root to turn sharply to the distal or mesial side in the apical third. A general rule is that most roots, if they do have an apical curvature, point toward the distal side. Although this rule applies to almost all single-rooted teeth, there are some exceptions. If an apical curvature is not present, the root itself has a tendency to point more often toward the distal side than to the mesial side.

Lingual Aspect (Fig. 13.3; also see Fig. 13.1B)

The root of a maxillary canine tapers toward the lingual surface. The lingual sides of both the crown and root are narrower than the labial sides.

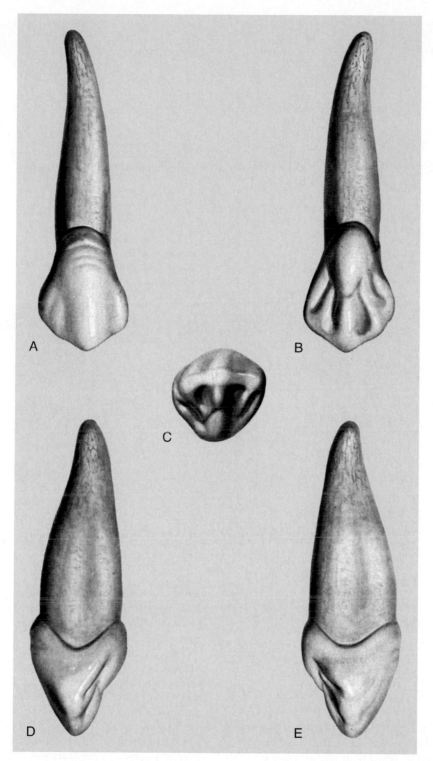

• **Figure 13.1** A maxillary right canine. **(A)** Labial view. **(B)** Lingual view. **(C)** Incisal view. **(D)** Mesial view. **(E)** Distal view. (Modified from Zeisz RC, Nuckolls J. *Dental Anatomy*. St. Louis, MO: Mosby; 1949.)

Compared with the facial line, the cervical line shows a more even curvature, and the crest is straighter and centered over the middle of the tooth.

The most obvious structure on the lingual surface of a maxillary canine is the well-developed cingulum. It is huge in comparison with those of all other anterior teeth.

Confluent to the cingulum and running from the cusp tip is a well-developed lingual ridge. This ridge runs from the cusp tip on the lingual side to the cingulum. Unlike other anterior teeth that have a lingual fossa, this area on a maxillary canine is occupied by a lingual ridge, which divides the lingual side of the three facial lobes, creating two separate lingual fossae, one on the mesial and one on the distal side of the lingual ridge. These fossae are bordered by a mesial and a distal marginal ridge, respectively. When present, these fossae are called the *mesial* and *distal lingual fossae*. The borders of the lingual fossae

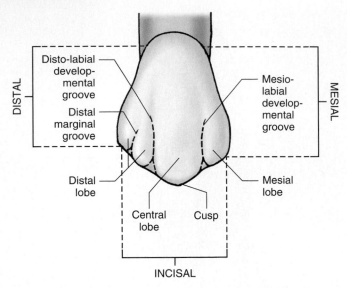

• **Figure 13.2** The labial surface of a maxillary right canine. (Modified from Zeisz RC, Nuckolls J. *Dental Anatomy*. St. Louis, MO: Mosby; 1949.)

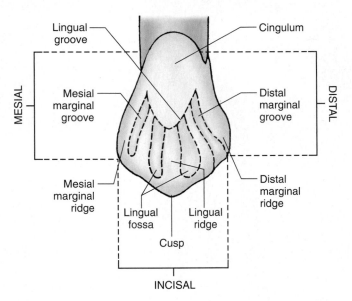

• **Figure 13.3** The lingual surface of a maxillary right canine. (Modified from Zeisz RC, Nuckolls J. *Dental Anatomy*. St. Louis, MO: Mosby; 1949.)

are the incisal ridge, lingual ridge, and mesial or distal marginal ridge.

Sometimes the lingual surface of a canine crown is so smooth that no concavities or fossae are present. Usually the cingulum and marginal ridges are less developed in these instances, with little evidence of developmental grooves.

The lingual side of the root is narrower than the labial side. A cross-sectional view of the root appears triangular, with the lingual portion more tapered than the labial portion.

Mesial Aspect

The functional form of a maxillary canine is evident on the mesial view (Fig. 13.4; see Fig. 13.1D). The wedge-shaped outline of the crown shows the canine to have greater labiolingual bulk compared with any other anterior tooth. The greatest measurement labiolingually is at the cervical third. This is because of the very large

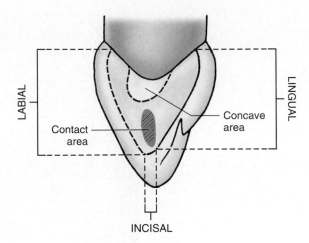

• **Figure 13.4** The mesial surface of a maxillary right canine. (Modified from Zeisz RC, Nuckolls J. *Dental Anatomy*. St. Louis, MO: Mosby; 1949.)

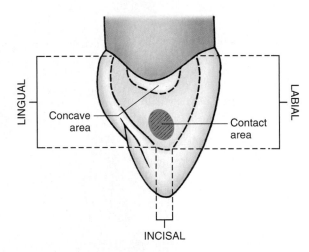

• **Figure 13.5** The distal surface of a maxillary right canine. (Modified from Zeisz RC, Nuckolls J. *Dental Anatomy*. St. Louis, MO: Mosby; 1949.)

cingulum on the lingual side and the more convex labial outline of the canine. The entire labial surface is more convex from the cervical line to the cusp tip than any other maxillary anterior tooth. The cervical line curves toward the cusp an average of 2.5 mm.

The root of a canine is broad labiolingually and is usually extremely long. The end of the root apex is blunt and may often curve to the lingual or distal lingual side. The mesial surface of the root shows much labiolingual development, with a shallow developmental depression extending from the cervical line halfway to the apex of the root. This developmental depression appears to almost divide the single root into two roots. In extremely well-developed roots, it helps anchor a canine in bone and prevents root rotation.

The mesial surface of a canine crown is entirely convex throughout except for a small area between the contact area and the cervical line, which may be flat.

Distal Aspect

The distal aspect (Fig. 13.5; see also Fig. 13.1E) of a maxillary canine shows the same form and outline as the mesial view does. However, the cervical line shows less curvature toward the cusp tip. The distal marginal ridge is more developed and heavier in outline compared with the mesial marginal ridge. Although both

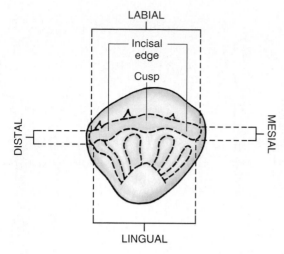

• **Figure 13.6** The incisal edge of a maxillary right canine. (Modified from Zeisz RC, Nuckolls J. *Dental Anatomy*. St. Louis, MO: Mosby; 1949.)

the mesial and the distal surfaces show a slightly flat or concave area cervical to the contact area, the distal surface displays much more concavity. The root surface on the distal aspect may show a more pronounced developmental depression compared with that on the mesial aspect.

Incisal Aspect

An incisal view (Fig. 13.6; see Fig. 13.1C) of a maxillary canine shows that the tooth is not only wide mesiodistally but also has

the thickest labiolingual measurement compared with any anterior tooth. Although these two measurements are about equal, the crown is usually larger in a labiolingual direction. The cusp tip is labial to the center of the crown labiolingually and mesial to the center mesiodistally.

The distal aspect of the crown appears thinner than the mesial aspect. Indeed, it seems to stretch out to make contact with the first premolars.

Root

The root of the maxillary canine is usually the longest compared with any tooth in the mouth. It is very strong and firmly embedded in the maxilla. In a cross-sectional view, the root appears to taper from the labial area toward the lingual area. From a proximal view, a longitudinal groove may be seen. The apical portion often points distally but seldom mesially (see Fig. 13.1).

Pulp Cavity

The pulp cavity of the maxillary canine (Fig. 13.7) consists of a large pulp chamber and a single root canal. The pulp chamber has one single pulp horn, which extends toward the tip of the cusp. The root canal is usually straight but can be tortuous when the root is curved.

Pertinent Data

Maxillary Canines

	Right	Left
Universal code	6	11
International code	13	23

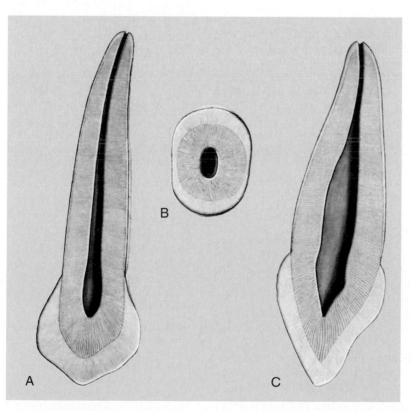

• **Figure 13.7** The pulp cavity of a maxillary right canine. **(A)** Distomesial section, lingual view. **(B)** Cross-section, incisal view. **(C)** Linguolabial section, mesial view. (Modified from Zeisz RC, Nuckolls J. *Dental Anatomy*. St. Louis, MO: Mosby; 1949.)

Palmer notation:
Number of roots: 1
Number of pulp horns: 1
Number of cusps: 1
Number of developmental lobes: 4

Location of Proximal Contact Areas
Mesial: Junction of incisal and middle thirds
Distal: Middle third

Height of Contour
Facial: Cervical third, 0.5 mm
Lingual: Cervical third, 0.5 mm

Identifying Characteristics
Maxillary canines are the longest teeth in the mouth. They have a single cusp, with mesial and distal ridges forming an incisal edge. The cingulum is prominent, and a prominent facial ridge is off center toward the mesial side. The facial and lingual ridges of its single cusp are more developed than corresponding ridges on any other tooth. This lingual ridge divides the mesial and distal fossae. The distofacial ridge is longer and more rounded compared with the mesiofacial ridge.

Mandibular Canines

Evidence of calcification: 4 months
Enamel completed: 7 years
Eruption: 9 to 10 years
Root completed: 13 years

Mandibular canines resemble maxillary canines in that they have the same wedge-shaped outline, long crown and root, and well-developed cingulum. They differ from the maxillary canines, however, in the following ways (Fig. 13.8):

1. A mandibular canine crown is narrower mesiodistally by about 0.5 mm.
2. A mandibular canine crown length is as long as that of a maxillary canine and sometimes longer.
3. The root may be as long as that of a maxillary canine but more often is shorter.
4. The labiolingual measurements of the crown and the root are usually fractions of a millimeter less compared with a maxillary canine. How then does the total length of a mandibular tooth (crown and root) compare with other teeth?
5. The lingual surface of a mandibular canine is smoother, the cingulum is less developed, and the marginal ridges are less prominent compared with those of a maxillary canine. The lingual surface of a mandibular canine resembles the lingual surface of other mandibular anterior teeth.
6. The cusp tip of a mandibular canine is not as well developed as that of a maxillary canine, and the cusp ridges are thinner labiolingually.
7. The cusp tip of a mandibular canine may be centered more lingually compared with a maxillary canine cusp tip.
8. An anomaly of a mandibular canine is bifurcation of roots; when a mandibular canine has two roots, one buccal and one lingual, usually only the apical third of the root is bifurcated.
9. The distal contact area is more incisal on the mandibular canine than on the maxillary canine.

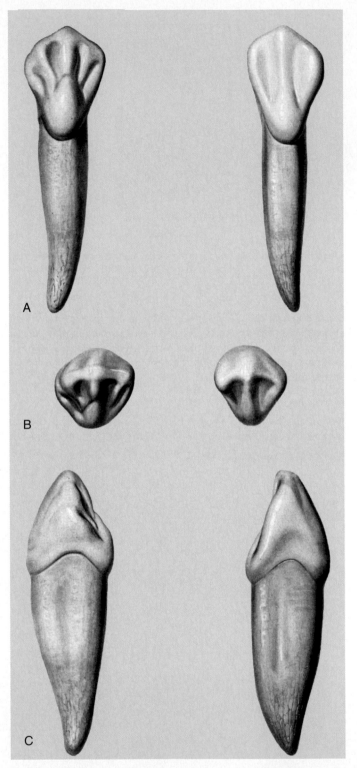

• **Figure 13.8** Comparison of maxillary (left column) and mandibular (right column) right canines. **(A)** Lingual view. **(B)** Incisal view. and **(C)** Distal view. The lengths of the teeth are about the same, but the maxillary root is longer whereas its crown is shorter than that of the mandibular canine. The maxillary lingual surface shows more convexity than the lingual surface of the mandibular canine, it protrudes more, and it is more pronounced. The lingual surface of the mandibular is smoother and shallower, and resembles the lingual surface of other mandibular incisors. The mandibular canine is narrower mesiodistally than the maxillary canine. The cusp tip of the mandibular canine is more lingually centered over its root. (Modified from Zeisz RC, Nuckolls J. *Dental Anatomy*. St. Louis, MO: Mosby; 1949.)

Labial Aspect

From the labial view (Fig. 13.9; see Fig. 13.14A), a mandibular canine shows a straighter mesial outline compared with a maxillary canine. The distal outline resembles that of a maxillary canine, which means that the mesial outline of a mandibular canine is less convex than is its distal outline. Which surface, mesial or distal, shows the greater convexity on a maxillary canine? Is it the same for a mandibular canine?

The distal contact area is more incisal on a mandibular canine compared with the same contact area on its maxillary counterpart and is located somewhat cervical to the junction of its incisal and middle thirds. Where is the distal contact on a maxillary canine? The mesial contact area of a mandibular canine is nearer the mesioincisal point angle compared with its maxillary counterpart, at the incisal third of the tooth. Where is the mesial contact area of a maxillary canine?

Facially, the cervical line of a mandibular canine is more symmetrically contoured compared with the cervical line of a maxillary canine. The cervical line of a maxillary canine is less uniform, cresting slightly mesial to the midline of the tooth.

Lingual Aspect

The lingual surface (Fig. 13.10; see Fig. 13.14B) of the crown of a mandibular canine is flatter than that of a maxillary canine. Lingual features are less prominent; the cingulum is relatively smooth, the marginal ridges are less distinct, and the lingual fossae and ridge are less pronounced.

The lingual surface of a mandibular canine resembles the other mandibular anterior teeth but has a larger cingulum and a pronounced lingual ridge. The cingulum is larger and more developed compared with those on other mandibular anterior teeth. Compared with a maxillary canine, a mandibular canine's cingulum tapers more lingually and is less developed.

The lingual ridge of a mandibular canine is less distinct than the same ridge on a maxillary canine except toward the cusp tip, where it is raised. No lingual pits are on the mandibular canines.

A mandibular canine resembles other mandibular teeth from a lingual view in that the marginal ridges and lingual fossae are

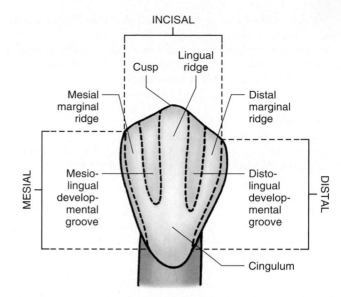

• **Figure 13.10** The lingual surface of a mandibular right canine. (Modified from Zeisz RC, Nuckolls J. *Dental Anatomy*. St. Louis, MO: Mosby; 1949.)

flatter than those of maxillary teeth. In fact, the lingual surfaces of all the mandibular teeth are smoother and more hollowed than those of their maxillary counterparts.

Mesial Aspect

A mandibular canine resembles its maxillary counterpart from a mesial view (Fig. 13.11; see Fig. 13.14D), having the same wedge-shaped and pointed cusp. It differs from a maxillary canine in that it has a less-developed cingulum and thinner marginal ridges. The cusp tip of a mandibular canine is more lingually inclined, whereas the cusp tip of a maxillary is centered slightly labially. As the canines become abraded with wear, this discrepancy in the centering of a canine cusp tip becomes more apparent. The reason for the lingual incline of the mandibular canine is apparent, given the position of a mandibular canine in relation to its maxillary counterpart when the two are touching.

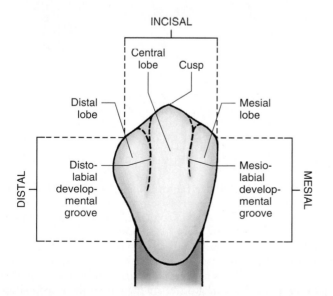

• **Figure 13.9** The labial surface of a mandibular right canine. (Modified from Zeisz RC, Nuckolls J. *Dental Anatomy*. St. Louis, MO: Mosby; 1949.)

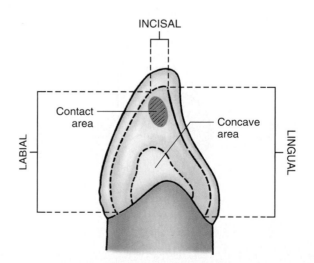

• **Figure 13.11** The mesial surface of a mandibular right canine. (Modified from Zeisz RC, Nuckolls J. *Dental Anatomy*. St. Louis, MO: Mosby; 1949.)

The cervical line curves more toward the incisal portion compared with the cervical line on a maxillary canine.

The roots of the mandibular and maxillary canines are similar except that a mandibular canine's root may be more pointed at the apex. The developmental depression on the root of a mandibular canine is more pronounced, and sometimes the root is bifurcated.

Distal Aspect

The distal aspect (Fig. 13.12; see Fig. 13.14E) of a mandibular canine resembles a maxillary canine except for those features mentioned in the discussion on the mesial aspects.

Incisal Aspect

From an incisal view (Fig. 13.13; see also Fig. 13.14C) the incisal edge of a mandibular canine slants toward the lingual side with the distal incisal ridge slanting more lingually compared with the mesial side. The cusp tip is located more lingually on a mandibular canine than on a maxillary canine. In all other ways, the mandibular canines resemble the maxillary canines. (Fig. 13.14 shows all views of a mandibular right canine.)

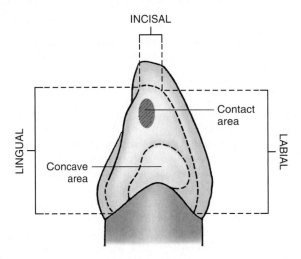

• **Figure 13.12** The distal surface of a mandibular right canine. (Modified from Zeisz RC, Nuckolls J. *Dental Anatomy*. St. Louis, MO: Mosby; 1949.)

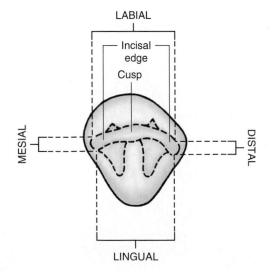

• **Figure 13.13** The incisal edge of a mandibular right canine. (Modified from Zeisz RC, Nuckolls J. *Dental Anatomy*. St. Louis, MO: Mosby; 1949.)

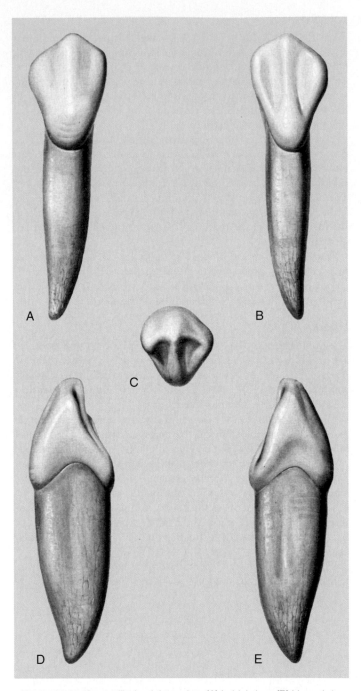

• **Figure 13.14** A mandibular right canine. **(A)** Labial view. **(B)** Lingual view. **(C)** Incisal view. **(D)** Mesial view. **(E)** Distal view. (Modified from Zeisz RC, Nuckolls J. *Dental Anatomy*. St. Louis, MO: Mosby; 1949.)

Root

The root of the mandibular canine is the longest mandibular root, and of all the tooth roots, it is second only to the root of the maxillary canine; it is wide labiolingually and narrow mesiodistally (see Fig. 13.8). Some specimens show a bifurcated root in the apical third. The anterior tooth root is the one most likely to be bifurcated. When the root is bifurcated, one branch is labial and the other lingual. The single-rooted form is much more common, and if deep longitudinal grooves are present on the proximal surfaces of the root, then a tendency exists for two root canals to form, even if these join together at the apex. Bifurcated or not, the

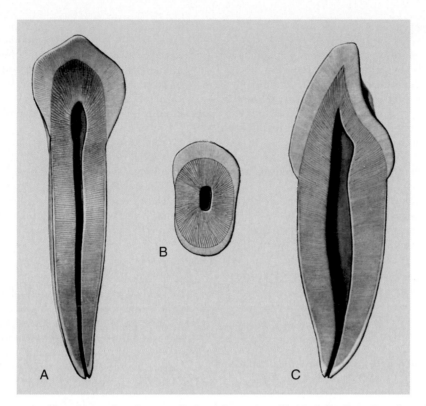

• **Figure 13.15** The pulp cavity of a mandibular right canine. **(A)** Mesiodistal section, lingual view. **(B)** Cross-section, incisal view. **(C)** Labiolingual section, mesial view. (Modified from Zeisz RC, Nuckolls J. *Dental Anatomy*. St. Louis, MO: Mosby; 1949.)

mandibular canine root is flatter than the maxillary canine root on the distal or mesial surface.

Pulp Cavity

The pulp cavity of the mandibular canine resembles that of the maxillary canine in that they both have a large pulp chamber and usually a single root canal. Only one pulp horn is present.

The major difference between the two teeth is that the mandibular canine may have two separate root canals. When this happens, one canal is to the labial side, and the other is to the lingual side. The canals may join at the apex or have separate apical foramina. When the root is bifurcated, two canals are almost always present, each with its own apical foramen (Fig. 13.15).

Pertinent Data

Mandibular Canines

	Right	Left
Universal code	27	22
International code	43	33

Palmer notation:
Number of roots: 1 or 2
Number of pulp horns. 1
Number of cusps: 1
Number of developmental lobes: 4

Location of Proximal Contact Areas

Mesial: Incisal third
Distal: Just cervical to the junction of incisal and middle thirds

Height of Contour

Facial: Cervical third, less than 0.5 mm
Lingual: Cervical third, less than 0.5 mm

Identifying Characteristics

The crown is similar to that of the maxillary canine but narrower and smoother. It has less prominent lingual features. From a proximal view, the cusp tip is inclined lingually. From an incisal view, the distal end of the incisal edge is rotated lingually. Mandibular canines have the longest roots in the mandibular arch; the maxillary canines are the only teeth with longer roots.

Review Questions

1. A maxillary canine can be distinguished from a mandibular canine by which of the following characteristics?
   a. A mandibular canine has a less prominent cingulum.
   b. The mesial side of a mandibular canine crown and root is relatively straight.
   c. The incisal edge of a mandibular canine is located lingual to the center of the tooth.
   d. All of the above.
2. Which of the following is characteristic of the root of a mandibular canine?
   a. It is longer than the root of a maxillary canine.
   b. The root is never bifurcated.
   c. It is flattened or slightly concave on the distal surface.
   d. The crown length can be longer than any other tooth in the mouth.
3. Generally, on the lingual surface of a maxillary canine, there is/are
   a. one fossa
   b. two fossae
   c. three fossae
   d. four fossae
4. Compared with other anterior teeth, a mandibular canine is the most likely to have
   a. longitudinal grooves
   b. a root that is narrow mesiodistally
   c. two root canals
   d. any or all of the above
5. A mandibular canine root sometimes bifurcates into the
   a. mesiofacial and distolingual roots
   b. facial and lingual roots
   c. mesial and distal roots
   d. none of the above; the mandibular canine root does not bifurcate
6. Canine teeth exhibit
   a. a facial ridge
   b. a lingual ridge
   c. a mesial marginal ridge
   d. all of the above
7. What is the bony projection that is a part of the support for canines?

True or False

8. Facially the cervical line crests slightly mesial to the center of the tooth.
9. The contact area of a canine is located more toward the junction of the mesial and middle thirds on the distal surface.
10. The mesial contact areas are located more cervically compared with the distal contact areas.
11. Identify this tooth (Fig. 13.16).

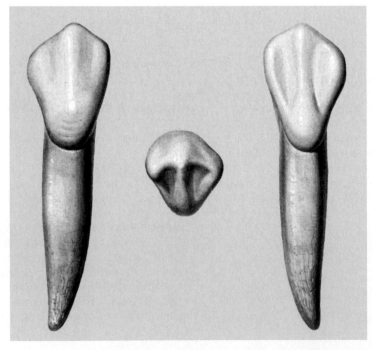

• **Figure 13.16** Identify this tooth. (Modified from Zeisz RC, Nuckolls J. *Dental Anatomy*. St. Louis, MO: Mosby; 1949.)

14

Premolars

OBJECTIVES

- To understand how development occurs through the formation and fusion of lobes
- To understand how the form of a tooth relates to its ultimate function
- To recognize and name the pertinent dental anatomic form of each tooth, such as cusps, ridges, developmental grooves, triangular grooves, pits, and developmental depressions
- To discuss the major differences and similarities between maxillary first and second premolars
- To identify an extracted premolar as maxillary or mandibular, first or second, right or left
- To make comparisons between maxillary and mandibular premolars
- To compare mandibular first premolars with mandibular second premolars (development, shape, and diversities of anatomic form)
- To describe briefly the various occlusal forms possible for a mandibular second premolar

Premolars succeed the deciduous molars. Eight premolar teeth are present, with two in each quadrant. The term *premolar* implies that these will be located immediately anterior to the permanent molars. In the study of human dentition the term *bicuspid* is often used in place of *premolar*. This is inaccurate because *bicuspid* presupposes that a tooth has only two cusps. In human dentition, however, mandibular premolars show variation from one to three in the number of cusps. Thus the use of the term *bicuspid* is discouraged in favor of the term *premolar*.

Maxillary first and second premolars and mandibular first premolars are developed from four lobes as in the case of anterior teeth. Mandibular second premolars usually develop from five lobes—three buccal and two lingual.

The buccal cusp of a premolar is developed from three labial lobes, as in anterior teeth. The primary difference in development is that the lingual cusp, which is extremely well formed, develops from the single lingual lobe. In anterior teeth, the lingual lobe forms the cingulum of incisors and canines. In premolars, this single lingual lobe forms an extremely well-developed lingual cusp.

In the case of the three-cusp form (the mandibular second premolar), two lingual lobes are present, each of which forms a separate small lingual cusp. A two-cusp form of the mandibular second premolar also develops from just four lobes. The lingual

cusps of the mandibular premolars are small and **afunctional** compared with the larger lingual cusps of maxillary premolars. The premolar crowns and roots are shorter compared with those of canines.

Maxillary first premolars are bifurcated 60% of the time; maxillary second premolars are bifurcated 25% of the time; and mandibular first premolars rarely bifurcate, even less frequently compared with canines. Mandibular second premolars almost never bifurcate, but all premolars show evidence of proximal root concavities whether they bifurcate or not.

Both maxillary premolars usually erupt earlier than their mandibular counterparts do. First premolars erupt earlier than second premolars.

At the back of this book there are flash cards to assist your study of teeth. A very effective way to compare the different premolars is by placing the flash cards side by side.

Refer to *Chapter 12*, Table 14.1, *is a chart showing various measurements associated with permanent teeth. This chart is also displayed at the end of Chapter 16.*

Maxillary Premolars

First Premolars

Evidence of calcification: 1.5 years
Enamel completed: 5 to 6 years
Eruption: 10 to 11 years
Root completed: 12 to 13 years

Maxillary first premolars (Fig. 14.1) have buccal and lingual cusps. The buccal cusp is usually 1 mm or more longer than the lingual cusp. These teeth are also the only premolars that normally have two roots, a buccal root and a lingual root, although occasionally only a single root is evident.

Most maxillary first premolars have two roots and two pulp canals. Even when only one root is present, two pulp canals can usually be found. It is not uncommon for maxillary second premolars to also have two roots; however, usually only one is evident.

Facial (Buccal) Aspect *(Fig. 14.2; see Fig. 14.1A)*

A maxillary first premolar is similar in appearance to a maxillary canine. However, the crown is shorter and narrower mesiodistally, and unlike in a canine, the mesial and distal contact areas are at approximately the same level. The mesial and distal marginal ridges are also sharper than are those of a canine.

The tip of the facial cusp is located distally to the midline and separates the occlusal border into a long, straight mesial ridge and a short, convex distal ridge. The mesial ridge may even have a slight indentation at the junction of the mesial and middle lobes. From the contact areas cervically, the distal border is straight,

TABLE 14.1 Comparison Chart of Premolars

Aspect	Maxillary First	Maxillary Second	Mandibular First	Mandibular Second
Crown	Larger than second	Cusps same length	Smaller than second	May have three cusps
Mesial	Mesial groove and depression	Larger lingual cusp	Mesiolingual groove	Shorter buccal cusp
Eruption	10–11	10–12	10–12	11–12
Occlusal	2 cusps	2 cusps same size	Smallest lingual cusp	Three cusps form
Roots	60% bifurcated	25% bifurcated	Single root	Single root
Lobes	4	4	4	4 or 5

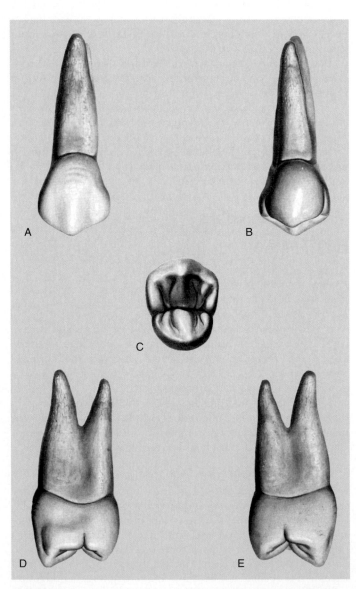

• **Figure 14.1** A maxillary right first premolar. **(A)** Buccal view. **(B)** Lingual view. **(C)** Occlusal view. **(D)** Mesial view. **(E)** Distal view. (Modified from Zeisz RC, Nuckolls J. *Dental Anatomy*. St. Louis, MO: Mosby; 1949.)

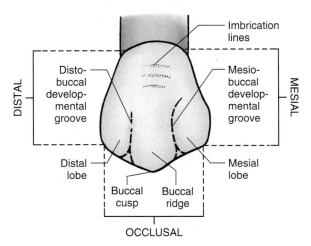

• **Figure 14.2** The buccal surface of a maxillary right first premolar. (Modified from Zeisz RC, Nuckolls J. *Dental Anatomy*. St. Louis, MO: Mosby; 1949.)

whereas the mesial border is more concave. Two developmental lines on the facial surface mark the coalescence of the developmental lobes. The facial surface of the crown is convex, and an extremely well-developed middle facial lobe is present.

Lingual Aspect

From the lingual view (Fig. 14.3; see Fig. 14.1B), the crown converges toward the lingual cusp, which is shorter than the facial cusp. The tip of the lingual cusp is located slightly toward the mesial side of the midline.

Mesial Aspect

On the mesial surface (Fig. 14.4; see Fig. 14.1C) of the crown, a groove extends from the mesial marginal ridge cervically. This groove is called the **mesial marginal groove**. It crosses the mesial marginal ridge and runs from the occlusal third to the middle third of the crown, lingual to the contact area. The mesial surface can also be identified by a **mesial developmental depression** located cervically to the mesial contact area. The concavity continues cervically from above the contact area across the cervical

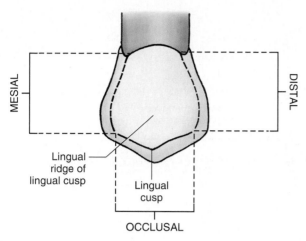

• **Figure 14.3** The lingual surface of a maxillary right first premolar. (Modified from Zeisz RC, Nuckolls J. *Dental Anatomy.* St. Louis, MO: Mosby; 1949.)

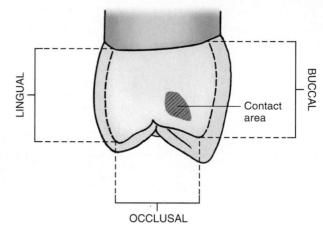

• **Figure 14.5** The distal surface of a maxillary right first premolar. (Modified from Zeisz RC, Nuckolls J. *Dental Anatomy.* St. Louis, MO: Mosby; 1949.)

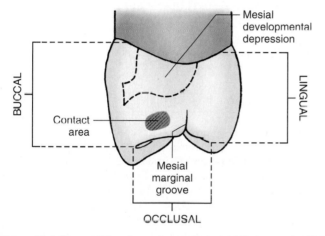

• **Figure 14.4** The mesial surface of a maxillary right first premolar. Note the mesial developmental depression. (Modified from Zeisz RC, Nuckolls J. *Dental Anatomy.* St. Louis, MO: Mosby; 1949.)

line, where it joins a deep **developmental depression** between the roots. The mesial marginal groove is not always present, but the mesial developmental depression usually is quite evident (Fig. 14.1D).

The facial outline is convex, with the crest of contour located within the cervical third of the crown. The lingual outline is also convex, with its crest of contour located within the middle third of the crown. The curvature of the cervical line is greater on the mesial surface than on the distal surface. Compare the cervical lines in Fig. 14.1D, and Fig. 14.1C.

Distal Aspect

From the distal view (Fig. 14.5; see Fig. 14.1E), a maxillary first premolar is similar to that on the mesial view, except no groove usually crosses the distal marginal ridge, and no developmental depression is present. Some specimens show a distinct distal **marginal groove**, but the mesial marginal groove is deeper and more obvious. The cervical line is less curved on the distal surface than on the mesial surface. The crown also appears more rounded and smooth. Both the buccal and lingual cusp tips are centered over

the root, and this is also true of the mesial view. All maxillary premolars have their cusp tips centered over their root.

Occlusal Aspect

The occlusal surface (Fig. 14.6; see Fig. 14.1C) shows two well-developed cusps. The lingual cusp is more pointed than the facial cusp, but the facial cusp is much larger and longer than the lingual cusp. Each cusp has four ridges emanating from it, and each ridge is named according to its location: facial, lingual, distal, and mesial.

On the facial cusp, the facial ridge descends from the cusp tip cervically onto the facial surface. The mesial and distal ridges descend from the cusp tip to their respective point angles. They are called the *mesial* and *distal cusp ridges.*

The lingual cusp ridge extends from the cusp tip lingually to the central area of the occlusal surface. Any ridge that runs from the cusp tip to the central groove of the occlusal surface is called a *triangular ridge.* Examples are the lingual cusp ridge of the buccal cusp and the buccal cusp ridge of the lingual cusp, which runs from the cusp tip of the lingual cusp to the central groove (Fig. 14.7).

Like its counterpart, the buccal cusp, the lingual cusp also has four ridges. The lingual cusp ridge of the lingual cusp extends onto the lingual surface. The mesial and distal cusp ridges extend from the cusp tip to their respective point angles and fuse into the mesial and distal marginal ridges.

When two triangular ridges join, after traversing the tooth buccolingually, they form a transverse ridge. Thus a transverse ridge exists on the occlusal surface of a maxillary first premolar. It is formed by the union of the two triangular ridges—the lingual cusp ridge of the buccal cusp and the facial cusp ridge of the lingual cusp. See Fig. 14.7 for the transverse ridge formed by the two joining triangular ridges.

From the occlusal aspect, close observation reveals that the crown is wider on the buccal surface than on the lingual surface. Note also that the buccolingual dimension of the crown is much greater than the mesiodistal dimension.

The primary anatomic features are composed of the major structures, grooves, and pits that are pertinent to teeth. They must occur regularly with uniformity in shape and size.

Thus primary grooves are sharp, deep, and "V" shaped. They occur consistently and mark the junction of major anatomic

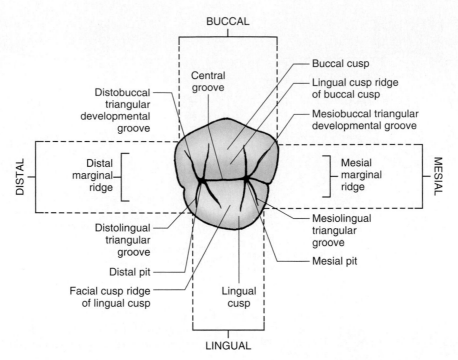

• **Figure 14.6** The occlusal surface of a maxillary right first premolar. Identify the mesial marginal groove (not labeled; see Fig. 14.4 for help). (Modified from Zeisz RC, Nuckolls J. *Dental Anatomy*. St. Louis, MO: Mosby; 1949.)

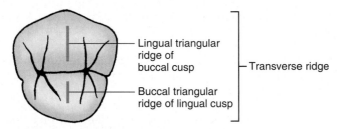

• **Figure 14.7** The occlusal surface of a maxillary right first premolar. (Modified from Zeisz RC, Nuckolls J. *Dental Anatomy*. St. Louis, MO: Mosby; 1949.)

boundaries. All developmental grooves are primary grooves because they occur routinely and are of major importance to anatomic development. What are these structures that are separated by developmental grooves?

Secondary grooves are of lesser importance. They differ from primary grooves in that they usually are more shallow and irregular in shape, giving the tooth a more wrinkled appearance. They are not always present.

As a general rule, first premolars and first molars have fewer secondary anatomic features. Second premolars and second molars will have more secondary grooves and pits. Third molars have even more secondary anatomic grooves, pits, and fissures. Therefore third molars appear more wrinkled because of the more numerous and shallow anatomic features.

Few secondary grooves are on the occlusal surface of a maxillary first premolar. In most instances, the surface is relatively smooth. A well-defined **central developmental groove** divides the tooth buccolingually. A **mesial marginal developmental groove** extends from the central developmental groove, across the mesial marginal ridge, and onto the mesial surface of the tooth.

Two developmental grooves connect to the central groove just inside the mesial and distal marginal ridges. These grooves are the **mesiobuccal developmental groove** and the **distobuccal developmental groove**. Each can connect at the opposite ends of the central developmental groove, at which point they usually end in a deep depression in the occlusal surface called *mesial* and *distal developmental pits*.

The triangular depression that harbors the mesiobuccal developmental groove is called the *mesial triangular fossa*. Likewise, the depression in which the distobuccal developmental groove lies is called the *distal triangular fossa*. The terms *mesiobuccal developmental groove* and *mesiobuccal triangular groove* are synonymous.

Root

The root of a maxillary first premolar may be either single or bifurcated. The bifurcated root form is far more common, but even in the single root form, two root canals are usually present. The number of pulp horns corresponds to the number of cusps, which, in this case, is two.

On the bifurcated root form, one buccal (facial) root and one **palatal root** (lingual root) are present. The buccal root is larger and longer than the palatal root (see Fig. 14.1D–E).

On the single-rooted form, grooves are usually present lengthwise in the middle of the root, giving the appearance of a root trying to divide itself. The mesial root surface has a more highly developed root groove.

Pulp Cavity

The pulp cavity (Fig. 14.8) of the maxillary first premolar has two pulp horns, one for each cusp, and two root canals, one for each root. Sometimes only one undivided root is present. When this occurs, usually two root canals are still evident, although they

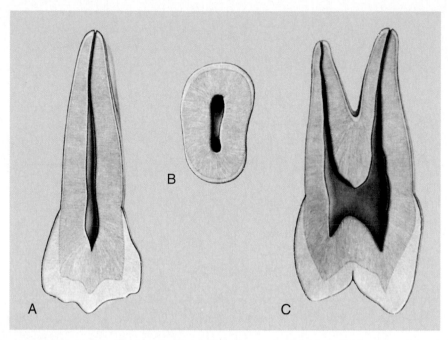

• **Figure 14.8** The pulp cavity of a maxillary right first premolar. **(A)** Mesiodistal section, buccal view. **(B)** Cross section, occlusal view. **(C)** Buccolingual section, distal view. (Modified from Zeisz RC, Nuckolls J. *Dental Anatomy.* St. Louis, MO: Mosby; 1949.)

often combine to form one apical foramen. In some specimens with only one root, only one single root canal is present.

General Characteristics

Maxillary first premolars exemplify the following characteristics that are common to all posterior teeth compared with anterior teeth:

1. Posterior teeth have a greater faciolingual measurement in relation to their mesiodistal measurements.
2. Mesial and distal contact areas are broader and closer to the same level on the tooth.
3. The mesial and distal curvature of the cervical line is less.
4. The crown measurements cervico-occlusally are less, giving the appearance of shorter crown length.

Second Premolars

Evidence of calcification: 2 years
Enamel completed: 6 to 7 years
Eruption: 10 to 12 years
Root completed: 12 to 14 years

Maxillary second premolars (Fig. 14.9) resemble maxillary first premolars in both form and function. The crown, however, has a less angular and more rounded appearance. Second premolars also vary from the first in that they usually have only one root. How many roots do maxillary first premolars have?

Second premolars vary individually more than first premolars do. A maxillary second premolar may have a crown that is noticeably smaller cervico-occlusally and mesiodistally. However, it may be larger in those dimensions and usually is.

Generally the root of a second premolar is longer than that of a first premolar. Although a second premolar usually has only one root, it is not unusual to find these premolars with two roots.

Facial (Buccal) Aspect

From the buccal view (Fig. 14.10; see Fig. 14.9A), it is evident that the buccal cusp of a second premolar is not as long as that of a first premolar, and it appears less pointed. A second premolar has the same general markings as the first, but they are not as well defined.

Lingual Aspect

Little variation can be seen from the lingual view (Fig. 14.11; see also Fig. 14.9B) except that the lingual cusp is almost the same length as the buccal cusp.

Mesial Aspect

The mesial view (Fig. 14.12; see Fig. 14.9D) shows the difference in cusp length between the maxillary first and second premolars. The buccal cusp of a second premolar is shorter than the buccal cusp of a first premolar, and the lingual cusp is almost as long; thus the buccal and lingual cusps are nearly the same length.

No deep developmental groove crosses the mesial marginal ridge, just as no deep developmental depression is on the mesial surface of the crown; instead, the crown surface is convex. A shallow developmental groove bisects the single root form, giving the appearance of two roots fused into one.

Distal Aspect

The distal view (see Fig. 14.9E) shows that the features of first and second premolars are the same, except that the buccal and lingual cusps of a second premolar are more even in length.

Occlusal Aspect

The occlusal outline (Fig. 14.13, p. 146; see also Fig. 14.9C) is more rounded than that of a first premolar, and the second premolar is ovoid rather than hexagonal.

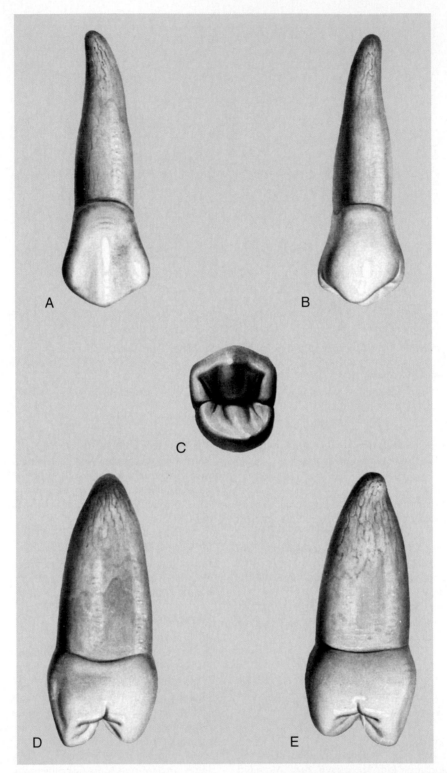

• **Figure 14.9** A maxillary right second premolar. **(A)** Buccal view. **(B)** Lingual view. **(C)** Occlusal view. **(D)** Mesial view. **(E)** Distal view. (Modified from Zeisz RC, Nuckolls J. *Dental Anatomy.* St. Louis, MO: Mosby; 1949.)

More distance is evident between the cusp tips buccolingually than on the first premolar, and the lingual cusp is almost as wide as the buccal cusp. Is this true of a first premolar?

The groove pattern is less distinct than in the first premolar, and the grooves are shorter, shallower, and more irregular. The central developmental groove is also shorter and more irregular,

with numerous supplemental grooves radiating from it, giving the occlusal surface a more wrinkled appearance.

Root

The root of a maxillary second premolar is usually single with a longitudinal groove on the mesial and distal surfaces. This groove

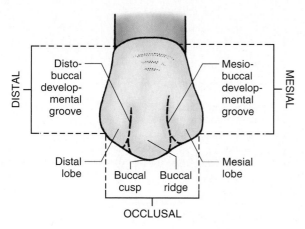

• **Figure 14.10** The buccal surface of a maxillary right second premolar. (Modified from Zeisz RC, Nuckolls J. *Dental Anatomy.* St. Louis, MO: Mosby; 1949.)

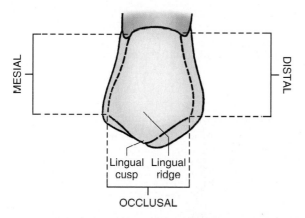

• **Figure 14.11** The lingual surface of a maxillary right second premolar. The buccal and lingual cusps are almost the same length. (Modified from Zeisz RC, Nuckolls J. *Dental Anatomy.* St. Louis, MO: Mosby; 1949.)

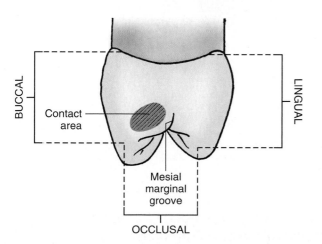

• **Figure 14.12** The mesial surface of a maxillary right second premolar. *Note:* Although mesial and distal marginal grooves are present in all drawings of maxillary second premolars, the actual grooves are shallower than the mesial marginal groove of a maxillary first premolar. (Modified from Zeisz RC, Nuckolls J. *Dental Anatomy.* St. Louis, MO: Mosby; 1949.)

gives the appearance of a single root dividing into two, buccally and lingually. Usually only one root canal is evident, but often a divided canal occurs in at least a portion of the root. A bifurcated root similar to that of a first premolar is common; this form has two root canals.

Pulp Cavity

The pulp cavity (Fig. 14.14) of the maxillary second premolar has two pulp horns and a single root canal. The single-rooted form and one root canal are more common. If two canals are present, they usually join to form one single apical foramen, although it is not rare to find two apical foramina. In the bifurcated root, two canals and two apical foramina may be present.

Pertinent Data

Maxillary First Premolars

	Right	Left
Universal code	5	12
International code	14	24
Palmer notation:	4⌋	⌊4

Number of roots: 2
Number of pulp horns: 2
Number of cusps: 2
Number of developmental lobes: 4

Location of Proximal Contact Areas
Mesial: Just cervical to the junction of occlusal and middle thirds
Distal: Just cervical to the junction of occlusal and middle thirds

Height of Contour
Facial: Cervical third, 0.5 mm
Lingual: Middle third, 0.5 mm

Identifying Characteristic
Maxillary first premolars have bifurcated roots, and a longitudinal groove is present on each root. The mesial surface shows a developmental fossa. The mesial marginal groove crosses the mesial marginal ridge and extends onto the mesial surface. The facial cusp is wider and longer than the lingual cusp. The mesial ridge of the facial cusp may have a slight concavity.

Maxillary Second Premolars

	Right	Left
Universal code	4	13
International code	15	25
Palmer notation:	5⌋	⌊5

Number of roots: 1
Number of pulp horns: 2
Number of cusps: 2
Number of developmental lobes: 4

Location of Proximal Contact Areas
Mesial: Just cervical to the junction of occlusal and middle thirds
Distal: Just cervical to the junction of occlusal and middle thirds

Height of Contour
Facial: Cervical third, 0.5 mm
Lingual: Middle third, 0.5 mm

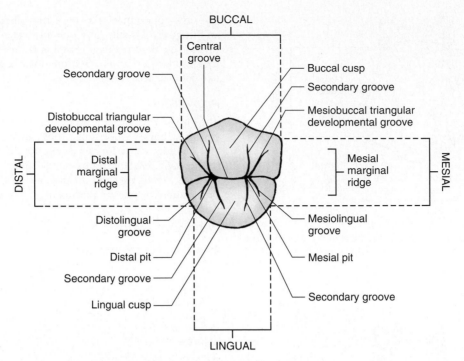

• **Figure 14.13** The occlusal surface of a maxillary right second premolar. (Modified from Zeisz RC, Nuckolls J. *Dental Anatomy.* St. Louis, MO: Mosby; 1949.)

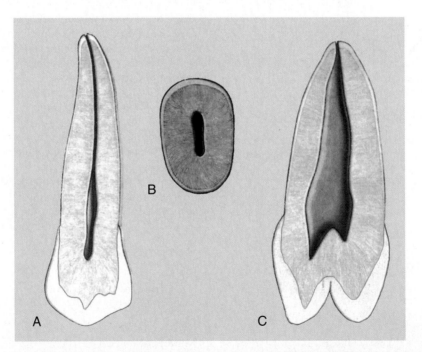

• **Figure 14.14** The pulp cavity of a right maxillary second premolar. **(A)** Mesiodistal section, buccal view. **(B)** Cross section, occlusal view. **(C)** Linguobuccal section, mesial view. (Modified from Zeisz RC, Nuckolls J. *Dental Anatomy.* St. Louis, MO: Mosby; 1949.)

Identifying Characteristics

Maxillary second premolars usually have a single root. About 40% have two root canals. The buccal and lingual cusps are nearly equal in length. The buccal cusp is shorter than that of a first premolar. The entire crown, especially the occlusal outline, is less angular and more rounded than that of a maxillary first premolar. The occlusal surface has more supplemental grooves. The occlusal developmental grooves are shorter, shallower, and more irregular.

Maxillary First Premolars Compared With Maxillary Second Premolars

The following features are truer of a maxillary first premolar than of a maxillary second premolar:

1. It usually has two roots.
2. It usually has two root canals, even if it has only one root.
3. It has a mesial developmental fossa.

4. Its mesial marginal ridge is crossed by a mesial marginal developmental groove.
5. The lingual and buccal cusps are not nearly the same height; the buccal cusp is longer.
6. The occlusal outline is less rounded in first premolars.
7. The facial contour is more angular.
8. The occlusal grooves are not as short, shallow, or irregular as those of second premolars.
9. It has fewer secondary anatomic features and supplemental grooves.
10. It has a more rounded and very slightly shorter buccal cusp.

Mandibular Premolars

First Premolars

Evidence of calcification: 2 years
Enamel completed: 5 to 6 years
Eruption: 10 to 12 years
Root completed: 12 to 13 years

Mandibular first premolars (Fig. 14.15) have many of the characteristics of mandibular canines. Like canines, they have a dominant facial cusp, which is the only part that occludes with maxillary teeth.

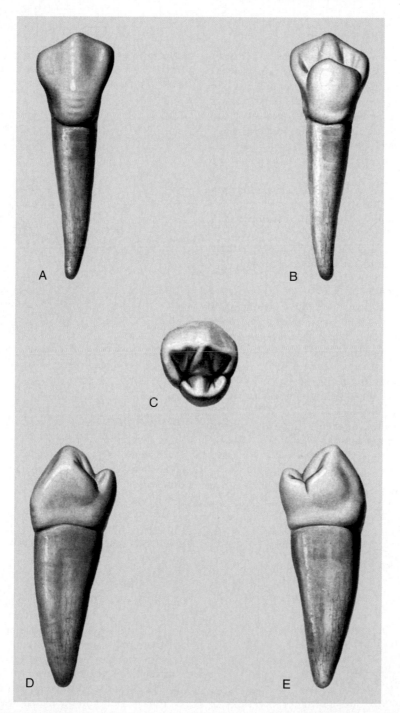

• **Figure 14.15** A mandibular right first premolar. **(A)** Buccal view. **(B)** Lingual view. **(C)** Occlusal view. **(D)** Mesial view. **(E)** Distal view. (Modified from Zeisz RC, Nuckolls J. *Dental Anatomy.* St. Louis, MO: Mosby; 1949.)

As a rule, mandibular first premolars are always smaller than mandibular second premolars. In most cases, this is not true of maxillary premolars.

Mandibular first premolars develop from four lobes, just like maxillary first and second premolars. The three facial lobes form the large buccal cusp, and the single lingual lobe forms into a lingual cusp. This lingual cusp is much smaller than the lingual cusp of maxillary premolars. It is so small in height and width that it does not occlude with any maxillary teeth. It is for this reason that the lingual cusp of mandibular first premolars is considered afunctional. As in the case of maxillary premolars, each cusp has its own pulp horn. How many pulp horns would mandibular first premolars have?

Facial (Buccal) Aspect

A mandibular first premolar resembles a mandibular canine from the facial view (Fig. 14.16; see Fig. 14.15A). This premolar has nearly the same buccolingual measurement as a canine, and like the canine, it has a sharp buccal cusp. The middle buccal lobe is well developed. The mesial cusp ridge is shorter than the distal cusp ridge, but the contact areas are almost at the same level mesially and distally. They are located slightly occlusal to the midpoint of the tooth cervico-incisally. In what third of the tooth are the contact areas located?

A mandibular premolar is more convex than a maxillary premolar at the cervical and middle thirds.

The root of this tooth is usually 3 mm (or more) shorter than that of a mandibular canine.

Developmental depressions are often seen between the three lobes. However, developmental lines are usually not present.

Lingual Aspect (Fig. 14.17; see Fig. 14.15B)

The crown and root of a mandibular first premolar taper lingually. Like a canine, a first premolar is broader mesiodistally on the buccal cusp portion of the tooth than on the part developed from the lingual lobe. The lingual cusp is small in comparison with the buccal cusp.

The occlusal surface slopes toward the lingual side in a cervical direction. On each side of the triangular ridge, mesial and distal occlusal pits can be seen within the fossae.

The most striking and characteristic identifying feature of this tooth is the mesiolingual developmental groove, which separates the mesial marginal ridge from the lingual cusp.

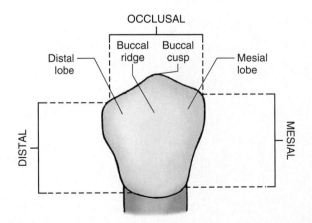

• **Figure 14.16** The buccal surface of a mandibular right first premolar. (Modified from Zeisz RC, Nuckolls J. *Dental Anatomy*. St. Louis, MO: Mosby; 1949.)

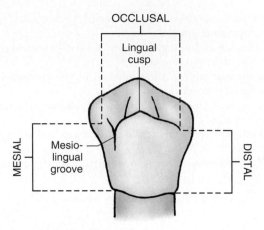

• **Figure 14.17** The lingual surface of a mandibular right first premolar. (Modified from Zeisz RC, Nuckolls J. *Dental Anatomy*. St. Louis, MO: Mosby; 1949.)

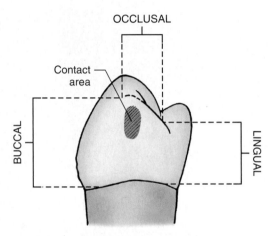

• **Figure 14.18** The mesial surface of a mandibular right first premolar. (Modified from Zeisz RC, Nuckolls J. *Dental Anatomy*. St. Louis, MO: Mosby; 1949.)

Mesial Aspect

From the mesial view (Fig. 14.18; see Fig. 14.15D), the buccal cusp overshadows the smaller lingual cusp. The tip of the buccal cusp is centered directly over the root, and the tip of the lingual cusp is centered lingually to the root. How does this differ from maxillary premolars?

The buccal crest of curvature is located in the cervical third of the crown, the lingual crest near the middle third. The mesiolingual developmental groove can be seen between the mesiobuccal and lingual lobes.

Distal Aspect

The distal view (Fig. 14.19; see Fig. 14.15E) resembles the mesial view, except for the following characteristics:
1. No mesiolingual developmental groove is evident.
2. The distal marginal ridge is much more developed compared with the mesial ridge, and its continuity is unbroken by any deep developmental lines.
3. The curvature of the cervical line is less than the 1 mm and usually found on the mesial line.
4. The distal contact area is broader than the mesial contact area, although it is centered in the same relationship to the crown.

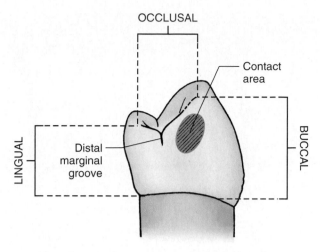

• **Figure 14.19** The distal surface of a mandibular right first premolar. (Modified from Zeisz RC, Nuckolls J. *Dental Anatomy*. St. Louis, MO: Mosby; 1949.)

5. The root exhibits more convexity distally than mesially and rarely shows a developmental groove.
6. A shallow developmental depression, less prominent than on the mesial side, is often found.

Occlusal Aspect

The occlusal aspect (Fig. 14.20; see Fig. 14.15C) displays considerable individual variation. Much more variation exists on either mandibular first or second premolars than on their maxillary counterparts.

The crown converges sharply toward the lingual side, marginal ridges are well developed, and the lingual cusp is small. The buccal cusp shows a heavy facial triangular ridge and a smaller lingual triangular ridge. Two depressions, the mesial and distal fossae, are visible, one on each side of the lingual triangular ridge of the buccal cusp.

Mandibular first premolars are the only premolars that may have a transverse ridge that does not cross an occlusal developmental groove. The mesial developmental groove extends from the mesial fossa lingually, between the mesial marginal ridge and the lingual cusp, and onto the lingual surface. Either fossa may contain a pit. What would the name of these pits be, if they occur? Does a mandibular first premolar always have a central developmental groove?

Root

A mandibular first premolar is normally single rooted. The mesial and distal surfaces are usually slightly convex. If a longitudinal groove is present, then the mesial and distal surfaces may be concave. Occasionally, the two roots present are buccal and lingual. A deep longitudinal groove separates the roots on the proximal sides in such cases.

Pulp Cavity

The pulp cavity of the mandibular first premolar is composed of two pulp horns, a pulp chamber, and a single root canal. The buccal pulp horn is dominant, and the lingual pulp horn is small and insignificant. Each pulp horn is located within a cusp (Fig. 14.21).

Second Premolars

Evidence of calcification: 2.5 years
Enamel completed: 6 to 7 years
Eruption: 11 to 12 years
Root completed: 13 to 14 years

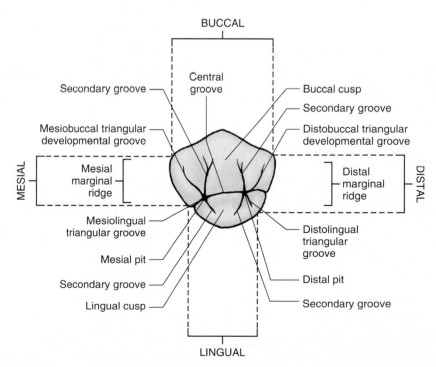

• **Figure 14.20** The occlusal surface of a mandibular right first premolar. A central groove is not always present. (Modified from Zeisz RC, Nuckolls J. *Dental Anatomy*. St. Louis, MO: Mosby; 1949.)

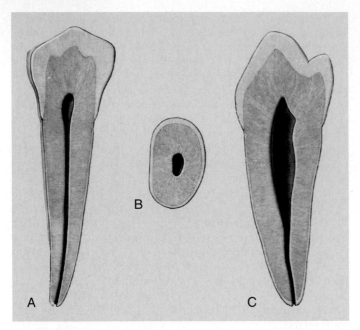

• **Figure 14.21** The pulp cavity of a mandibular right first premolar. **(A)** Mesiodistal section, buccal view. **(B)** Cross section, occlusal view. **(C)** Buccolingual section, mesial view. (Modified from Zeisz RC, Nuckolls J. *Dental Anatomy.* St. Louis, MO: Mosby; 1949.)

A mandibular second premolar (Fig. 14.22) is always larger than a mandibular first premolar. From the labial view, the crown resembles a first premolar in its general shape and in the fact that the contact areas, mesially and distally, are near the same level. The buccal cusp is shorter, however, and the root is longer.

The lingual cusps of a second premolar are much more developed, and both marginal ridges are higher. This produces a more efficient occlusion with its maxillary antagonist. Therefore a mandibular second premolar functions more like a molar than a canine. How does this differ from a mandibular first premolar?

The two common forms of this tooth are the three-cusp and two-cusp types, with one pulp horn in each cusp. The three-cusp form resembles mandibular molars in the following ways:

1. It has two lingual cusps formed from two separate developmental lobes.
2. It has two lingual pulp canals.
3. It has afunctional lingual cusps.
4. It has higher mesial and distal marginal ridges.
5. The marginal ridges function in occlusion, offering more efficient contact and intercuspation of the teeth even though lingual cusps are afunctional.

The single root of a second premolar is larger and longer than that of the first. It is sometimes bifurcated, but this is rare.

Facial (Buccal) Aspect

From the buccal view (Fig. 14.23; see Fig. 14.22A), a mandibular second premolar appears to have a shorter buccal cusp than that of a first premolar. The mesiobuccal and distobuccal cusp ridges are more rounded. The mesial and distal contact areas are broad, and they are located just cervical to the junction of the middle cervical third of the crown. The root is wider mesiodistally and slightly longer, with a blunter apex.

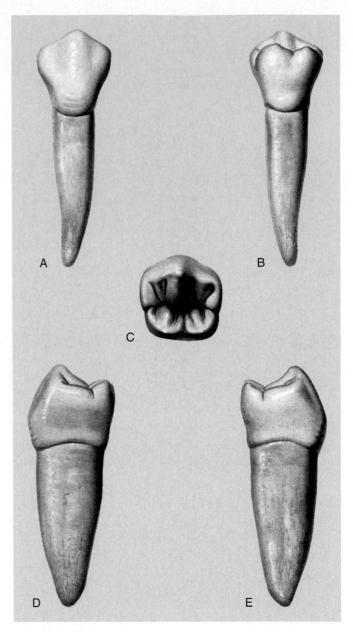

• **Figure 14.22** A mandibular right second premolar. **(A)** Buccal view. **(B)** Lingual view. **(C)** Occlusal view. **(D)** Mesial view. **(E)** Distal view. (Modified from Zeisz RC, Nuckolls J. *Dental Anatomy.* St. Louis, MO: Mosby; 1949.)

Lingual Aspect

The lingual view (Fig. 14.24; see Fig. 14.22B) of a second premolar shows much variation because of the two different cusp forms. In general, however, the following statements are true of a mandibular second premolar compared with the first premolar:

1. The lingual lobes are developed to a greater degree. At least one lingual cusp is longer than a lingual cusp of a first premolar.
2. In the three-cusp form, a **mesiolingual cusp** and a **distolingual cusp** are present. The mesiolingual cusp is usually the wider and longer of the two cusps, which are divided by a lingual groove. Neither of these two cusps comes close to the size of the much larger buccal cusp.
3. In the two-cusp form, the single lingual lobe is higher than on a mandibular first premolar. No groove is on the lingual lobe, as in the three-cusp form, but a developmental depression can

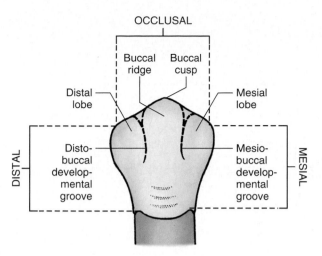

• **Figure 14.23** The buccal surface of a mandibular right second premolar. (Modified from Zeisz RC, Nuckolls J. *Dental Anatomy*. St. Louis, MO: Mosby; 1949.)

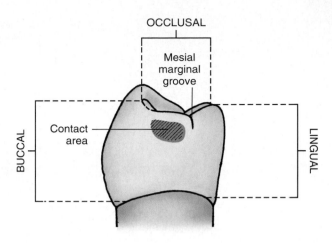

• **Figure 14.25** The mesial surface of a mandibular right second premolar. (Modified from Zeisz RC, Nuckolls J. *Dental Anatomy*. St. Louis, MO: Mosby; 1949.)

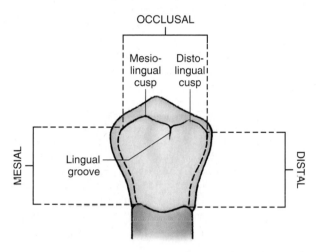

• **Figure 14.24** The lingual surface of a mandibular right second premolar. (Modified from Zeisz RC, Nuckolls J. *Dental Anatomy*. St. Louis, MO: Mosby; 1949.)

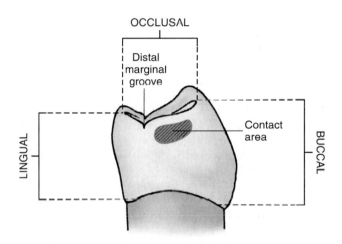

• **Figure 14.26** The distal surface of a mandibular right second premolar. (Modified from Zeisz RC, Nuckolls J. *Dental Anatomy*. St. Louis, MO: Mosby; 1949.)

be seen distolingually where the lingual cusp ridge joins the distal marginal ridge.

4. The lingual surface of the root is wider than that of a first premolar. Thus the convergence of the root toward the lingual side is less. This is true even though the root is wider buccally because the root is much wider lingually than on a first premolar, resulting in less convergence toward the lingual side.

The lingual portions of the crown and the root are slightly convex.

Mesial Aspect (Fig. 14.25; see Fig. 14.22D)

A second premolar differs mesially from a first premolar in the following ways:

1. The buccal cusp is shorter, and its tip is located more to the buccal side.
2. The crown and root are wider buccolingually.
3. The lingual lobe shows more development.
4. The marginal ridge is at a right angle to the long axis of the tooth.

5. No mesiolingual developmental groove is evident.
6. The root is longer, and the apex is blunter.

Distal Aspect

From the distal view (Fig. 14.26; see also Fig. 14.22E) more of the occlusal surface can be seen because the distal marginal ridge is at a lower level compared with the mesial marginal ridge.

As a general rule, the crowns of all posterior teeth, maxillary or mandibular, are tipped distally to the long axis of the root. Thus if a specimen is held vertically, more of the occlusal surface of a posterior tooth can be seen from the distal aspect. Another general rule is that more roots of posterior teeth tip toward the distal side. In other words, the apex of the root curves distally.

Occlusal Aspect (Fig. 14.27; see also Fig. 14.22C)

In both the two- and three-cusp forms, the buccal cusp is similar. In the three-cusp form, the buccal cusp is the largest, the mesiolingual cusp the next largest, and the distolingual cusp the smallest.

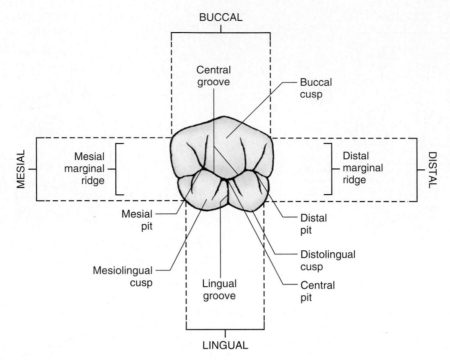

BUCCAL

Central groove

Buccal cusp

MESIAL

Mesial marginal ridge

Distal marginal ridge

DISTAL

Mesial pit

Distal pit

Distolingual cusp

Mesiolingual cusp

Lingual groove

Central pit

LINGUAL

• **Figure 14.27** The occlusal surface of a mandibular right second premolar (three-cusp variety). (Modified from Zeisz RC, Nuckolls J. *Dental Anatomy.* St. Louis, MO: Mosby; 1949.)

Each of the three cusps has a well-developed triangular ridge separated by deep developmental grooves. These grooves form a wide pattern on the occlusal surface. The three developmental grooves are the mesial, distal, and lingual grooves. Three pits may be present: central, mesial, and distal. Of the three, the central pit is the most likely to be present. Mesial and distal **triangular fossae** are also present.

Supplemental grooves are more commonly found on a second premolar than on a first, and the developmental grooves are usually not so deep.

In the two-cusp type, compared with the three-cusp type, the following can be observed:

1. The occlusal outline of the crown is more rounded.
2. The lingual surface of the crown is more convex and tapers toward lingually.
3. No lingual developmental groove is present.
4. Only one well-developed lingual cusp is on the two-cusp form, and it is located directly opposite the buccal cusp in a lingual direction.
5. Usually, no central pit is present; a mesial or distal pit is much more likely.

In the three-cusp type, the groove pattern is commonly called a *Y-groove pattern*. In the two-cusp type, the groove pattern can be either a *U-groove pattern* (sometimes called a *C-groove pattern*) or *H-groove pattern* (Figs. 14.28 through 14.30), depending on whether the central developmental groove is straight mesiodistally or curves buccally at its ends. The central groove of the two-cusp form terminates in the mesial and distal fossae. If lingual triangular grooves radiate from these fossae, the H-groove pattern is present.

The Y-groove pattern as seen in the three-cusp form is, by far, the most dominant form, occurring with much more frequency compared with the two-cusp forms. Of the less prevalent two-cusp forms, the H-groove pattern is more common than the U-groove pattern.

According to Julian Woelfel, as discussed in his text *Dental Anatomy: Its Relevance to Dentistry,* 43% of mandibular second premolars have two cusps, 54.2% have three cusps, and 2.8% have four cusps. His sample comprised 1532 specimens.

As a rule, second premolars and second molars have shallower developmental grooves compared with first premolars and first molars. They also have more secondary grooves. In general, the more posterior the tooth, the more wrinkled it appears.

Root

The root of the mandibular second premolar is similar to that of the first premolar. It is longer and wider buccolingually. It has no tendency to bifurcate, as the mandibular first premolar sometimes does.

The distal surface of the root of both premolars, first and second, is more likely to have a longitudinal depression in the middle third. The mesial surface is far less likely to have such a longitudinal depression. This is just the reverse of maxillary premolars.

Pulp Cavity

The pulp cavity (Fig. 14.31) of the mandibular second premolar shows two pointed pulp horns and three in the three-cusp variety. The pulp horns are more pointed than in the mandibular first premolar. A single root canal is present, with even less tendency to have divided root canals than in the first premolar.

Pertinent Data

Mandibular First Premolars

	Right	Left
Universal code	28	21
International code	44	34
Palmer notation:	4⌋	⌊4

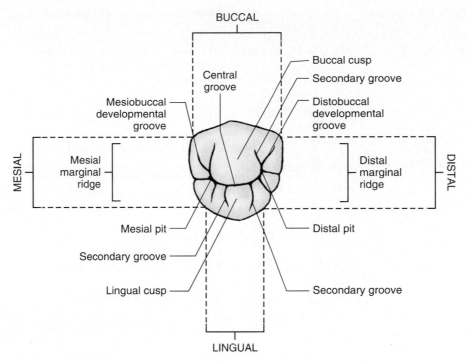

• **Figure 14.28** Occlusal surface, U-groove (two-cusp variety). (Modified from Zeisz RC, Nuckolls J. *Dental Anatomy.* St. Louis, MO: Mosby; 1949.)

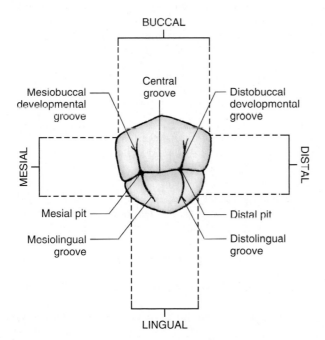

• **Figure 14.29** Occlusal surface, H-groove (two-cusp variety). (Modified from Zeisz RC, Nuckolls J. *Dental Anatomy.* St. Louis, MO: Mosby; 1949.)

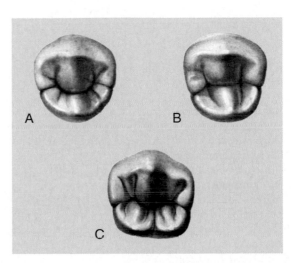

• **Figure 14.30** Occlusal views. **(A)** U-groove. **(B)** H-groove. **(C)** Y-groove. (Modified from Zeisz RC, Nuckolls J. *Dental Anatomy.* St. Louis, MO: Mosby; 1949.)

Number of roots: 1
Number of pulp horns: 1 or 2
Number of cusps: 2
Number of developmental lobes: 4

Location of Proximal Contact Areas

Mesial: Just cervical to junction of occlusal and middle thirds
Distal: Just cervical to junction of occlusal and middle thirds

Height of Contour

Facial: Cervical third, 0.5 mm
Lingual: Middle third, 1 mm

Identifying Characteristics

Mandibular first premolars have two cusps—one large buccal cusp and one small lingual cusp. The buccal cusp is centered directly over the root. The lingual cusp is centered lingual to the root and is afunctional and nonoccluding. The occlusal surface slopes sharply lingual in a cervical direction. The mesiobuccal cusp ridge is shorter than the distobuccal cusp ridge. It has a mesiolingual developmental groove and one root.

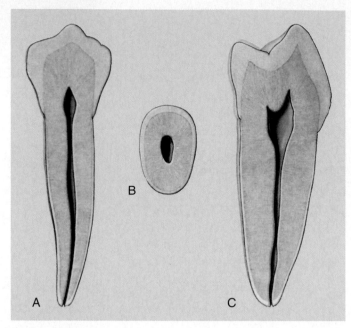

• **Figure 14.31** The pulp cavity of a mandibular right second premolar. **(A)** Mesiodistal section, buccal view. **(B)** Cross section, occlusal view. **(C)** Buccolingual section, mesial view. (Modified from Zeisz RC, Nuckolls J. *Dental Anatomy*. St. Louis, MO: Mosby; 1949.)

Mandibular Second Premolars

	Right	Left
Universal code	29	20
International code	45	35
Palmer notation:	5⌋	⌊5

Number of roots: 1
Number of pulp horns: 2 or 3
Number of cusps: 2 or 3
Number of developmental lobes: 4 or 5

Location of Proximal Contact Areas
Mesial: Just cervical to junction of occlusal and middle thirds
Distal: Just cervical to junction of occlusal and middle thirds

Height of Contour
Facial: Cervical third, 0.5 mm
Lingual: Middle third, 1 mm

Identifying Characteristics
Mandibular second premolars have two or three cusps. The buccal cusp is very large. If two lingual cusps are present, the mesiolingual is the larger of the two. Although the lingual cusps are larger than on the first premolar, they are afunctional and do not occlude with maxillary teeth. A second premolar has more secondary anatomic features and more variation than any other tooth except a third molar. The two-cusp form has a U-groove or H-groove pattern. A mesiolingual groove is rare and poorly developed if present. The three-cusp form has a lingual developmental groove between the two lingual cusps. The single root is longer and larger than that of a first premolar.

Review Questions

1. In which way is a maxillary second premolar different from a maxillary first premolar?
   a. number of developmental lobes
   b. size of cusps and number of roots
   c. existence of a central groove
   d. location of proximal contacts
2. Which of the following *best* describes the functional cusp(s) of a mandibular first premolar?
   a. both facial and lingual
   b. facial
   c. lingual
   d. neither facial nor lingual
3. Which tooth in the human dentition is most likely to be derived from five developmental lobes?
   a. maxillary right first premolar
   b. maxillary right second premolar
   c. mandibular left first premolar
   d. mandibular right second premolar
4. In comparing mandibular and maxillary first premolars
   a. the facial cusp of a mandibular premolar is more lingually located
   b. the lingual cusp is more facially located
   c. the occlusal surface of a mandibular first premolar is relatively large
   d. the occlusal outline is wider mesiodistally in the lingual portion of the mandibular first premolar
5. A maxillary first premolar may be identified by
   a. a noticeable mesial concavity in the cervical area
   b. rounded cusps of nearly equal height
   c. long supplemental grooves
   d. a single root canal
6. Which of the following *best* describes the location of the proximal contacts of a maxillary second premolar?
   a. just cervical to the junction of the occlusal and middle thirds
   b. just occlusal to the junction of the cervical and middle thirds
   c. just cervical to the junction of the cervical and middle thirds
   d. just occlusal to the junction of the occlusal and middle thirds
7. Mandibular first and second premolars are distinguished with respect to
   a. the usual number of cusps
   b. the average number of root canals in 100 specimens
   c. the cervico-incisal location of proximal contacts
   d. the number of developmental lobes forming the facial portion
8. Usually, the most striking identifying characteristic of a mandibular first premolar is which of the following grooves?
   a. central
   b. mesiolingual
   c. faciolingual
   d. mesial

9. Which of the following groove patterns is the most dominant form of mandibular second premolars?
   a. Y-groove
   b. C-groove
   c. H-groove
   d. U-groove
10. When the triangular ridge of the buccal cusp joins the triangular ridge of the lingual cusp, it is known as
   a. triangular ridge
   b. marginal ridge
   c. transverse ridge
   d. occlusal ridge
11. One permanent premolar has the most pronounced cervical concavity of any of the premolars, which requires special consideration when restoring it. The premolar and the proximal surface where the concavity is located is the
   a. distal surface of a mandibular second premolar
   b. mesial surface of a maxillary first premolar
   c. distal surface of a maxillary second premolar
   d. mesial surface of a maxillary second premolar
12. Which of the permanent premolars often has fewer pulp horns than the other premolars?
   a. maxillary first premolar
   b. maxillary second premolar
   c. mandibular first premolar
   d. mandibular second premolar
13. A cusp has how many ridges?
   a. 2
   b. 3
   c. 4
   d. 5
14. If you examined an extracted premolar tooth and found a single root, a symmetric rounded effect of the crown in all aspects, and many secondary grooves arising from the central groove, you could assume it to be a
   a. maxillary first premolar
   b. maxillary second premolar
   c. mandibular first premolar
   d. mandibular second premolar
15. A premolar with a root that is most commonly bifurcated is a
   a. maxillary first premolar
   b. mandibular first premolar
   c. maxillary second premolar
   d. mandibular second premolar
16. Which of the following is true concerning longitudinal grooves?
   a. They are often present on the mesial and distal sides of maxillary second premolars.
   b. They are more common on the distal side of mandibular premolars than the mesial side.
   c. They are usually present on maxillary premolars.
   d. All of the above.

True or False

17. Posterior teeth are wider buccolingually compared with anterior teeth.
18. Mandibular premolars have functional lingual cusps.
19. Posterior teeth are higher cervico-occlusally compared with anterior teeth.
20. Mesial and distal contact areas of premolars are broader than the contact areas of anterior teeth.

15

Molars

OBJECTIVES

- To understand the lobe formations of the crowns of molars
- To compare the formations of first, second, and third molars
- To understand the anchorage of the roots as resistance to forces of displacement
- To describe the details of the various molars
- To make comparisons among the various molars: maxillary and mandibular molars, as well as first, second, and third molars
- To identify each molar

The 12 permanent molars are the largest and strongest teeth in the mouth by virtue of their crown bulk size and root anchorage in bone (Fig. 15.1). Their primary function is to grind or crush food.

Permanent molars erupt long after all deciduous teeth have already erupted. First permanent molars erupt distal to the primary second molars. In humans, usually the first permanent teeth to erupt are first molars. It is only after these molars have erupted that permanent incisors begin replacing deciduous incisors.

The following chart shows the approximate eruption time for molars. However, much individual variation occurs. Which teeth usually erupt first, mandibular teeth or maxillary teeth? Usually mandibular teeth develop and erupt slightly before maxillary teeth. The maxillary third molar is usually the last to complete formation.

Eruption Times of Molars

	Eruption	Enamel Completion	Root Completion	Begins Calcification	Lobes
First molar	6–7 years	2.5–4 years	9–10 years	Birth	5
Second molar	11–13 years	7–8 years	14–16 years	2.5 years	4
Third molar	17–22 years	12–16 years	18–25 years	7–10 years	4

Molars are nonsuccedaneous teeth—that is, they do not replace any primary teeth. They are referred to as **accessional**, or nonsuccedaneous, as opposed to succedaneous teeth, which do replace deciduous teeth.

Generally, first molars are formed from five lobes, but some second and third molars may have only four lobes. Five lobes are numbered in Fig. 15.2. These lobes vary in size; the smallest one is absent on second molars.

In general, each cusp of a molar is formed from its own lobe. For instance, a maxillary first molar forms from five lobes, three of which form major cusps. These major cusps are large and well developed, characteristic of, and usually present on, all maxillary molars: first, second, and third. The fourth lobe on a maxillary first molar forms a minor cusp. A minor cusp has smaller proportions and less development. It is less functional than the major cusps and is not always present on second and third molars. Maxillary first molars have a fifth lobe, which develops into a supplementary cusp. A supplementary cusp is completely afunctional and is not usually present on either second or third molars. First molars are the most highly developed and largest of molars and are more likely to have minor and supplementary cusps in addition to their major cusp.

Maxillary molars have only three major cusps, one minor cusp, and sometimes one supplementary cusp. Mandibular molars usually have four major cusps and sometimes one minor cusp (see Chapter 10, Figs. 10.34 and Fig. 10.35 as well as Fig. 10.40).

The distolingual cusps are the minor cusps of maxillary teeth; but, an even smaller fifth cusp, a supplemental cusp (cusp of Carabelli), occurs on a maxillary first molar. However, it may not be present at all or it may exhibit a smaller presence on second and third maxillary molars as well.

The minor cusps of mandibular molars are the distal cusps. The minor cusps are usually present in both maxillary and mandibular first molars. However, these minor cusps are not always present on second and third molars.

The fifth cusp of maxillary molars, which is a supplemental cusp (actually a tubercle rather than a full cusp), is also more prominent on maxillary first molars. It diminishes in size on second and third molars, if present at all. The difference between a minor cusp and a supplemental cusp is that the minor cusp is an actual cusp, not a tubercle. Minor cusps are not always present on second and third molars, but when they are, they are actual cusps.

In review, the most developed of molars are first molars, whether maxillary or mandibular. Second molars usually have no supplementary cusps, and minor cusps are even more minor in relation to major cusps. Third molars may not develop minor cusps at all. A maxillary third molar may have only three major cusps, or a mandibular third molar may have four major cusps.

Maxillary Molars

First Molars

Evidence of calcification: Birth
Enamel completed: 3 to 4 years
Eruption: 6 to 7 years
Root completed: 9 to 10 years

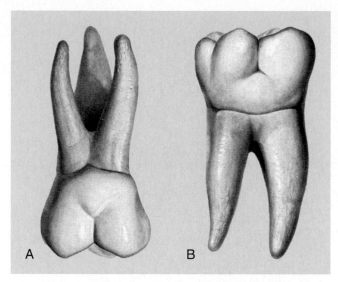

• **Figure 15.1** **(A)** Maxillary first molar. **(B)** Mandibular first molar. (Modified from Zeisz RC, Nuckolls J. *Dental Anatomy*. St. Louis, MO: Mosby; 1949.)

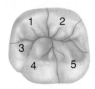

• **Figure 15.2** Lobes of permanent first molars. (From Nelson SJ, Ash M. *Wheeler's Dental Anatomy*. 9th ed. St. Louis, MO: Saunders; 2010.)

Maxillary first molars (Fig. 15.3) are normally the largest teeth in the maxillary arch. The three molars on each side are first, second, and third maxillary molars. Each has three well-developed major cusps and one minor cusp, all of which are functional. The fifth or supplemental cusp, which is afunctional, is called the *cusp* or *tubercle of Carabelli*. This fifth cusp is usually found on all maxillary first molars. The five cusps are formed from five lobes.

The crown of a first molar is broad mesiodistally and buccolingually and just slightly wider buccolingually than mesiodistally. Of the four functional cusps, two are on the buccal side and two are on the lingual side.

Facial (Buccal) Aspect

From the buccal view (Fig. 15.4; see Fig. 15.3A), four cusps can usually be seen: mesiobuccal, distobuccal, mesiolingual, and distolingual. The two lingual cusps are not located directly behind the buccal cusps but are distal and lingual to them. Although the mesiobuccal cusp is broader than the distobuccal cusp, the latter is usually sharper and longer.

The buccal developmental groove divides the two buccal cusps. This groove runs in a line parallel to the long axis of the tooth, terminating halfway from its point of origin to the cervical line of the crown. Although not very deep at any point, at its terminal end, it splits into a buccal pit, with two small grooves radiating from it. The cervical line is irregular and curved, generally toward the occlusal side at the mesial and distal ends.

The mesial outline is straight from the cervical line to the mesial contact area. Below the contact area, it curves distally until it reaches the mesiobuccal cusp tip. The height of curvature is just cervical to the junction of the middle and occlusal thirds. Distally, the outline of the crown is convex, and the contact area is in the center of the middle third.

Lingual Aspect

The lingual cusps alone can be seen from the lingual aspect (Fig. 15.5; see Fig. 15.3B). The mesiolingual cusp is much longer and larger than either of the buccal cusps. Wider mesiodistally and buccolingually, the mesiofacial cusp is the next largest, although it is not as long as the distofacial cusp. The distolingual cusp is the smallest and the shortest of the functional cusps. Of course, the cusp of Carabelli is the shortest and smallest of all five cusps, but it is afunctional. In fact, the cusp of Carabelli is not a cusp at all but rather a tubercle. A **fifth-cusp developmental groove**, called the **mesiolingual groove**, separates the cusp of Carabelli from the mesiolingual cusp. To review, the mesiolingual cusps are the largest; the mesiofacial next largest; then the distofacial cusps; finally the cusp of Carabelli, if present at all.

The outline of the crown is as straight mesially as it is buccally. The distal outline is more convex because of the roundness of the distolingual cusp. The **lingual developmental groove** extends from the center of the lingual surface occlusally, between the two lingual cusps, where it curves sharply to the distal side and becomes the **distal oblique groove**. These two grooves (lingual and distal oblique grooves) are sometimes considered to be one and are then referred to as the **distolingual developmental groove**.

The distolingual cusp of a maxillary first molar is functional, even though it is small. On a first molar, the distolingual cusp occupies approximately 40% of the lingual surface, and the mesiolingual cusp occupies the other 60%. The distolingual cusp is progressively smaller on maxillary second and third molars.

All three roots can be seen from the lingual aspect. On average, roots are almost twice as long as the crown. The lingual root is usually longer than either of the two buccal roots, which are the same length.

Mesial Aspect

The mesial aspect (Fig. 15.6; see Fig. 15.3D) of a maxillary first molar usually shows a clear profile of the cusp of Carabelli. The lingual crest of curvature is at the center of the middle third of the crown, the buccal crest at the cervical third. The cervical line is slightly convex mesially.

Distal Aspect (Fig. 15.7; see Fig. 15.3E)

The crown has a tendency to taper distally. The buccolingual measurement of the crown on the mesial side is greater than the same measurement distally. The distal cervical line is usually straighter and less curved than that on the mesial side. Although the distal surface of the crown is convex and smooth, a slight concavity is evident on the distal surface of the root trunk from the cervical line to the distobuccal root.

The distal marginal ridge is shorter and less prominent than the mesial marginal ridge, and more of the occlusal surface, in general, can be seen from the distal view. The distobuccal root is the narrowest of all three roots.

Occlusal Aspect

A maxillary first molar has a rhomboidal occlusal outline (Fig. 15.8; see Fig. 15.3C). The molar crown is wider mesially than distally; it is also wider lingually than buccally. This is the only tooth that is wider lingually than buccally. Is the occlusal outline of a maxillary first molar more like a square or more like

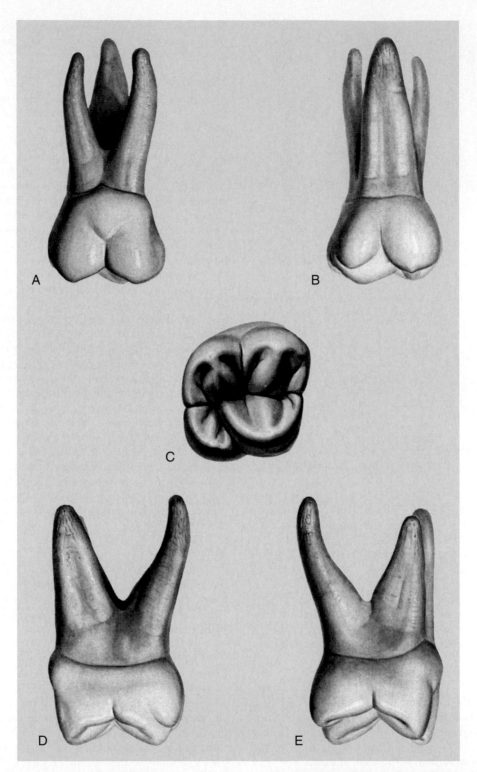

• **Figure 15.3**   A maxillary right first molar. **(A)** Buccal view. **(B)** Lingual view. **(C)** Occlusal view. **(D)** Mesial view. **(E)** Distal view. (Modified from Zeisz RC, Nuckolls J. *Dental Anatomy.* St. Louis, MO: Mosby; 1949.)

a square that has been squashed sideways? What is the difference between a rhomboidal form and a square form?

Other Anatomic Structures

Two major fossae and two minor fossae are found on maxillary first molars. The major fossae are the **central fossa**, which is mesial to the oblique ridge, and the **distal fossa**, which is distal to the oblique ridge. The minor fossae are the **mesial fossa** and the **distal triangular fossa**, both of which are located on the inside of their respective marginal ridges.

The **central developmental pit** lies in the central fossa. The **buccal developmental groove** radiates from this pit buccally between the two buccal cusps. The central developmental groove lies in a mesial direction, originating in the central developmental pit

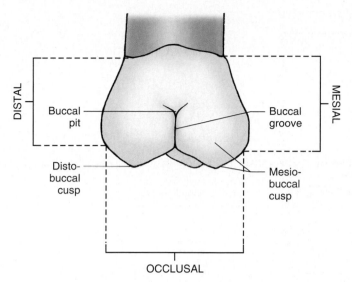

• **Figure 15.4** The buccal surface of a maxillary right first molar. (Modified from Zeisz RC, Nuckolls J. *Dental Anatomy.* St. Louis, MO: Mosby; 1949.)

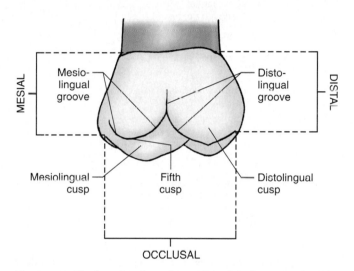

• **Figure 15.5** The lingual surface of a maxillary right first molar. A triangular groove is a developmental groove that separates a marginal ridge from the triangular ridge of a cusp. (Modified from Zeisz RC, Nuckolls J. *Dental Anatomy.* St. Louis, MO: Mosby; 1949.)

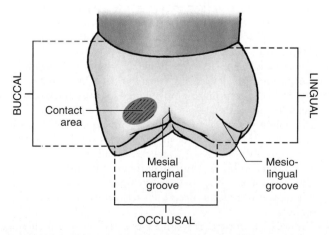

• **Figure 15.6** The mesial surface of a maxillary right first molar. (Modified from Zeisz RC, Nuckolls J. *Dental Anatomy.* St. Louis, MO: Mosby; 1949.)

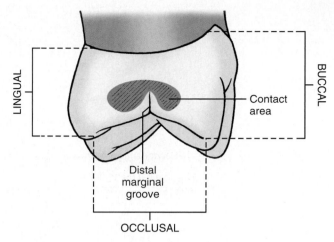

• **Figure 15.7** The distal surface of a maxillary right first molar. (Modified from Zeisz RC, Nuckolls J. *Dental Anatomy.* St. Louis, MO: Mosby; 1949.)

and terminating at the mesial triangular fossa. Here it is joined by the mesiofacial and mesiolingual triangular grooves, which appear as branches of the **central groove**. The mesial marginal groove, a branch of the central groove, lies between these two triangular grooves and may cross the mesial marginal ridge of the crown. The **mesial pit** is found in the mesial triangular fossa.

Sometimes a secondary developmental groove radiates from the central pit in a distal direction. If it crosses the oblique ridge, joining the central and distal fossae, it is called the **transverse groove of the oblique ridge** or the distal groove and it joins the central and distal pits.

The **oblique ridge** is a transverse ridge and is unique to maxillary molars. A transverse ridge is formed by two triangular ridges joining together and crossing the surface of a posterior tooth diagonally rather than straight across buccolingually. In this case the triangular ridge of the mesiolingual cusp joins the triangular ridge of the distobuccal cusp. This cannot happen unless the ridges cross the tooth transversely, as opposed to buccolingually. Therefore the oblique ridge runs from the tip of the mesiolingual cusp to the tip of the distobuccal cusp.

The distal fossa of a maxillary first molar runs parallel with and distal to the oblique ridge. This fossa is long and narrow rather than circular. In this fossa lies the distal oblique groove from which it takes its shape. The **distal pit** is found in the distal fossa.

The distal triangular fossa is mesial to the distal marginal ridge. The distal oblique groove terminates in the distal triangular fossa, where the distal oblique groove gives off three branches: the distofacial triangular groove, the distolingual triangular groove, and the **distal marginal groove**.

The primary grooves of maxillary first molars are as follows:
1. Facial groove
2. Central groove (two parts: mesial and distal)
3. Distolingual groove (two parts: lingual and distal oblique grooves)
4. Mesiolingual groove (cusp of Carabelli groove)
5. Mesial marginal groove
6. Distal marginal groove
7. Mesiofacial triangular groove
8. Mesiolingual triangular groove
9. Distolingual triangular groove
10. Distofacial triangular groove

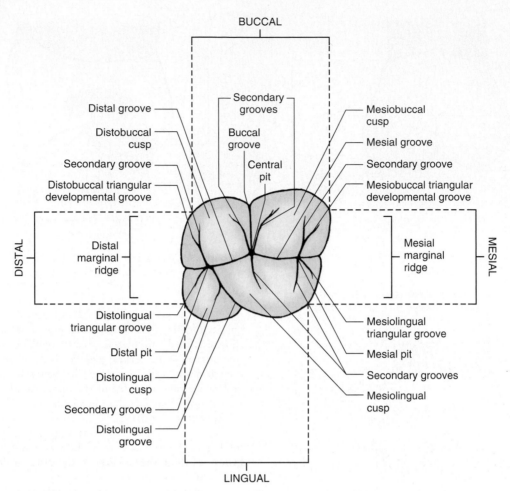

BUCCAL

Distal groove

Distobuccal
cusp

Secondary groove

Distobuccal triangular
developmental groove

Secondary
grooves

Buccal
groove

Central
pit

Mesiobuccal
cusp

Mesial groove

Secondary groove

Mesiobuccal triangular
developmental groove

DISTAL

MESIAL

Distal
marginal
ridge

Mesial
marginal
ridge

Distolingual
triangular groove

Distal pit

Distolingual
cusp

Secondary groove

Distolingual
groove

Mesiolingual
triangular groove

Mesial pit

Secondary grooves

Mesiolingual
cusp

LINGUAL

• **Figure 15.8** The occlusal surface of a maxillary right first molar. The mesial marginal groove crosses the mesial marginal ridge above. (Modified from Zeisz RC, Nuckolls J. *Dental Anatomy.* St. Louis, MO: Mosby; 1949.)

As a point of clarification, it should be mentioned that triangular grooves are primary grooves that separate a marginal ridge from the triangular ridge of a cusp. These triangular grooves end in a triangular fossa. When studying the central groove, note that the triangular groove is a continuation of the central groove. As the central groove goes toward the marginal ridge, it separates into two or three branches. The two outer Y-shaped branches curve between the marginal ridge and triangular ridges of the buccal and lingual cusps. The part of the groove that lies between the cusp ridge and marginal ridge is the triangular groove. The two triangular grooves are bisected by a third groove, which lies between them. This groove connects with the marginal ridge and is called the *marginal groove. If this is not clear, review Chapter 2 (see Fig. 2.31).*

Second Molars

Evidence of calcification: to 3 years
Enamel completed: 7 to 8 years
Eruption: 12 to 13 years
Root completed: 14 to 16 years
A maxillary second molar (Fig. 15.9) supplements a first molar's function. Generally, the differences that occur between first and second molars are even more accentuated between first and third

molars. In other words, certain characteristics in form and development that occur in a first molar occur to a lesser degree in a second molar and possibly not at all in a third molar. What are these characteristics? Following is a list of several traits that may occur, but in general, they tend to be more accentuated in a second molar and most accentuated in a third molar.

1. The crowns of maxillary molars are shorter occlusocervically and narrower mesiodistally in second molars than in first molars. Third molars continue to be smaller in all crown proportions, including buccolingually.
2. The crowns of molars show more **supplemental (secondary) grooves** and pits on second molars than on first molars. Third molars show even more supplemental grooves and **accidental (tertiary) grooves** and pits.
3. The oblique ridge is less prominent on second molars and, in some instances, disappears almost entirely on third molars.
4. The fifth lobe, or cusp of Carabelli, usually disappears on second molars and occurs infrequently on third molars.
5. The distolingual cusp is less developed on maxillary second molars and disappears almost entirely on most maxillary third molars.
6. The occlusal outline of second molars is less rhomboidal and more heart shaped. A third molar is even more heart shaped in occlusal outline.

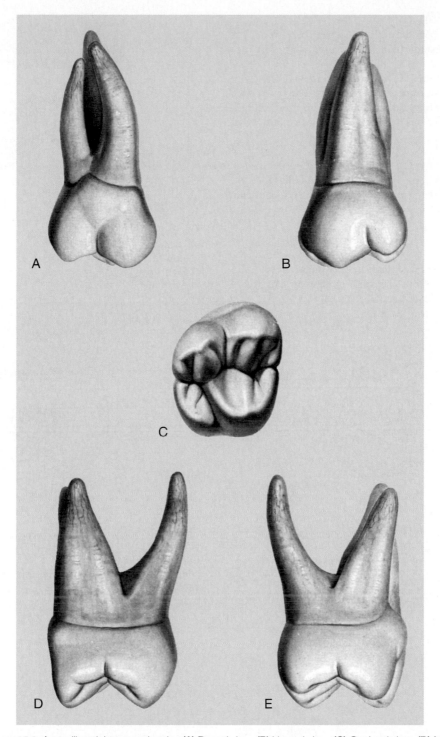

• **Figure 15.9** A maxillary right second molar. **(A)** Buccal view. **(B)** Lingual view. **(C)** Occlusal view. **(D)** Mesial view. **(E)** Distal view. (Modified from Zeisz RC, Nuckolls J. *Dental Anatomy.* St. Louis, MO: Mosby; 1949.)

7. The roots of second molars tend to lie closer together and may even be fused.
8. The mesiobuccal roots of second and third molars have a greater tendency to curve distally in their apical third. The distobuccal root of a maxillary second molar is straighter than that of a maxillary first molar, with little or no mesial curvature. The third molar's distobuccal root tends to curve distally in its apical third.

9. The roots of second molars are almost as long and sometimes even longer than those of first molars. The roots of third molars are almost always smaller than those of either first or second molars.
10. Second molars show more variety of form than first molars, not only in the crown but also in root development. The third molars show unlimited variety in crown and root formations and are often congenitally missing.

Facial (Buccal) Aspect *(Fig. 15.10; see Fig. 15.9A)*

The crown of a maxillary second molar is shorter cervico-occlusally and narrower mesiodistally than that of a maxillary first molar. The distobuccal cusp also is smaller.

The buccal roots are about the same length as each other and are closer together. The distobuccal root is straighter up and down than that of the maxillary first molar, and it has no mesial curvature. The mesiobuccal root has a greater curvature distally at its apical third.

Lingual Aspect

The lingual view (Fig. 15.11; see Fig. 15.9B) of a maxillary second molar shows no fifth cusp (cusp of Carabelli). The distolingual cusp is smaller than that of first molars.

Mesial Aspect

The mesial view (Fig. 15.12; see also Fig. 15.9D) shows the second molar crown to be shorter than the first molar, but its buccolingual measurement is about the same as that of a maxillary first molar. The roots are closer together.

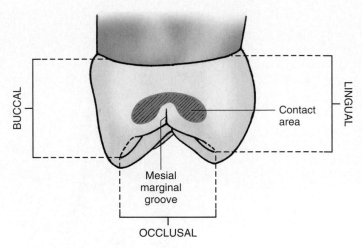

• **Figure 15.12** The mesial surface of a maxillary right second molar. (Modified from Zeisz RC, Nuckolls J. *Dental Anatomy*. St. Louis, MO: Mosby; 1949.)

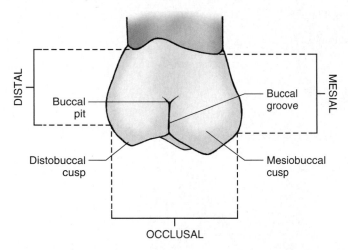

• **Figure 15.10** The buccal surface of a maxillary right second molar. (Modified from Zeisz RC, Nuckolls J. *Dental Anatomy*. St. Louis, MO: Mosby; 1949.)

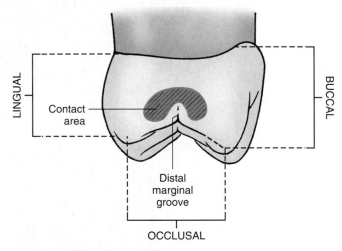

• **Figure 15.13** The distal surface of a maxillary right second molar. (Modified from Zeisz RC, Nuckolls J. *Dental Anatomy*. St. Louis, MO: Mosby; 1949.)

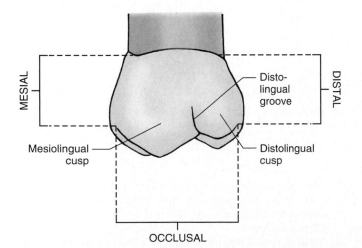

• **Figure 15.11** The lingual surface of a maxillary right second molar. Usually no cusp of Carabelli is present. (Modified from Zeisz RC, Nuckolls J. *Dental Anatomy*. St. Louis, MO: Mosby; 1949.)

Distal Aspect

The distobuccal cusp is smaller than the mesiobuccal cusp, thus more of the mesiobuccal cusp can be seen from the distal view (Fig. 15.13; see Fig. 15.9E).

Occlusal Aspect

The occlusal outline (Fig. 15.14; see Fig. 15.9C) of the crown of a maxillary second molar is less rhomboidal than that of a maxillary first molar. The increase in the size of the mesiolingual cusp and the absence of the cusp of Carabelli make this possible. Another reason is that the distolingual cusp is smaller.

The mesiodistal diameter of the crown is smaller, but the buccolingual diameter is about the same as that of a maxillary first molar.

Mesiobuccal and mesiolingual cusps are just as developed as in a first molar. The distobuccal cusp is just barely smaller, and the distolingual cusp is noticeably smaller.

More supplemental grooves and pits are present on a maxillary second molar than on a maxillary first molar.

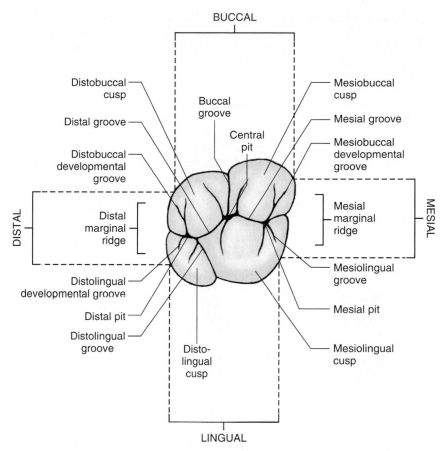

BUCCAL

Distobuccal cusp

Distal groove

Distobuccal developmental groove

DISTAL

Distal marginal ridge

Distolingual developmental groove

Distal pit

Distolingual groove

Disto-lingual cusp

Buccal groove

Central pit

Mesiobuccal cusp

Mesial groove

Mesiobuccal developmental groove

Mesial marginal ridge

MESIAL

Mesiolingual groove

Mesial pit

Mesiolingual cusp

LINGUAL

• **Figure 15.14** An occlusal view of a maxillary second molar. Usually shows a much less prominent oblique ridge if present at all. (Modified from Zeisz RC, Nuckolls J. *Dental Anatomy.* St. Louis, MO: Mosby; 1949.)

Third Molars

Evidence of calcification: 7 to 9 years
Enamel completed: 12 to 16 years
Eruption: 17 to 22 years
Root completed: 18 to 25 years

A maxillary third molar varies more than any other maxillary tooth in size, shape, and relative position to other teeth. Rarely is it as well developed as a maxillary second molar. It often appears as a developmental anomaly or does not form at all. What term is descriptive of the latter situation?

The crown of a third molar is shorter than that of a second molar, and the roots tend to fuse into one. The occlusal outline of a maxillary third molar is heart shaped. The distolingual cusp is poorly developed or even absent (Fig. 15.15).

Third molars tend to become impacted. If a tooth does not erupt because it is obstructed by bone or another tooth, or if it is prevented from eruption because of the angle at which it is situated within bone, it is said to be impacted. Third molars, maxillary or mandibular, have a greater tendency to be impacted than any other teeth. The impaction of third molars is, to a large extent, caused by an underdeveloped jaw, which has insufficient space to accommodate them. Thus they are blocked out and prevented from erupting.

The need for third molars was critical in our human ancestors. The eruption of third molars helped push together the remaining teeth, which was especially necessary if a portion of a tooth or a whole tooth was lost through attrition or accident. Prehistoric

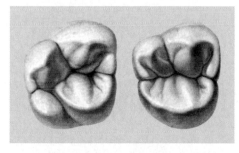

• **Figure 15.15** Occlusal surfaces of maxillary right third molars. (Modified from Zeisz RC, Nuckolls J. *Dental Anatomy.* St. Louis, MO: Mosby; 1949.)

humans wore down the occlusal surfaces of their crowns to a flat plane without cusps. This not only shortened the height of their crowns, but it made their teeth narrower mesiodistally. When wear occurred past their proximal contacts, their teeth accumulatively occupied less space and allowed more room for the eruption of their third molars. This wear and attrition was caused by primitive human's very coarse diet, which contained grit, sand, and bone fragments. This also required a lot more muscular action as well, and thus their jaws were more developed and their arch length was greater, allowing more space to accommodate more space for the erupted teeth. This extra space allowed third molars more room to erupt. In prehistoric times, impacted molars could easily lead to fatal outcomes.

With advancing civilization, survival became less dependent on preserving one's teeth. More and more humans survived without third molars. Today the congenital absence of third molars presents no problem whatsoever. Congenitally missing third molars are a modern genetic trend and an increasingly dominant feature in humans. More and more humans will never have one or more third molars formed, and they will experience no adverse consequences because of it.

Roots

Maxillary molars are trifurcated and have three roots—mesiobuccal, distobuccal, and lingual—connected to a single **root trunk** (Figs. 15.16 and 15.17). **Trifurcation** gives maxillary molars sturdy anchorage against forces that would tend to displace them. The lingual root is the longest, and the distobuccal is the shortest.

All three roots are usually visible from the buccal view (see Fig. 15.16). The two buccal roots incline distally, with the mesiobuccal root starting to curve at its middle third. The distal root is usually straighter and tends to curve mesially at its middle third.

A deep developmental groove runs buccally between the bifurcation and the cervical line. The point of bifurcation of the two buccal roots is located about 4 mm apical to the cervical line.

The point of bifurcation for deciduous molars is much less. Deciduous molars have a shorter root trunk compared with permanent molars. The buccal roots of deciduous molars flare apart rather than curving toward each other.

The following are several characteristics of the roots of maxillary molars:

1. Roots become shorter as the maxillary molar is more posterior. The maxillary first molar has the longest roots and the third molar the shortest.

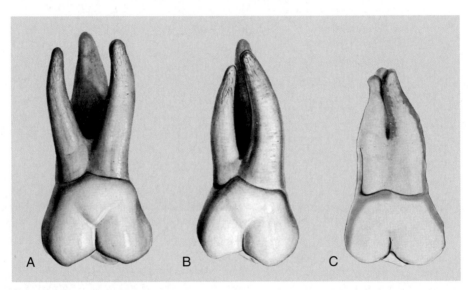

• **Figure 15.16** A buccal view of maxillary right molars. **(A)** First molar. **(B)** Second molar. **(C)** Third molar. Note how the roots tend to be closer together when the molars are farther distally. The roots of third molars are often fused. (Modified from Zeisz RC, Nuckolls J. *Dental Anatomy.* St. Louis, MO: Mosby; 1949.)

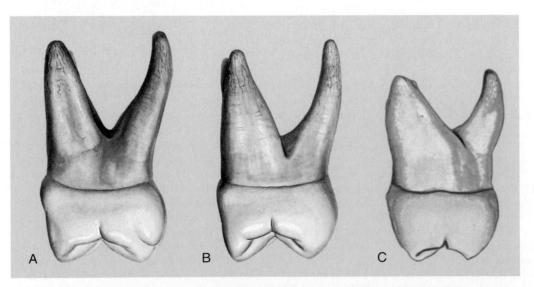

• **Figure 15.17** A mesial view of maxillary right molars. **(A)** First molar. **(B)** Second molar. **(C)** Third molar. The first molar has the longest roots, and the third molar has the shortest. (Modified from Zeisz RC, Nuckolls J. *Dental Anatomy.* St. Louis, MO: Mosby; 1949.)

2. Roots become less divided as the maxillary molar is more posterior. The roots of the maxillary first molar are much more divided than those of the second or third molar. The third molar often has fused roots.

3. Roots become more varied in shape, size, and direction of curvature as the maxillary molar is more posterior.

Pulp Cavity

The pulp cavity of a maxillary molar (Figs. 15.18 and 15.19) consists of a pulp chamber and three main pulp canals, one for each root. The lingual root canal is, by far, the largest; the distobuccal is the smallest; and the mesiobuccal is slightly larger than the distobuccal.

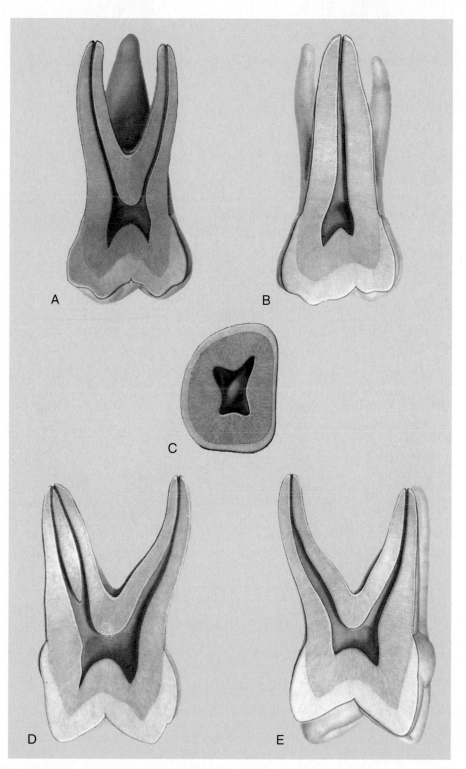

• **Figure 15.18** The pulp cavity of a maxillary right first molar. **(A)** Mesiodistal section, buccal view. **(B)** Distomesial section, lingual view. **(C)** Cross section, occlusal view. **(D)** Linguobuccal section, mesial view. **(E)** Buccolingual section, distal view. Note that there are two root canals within the mesiobuccal root. (Modified from Zeisz RC, Nuckolls J. *Dental Anatomy.* St. Louis, MO: Mosby; 1949.)

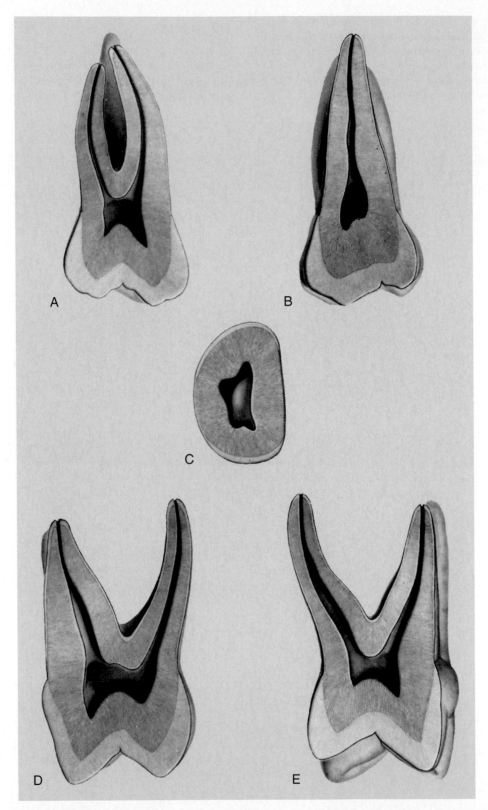

• **Figure 15.19** The pulp cavity of a maxillary right second molar. **(A)** Mesiodistal section, buccal view. **(B)** Distomesial section, lingual view. **(C)** Cross section, occlusal view. **(D)** Linguobuccal section, mesial view. **(E)** Buccolingual section, distal view. Note that there is only one root canal present within its mesiobuccal root. This tooth often has two root canals in its mesiobuccal root, but not as often as the first molar which most frequently has two. (Modified from Zeisz RC, Nuckolls J. *Dental Anatomy.* St. Louis, MO: Mosby; 1949.)

The maxillary first molar tends to have four root canals, with two canals in the mesiobuccal root. If four roots are present, as in some maxillary third molars, four root canals may be present too—one for each root. In the fused-root form, only one large root with one root canal may be evident.

While the maxillary first molar tends to have two root canals in its mesiobuccal root, the maxillary second molar tends to have just one root canal in its mesiobuccal root. Yet it is not uncommon for any maxillary molar to have one or two root canals in its mesiobuccal root—for first, second, or even third molars.

Each cusp has one pulp horn. The maxillary molars would then have four pulp horns—mesiobuccal, distobuccal, mesiolingual, and distolingual. (The exception is a three-cusped third molar, which then would have only three pulp horns.)

Pertinent Data

Maxillary First Molars

	Right	Left
Universal code	3	14
International code	16	26
Palmer notation:	6⌋	⌊6

Number of roots: 3
Number of pulp horns: 4
Number of cusps: 4, 5 if a well-developed cusp of Carabelli
Number of developmental lobes: 5

Location of Proximal Contact Areas
Mesial: Middle third
Distal: Middle third

Height of Contour
Facial: Cervical third, 0.5 mm
Lingual: Middle third, 0.5 mm

Identifying Characteristics
A cusp of Carabelli may be present. The occlusal outline is square or rhomboidal rather than triangular, and the distolingual cusp is well developed. A prominent oblique ridge and distolingual grooves are evident. The crown is wider buccolingually than mesiodistally and the three roots are widely separated.

Maxillary Second Molars

	Right	Left
Universal code	2	15
International code	17	27
Palmer notation:	7⌋	⌊7

Number of roots: 3
Number of pulp horns: 4
Number of cusps: 4
Number of developmental lobes: 4

Location of Proximal Contact Areas
Mesial: Middle third
Distal: Middle third

Height of Contour
Facial: Cervical third, 0.5 mm
Lingual: Middle third, 0.5 mm

Identifying Characteristics
These teeth are similar to maxillary first molars except that the fifth cusp is usually absent and the distolingual cusp is not as developed. The oblique ridge is less prominent. The crown is shorter occlusocervically and narrower mesiodistally. It is just as wide buccolingually. The occlusal outline of the crown is rhomboidal to heart shaped. The three roots are less separated.

Maxillary Third Molars

	Right	Left
Universal code	1	16
International code	18	28
Palmer notation:	8⌋	⌊8

Number of roots: 1 to 4
Number of pulp horns: 1 to 4
Number of cusps: 3 to 5
Number of developmental lobes: 4

Location of Proximal Contact Areas
Mesial: Middle third
Distal: None

Height of Contour
Facial: Cervical third, 0.5 mm
Lingual: Middle third, 0.5 mm

Identifying Characteristics
These teeth vary more in form compared with any others. They usually do not have a distolingual cusp. The occlusal outline is heart shaped with three cusps. The roots, usually three, tend to be very close together or to fuse with an extreme distal inclination.

Comparison of Maxillary Molars

Aspect	First Molar	Second Molar	Third Molar
Buccal	Widest of the three mesiodistally	Intermediate in width mesiodistally	Smallest in width
	Buccal cusps equal in height	Distobuccal cusps slightly shorter than mesiobuccal	Distobuccal cusps much shorter than mesiobuccal
	Distobuccal root apex curves mesially	Distobuccal root straight	All roots show pronounced distal inclination
Lingual	Distolingual cusp well formed	Distolingual cusps smaller in width and height	Distolingual cusp usually missing
Mesial	Cusp of Carabelli is very prominent	Cusp of Carabelli is less prominent and often absent	Cusp of Carabelli is absent
Occlusal	Crown outline square to rhomboidal	Rhomboidal form more pronounced in crown outline	Triangular or heart-shaped crown outline
	Oblique ridge prominent	Oblique ridge smaller	Oblique ridge often absent
Roots	Wide apart	Closer together	Usually fused

Mandibular Molars

Mandibular permanent molars are larger than any other mandibular teeth. They function as chewing or grinding tools. Three are on each side—mandibular first, second, and third molars. They occupy the posterior segment of each mandibular quadrant. Like their maxillary counterparts, the more posterior the teeth, the smaller they are in size. Which molars are therefore the smallest? Third molars are usually the smallest. If the second molar is lost early, that is, before 13 years of age, the third molar can develop into a molar that is almost the size that the second molar was. Both in the mandible and the maxilla, extra space for a third molar to develop can occur when the tooth bud is less compressed and thus has more room to develop and become larger.

The crowns of mandibular molars are shorter cervico-occlusally than those of teeth anterior to them, but in all other dimensions, molars are larger. Roots are not as long as some mandibular roots, but their bifurcation results in excellent anchorage.

The crowns of mandibular molars are wider mesiodistally than buccolingually. Is this also true of maxillary molars? If not, how are they different? Certain traits distinguish mandibular molars from maxillary molars.

1. Mandibular molars, as a rule, have only two roots—one mesial and one distal. How many roots do maxillary molars have?
2. Generally, four major cusps are found on mandibular molars; if a fifth cusp is present, it is a minor cusp.
3. The crowns are always broader mesiodistally than buccolingually.
4. Mandibular molars have two buccal cusps that are nearly equal in size. They also have two lingual cusps that are almost equal in size.

First Molars

Evidence of calcification: Birth
Enamel completed: 2½ to 3 years
Eruption: 6 years
Root completed: 9 to 10 years

Mandibular first molars (Fig. 15.20) are usually the first permanent teeth to erupt, with eruption occurring around 6 years of age. They are the only mandibular molars that usually have five cusps—two buccal and two lingual, which are major, and one distal, which is minor. Mandibular first molars are normally the largest teeth in the mandibular arch, with a crown usually about 1 mm longer mesiodistally than buccolingually.

Mandibular molars generally have two roots—one mesial and one distal. What other teeth have two roots? Are the roots mesial and distal or buccal and lingual?

Facial (Buccal) Aspect

From the buccal view (Fig. 15.21; see Fig. 15.20A), one distal and two buccal cusps can be seen. The mesiobuccal cusp is the widest of the three; the distal cusp is the smallest. The mesiobuccal and distobuccal cusps are approximately equal in height and are separated by the mesiobuccal groove. This mesiobuccal groove often ends in a buccal pit. The distal cusp is much more conical in shape and is smaller in height and width than the other two. It is separated from a distobuccal cusp by a distobuccal groove. The cervical line on a mandibular first molar dips apically toward the root bifurcation. The entire distal profile of the crown is convex, whereas only the mesial profile of the crown is convex at the middle and occlusal thirds; the cervical third is concave. Both the mesial and distal crown profiles converge toward the cervical side so that the cervical third of the crown is narrower than the occlusal third.

The roots of this tooth are well formed. The mesial root is almost perpendicular to the middle third of the root. From this point, it curves distally toward its apex, which is located directly below and in line with the mesiobuccal cusp. The distal root shows little curvature and projects distally from the root base. The two roots are widely separated at their apices but share a common root base.

Lingual Aspect

Two cusps of almost equal size, mesiolingual and distolingual cusps, make up the lingual profile (Fig. 15.22; see Fig. 15.20B). The lingual developmental groove separates these two cusps. The lingual cusps are higher and more pointed than the two buccal cusps.

The tooth is wider on the buccal side than on the lingual side. From the lingual view, the convergence from the buccal side toward the lingual can be noted.

The mesial and distal profiles of the lingual aspect are both convex. The crest of contour, which represents the contact area, is somewhat higher on the mesial side than on the distal side; however, both are in the middle third of the tooth.

The bifurcation of the two roots begins with the bifurcation groove on the root trunk located directly in line with the lingual developmental groove. The lingual surface of the crown is rather flat in comparison with the convex buccal surface. The cervical line is straight mesiodistally.

Mesial Aspect

From the mesial aspect (Fig. 15.23; see Fig. 15.20D), two cusps can be seen—mesiolingual and mesiobuccal cusps. The mesiolingual cusp is the higher and more conical of the two.

Only one root, the mesial root, can be seen from the mesial view.

The mesial marginal ridge has a prominent crest, which is divided by the mesial marginal groove, located lingual to the center of the crown. The buccal profile is marked by the buccocervical ridge, a slight bulge in the cervical third of the buccal surface. The lingual height of contour is located at the center of the middle third of the tooth on the lingual surface. The cervical line tends to curve occlusally about 1 mm in the center of the mesial surface. It is located higher on the lingual side than on the buccal side by almost 1 mm.

The buccolingual measurements of the crown, root, and cusps are all greater the mesial surface than on the distal surface. The mesial cusps are also higher than the distal cusps.

Distal Aspect

The distolingual cusp is the largest of the three cusps visible from the distal aspect (Fig. 15.24; see Fig. 15.20E). The distobuccal cusp is next in size, and the distal cusp is the smallest. The distobuccal groove can be seen separating the latter two cusps. The distal marginal ridge, not as wide as the mesial marginal ridge, is bisected by the distal marginal groove. This groove is lingual to the center of the tooth.

The crown of a first molar tapers and converges distally; if a specimen of the tooth is held with the distal surface of the crown at a right angle to the line of vision, one can see the crown taper from mesial toward the distal. The distal contact area is located on the distal cusp and is centered over the distal root.

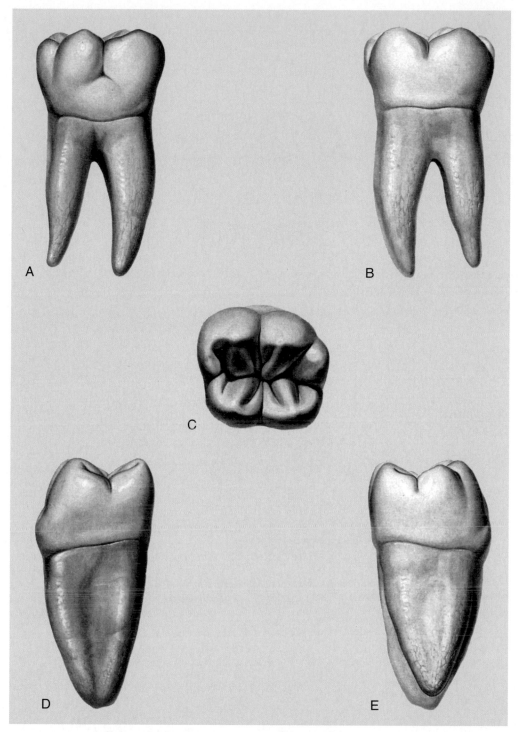

• **Figure 15.20** A mandibular right first molar. **(A)** Buccal view. **(B)** Lingual view. **(C)** Occlusal view. **(D)** Mesial view. **(E)** Distal view. (Modified from Zeisz RC, Nuckolls J. *Dental Anatomy.* St. Louis, MO: Mosby; 1949.)

Occlusal Aspect

The occlusal view (Fig. 15.25; see Fig. 15.20C) of a mandibular first molar shows five cusps—four major and one minor. All five are functional. Which one is the minor cusp? What differentiates a major cusp from a minor cusp?

The occlusal outline of the tooth is pentagonal and shows a tapering convergence toward the distal and lingual sides. Not only are the mesial cusps wider buccolingually compared with the distal cusps, but the mesiodistal measurement of the three buccal cusps together is much larger than the same measurement for two lingual cusps combined.

The mesiobuccal cusp is wider than either of the lingual cusps, which are about the same size.

The distobuccal cusp is the smallest of the four major cusps, and the distal is the smallest of all five.

The developmental grooves that separate these cusps are the **central developmental groove**, the **mesiobuccal developmental groove**, the **distobuccal developmental groove**, and the lingual

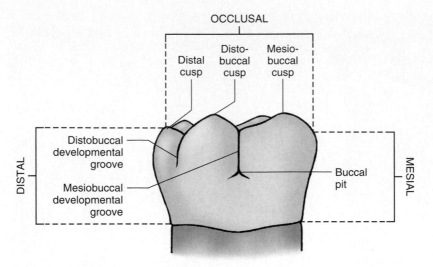

• **Figure 15.21** The buccal surface of a mandibular right first molar. (Modified from Zeisz RC, Nuckolls J. *Dental Anatomy.* St. Louis, MO: Mosby; 1949.)

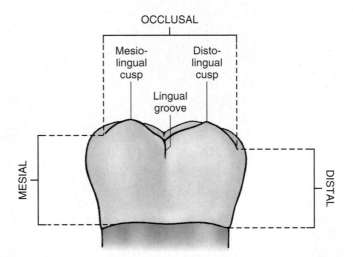

• **Figure 15.22** The lingual surface of a mandibular right first molar. (Modified from Zeisz RC, Nuckolls J. *Dental Anatomy.* St. Louis, MO: Mosby; 1949.)

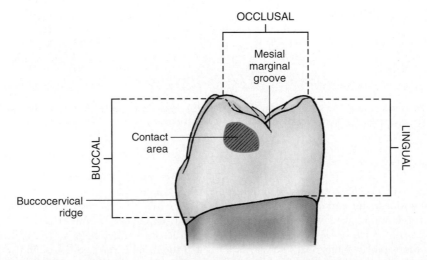

• **Figure 15.23** The mesial surface of a mandibular right first molar. (Modified from Zeisz RC, Nuckolls J. *Dental Anatomy.* St. Louis, MO: Mosby; 1949.)

developmental groove. All the developmental grooves converge at the central pit in the center of the central fossa. The central fossa of the occlusal surface is a concave area bordered by the distal slope of the mesiofacial cusp, the mesial and distal slopes of the distofacial cusp, the mesial slope of the distal cusp, the distal slope of the mesiolingual cusps, and the mesial slope of the distolingual cusp. Two other fossae are present, the mesial triangular fossa (just inside the mesiodistal marginal ridge) and the distal triangular fossa (a slight depression just mesial to the central portion of the distal marginal ridge).

The mesiobuccal groove separates the mesiofacial and distofacial cusps and extends onto the buccal surface. The distobuccal groove separates the distofacial and distal cusps. The lingual groove separates the two lingual cusps and continues onto the lingual surface. The two buccal grooves and the lingual groove form a Y-shaped pattern on the occlusal surface of the crown.

Mesial and distal marginal ridge grooves may also be present. Several supplemental grooves radiate from the mesial and distal pits, which are usually found in the mesial and distal triangular fossae, respectively.

Second Molars

Evidence of calcification: 2 to 3 years
Enamel completed: 7 to 8 years
Eruption: 11 to 13 years
Root completed: 14 to 15 years

Mandibular second molars (Fig. 15.26) resemble mandibular first molars buccally and lingually, except that usually no fifth or distal cusp is present. The roots of a second molar are shorter, closer together, and more distally inclined than those of a first molar.

All four cusps of the mandibular second molars are nearly equal in size. Occlusally, the second molars have a more rectangular shape compared with first molars.

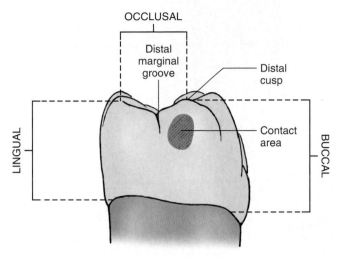

• **Figure 15.24** The distal surface of a mandibular right first molar. (Modified from Zeisz RC, Nuckolls J. *Dental Anatomy.* St. Louis, MO: Mosby; 1949.)

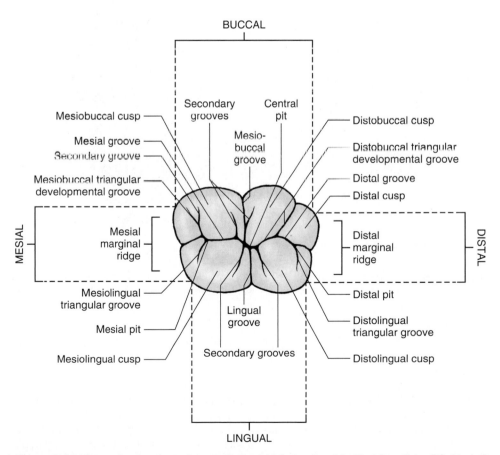

• **Figure 15.25** The occlusal surface of a mandibular right first molar. (Modified from Zeisz RC, Nuckolls J. *Dental Anatomy.* St. Louis, MO: Mosby; 1949.)

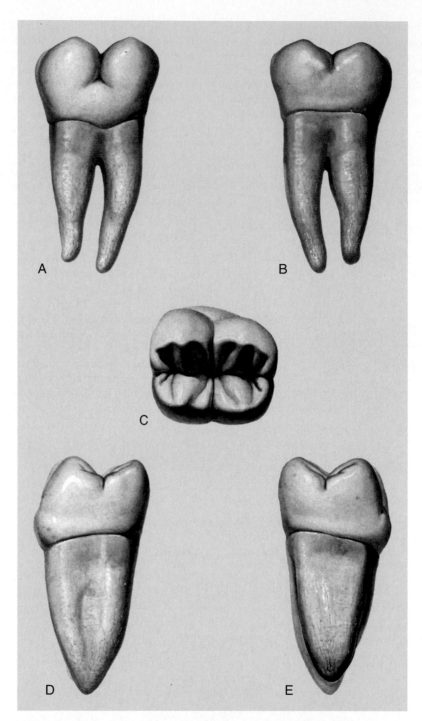

• **Figure 15.26** A mandibular right second molar. **(A)** Buccal view. **(B)** Lingual view. **(C)** Occlusal view. **(D)** Mesial view. **(E)** Distal view. (Modified from Zeisz RC, Nuckolls J. *Dental Anatomy.* St. Louis, MO: Mosby; 1949.)

Facial (Buccal) Aspect *(Fig. 15.27; see Fig. 15.26A)*

Facially, first and second molars are similar, except that the crown of a second molar is not as long mesiodistally and is slightly shorter cervico-occlusally. A second molar has only two buccal cusps separated by a single buccal groove. These two cusps, the mesiobuccal and distobuccal cusps, are equal in their mesiodistal measurements. The distal, a minor cusp, is usually absent.

The roots of a second molar may be somewhat shorter and are usually located closer together than the roots of a first molar. They

are also more distally inclined in relation to the occlusal plane of the crown.

Lingual Aspect *(Fig. 15.28; see Fig. 15.26B)*

The crown of a mandibular second molar converges far less lingually than that of a first molar because no distal cusp is present. The two lingual cusps, the mesiolingual and distolingual cusps, are nearly the same size and are separated by a lingual groove, which sometimes terminates in a lingual pit. The contact areas are at a lower level mesially and especially distally.

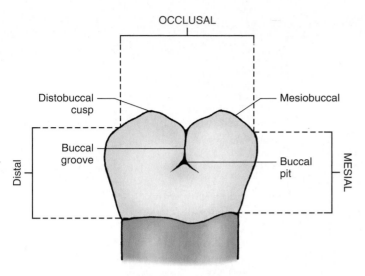

• **Figure 15.27** The buccal surface of a mandibular right second molar. (Modified from Zeisz RC, Nuckolls J. *Dental Anatomy.* St. Louis, MO: Mosby; 1949.)

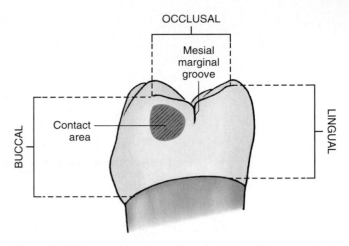

• **Figure 15.29** The mesial surface of a mandibular right second molar. (Modified from Zeisz RC, Nuckolls J. *Dental Anatomy.* St. Louis, MO: Mosby; 1949.)

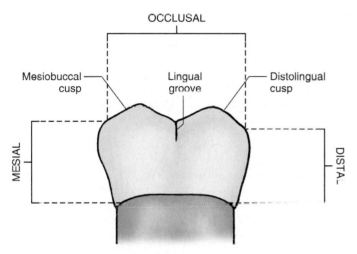

• **Figure 15.28** The lingual surface of a mandibular right second molar. (Modified from Zeisz RC, Nuckolls J. *Dental Anatomy.* St. Louis, MO: Mosby; 1949.)

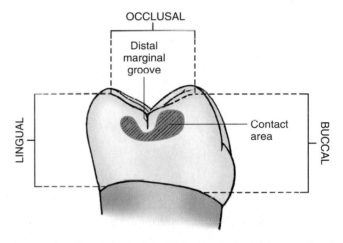

• **Figure 15.30** The distal surface of a mandibular right second molar. (Modified from Zeisz RC, Nuckolls J. *Dental Anatomy.* St. Louis, MO: Mosby; 1949.)

Mesial Aspect

From the mesial view of the mandibular second molar (Fig. 15.29; see Fig. 15.28D), the cervical line shows less curvature compared with a first molar, and the mesial root is less broad. Otherwise the mesial view is the same for both molars.

Distal Aspect

On the distal view (Fig. 15.30; see Fig. 15.26E), the most noticeable difference between first and second molars is the absence of a distal cusp. The contact area is therefore centered both buccolingually and cervico-occlusally.

Occlusal Aspect

The occlusal outline (Fig. 15.31; see Fig. 15.26C) of a second molar is rectangular. All four cusps are equal in size. The developmental grooves are the buccal groove, the lingual groove, and the central developmental groove, and they traverse the occlusal surface in a cross pattern. More secondary grooves are present than

on a first molar. The four triangular grooves include the distofacial, distolingual, mesiofacial, and mesiolingual grooves. Three pits may be present—mesial, distal, and central.

Third Molars

Evidence of calcification: 8 to 10 years
Enamel completed: 12 to 16 years
Eruption: 17 to 21 years
Root completed: 18 to 24 years

Like maxillary third molars, mandibular third molars are irregular and unpredictable. The crown is usually shorter in all dimensions compared with second molars, although it is possible to find a third molar larger than even a first molar. This, however, is an exception and not the rule.

The occlusal outline of the crown is more oval than rectangular, although the crown usually resembles that of a mandibular second molar. The combined measurement of the buccal cusps is greater than that of the lingual cusps. The two mesial cusps are larger than the two distal cusps. The occlusal surface

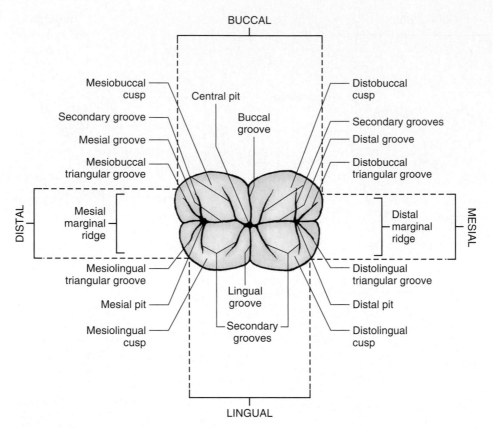

• **Figure 15.31** The occlusal surface of a mandibular right second molar. (Modified from Zeisz RC, Nuckolls J. *Dental Anatomy*. St. Louis, MO: Mosby; 1949.)

tapers toward the lingual and the distal and has a very wrinkled appearance, with an irregular groove pattern and numerous pits (Fig. 15.32).

The roots of third molars are usually shorter than those of second molars and are inclined acutely to the distal side. They are also very close together and often fused.

Roots

Mandibular molars have two roots (Figs. 15.33 and 15.34)—one mesial and one distal–with a single root trunk (bifurcated root). The mesial root is the longer and stronger of the two. It curves mesially and then turns distally in the apical portion. The distal root is usually quite straight and may curve mesially or distally at its apical third.

Comparison of Mandibular Molars

Aspect	First Molar	Second Molar	Third Molar
Buccal	Crown has widest mesiodistal diameter	Smaller crown than first molar	Smallest crown
	Three buccal cusps: mesiobuccal, distobuccal, and distal	Two buccal cusps: mesiobuccal and distobuccal	Two buccal cusps—mesiobuccal and distobuccal
	Two buccal grooves	One buccal groove	One buccal groove
	Roots widely separated and relatively vertical	Roots closer together and inclined distally	Roots short and fused, with pronounced distal inclination
Mesial	Mesial root broad	Mesial root not as broad	Same as second molar
Occlusal	Pentagonal outline	Rectangular outline	Ovoid outline
	Mesial and distal profiles straight, converging lingually and distally	Mesial and distal profiles curved; no lingual convergence	Mesial and distal profiles highly curved; slight lingual convergence
	Main grooves form Y pattern	Main grooves form a cross (+)	Grooves show no set pattern
	Large occlusal surface relative to total crown area seen from occlusal side	Occlusal table same as in first molar	More supplementary and accessory grooves
Roots	Wide apart and longest	Closer together	Usually fused, curved, and shorter

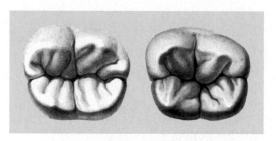

• **Figure 15.32** Occlusal view of two mandibular right third molars. (Modified from Zeisz RC, Nuckolls J. *Dental Anatomy*. St. Louis, MO: Mosby; 1949.)

The root trunk is bifurcated very close to the cervical line. The trunk is short and is grooved on the buccal and lingual surfaces toward the bifurcation. The following are characteristics of the roots of mandibular molars:

1. The roots become shorter as the molar is more posterior; the mandibular first molar is therefore the longest.
2. The roots are less divided as the molar is further posterior.
3. The roots become more varied in shape, size, and direction as the tooth is more posterior.

Pulp Cavity

The pulp cavity of the mandibular molars (Figs. 15.35 and 15.36) consists of a pulp chamber and three pulp canals—distal, mesiobuccal, and mesiolingual.

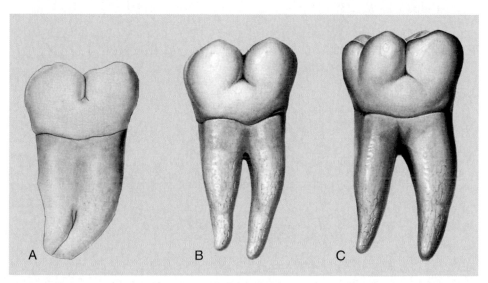

• **Figure 15.33** A buccal view of mandibular right molars. **(A)** Third molar. **(B)** Second molar. **(C)** First molar. Note how the roots get closer together and become shorter from the first molar to the third molar. Third molar roots are often fused. (Modified from Zeisz RC, Nuckolls J. *Dental Anatomy*. St. Louis, MO: Mosby; 1949.)

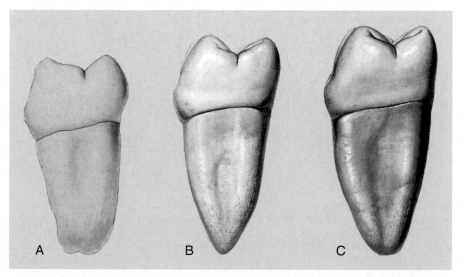

• **Figure 15.34** A mesial view of mandibular right molars. **(A)** Third molar. **(B)** Second molar. **(C)** First molar. (Modified from Zeisz RC, Nuckolls J. *Dental Anatomy*. St. Louis, MO: Mosby; 1949.)

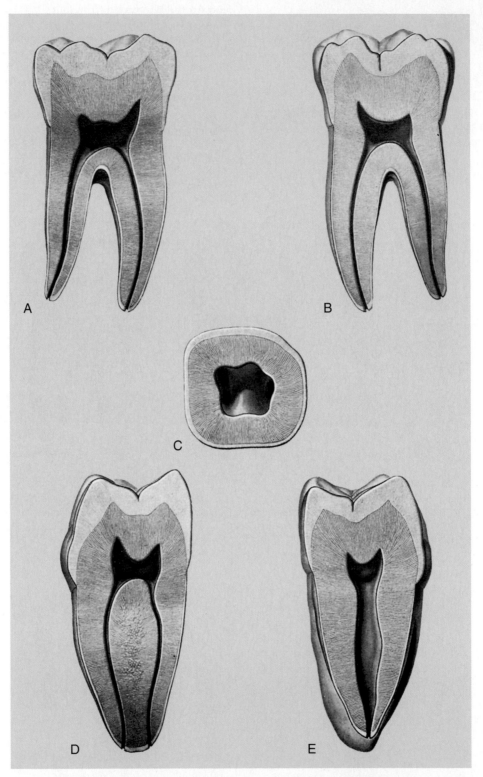

• **Figure 15.35** The pulp cavity of a mandibular right first molar. **(A)** Mesiodistal section, buccal view. **(B)** Distomesial section, lingual view. **(C)** Cross section, occlusal view. **(D)** Linguobuccal section, mesial view. **(E)** Buccolingual section, distal view. The mesial root can have just one root canal, but more often, like above, has two. (Modified from Zeisz RC, Nuckolls J. *Dental Anatomy.* St. Louis, MO: Mosby; 1949.)

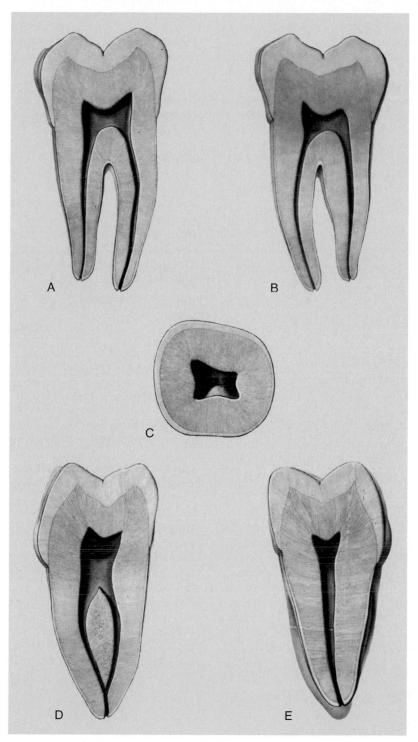

• **Figure 15.36** The pulp cavity of a mandibular right second molar. **(A)** Distomesial section, buccal view. **(B)** Mesiodistal section, lingual view. **(C)** Cross section, occlusal view. **(D)** Buccolingual section, mesial view. **(E)** Linguobuccal section, distal view. Although panel (D) shows two root canals in its mesial root, very frequently there is only one root canal in the mesial root. (Modified from Zeisz RC, Nuckolls J. *Dental Anatomy.* St. Louis, MO: Mosby; 1949.)

The distal root canal is much larger than the other two canals and is the only canal in the distal root. The mesial root houses two root canals—mesiobuccal and mesiolingual. Often these two canals join into one single apical foramen; sometimes only one canal is in the mesial root. On rare occasions, two canals are in the distal root, just as in the mesial root. The mandibular first molar is most likely to have two root canals in its mesial root, the second molar less likely, and the third molar the least likely to have two root canals in its mesial root.

Five pulp horns can be found—one for each cusp. In the four-cusp form, only four pulp horns are present. Which pulp horn is missing? (Hint: In the four-cusp form, which cusp is missing?)

The first molar is more likely to have three root canals (distal, mesiobuccal, and mesiolingual) and five pulp horns. Although the second molar may have two canals (the mesial and the distal, one in each root), it is more likely to have three root canals. The second molar has only four pulp horns. Third molars resemble second molars in pulpal anatomy.

Pertinent Data

Mandibular First Molars

	Right	Left
Universal code	30	19
International code	46	36
Palmer notation:	6⌋	⌊6

Number of roots: 2
Number of pulp horns: 5
Number of cusps: 5
Number of developmental lobes: 5

Location of Proximal Contact Areas
Mesial: Middle third
Distal: Middle third

Height of Contour
Facial: Cervical third, 0.5 mm
Lingual: Middle third, 1 mm

Identifying Characteristics
The five cusps make these the largest mandibular teeth. They are wider mesiodistally than buccolingually. The crown converges lingually and slightly distally. The three buccal cusps are separated by two buccal grooves, and the two lingual cusps are separated by one lingual groove. These three grooves converge to form a Y-shaped pattern. The two roots are mesial and distal, and three root canals (the mesial root has two root canals) are present.

Mandibular Second Molars

	Right	Left
Universal code	31	18
International code	47	37
Palmer notation:	7⌋	⌊7

Number of roots: 2
Number of pulp horns: 4
Number of cusps: 4
Number of developmental lobes: 4

Location of Proximal Contact Areas
Mesial: Middle third
Distal: Middle third

Height of Contour
Facial: Cervical third, 0.5 mm
Lingual: Middle third, 1 mm

Identifying Characteristics
These molars have four cusps of nearly equal size. The crown is smaller in all dimensions and has less lingual convergence. Only one buccal groove and one lingual groove are evident, which join on the occlusal surface as they bisect the central developmental groove; the groove therefore has a cross pattern. The two roots are closer together and incline slightly distally. One root canal is in the distal root. The mesial root can have one or two root canals.

Mandibular Third Molars

	Right	Left
Universal code	32	17
International code	48	38
Palmer notation:	8⌋	⌊8

Number of roots: 2 (fused into 1)
Number of pulp horns: 4 or 5
Number of cusps: 4 or 5
Number of developmental lobes: 4 or 5

Location of Proximal Contact Areas
Mesial: Middle third
Distal: Middle third

Height of Contour
Facial: Cervical third, 0.5 mm
Lingual: Middle third, 1 mm

Identifying Characteristics
These mandibular teeth are the most variable in form. They usually resemble the mandibular second molars, with four cusps; a shallower, smaller central fossa; and more secondary and tertiary grooves. A five-cusp form is not unusual. The two roots (mesial and distal) are often fused and inclined distally.

Review Questions

1. Which cusp of a maxillary first molar has the widest mesio-distal measurement?
2. Which two cusps join to form the oblique ridge?
3. Which of the five cusps of a maxillary first molar is least developed?
4. Which of the four functional lobes is least developed?
5. On which cusp is the tubercle of Carabelli located?
6. Which cusps surround the central fossa?
7. Are the terms *mesiolingual triangular groove* and *developmental groove of the cusp of Carabelli* synonymous?
8. What is the longest root on maxillary molars?
9. Are the terms *distolingual groove* and *distal oblique groove* synonymous?
10. Does the distal oblique groove separate the distolingual cusp from the mesiolingual cusp?
11. Are the terms *mesiolingual triangular groove* and *mesiolingual groove* synonymous?
12. Of the three roots of a maxillary molar, which is most likely to help differentiate maxillary first, second, and third molars from each other?
13. Which of the following is more likely to be present only on maxillary first molars?
    a. oblique ridge
    b. distolingual cusp
    c. cusp of Carabelli
    d. distobuccal root with its apex curved slightly mesially
14. The roots of a maxillary second molar lie closer together than the roots of which tooth?
    a. maxillary first molar
    b. maxillary third molar
15. Which two cusp ridges make up the transverse oblique ridge?
16. Identify the molar in Fig. 15.37.
17. Maxillary molars often have three root canals, but if four root canals are present, which maxillary molar is most likely to have four root canals?
    a. none of them
    b. maxillary first molar
    c. maxillary second molar
    d. maxillary third molar
18. A 6-year-old patient is given tetracycline antibiotics. If tetracycline can discolor teeth that are in their formative stages, which molars might be affected?
    a. maxillary permanent first molars
    b. first and second permanent molars
    c. second and third permanent molars
    d. only third molars

19. If a maxillary third molar only has three cusps, which three cusps are they most likely to be?
    a. mesiobuccal
    b. mesiolingual
    c. distolingual
    d. distobuccal
    e. cusp of Carabelli
20. A tooth that is an obvious maxillary molar is found with four roots fused to each other but is severely dilacerated at the apical third. Which molar is the tooth most likely to be?
    a. first
    b. second
    c. third
    d. first or second
21. When the first and second molars of the mandibular arch are compared, which of the following is *not* true?
    a. Only one groove is visible from the facial surface on a second molar.
    b. The crown is larger both mesiodistally and faciolingually on a second molar.
    c. Less lingual convergence is on a second molar.
    d. Both have two roots.
22. When the mandibular first and second molars are compared, in what way are the two different?
    a. The first has more roots and root canals.
    b. The second has more pulp horns.
    c. The second does not have a distal cusp.
    d. The first has a different height of contour.
23. The lingual height of contour on all mandibular molars
    a. measures 0.5 mm
    b. measures more than 0.5 mm
    c. measures less than 0.5 mm
    d. varies considerably from the first to the third molar
24. An important factor concerning personal oral hygiene is that the mandibular molars
    a. do not have an oblique ridge, which helps deflect the food onto the gums
    b. are more difficult to clean because of their lingual contours
    c. are equal with consideration to oral hygiene practice
25. Which of the following is not true of a mandibular second molar?
    a. It has four cusps of nearly equal size.
    b. It may have three root canals, with two in the mesial root.
    c. It has a cusp of Carabelli.
    d. It has four developmental lobes.
26. Which of the following is a list of correct names for the cusps of a mandibular first molar?
    a. mesiolingual, mesiofacial, distolingual, distofacial, cusp of Carabelli
    b. central, mesial, distal, facial, lingual
    c. mesiolingual, mesiofacial, distolingual, distofacial, distal
    d. distolingual, distofacial, mesiolingual, mesiofacial
27. The roots of a mandibular first molar are
    a. facial and lingual
    b. mesial, distal, and central
    c. facial, lingual, and middle
    d. mesial and distal

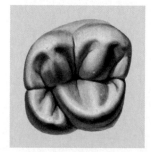

• **Figure 15.37**

28. When comparing all maxillary and mandibular molars, fused roots would most likely be found on which of the following?
    a. first molars
    b. second molars
    c. third molars
    d. all of the above
29. What is a major difference between first and second molars, whether maxillary or mandibular?
    a. First molars usually have four cusps, and second molars have three.
    b. First molars usually have five cusps, and second molars have four.
    c. First molars have more supplemental grooves.
    d. Second molars are wider mesiodistally.
30. Which of the following is true concerning maxillary and mandibular molars?
    a. Both have oblique ridges.
    b. Only maxillary molars have oblique ridges.
    c. Both do not have oblique ridges.
    d. Only mandibular molars have oblique ridges.
31. Two root canals are commonly found in
    a. the lingual root of maxillary first molars.
    b. the distal root of mandibular first molars.
    c. the mesial root of mandibular first molars.
    d. none of the above.

32. Furcation refers to
    a. the absence of a particular characteristic of the root anatomy.
    b. the splitting of a root trunk into terminal roots.
    c. the division of root canals from the root trunk.
    d. the action of movement of molars during mastication.
33. Name the smallest cusp of permanent mandibular molars.
34. A buccal pit is found at the end of the
    a. buccal groove of a mandibular second molar.
    b. mesiobuccal developmental groove of a mandibular first molar.
    c. distobuccal developmental groove of a mandibular first molar.
    d. distobuccal groove of a mandibular second molar.
    e. a and b
    f. a and d
35. Name the occlusal pits of mandibular first molars.
    a. mesial
    b. distal
    c. central
    d. all of the above

16

Deciduous Dentition

OBJECTIVES

- To identify various deciduous teeth
- To recognize whether a tooth is primary or secondary
- To know the eruption dates of primary and secondary teeth
- To understand the essential differences between deciduous and permanent teeth
- To understand the importance and functions of deciduous teeth
- To compare the dental anatomic features of deciduous teeth with other deciduous teeth and with their permanent counterparts

The deciduous dentition in humans is made up of 20 primary teeth. These teeth are shed and then replaced by permanent successors. This process of shedding deciduous teeth and replacement by permanent teeth is called *exfoliation.* Exfoliation begins 2 or 3 years after the deciduous root is completely formed. At this time the root begins to resorb at its apical end, and resorption continues in the direction of the crown until the entire root is resorbed and the tooth finally falls out.

The primary or deciduous dentition consists of 20 teeth, each quadrant containing two incisors, one canine, and two molars (Fig. 16.1).

The first deciduous teeth to erupt, about 8 months after birth, are usually mandibular central incisors. Maxillary central incisors usually erupt about a month after mandibular. In both permanent and primary teeth the mandibular usually erupt before the maxillary. The following is an approximate eruption schedule of deciduous teeth in chronologic order (also see Fig. 5.1).

Primary teeth begin to calcify *in utero* at 13 to 16 weeks. No deciduous teeth are present in the mouth at birth. In those rare instances when teeth are present, they are extremely small toothlike structures that are not real deciduous teeth. They are lost soon after birth.

The deciduous dentition begins with the eruption of a central incisor. Usually the mandibular centrals erupt before the maxillary centrals. The rest of the teeth erupt in the order given previously. It takes 2 to 3 years for eruption of the deciduous dentition to be completed. There is a lot of variation in eruption times, and a 4-month leeway is still considered normal. In general, when taken as a group average, eruption of teeth tends to be a little earlier in girls than in boys.

Deciduous teeth resemble permanent teeth except that their crowns are shorter and more constricted. In addition to being a shorter version of permanent teeth, deciduous teeth are also whiter in color.

The deciduous dentition has spaces between the primary teeth. These spaces get larger as the jaws grow, but teeth stay the same size. When permanent teeth start to erupt, these spaces are closed because permanent anterior succedaneous teeth require more space than the space necessary for the deciduous anterior teeth if no spaces were present.

Deciduous molar teeth are wider mesio-distally than the succedaneous premolar teeth that replace them (see Table 5.10; also Table 16.1). The extra space is needed for these succedaneous teeth because they sometimes erupt slightly rotated, thus requiring more space than their actual size. Therefore spaces are present throughout the mixed dentition as well. Clinically these spaces are necessary. Without this extra room, the permanent teeth would not have enough room to erupt. When this happens permanent teeth are blocked from erupting. This causes overcrowding, tipped and shifted alignment of teeth, and sometimes the prevention of a permanent tooth from erupting at all.

CLINICAL NOTE If a deciduous second molar has a large carious lesion on its distal surface, the permanent first molar most likely will move mesially into this decayed space (see Chapter 5). The loss of this small amount of space may be enough to block out the eruption of the permanent premolar that was supposed to replace the deciduous molar.

In rare instances a deciduous tooth will have no permanent replacement. In that case the deciduous tooth will have to last as long as possible. A deciduous tooth, by design, usually is needed to last no longer than 6 to 10 years depending on the tooth. If there is no permanent replacement the deciduous tooth might last 20 or even 30 years. Retained deciduous teeth usually last no longer than that. They do not last a lifetime.

A deciduous tooth may have no replacement for a variety of reasons: no congenital replacement; the permanent molar, taking advantage of the loss of space due to decay on the deciduous tooth mesial to it, may block it out; the deciduous tooth may become impacted in the bone. In the latter case the permanent tooth is not able to follow the deciduous root and does not erupt.

Essential Differences Between Deciduous and Permanent Teeth

1. Deciduous anterior teeth are *smaller* than their permanent successors in both their crown and root proportions. Deciduous molars are wider mesiodistally than permanent premolars, which will take their place.
2. The roots of deciduous anterior teeth appear longer and more slender proportionately in comparison with permanent teeth. All permanent teeth have much longer roots, but the crowns of deciduous teeth are so short that proportionately their roots appear to be long and slender.

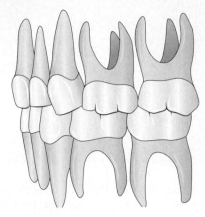

• **Figure 16.1** Deciduous teeth.

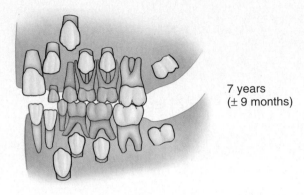

7 years
(± 9 months)

• **Figure 16.2** Premolars rest between deciduous molar roots. Gray teeth are primary; white teeth are secondary.

3. The roots of deciduous posterior teeth are very narrow at their cementoenamel junctions (CEJs), where the crowns join the roots. In addition, the root trunks of deciduous molars are very short.
4. The **cervical ridge** of enamel at the cervical third of the anterior crown, labially and lingually, is much more prominent in deciduous dentition. These bulky ridges extend out from the very narrow cervical necks of teeth.
5. The buccocervical ridges on deciduous molars are much more pronounced, especially on first molars. These cervical prominences give deciduous crowns a bulbous appearance and accentuate the narrow cervical portion of deciduous roots.
6. The buccal and lingual surfaces of deciduous molars taper occlusally above the cervical curvatures much more so than the permanent molar buccal and lingual surfaces. This results in a much narrower **occlusal table** of the occlusal surface buccolingually.
7. The roots of deciduous molars, compared with permanent molars, are also proportionately longer and narrower because the crowns of deciduous teeth are very short. These roots also flare apically to allow room for permanent teeth to develop between them (Fig. 16.2).
8. Deciduous teeth are usually lighter in color compared with permanent teeth. They are whiter in color, with a bluish cast. Permanent teeth have more yellow, gray, or brown tones.
9. The pulp chambers of deciduous teeth are relatively large in comparison with the crowns that envelop them.
10. The pulp horns of deciduous teeth extend rather high occlusally, placing them much closer to enamel than the pulp horns in permanent teeth.
11. The thickness of dentin between the pulp chambers and enamel is much thinner than in permanent teeth.
12. The enamel of deciduous teeth is relatively thin and has a consistent depth; in spite of this, the opacity of enamel makes it appear whiter (Fig. 16.3).

The Importance of Deciduous Teeth

The importance of deciduous teeth cannot be stressed enough. These teeth are extremely important for the proper development of the muscles of mastication; the formation of the bones of the jaws; and the eventual location, alignment, and occlusion of permanent teeth. Indeed, succedaneous teeth develop as buds from the tooth buds of deciduous teeth.

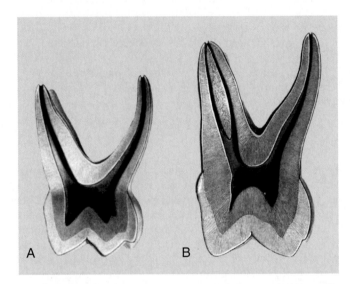

A   B

• **Figure 16.3** **(A)** A deciduous maxillary molar. **(B)** A permanent maxillary molar. (Modified from Zeisz RC, Nuckolls J. *Dental Anatomy*. St. Louis: Mosby; 1949.)

Clinical Considerations

If a deciduous tooth is congenitally missing its permanent placement cannot develop from the deciduous tooth bud. The congenital absence of the deciduous tooth means its permanent replacement is also missing.

Deciduous teeth maintain a place for permanent teeth. It is their function to allow for bone growth of the dental arches. As bone continues to grow, deciduous teeth develop spaces between them. It is normal and essential to have spaces, diastemae, between primary teeth. The diastema is called a **primate space** if it is between the primary maxillary lateral incisor and canine or if the space is between the mandibular canine and first molar. Primates, such as apes, chimps, and gorillas, also exhibit these spaces, hence the term *primate space* (Fig. 16.4).

The spaces between deciduous canines and first molars and those between first and second molars are called **leeway spaces**. They allow an extra margin of space for the eruption of permanent canines, as well as first and second premolars. Leeway space is formed because the mesiodistal measurement of two permanent

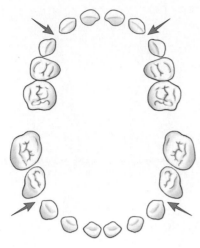

© Elsevier Collection

• **Figure 16.4** The primate spaces are diastemae mesial to maxillary canines and distal to the mandibular canines.

premolars combined is less than the sum of the mesiodistal measurements of deciduous molars. This allows extra room for premolars, but the permanent canine requires more room than the deciduous canine. This extra space is gained by the lateral bone growth formed when the canine erupts. As the canine erupts it brings with it extra bone on the lateral side of the developing dental arch. This extra bone forms the canine eminence. Leeway space is generated from this increase in arch length (see Chapter 6).

TABLE 16.1	Primary Tooth Development.			
Teeth	First Evidence of Calcification (*in utero*)	Crown Complete	Eruption (Mean Age)	Root Complete
Upper				
Central incisors	14 weeks	1½ months	10 months	1½ years
Lateral incisors	16 weeks	2½ months	11 months	2 years
Canines	17 weeks	9 months	19 months	3¼ years
First molars	15 weeks	6 months	16 months	2½ years
Second molars	19 weeks	11 months	29 months	3 years
Lower				
Central incisors	14 weeks	2½ months	8 months	1½ years
Lateral incisors	16 weeks	3 months	13 months	1½ years
Canines	17 weeks	9 months	20 months	3¼ years
First molars	15½ weeks	5½ months	16 months	2½ years
Second molars	18 weeks	10 months	27 months	3½ years

Note the eruption sequence is listed from the earliest to the latest, with the canines erupting after the first molars but before the second molars. The first evidence of calcification and root completion is a different sequence.

This data is an approximation gathered from Nelson S. Wheeler's *Dental Anatomy: Physiology and Occlusion*. 11th Edition, St. Louis. Elsevier; 2020.

The resorption of the deciduous roots helps guide their erupting permanent replacements into the proper location. Succedaneous teeth follow the resorbing root through bone until the deciduous tooth exfoliates as a result of lack of root anchorage. When a deciduous tooth exfoliates, its permanent replacement can often be seen directly underneath it. Sometimes a thin layer of gum may be covering it; usually it is not completely impacted with bone.

> ### Clinical Considerations
>
> If a deciduous molar is prematurely lost, a space maintainer can be placed. This will preserve the space necessary for the permanent tooth to erupt.

Maxillary Central Incisors (Fig. 16.5)

Labial Aspect (Fig. 16.6; see Fig. 16.5A)

A deciduous central incisor's mesiodistal diameter is greater than its cervico-incisal length, whereas a permanent central incisor's cervico-incisal length is greater than its mesiodistal diameter. No mamelons are visible on the deciduous tooth.

Lingual Aspect

From the lingual aspect (Fig. 16.7; see Fig. 16.5B), the crown shows well-developed marginal ridges and a highly developed cingulum.

Mesial and Distal Aspects

From the proximal aspects (Fig. 16.8; see Fig. 16.5D, E) the crown appears wide in relation to its total length. Because of its short length, the labiolingual measurements make the crown appear thick, even at the incisal third. The mesiocervical curvature is greater than the distal curvature.

Incisal Aspect

From the incisal surface (see Fig. 16.5C), the crown appears much wider mesiodistally than labiolingually. The incisal edge appears nearly straight.

Maxillary Lateral Incisors

A lateral incisor's crown is smaller than a central incisor's crown in all dimensions, except that the cervico-incisal length is greater than its mesiodistal width. In all other ways, it appears similar to a central incisor. The root appears much longer in proportion to the crown compared with the central incisor (Fig. 16.9).

Roots of Maxillary Incisors

The root of a deciduous maxillary incisor appears constricted at its cervical third. It is twice as long as the crown and tapers evenly toward a blunt apex. A mesial concavity is on the root surface, but the distal surface is generally convex. The lateral incisor surface is longer and more tapered than that of the central incisor.

Mandibular Central Incisors (Fig. 16.10)

Labial Aspect

Remnants of mamelons or grooves may be visible in the labial view of a deciduous mandibular incisor (Fig. 16.11; see

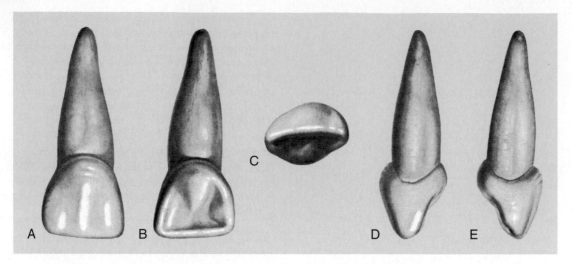

• **Figure 16.5** A maxillary right central incisor. **(A)** Labial view. **(B)** Lingual view. **(C)** Incisal view. **(D)** Mesial view. **(E)** Distal view. (Modified from Zeisz RC, Nuckolls J. *Dental Anatomy.* St. Louis: Mosby; 1949.)

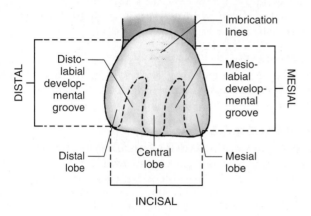

• **Figure 16.6** The labial surface of a maxillary right central incisor. (Modified from Zeisz RC, Nuckolls J. *Dental Anatomy.* St. Louis: Mosby; 1949.)

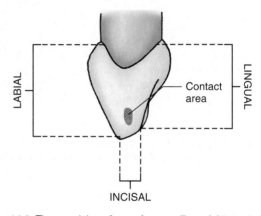

• **Figure 16.8** The mesial surface of a maxillary right central incisor. (Modified from Zeisz RC, Nuckolls J. *Dental Anatomy.* St. Louis: Mosby; 1949.)

Lingual Aspect

The lingual surface (Fig. 16.12; see also Fig. 16.10B) appears smoothly contoured and tapers toward the cingulum. The marginal ridges are less pronounced than those of the primary maxillary incisors.

Mesial and Distal Aspects

From the mesial aspect, the incisal ridge is centered over the root. The labial and lingual cervical contours are quite convex, much more so than those of permanent mandibular incisors. Cervical curvature is greater on the mesial side than on the distal side (Fig. 16.13; see Fig. 16.10D, E).

Incisal Aspect

The incisal view (Fig. 16.14; see Fig.16.10C) shows the incisal ridge centered over the crown of the tooth. The labial surface appears flat with a slight convexity, whereas the lingual surface appears concave.

Mandibular Lateral Incisors

Mandibular lateral incisors (Fig. 16.15) are wider and longer than the central incisors, and their cingula are more developed. Lateral

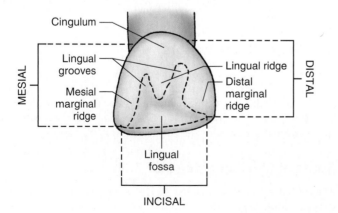

• **Figure 16.7** The lingual surface of a maxillary right central incisor. (Modified from Zeisz RC, Nuckolls J. *Dental Anatomy.* St. Louis: Mosby; 1949.)

Fig. 16.10A). The crown appears wide in comparison with its permanent successor. The mesial and distal sides of the crown taper evenly from the contact areas. The root may be two to three times the height of the crown. It is very narrow and is conical in shape.

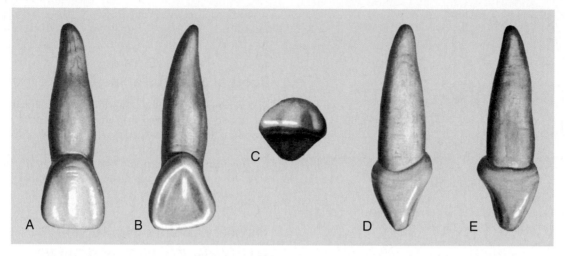

• **Figure 16.9** A maxillary right lateral incisor. **(A)** Labial view. **(B)** Lingual view. **(C)** Incisal view. **(D)** Mesial view. **(E)** Distal view. (Modified from Zeisz RC, Nuckolls J. *Dental Anatomy.* St. Louis: Mosby; 1949.)

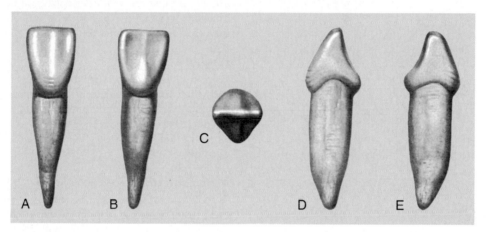

• **Figure 16.10** A mandibular right central incisor. **(A)** Labial view. **(B)** Lingual view. **(C)** Incisal view. **(D)** Mesial view. **(E)** Distal view. (Modified from Zeisz RC, Nuckolls J. *Dental Anatomy.* St. Louis: Mosby; 1949.)

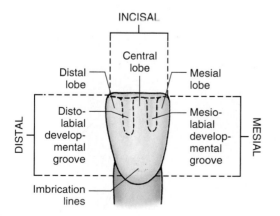

• **Figure 16.11** The labial surface of a mandibular right central incisor. (Modified from Zeisz RC, Nuckolls J. *Dental Anatomy.* St. Louis: Mosby; 1949.)

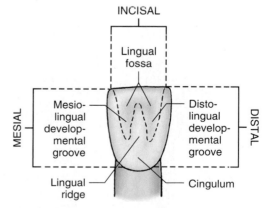

• **Figure 16.12** The lingual surface of a mandibular right central incisor. (Modified from Zeisz RC, Nuckolls J. *Dental Anatomy.* St. Louis: Mosby; 1949.)

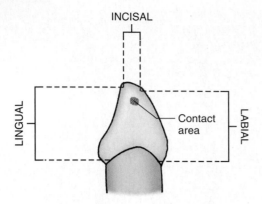

INCISAL

LINGUAL

Contact area

LABIAL

• **Figure 16.13** The distal surface of a mandibular right central incisor. (Modified from Zeisz RC, Nuckolls J. *Dental Anatomy*. St. Louis: Mosby; 1949.)

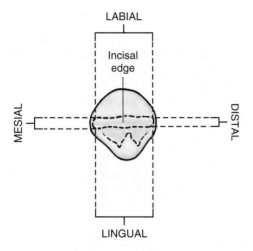

LABIAL

Incisal edge

MESIAL

DISTAL

LINGUAL

• **Figure 16.14** The incisal edge of a mandibular right central incisor. (Modified from Zeisz RC, Nuckolls J. *Dental Anatomy*. St. Louis: Mosby; 1949.)

incisors are also wider labiolingually. There is a tendency for the incisal ridge to slope distally, and its distal margin is more rounded.

Roots of Mandibular Incisors

The root of the deciduous mandibular lateral incisor is longer, narrower, and more tapered than that of the central incisor. It is also less blunt at the apex. The lateral incisor has a distal longitudinal groove and a mesial depression running lengthwise.

The mandibular central incisor's root is just a little shorter and does not have any grooves or depressions on its root surfaces.

Maxillary Canines (Fig. 16.16)

Labial Aspect (Fig. 16.17; see Fig. 16.16A)

A primary canine is bulkier than primary incisors in every aspect. The crown is more constricted at the cervix in relation to its mesiodistal width and more convex on its mesial and distal surfaces. The facial lobes are well developed, and a sharp cusp is evident. The root is about twice as long as the crown and more slender than that of its permanent successor.

Lingual Aspect

From the lingual view (Fig. 16.18; see Fig. 16.16B), the mesial and distal marginal ridges, incisal ridges, and cingulum are all very pronounced. A tubercle may extend from the cusp tip to the lingual ridge. The lingual ridge extends from the cusp tip to the cingulum and divides the lingual surface into mesiolingual and distolingual fossae.

Mesial and Distal Aspects (Fig. 16.19; see Fig. 16.16D, E)

The outline form is similar to that of a lateral or central incisor, except that a canine is much wider at the cervical third of the crown. Both the crown and the root at the cervical third are wider labiolingually compared with incisors.

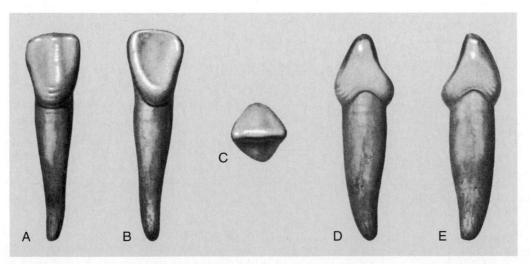

A   B   C   D   E

• **Figure 16.15** A mandibular right lateral incisor. **(A)** Labial view. **(B)** Lingual view. **(C)** Incisal view. **(D)** Mesial view. **(E)** Distal view. (Modified from Zeisz RC, Nuckolls J. *Dental Anatomy*. St. Louis: Mosby; 1949.)

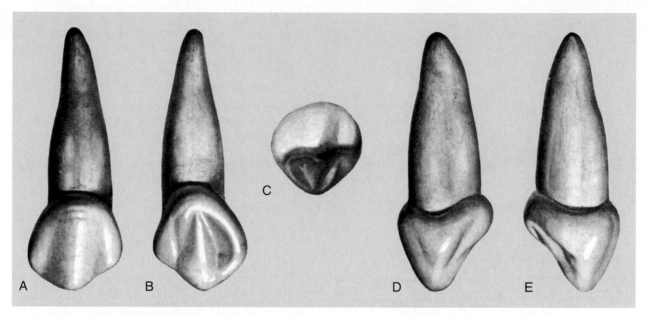

• **Figure 16.16** A maxillary right canine. **(A)** Labial view. **(B)** Lingual view. **(C)** Incisal view. **(D)** Mesial view. **(E)** Distal view. (Modified from Zeisz RC, Nuckolls J. *Dental Anatomy*. St. Louis: Mosby; 1949.)

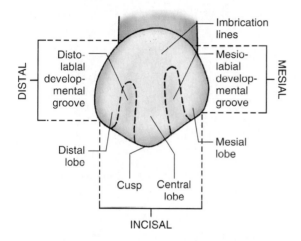

• **Figure 16.17** The labial surface of a maxillary right canine. (Modified from Zeisz RC, Nuckolls J. *Dental Anatomy*. St. Louis: Mosby; 1949.)

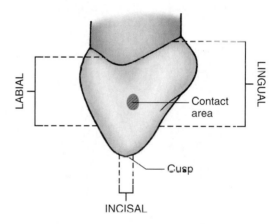

• **Figure 16.19** The mesial surface of a maxillary right canine. (Modified from Zeisz RC, Nuckolls J. *Dental Anatomy*. St. Louis: Mosby; 1949.)

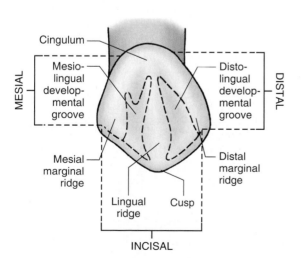

• **Figure 16.18** The lingual surface of a maxillary right canine. (Modified from Zeisz RC, Nuckolls J. *Dental Anatomy*. St. Louis: Mosby; 1949.)

Incisal Aspect

From the incisal view (Fig. 16.20; see Fig. 16.16C), the crown is rhomboidal—like a square that has been slightly shifted. The labial ridge is relatively pronounced, and the cingulum is obvious. The tip of the cusp is slightly distal to the center of the tooth.

Mandibular Canines (Fig. 16.21)

Labial Aspect

Compared with a maxillary canine, the labial surface of a mandibular canine (Fig. 16.22; see Fig. 16.21A) is much flatter, with shallow developmental grooves. The distal cusp ridge is longer than that of a maxillary canine. The root is long, narrow, and almost twice the length of the crown, although it is shorter and more tapered than that of a maxillary canine.

Lingual Aspect

The most obvious difference between maxillary and mandibular canines is the presence of a slight concavity called the *lingual fossa*.

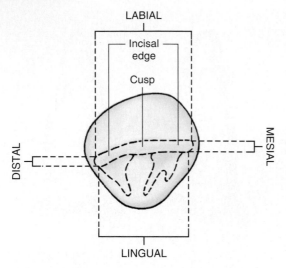

• **Figure 16.20** The incisal edge of a maxillary right canine. (Modified from Zeisz RC, Nuckolls J. *Dental Anatomy.* St. Louis: Mosby; 1949.)

Instead of two lingual fossae, only one is present. The lingual surface (Fig. 16.23; see Fig. 16.21B) is less prominent than that of a maxillary canine, and the crown converges lingually so that it is narrower on the lingual side than on the labial.

Mesial and Distal Aspects (Fig. 16.24; see Fig. 16.21D, E)

The outline form of a mandibular canine resembles that of an incisor, with the incisal ridge centered over the crown labiolingually. The labiolingual measurements are smaller than are those of a maxillary canine.

Incisal Aspect

The incisal ridge (Fig. 16.25; see Fig. 16.21C) is straight and centers over the crown labiolingually. The lingual surface shows a definite tapering toward the cingulum. The labial surface from this aspect presents a flat surface with a slight convexity, whereas the lingual surface presents a flattened surface that is slightly concave.

Roots of Canines

The roots of deciduous canines are almost twice as long as their crowns, they are thicker than the roots of incisors, and their apices

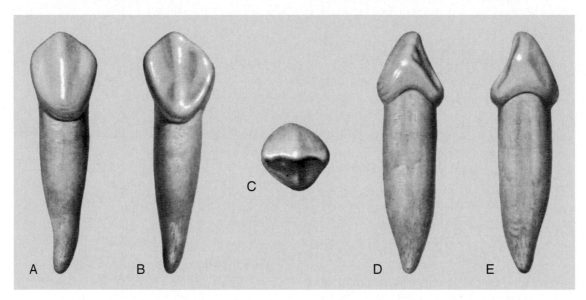

• **Figure 16.21** A mandibular right canine. **(A)** Labial view. **(B)** Lingual view. **(C)** Incisal view. **(D)** Mesial view. **(E)** Distal view. (Modified from Zeisz RC, Nuckolls J. *Dental Anatomy.* St. Louis: Mosby; 1949.)

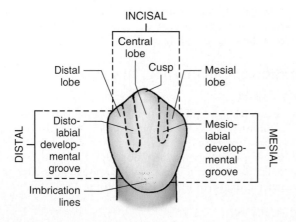

• **Figure 16.22** The labial surface of a mandibular right canine. (Modified from Zeisz RC, Nuckolls J. *Dental Anatomy.* St. Louis: Mosby; 1949.)

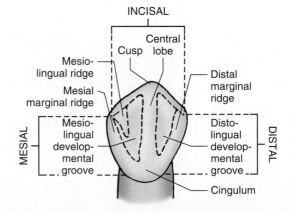

• **Figure 16.23** The lingual surface of a mandibular right canine. (Modified from Zeisz RC, Nuckolls J. *Dental Anatomy.* St. Louis: Mosby; 1949.)

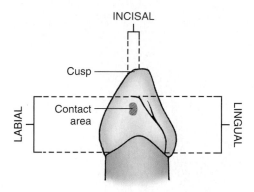

• **Figure 16.24** The mesial surface of a mandibular right canine. (Modified from Zeisz RC, Nuckolls J. *Dental Anatomy*. St. Louis: Mosby; 1949.)

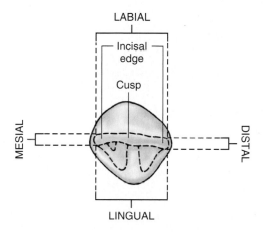

• **Figure 16.25** The incisal edge of a mandibular right canine. (Modified from Zeisz RC, Nuckolls J. *Dental Anatomy*. St. Louis: Mosby; 1949.)

are blunter. The mandibular root is slightly shorter than the maxillary root and is more tapered. Both have roots that taper lingually and apically. They are triangular in cross section.

Maxillary First Molars (Fig. 16.26)

Buccal Aspect (Fig. 16.27; see Fig. 16.26A)

The deciduous maxillary first molar is a blend of a premolar and a molar. It does not resemble any other tooth, deciduous or permanent. This is the most atypical of all maxillary molars. However, like all other maxillary molars, it is wider buccolingually than mesiodistally.

It has two major cusps—mesiobuccal and mesiolingual cusps. A distobuccal cusp is present, but it is only about half as large as the mesiobuccal cusp.

Lingual Aspect

The lingual view (Fig. 16.28; see Fig. 16.26B) shows that the crown of a deciduous maxillary first molar converges toward the lingual surface.

The mesiolingual cusp is the longest and sharpest cusp on this tooth. The distolingual cusp is small and rounded, if present at all. A type of deciduous maxillary first molar has only three cusps— one lingual and two buccal.

The lingual root is larger than the other two roots. A tiny tubercle can sometimes be seen on the mesiolingual cusps, but it cannot be called a *cusp of Carabelli*.

Mesial Aspect (Fig. 16.29; see also Fig. 16.26D)

The buccolingual measurement of a deciduous maxillary first molar at the cervical third is greater than the same measurement at the occlusal third. This is true of all molar teeth but is more evident on deciduous teeth. The mesiolingual cusp is more pronounced and longer in size compared with the mesiobuccal cusp. The most obvious difference between deciduous and permanent molars is that deciduous first molars have an extreme convexity in the cervical third of the buccal surface (buccocervical ridge). This convexity appears to be overdeveloped compared with that of permanent teeth. It is a major characteristic of deciduous maxillary first molars. The cervical line curves slightly toward the occlusal side.

Distal Aspect (Fig. 16.30; see Fig. 16.26E)

The crown appears to be narrower distally than mesially. The distobuccal cusp is more developed than the distolingual cusp, which is not always present. The cervical convexity (buccocervical ridge) on the buccal surface does not continue onto the distal surface.

Occlusal Aspect

The occlusal view (Fig. 16.31; see Fig. 16.26C) shows that the crown converges in a lingual direction so that the occlusal table appears triangular. The crown may have three or four cusps. If four are present, then two are on the buccal side and two are on the lingual side. If three cusps develop, only one is a lingual cusp.

The occlusal surface is similar to that of permanent molars except that the occlusal table is smaller in comparison. On the three-cusp form, only a central pit and a mesial pit (no distal pit) are evident, and an oblique ridge often unites the mesiolingual cusp with the distofacial cusp. The central groove connects the two fossae—the central fossa and the mesial triangular fossa. The buccal developmental groove is well developed and divides the two buccal cusps occlusally. The mesial, mesiofacial triangular, mesial marginal, and mesiolingual triangular grooves originate in the mesial pit. The distal, facial, and mesial developmental grooves radiate from the central pit.

The three fossae on four-cusp form are the mesial, central, and distal fossae. A small pit is usually present in each fossa. Grooves originating at the distal pit are the distofacial triangular, the distolingual, and the distal marginal grooves. An oblique ridge runs from the distobuccal cusp to the mesiolingual cusp.

Roots of Maxillary First Molars

Maxillary first molars have three roots—two buccal and one lingual. They are long, slender, and very flared. The lingual root is longer and more curved and tips back buccally at the apex. The mesiobuccal root is the next longest; the distobuccal is the shortest and straightest. The root trunk becomes trifurcated immediately above the cervical line. The root trunk is proportionately small compared with the length of the roots. Each root has a single root canal.

Clinical Considerations

When deciduous teeth exfoliate they do not just become loose and fall out. In fact they loosen but tighten back up. They repeat this cycle several times. If one attempts to remove a deciduous molar just because it is slightly loose, she or he must remember that deciduous molar roots wrap their roots around the crowns of their permanent replacements. Not until these roots are sufficiently resorbed is it really safe to remove the deciduous molar. Otherwise the permanent tooth bud that was meant to replace the deciduous tooth can be extracted with the deciduous tooth (see Table 5.10).

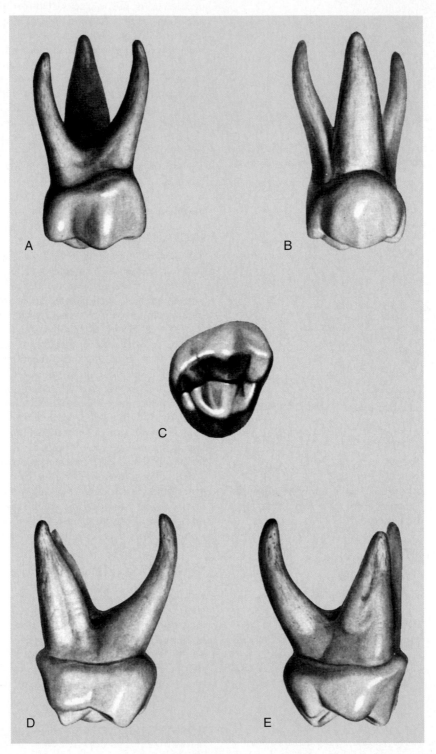

• **Figure 16.26** A maxillary right first molar. **(A)** Buccal view. **(B)** Lingual view. **(C)** Occlusal view. **(D)** Mesial view. **(E)** Distal view. (Modified from Zeisz RC, Nuckolls J. *Dental Anatomy*. St. Louis: Mosby; 1949.)

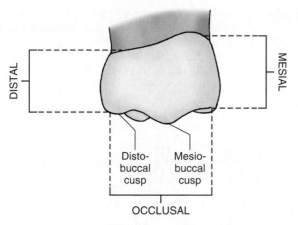

• **Figure 16.27** The buccal surface of a maxillary right first molar. (Modified from Zeisz RC, Nuckolls J. *Dental Anatomy.* St. Louis: Mosby; 1949.)

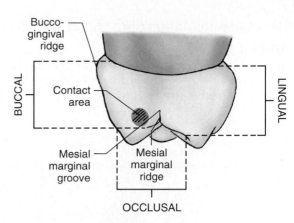

• **Figure 16.29** The mesial surface of a maxillary right first molar. (Modified from Zeisz RC, Nuckolls J. *Dental Anatomy.* St. Louis: Mosby; 1949.)

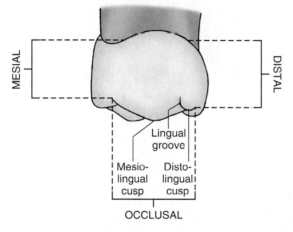

• **Figure 16.28** The lingual surface of a maxillary right first molar. (Modified from Zeisz RC, Nuckolls J. *Dental Anatomy.* St. Louis: Mosby; 1949.)

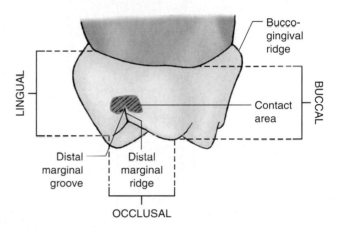

• **Figure 16.30** The distal surface of a maxillary right first molar. (Modified from Zeisz RC, Nuckolls J. *Dental Anatomy.* St. Louis: Mosby; 1949.)

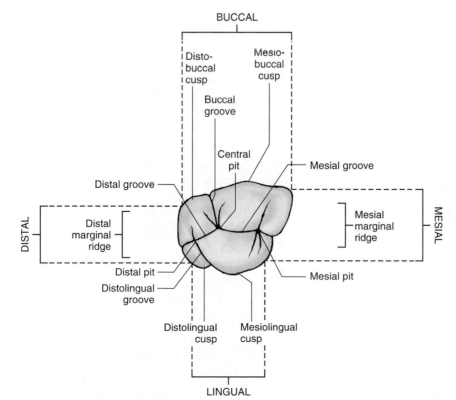

• **Figure 16.31** The occlusal surface of a maxillary right first molar. (Modified from Zeisz RC, Nuckolls J. *Dental Anatomy.* St. Louis: Mosby; 1949.)

Maxillary Second Molars (Fig. 16.32)

Buccal Aspect

A deciduous maxillary second molar resembles a permanent maxillary first molar, although it is much smaller. From the buccal view (Fig. 16.33; see Fig. 16.32A), two equal-sized buccal cusps with a buccal groove between them are visible. As on a deciduous first molar, the crown is narrow at its cervix, compared with its mesiodistal measurement at the contact area. A deciduous second molar is much larger than a deciduous first molar both in crown and root formation. The two buccal cusps are about equal in size. How is this different from the cusps of a deciduous first molar?

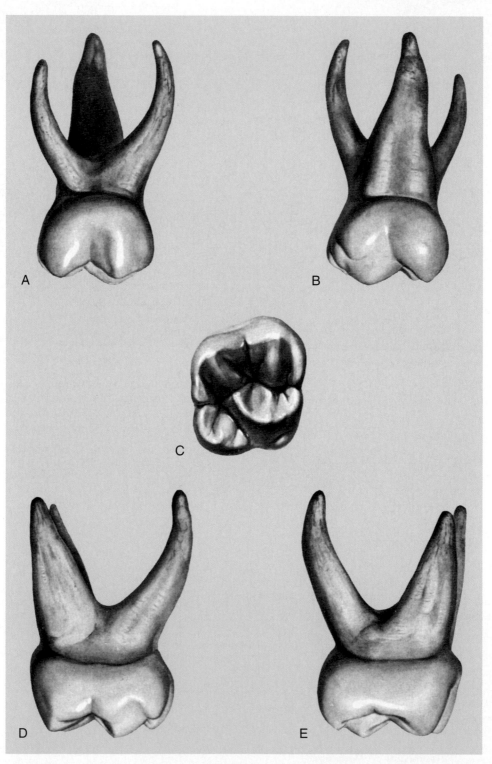

• **Figure 16.32** A maxillary right second molar. **(A)** Buccal view. **(B)** Lingual view. **(C)** Occlusal view. **(D)** Mesial view. **(E)** Distal view. (Modified from Zeisz RC, Nuckolls J. *Dental Anatomy.* St. Louis: Mosby; 1949.)

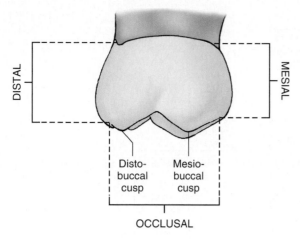

• **Figure 16.33** The buccal surface of a maxillary right second molar. (Modified from Zeisz RC, Nuckolls J. *Dental Anatomy*. St. Louis: Mosby; 1949.)

Lingual Aspect

From the lingual view (Fig. 16.34; see Fig. 16.32B), the crown shows three cusps—a mesiolingual cusp, a distolingual cusp, and the tubercle of Carabelli. The mesiolingual cusp is large and well developed. The distolingual cusp is more developed than that of a deciduous first molar but still small in comparison with the two buccal cusps and the mesiolingual cusp. The cusp of Carabelli, also called the tubercle of Carabelli or fifth cusp, is more of a tubercle than a cusp. It is less developed and is located on the lingual surface of the mesiolingual cusp. It is separated from the mesiolingual cusp by a developmental groove. A lingual developmental groove separates the mesiolingual and distolingual cusps.

Mesial Aspect

From the mesial view (Fig. 16.35; see Fig. 16.32D), this tooth resembles a permanent molar but is smaller. In comparison with a deciduous first molar, the crown is 0.5 mm longer and about 2 mm wider buccolingually, and the roots are up to 2 mm longer. The lingual root curves much the same way as those of first molars. The cusp of Carabelli is visible lingual and apical to the mesiolingual cusp, which is large in comparison with the mesiobuccal cusp.

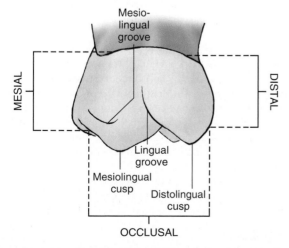

• **Figure 16.34** The lingual surface of a maxillary right second molar. (Modified from Zeisz RC, Nuckolls J. *Dental Anatomy*. St. Louis: Mosby; 1949.)

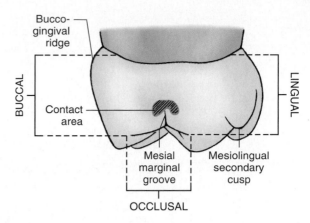

• **Figure 16.35** The mesial surface of a maxillary right second molar. (Modified from Zeisz RC, Nuckolls J. *Dental Anatomy*. St. Louis, MO: Mosby; 1949.)

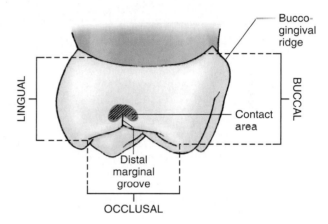

• **Figure 16.36** The distal surface of a maxillary right second molar. (Modified from Zeisz RC, Nuckolls J. *Dental Anatomy*. St. Louis: Mosby; 1949.)

Distal Aspect

From the distal view (Fig. 16.36; see Fig. 16.32E), the crown appears smaller than from a mesial aspect, but not to the same degree as found on a deciduous maxillary first molar. The distobuccal and distolingual cusps are about the same length. A rather straight cervical line is evident both distally and mesially.

Occlusal Aspect

From the occlusal view (Fig. 16.37; see Fig. 16.32C), the deciduous maxillary second molar resembles a permanent first molar. It has four well-developed cusps—the mesiobuccal, distobuccal, mesiolingual, distolingual cusps—and the cusp of Carabelli. The developmental grooves, although less defined, are almost identical to those found on a permanent first molar. The mesiolingual cusp is the largest, and the distolingual is the smallest, except for the fifth cusp.

Roots of Maxillary Second Molars

The three roots include two buccal roots and one lingual root. Like the deciduous first molar, the deciduous maxillary second molar's longest root is the lingual root, and its shortest is the distobuccal root. Unlike in the first molar, the mesiobuccal root

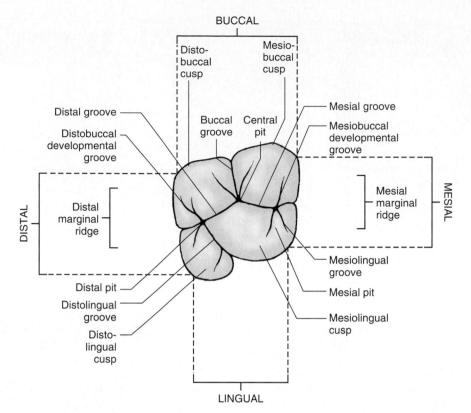

BUCCAL

Disto-
buccal
cusp

Mesio-
buccal
cusp

Distal groove

Distobuccal
developmental
groove

Buccal
groove

Central
pit

Mesial groove

Mesiobuccal
developmental
groove

DISTAL

MESIAL

Distal
marginal
ridge

Mesial
marginal
ridge

Distal pit

Distolingual
groove

Disto-
lingual
cusp

Mesiolingual
groove

Mesial pit

Mesiolingual
cusp

LINGUAL

• **Figure 16.37** The occlusal surface of a maxillary right second molar. (Modified from Zeisz RC, Nuckolls J. *Dental Anatomy*. St. Louis: Mosby; 1949.)

may be as long as the lingual root. The root trunk is short, and each of the roots has only one root canal.

Mandibular First Molars (Fig. 16.38)

Buccal Aspect (Fig. 16.39; see Fig. 16.38A)

A primary mandibular first molar does not resemble any other teeth, deciduous or permanent. Its mesial outline is rather flat straight up and down, whereas the distal outline is convex, converging sharply toward the cervical line. This makes the distal contact area fairly convex. The distal portion of the crown is shorter than the mesial portion.

Two distinct buccal cusps are present, but the developmental groove between them is not always evident. The mesial cusp is larger than the distal cusp. The crown is wider mesiodistally than buccolingually.

The roots are long, slender, and flared, with the mesial root curving slightly distally in its apical third. The point of bifurcation is very close to the cervical line of the crown, a characteristic of all deciduous molars. Observe the curvature of the cervical line (see Fig. 16.39).

Lingual Aspect (Fig. 16.40; see Fig. 16.38B)

The crown and root converge lingually on the mesial half of the crown; distally, they do not converge. The mesiolingual cusp is long and sharp, whereas the distolingual cusp is more rounded and not as long. The mesial marginal ridge is so well developed that it almost appears to be another cusp.

The cervical line is almost straight across, being quite different from the cervical line on the buccal aspect. Buccally, the cervical line curves apically on the mesial half of the tooth.

Mesial Aspect

The most characteristic feature of this tooth is an extremely bulbous curvature on its buccal surface at the cervical third. This buccocervical convexity can easily be seen from the mesial view (Fig. 16.41; see Fig. 16.38D) and causes the occlusal table to appear rather narrow from cusp tip to cusp tip.

The mesiobuccal cusp is longer than the mesiolingual cusp because the cervical line curves up from the buccal to the lingual side. The buccal surface is flat from the tip of the mesiobuccal cusp to the crest of the buccocervical curvature. Although this buccocervical curvature is quite pronounced, the remainder of the buccal surface above the curvature is rather flat and tipped at a sharp angle toward the buccal cusp.

Distal Aspect

The distal aspect (Fig. 16.42; see also Fig. 16.38D) of the crown does not display such an extreme buccocervical curvature. The height of the cusps, buccal and lingual, appears more uniform, and the cervical line is almost straight across buccolingually. The distobuccal and distolingual cusps are not as developed as the two mesial cusps. Furthermore, the distal marginal ridge is not as well defined as the mesial marginal ridge. The distal root is rounder and shorter than the mesial root, tapers apically, and houses only one root canal.

The distal surface is more convex than the mesial surface; therefore the distal contact area is more rounded and convex than the mesial contact area.

Occlusal Aspect

The occlusal outline (Fig. 16.43; see Fig. 16.38C) of the crown is rhomboidal in shape. From this view, the prominence of the

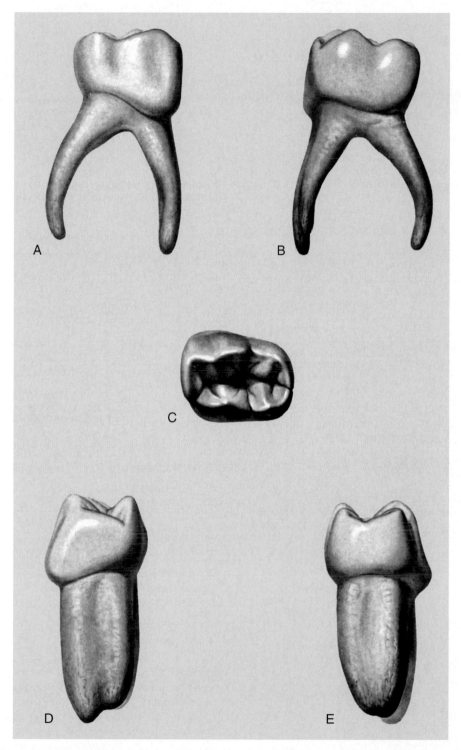

• **Figure 16.38** A mandibular right first molar. **(A)** Buccal view. **(B)** Lingual view. **(C)** Occlusal view. **(D)** Mesial view. **(E)** Distal view. (Modified from Zeisz RC, Nuckolls J. *Dental Anatomy.* St. Louis: Mosby; 1949.)

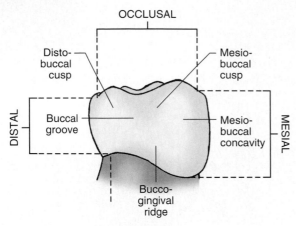

• **Figure 16.39** The buccal surface of a mandibular right first molar. (Modified from Zeisz RC, Nuckolls J. *Dental Anatomy.* St. Louis: Mosby; 1949.)

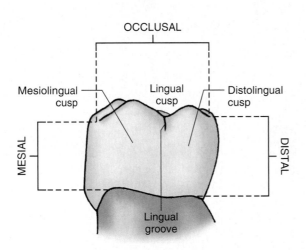

• **Figure 16.40** The lingual surface of a mandibular right first molar. (Modified from Zeisz RC, Nuckolls J. *Dental Anatomy.* St. Louis, MO: Mosby; 1949.)

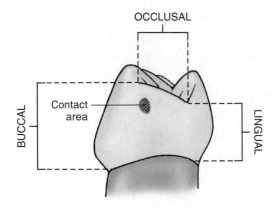

• **Figure 16.41** The mesial surface of a mandibular right first molar. (Modified from Zeisz RC, Nuckolls J. *Dental Anatomy.* St. Louis: Mosby; 1949.)

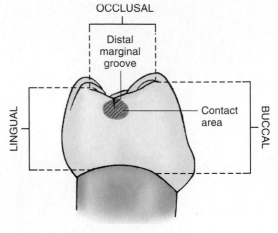

• **Figure 16.42** The distal surface of a mandibular right first molar. (Modified from Zeisz RC, Nuckolls J. *Dental Anatomy.* St. Louis: Mosby; 1949.)

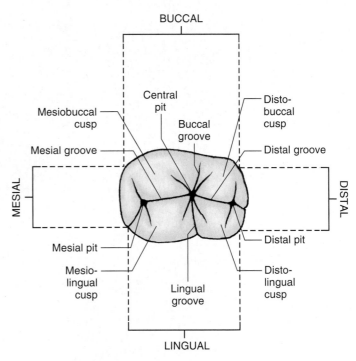

• **Figure 16.43** The occlusal surface of a mandibular right first molar. (Modified from Zeisz RC, Nuckolls J. *Dental Anatomy.* St. Louis: Mosby; 1949.)

mesiobuccal surface is evident. The mesiobuccal cervical ridge is also pronounced and gives the tooth its rhomboidal shape that tapers distally. The mesiolingual cusp appears to be the widest cusp, and the mesial marginal ridge is well developed. A buccal developmental groove may be present. A distinct transverse ridge runs between the mesiofacial and mesiolingual cusps. This ridge divides the occlusal surface into two fossae—one contains the mesial pit, and the other contains the central and distal pits. All are joined by a central developmental groove. A lingual groove radiates from the central pit between the two lingual cusps. A facial groove runs from the central pit to the buccal surface between the two buccal cusps. Mesial and distal triangular fossae and mesial and distal marginal and triangular grooves can be seen in Fig. 16.38C.

Roots of Mandibular First Molars

The deciduous mandibular first molar has two roots—mesial and distal. They are flat, broad, and flare apart widely. The mesial root has a longitudinal developmental groove running its length, and it has two root canals. The distal root is the shorter and thinner of the two; it has only one canal.

Mandibular Second Molars (Fig. 16.44)

Buccal Aspect (Fig. 16.45; see Fig. 16.44A)

A deciduous mandibular second molar resembles a permanent mandibular first molar except that the former is smaller than the latter and has the typical deciduous molar constriction at the cervix of the crown.

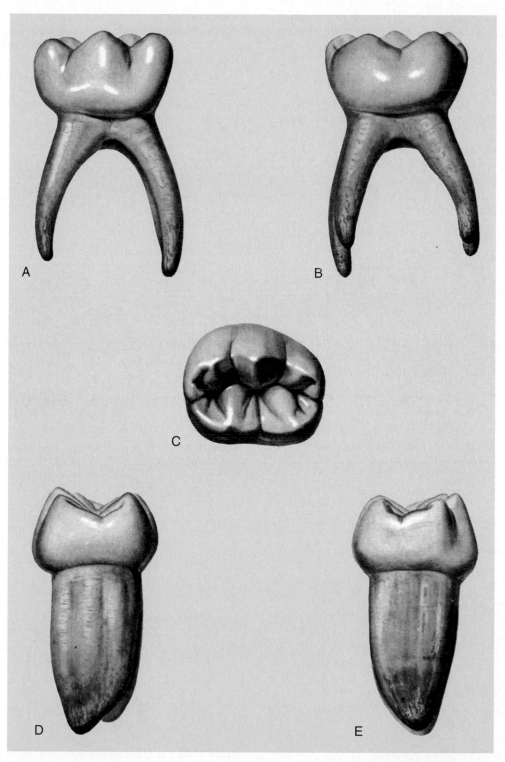

• **Figure 16.44** A mandibular right second molar. **(A)** Buccal view. **(B)** Lingual view. **(C)** Occlusal view. **(D)** Mesial view. **(E)** Distal view. (Modified from Zeisz RC, Nuckolls J. *Dental Anatomy*. St. Louis: Mosby; 1949.)

The mesiobuccal and distobuccal developmental grooves divide the buccal surface occlusally into three cusps. The three buccal cusps are the mesiofacial, distofacial, and distal cusps. The term *buccal* can be substituted for *facial*. What would the names of the three cusps then be? These cusps are about equal in length and width; the distobuccal (distofacial) cusp is slightly longer than the other two.

Characteristically, the roots of a second molar are long and slender, flaring mesiodistally at their middle and apical thirds. These roots are often twice as long as or longer than the crown. The point of bifurcation of the roots starts immediately below the cervical line of the crown. How is this different from the roots of a permanent first molar?

Lingual Aspect

From the lingual view (Fig. 16.46; see Fig. 16.44B), a short lingual groove can be seen dividing two cusps of about equal dimensions.

The two lingual cusps, the mesiolingual and distolingual cusps, are not as wide as the three buccal cusps. The tooth therefore converges lingually. The cervical line is straight.

Mesial Aspect

The mesial view (Fig. 16.47; see Fig. 16.44D) of the crown resembles that of a permanent mandibular first molar. However, its buccal surface shows a cervical bulge typical of deciduous molars. This crest of contour on the buccal side is notably less than that of a deciduous first molar. Like a deciduous first molar, a flattened buccal surface angles occlusally from this crest of contour, which presents a proportionately smaller occlusal table than that on permanent mandibular molars.

The mesial marginal ridge is rather high, giving the cusp the appearance of being shorter. The lingual cusp is longer than the buccal cusp because the cervical line extends up from the buccal side to the lingual side.

The mesial root is broad, flat, blunted at its apex, and houses two canals.

Distal Aspect (Fig. 16.48; see Fig. 16.44E)

The crown is not as wide distally as it is mesially, nor is the distal marginal ridge as high or as long as the mesial marginal ridge.

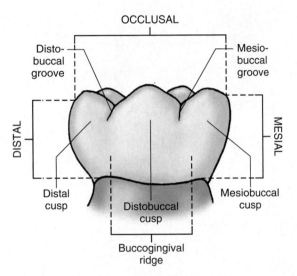

• **Figure 16.45** The buccal surface of a mandibular right second molar. (Modified from Zeisz RC, Nuckolls J. *Dental Anatomy.* St. Louis: Mosby; 1949.)

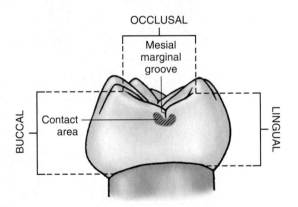

• **Figure 16.47** The mesial surface of a mandibular right second molar. (Modified from Zeisz RC, Nuckolls J. *Dental Anatomy.* St. Louis: Mosby; 1949.)

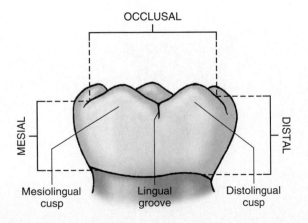

• **Figure 16.46** The lingual surface of a mandibular right second molar. (Modified from Zeisz RC, Nuckolls J. *Dental Anatomy.* St. Louis: Mosby; 1949.)

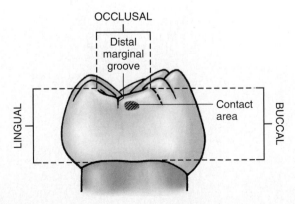

• **Figure 16.48** The distal surface of a mandibular right second molar. (Modified from Zeisz RC, Nuckolls J. *Dental Anatomy.* St. Louis, MO: Mosby; 1949.)

Similar to the mesiocervical line, the cervical line has an upper inclination buccolingually.

Three cusps can be seen from the distal view—the distofacial, distal, and distolingual cusps. Because the tooth converges distally, portions of the mesiofacial and mesiolingual cusps are also visible from the distal view.

Although the distal root is more tapered than the mesial root at its apical end, it does resemble the mesial root with its broad, flattened surface. The distal root has one canal. Does this differ from the distal root of a deciduous mandibular first molar?

Occlusal Aspect (Fig. 16.49; see Fig. 16.44C)

The three buccal cusps are similar in size, as are the two lingual cusps. However, the total mesiodistal width of the three buccal cusps is much more than the total mesiodistal width of the two lingual cusps. This allows the tooth to converge lingually.

The mesiofacial, distofacial, and lingual grooves radiate from the central pit in a "Y" shape. A central developmental groove joins the mesial triangular fossa and pit. Scattered over the occlusal surface are supplemental grooves located on the triangular ridges and fossae. The mesial marginal ridge is more pronounced than the distal marginal ridge.

The crown converges both distally and lingually. This convergence is similar to that seen in a permanent first molar, but the distal cusp in a permanent molar is much smaller than the two other buccal cusps. On a deciduous molar, the three buccal cusps are almost equal in size and development. All three buccal cusps of the deciduous molars are small in comparison with those of permanent molars. This gives the crown of the deciduous tooth a narrower buccolingual dimension in comparison with its mesiodistal dimensions.

Roots of Mandibular Second Molars

The roots of the deciduous mandibular second molar are twice as long as the crown. They are long, slender, and flared. The root trunk, as in all deciduous molars, is short, bifurcating immediately below the cervix of the tooth.

The two roots are the mesial and distal roots. The mesial root has two root canals and may have a longitudinal groove dividing it buccolingually. The distal root has only one root canal, and no grooves divide the root surface itself.

Pulp Cavities of Deciduous Teeth

The pulp cavities of deciduous teeth mirror the outer form of the teeth except that the pulp horns are longer and more pointed (Figs. 16.50 and 16.51). Compared with the pulp chambers of permanent teeth, the pulp chambers of deciduous teeth are large in proportion to the tooth size, and the pulp horns are more extreme. Mandibular deciduous molars are like miniature permanent teeth with larger-sized pulp chambers, root canals, and pulp horns (Fig. 16.52).

Clinical Considerations

The combination of short crowns with relatively large pulp chambers leads to a special clinical problem with deciduous teeth. Small carious lesions in deciduous teeth can open into their pulp chambers much faster than this same-sized carious lesion in permanent teeth.

Deciduous teeth have much shallower layers of dentin protecting their pulp cavities, and the deciduous pulp horns are much higher than in permanent teeth. The pulp horns are much closer to enamel and can be exposed easier. Such exposures could result in infection and eventual loss of the tooth.

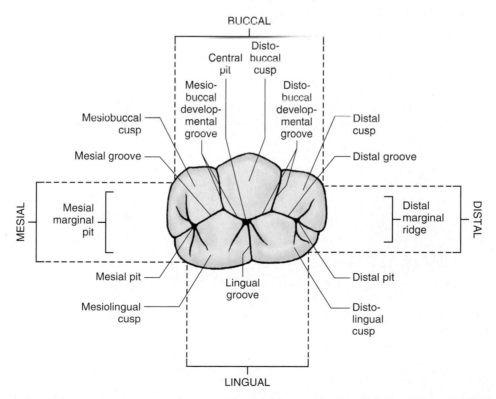

• **Figure 16.49** The occlusal surface of a mandibular right second molar. (Modified from Zeisz RC, Nuckolls J. *Dental Anatomy*. St. Louis: Mosby; 1949.)

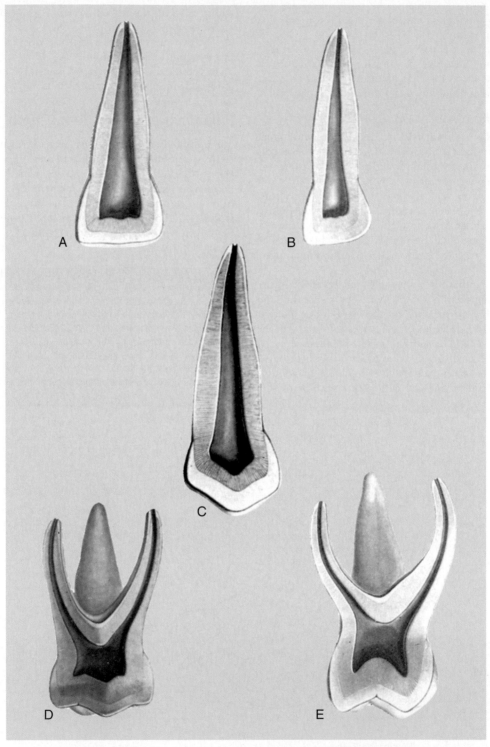

• **Figure 16.50** Maxillary right deciduous teeth, facial views. **(A)** Central incisor. **(B)** Lateral incisor. **(C)** Canine. **(D)** First molar. **(E)** Second molar. (Modified from Zeisz RC, Nuckolls J. *Dental Anatomy.* St. Louis: Mosby; 1949.)

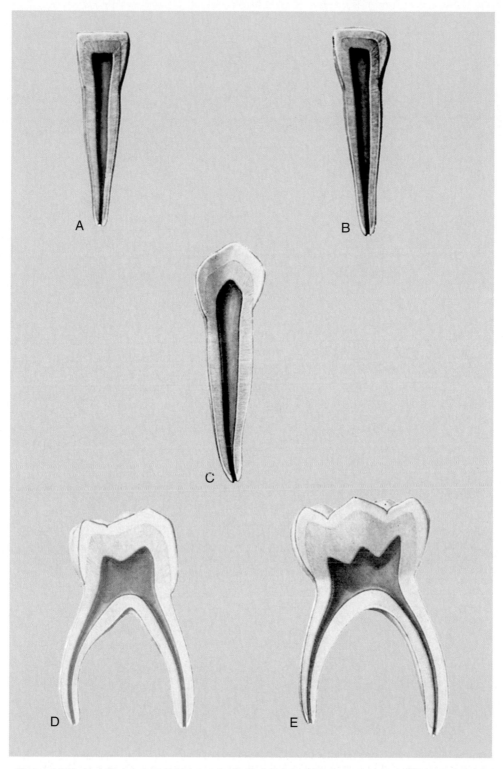

• **Figure 16.51** Mandibular right deciduous teeth, facial views. **(A)** Central incisor. **(B)** Lateral incisor. **(C)** Canine. **(D)** First molar. **(E)** Second molar. (Modified from Zeisz RC, Nuckolls J. *Dental Anatomy.* St. Louis: Mosby; 1949.)

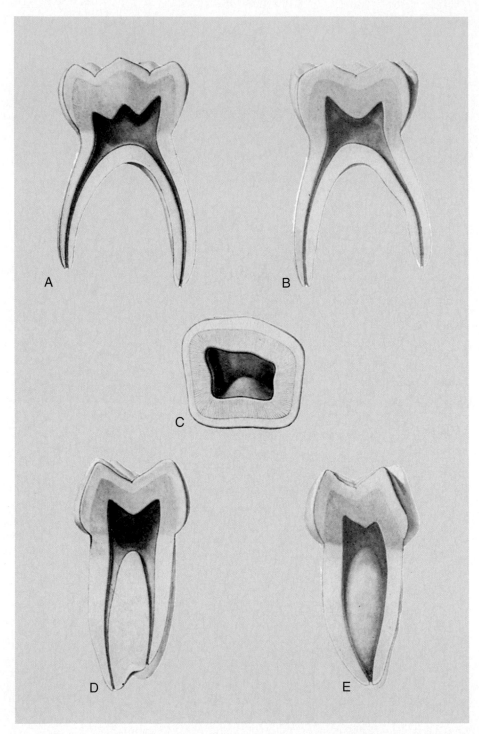

• **Figure 16.52** A mandibular right deciduous second molar. **(A)** Buccal view. **(B)** Lingual view. **(C)** Occlusal view. **(D)** Mesial view. **(E)** Distal view. (Modified from Zeisz RC, Nuckolls J. *Dental Anatomy.* St. Louis: Mosby; 1949.)

Review Questions

1. Give two terms that are synonymous with the commonly used term *baby teeth*.
2. How does exfoliation occur?
3. How many incisors, canines, premolars, and molars are in the primary dentition?
4. What are the eruption dates of the following?
   a. deciduous maxillary incisors
   b. deciduous mandibular incisors
   c. deciduous canines
   d. deciduous first molars
5. Which teeth usually erupt first, maxillary or mandibular?
6. What cervical bulge of enamel is more pronounced on deciduous teeth than on permanent teeth?
7. Which deciduous tooth is least like any in the permanent dentition?
   a. primary maxillary second molar
   b. primary mandibular first molar
   c. primary mandibular second molar
8. Give one special characteristic that is unique to each type of deciduous molar.
9. What are the 12 essential differences between deciduous and permanent teeth?
10. Caries in deciduous teeth can lead to nerve involvement more easily than that in permanent teeth. Which of the reasons for this are true?
    a. There is less thickness of dentin between enamel and the pulp chamber in deciduous teeth.
    b. The pulp horns extend rather high occlusally in deciduous teeth.
    c. The pulp chambers of deciduous teeth are relatively large compared with their crowns.
    d. a, b, and c
11. The cervical ridges of deciduous teeth are _____ compared with permanent teeth.
    a. more prominent
    b. less bulky
    c. thinner
12. What is the function of primate spaces between deciduous teeth?

True or False

13. The roots of deciduous teeth are wider than those of permanent teeth.
14. The roots of deciduous teeth are longer in comparison with the crowns than those in permanent teeth.
15. The roots of deciduous teeth are bulkier and thicker at their cervical junction.
16. The roots of deciduous molars flare more than those of permanent molars.
17. The smallest tooth in the human dentition is the deciduous mandibular central incisor.
18. Deciduous molars do not have a tubercle (cusp) of Carabelli.

Average Permanent Teeth Dimensions as Recorded by Dr. Russell C. Wheeler

	Length of Crown	Length of Root	Mesiodistal Diameter of Crown*	Mesiodistal Diameter at Cervix	Labio- or Buccolingual Diameter	Labio- or Buccolingual Diameter at Cervix	Curvature of Cervical Line (Mesial)	Curvature of Cervical Line (Distal)
Maxillary Teeth								
Central incisor	10.5	13.0	8.5	7.0	7.0	6.0	3.5	2.5
Lateral incisor	9.0	13.0	6.5	5.0	6.0	5.0	3.0	2.0
Canine	10.0	17.0	7.5	5.5	8.0	7.0	2.5	1.5
First premolar	8.5	14.0	7.0	5.0	9.0	8.0	1.0	0.0
Second premolar	8.5	14.0	7.0	5.0	9.0	8.0	1.0	0.0
First molar	7.5	B 12 L 13	10.0	8.0	11.0	10.0	1.0	0.0
Second molar	7.0	B 11 L 12	9.0	7.0	11.0	10.0	1.0	0.0
Third molar	6.5	11.0	8.5	6.5	10.0	9.5	1.0	0.0
Mandibular Teeth								
Central incisor	9.0†	12.5	5.0	3.5	6.0	5.3	3.0	2.0
Lateral incisor	9.5†	14.0	5.5	4.0	6.5	5.8	3.0	2.0
Canine	11.0	16.0	7.0	5.5	7.5	7.0	2.5	1.0
First premolar	8.5	14.0	7.0	5.0	7.5	6.5	1.0	0.0
Second premolar	8.0	14.5	7.0	5.0	8.0	7.0	1.0	0.0
First molar	7.5	14.0	11.0	9.0	10.5	9.0	1.0	0.0
Second molar	7.0	13.0	10.5	8.0	10.0	9.0	1.0	0.0
Third molar	7.0	11.0	10.0	7.5	9.5	9.0	1.0	0.0

*The sum of the mesiodistal diameters, both right and left, which gives the arch length, is 128 mm for maxillary teeth and 126 mm for mandibular teeth.
†Lingual measurement is approximately 0.5 mm longer.
Wheeler RC. *A Textbook of Dental Anatomy and Physiology*. 4th ed. Philadelphia: WB Saunders; 1965.

Unit II Test

1. A small elevation of enamel that may be found on the surface of a tooth is a
   a. cusp
   b. tubercle
   c. sulcus
   d. fossa

2. The permanent premolar most likely to have two root canals is the
   a. maxillary first premolar
   b. maxillary second premolar
   c. mandibular first premolar
   d. mandibular second premolar

3. Which of the following is *least* typical for the maxillary second premolar?
   a. The lingual cusp is slightly shorter than the facial cusp.
   b. The facial cusp is slightly larger than the lingual cusp.
   c. The two cusps are approximately the same length.
   d. The facial cusp is shorter and blunter compared with the lingual cusp.

4. When the two cusps of the maxillary first premolars are compared,
   a. the facial cusp is longer but not wider
   b. the lingual cusp is both shorter and narrower
   c. the facial cusp is shorter but wider
   d. the lingual cusp is both longer and wider

5. Which of the following is *not* true of maxillary first premolars?
   a. commonly bifurcated root
   b. single root trunk
   c. facial cusp tip displaced to the distal from midline
   d. the roots are the mesial and distal

6. Which of the following teeth erupt last?
   a. mandibular first premolars
   b. maxillary canines
   c. maxillary first premolars
   d. mandibular canines

7. Which of the following teeth are the *least* likely to be bifurcated?
   a. maxillary second premolar
   b. mandibular canine
   c. mandibular first premolar
   d. mandibular second premolar

8. Which of the following is the *least* likely to have two root canals?
   a. mesiobuccal root of a maxillary molar
   b. mesial root of the mandibular molar
   c. maxillary premolar
   d. mandibular canine

9. Which of the following are the first permanent teeth to erupt?
   a. maxillary first molars
   b. mandibular first molars
   c. mandibular central incisors
   d. maxillary central incisors

10. Which of the following have the fewest proximal contact areas?
    a. central incisors
    b. third molars
    c. canines
    d. premolars

11. Which of the following are class traits of all molars?
    a. Molars have the largest occlusal surfaces of any teeth in the dentition.
    b. Molars have three to five major cusps.
    c. Molars have two or three roots.
    d. All of the above.

12. The distobuccal and mesiolingual cusps on the occlusal table of a maxillary molar are usually connected by a ridge. This ridge is termed
    a. the mesiolingual ridge
    b. the triangular ridge
    c. the Carabellian ridge
    d. the oblique ridge

13. In a Class II, Division II malocclusion, the maxillary incisors are
    a. retruded
    b. protruded
    c. edge to edge
    d. in crossbite

14. Maxillary laterals exhibit
    a. the same number of lobes as first molars
    b. the same number of lobes as first premolars
    c. two labial and two lingual lobes
    d. three lobes only

Use the following information to answer questions 15 to 17: A 9-year-old boy presents himself with a large gingival abscess at the gingival crest of his deciduous maxillary first right molar. The tooth is loose and painful upon percussion.

15. We could expect this 9-year-old patient to exhibit
    a. no permanent teeth other than first molars
    b. a mixed dentition
    c. evidence of facial trauma
    d. evidence of severe periodontal disease

16. What treatment option seems appropriate for an abscessed deciduous second molar in a 9-year-old patient?
    a. root resection
    b. periodontal surgery
    c. extraction of the affected tooth
    d. splinting the deciduous molars together

17. If this molar was removed, which of the following would *not* be true?
    a. A space maintainer is probably not necessary.
    b. The permanent replacement should erupt soon.
    c. His eruption pattern is earlier compared with most children his age.
    d. The deciduous root, if still present, would be very small.

18. From the occlusal view, which tooth is wider on the lingual side than on the buccal side?
    a. maxillary central incisor
    b. mandibular first molar
    c. maxillary first molar
    d. mandibular first premolar
    e. mandibular second premolar

19. The cusp of Carabelli of the permanent maxillary first molar may be
    a. absent
    b. located lingual to the distolingual cusp
    c. the third largest cusp
    d. All of the above.

20. The longest and shortest cusps of the maxillary first molar are the
    a. mesiofacial and distofacial
    b. mesiolingual and distofacial
    c. mesiolingual and distolingual
    d. distofacial and distolingual
21. In Class I occlusion, the mandibular lateral incisor
    a. opposes the maxillary lateral incisor and canine
    b. opposes only the maxillary lateral incisor
    c. opposes maxillary central and lateral incisors
    d. is free of contact with opposing teeth
22. Compared with the permanent mandibular central incisor, the root of the mandibular lateral incisor is
    a. larger in all dimensions
    b. longer but not wider
    c. wider but not longer
    d. the same size
23. Morphologically, the mandibular lateral incisor and the mandibular central incisor are almost identical. Which of the following describes a slight difference between these two teeth?
    a. The mandibular lateral incisor is usually slightly larger.
    b. The mandibular lateral incisor has an elongation of the distoincisal angle distolingually.
    c. When the mandibular lateral incisor is viewed incisally, the crown appears to be slightly rotated on its base.
    d. All of the above.
24. In comparison with the permanent maxillary canine, the permanent mandibular canine has a mesiodistal crown width that is
    a. somewhat wider
    b. somewhat narrower
    c. identical
    d. a great deal wider
25. In comparison with the mandibular canine, the maxillary canine
    a. has a relatively longer crown
    b. is less likely to be bifurcated
    c. has a less pronounced cingulum
    d. has less prominent lingual features
26. Which of the following anterior teeth exhibits the *most* deviation in tooth morphology?
    a. mandibular central incisor
    b. maxillary canine
    c. maxillary lateral incisor
    d. mandibular lateral incisor
27. The smallest permanent tooth in the mouth is the
    a. maxillary central incisor
    b. mandibular central incisor
    c. maxillary lateral incisor
    d. mandibular lateral incisor
28. Which of the following anterior teeth is *most* likely to have two root canals?
    a. mandibular lateral incisor
    b. maxillary canine
    c. maxillary central incisor
    d. mandibular canine
29. Mesiodistal measurements of the crowns of anterior teeth as seen from an incisal view indicate that the crowns are
    a. wider at the mesial than the distal
    b. wider at the distal than the mesial
    c. wider at the lingual than the facial
    d. wider at the facial than the lingual

30. Which of the following is the largest, longest, and strongest root of the maxillary molar?
    a. facial
    b. lingual
    c. mesiofacial
    d. distofacial
31. Which of the following cusps is frequently missing from the maxillary third molar?
    a. mesiofacial
    b. distofacial
    c. distolingual
    d. mesiolingual
32. The oblique ridge of maxillary molars crosses the occlusal surface obliquely from the _____ cusps.
    a. mesiofacial to mesiolingual
    b. mesiolingual to distofacial
    c. distofacial to distolingual
    d. mesiofacial to distolingual
33. Where is the lingual height of contour located on the mandibular molars?
    a. middle third
    b. occlusal third
    c. cervical third
    d. at the junction of occlusal and middle thirds
34. The mandibular molars are aligned in the alveolar bone in such a way that their crowns are
    a. tilted to the distal and facial side
    b. tilted to the lingual side but upright otherwise
    c. upright in all directions
    d. tilted toward the mesial and lingual
35. The permanent mandibular first molar usually has
    a. two root canals in the mesial root, one in the distal
    b. one root canal in the lingual root, one in the facial
    c. two root canals in both the mesial and distal roots
    d. one root canal in each root
36. The four *most* frequently found congenitally missing teeth are
    a. maxillary first premolar, maxillary lateral incisor, mandibular lateral incisor, and mandibular third molar
    b. maxillary third molar, maxillary lateral incisor, mandibular canine, and mandibular third molar
    c. maxillary third molar, mandibular third molar, maxillary lateral incisor, and mandibular second premolar
    d. maxillary third molar, and maxillary first premolar, mandibular third molar, and mandibular canine
37. The greatest convexity of the facial surface of anterior teeth is
    a. different from that of posterior teeth
    b. the cervical third
    c. the middle third
    d. the junction of middle and incisal thirds
38. Which of the following is *not* a set trait of the deciduous dentition?
    a. Most primary teeth are smaller than their succedaneous permanent teeth.
    b. The crowns of primary teeth seem long relative to their total length compared with permanent teeth.
    c. In anterior primary teeth, the labial and lingual surfaces bulge conspicuously in the cervical third.
    d. Primary crowns are milk white in color.
    e. The enamel is thinner in primary teeth and the pulp chamber is larger.

39. Which is the most distinguishing feature of the maxillary first deciduous molar?
    a. cusp relationship
    b. buccal cervical ridge
    c. mesial profile
    d. all of the above

40. A child 14 months of age should normally have which deciduous teeth present in the mouth (all four quadrants)?
    a. central incisors, lateral incisors, canines, first molars, second molars
    b. central incisors, lateral incisors, canines, first molars
    c. central incisors, lateral incisors, first molars, second molars
    d. central incisors, lateral incisors, canines
    e. central incisors, lateral incisors, first molars

41. Which of the following deciduous teeth do *not* resemble any other deciduous teeth or permanent teeth?
    a. deciduous mandibular first molar
    b. deciduous mandibular second molar
    c. deciduous maxillary first molar
    d. deciduous maxillary second molar
    e. a and c

42. Which of the following have three roots?
    a. permanent mandibular molars
    b. permanent maxillary premolars
    c. deciduous maxillary molars
    d. permanent maxillary molars
    e. a, c, and d
    f. c and d

43. The cusp of Carabelli of the permanent maxillary first molar is sometimes
    a. located on the distolingual cusp
    b. missing entirely
    c. located on the lingual surface
    d. located on the mesiolingual cusp
    e. a, c, and d
    f. b, c, and d

44. The smallest tooth in the human dentition is the
    a. deciduous mandibular central incisor
    b. deciduous mandibular lateral incisor
    c. permanent mandibular central incisor
    d. permanent mandibular lateral incisor

45. How do the permanent mandibular incisors differ from the permanent maxillary incisors?
    a. Maxillary incisors are smaller.
    b. The mandibular lateral incisor is larger than the central incisor.
    c. Maxillary incisors have fewer pits and less-developed marginal ridges.
    d. Mandibular incisors have more developed cingula.

46. What are the excess spaces in the deciduous dentition that is available for permanent canines and premolars called?
    a. freeway space
    b. primate space
    c. interdental space
    d. leeway space
    e. b and d

47. Which permanent tooth is *most* likely to have two root canals?
    a. maxillary second premolar
    b. mandibular central incisor
    c. maxillary lateral incisor
    d. maxillary central incisor
    e. maxillary canine

48. Which of the following are possible if a dark radiolucent area is seen at the apex of a mandibular second premolar?
    a. an endodontic abscess
    b. a cementoma at the apex of the tooth
    c. the mental foramen
    d. a, b, or c

49. An abscessed tooth frequently responds to heat stimulation. This occurs because a dying nerve within the root canal is especially able to discern hot from cold temperatures.
    a. Both statements are true.
    b. Both statements are false.
    c. The first statement is true; the second is false.
    d. The first statement is false; the second is true.

50. If lost 1 year prematurely, which deciduous tooth would most likely necessitate the placement of a space maintainer?
    a. deciduous mandibular canine
    b. deciduous mandibular first molar
    c. deciduous mandibular second molar
    d. deciduous maxillary first molar

Unit II Suggested Readings

Andrews LF. The six keys to normal occlusion. *Am J Orthod*. 1972;62(3):296.

Angle EH. *Treatment of Malocclusion of the Teeth and Fractures of the Maxillae: Angle's System*. 6th ed. Philadelphia: SS White Dental Manufacturing Co.; 1900.

Ash MM. *Wheeler's Atlas of Tooth Form*. 5th ed. Philadelphia: WB Saunders Co.; 1984.

Ash MM. *Wheeler's Dental Anatomy, Physiology, and Occlusion*. 6th ed. Philadelphia: WB Saunders Co.; 1984.

Atkinson ME, White FH. *Principles of Anatomy and Oral Anatomy for Dental Students*. Edinburgh, UK: Longman Group UK; 1992.

Ayer WA. Thumb-finger sucking and bruxing habits in children. In: Bryant P, Gale E, Rugh J, eds. *Oral Motor Behavior: Impact on Oral Conditions and Dental Treatment*. NIH Publications No. 79-1845, Washington, DC: US Government Printing Office; 1979.

Begg PR. Stone age man's dentition. *Am J Orthod*. 1954;40:298.

Begg PR. Stone age man's dentition. *Am J Orthod*. 1954;40:373.

Begg PR. Stone age man's dentition. *Am J Orthod*. 1954;40:462.

Begg PR. Stone age man's dentition. *Am J Orthod*. 1954;40:517.

Begg PR, Kesling PC. *Begg Orthodontic Theory and Technique*. Philadelphia: WB Saunders; 1977.

Berkovitz BK, Moxham BL. *Color Atlas and Textbook of Oral Anatomy and Embryology*. 2nd ed. London: Mosby; 1992.

Berry DC, Singh BP. Effect of electromyographic biofeedback therapy on occlusion contacts. *J Prosthet Dent*. 1984;51:397.

Bohsali K, Shabahang S, Pertot WJ. Canal configuration of the mesiobuccal root of the maxillary molar. *Gen Dent*. 1999;490–495.

Chiego D. *Essentials of Oral Histology and Embryology*. 4th ed. St. Louis: Mosby; 2014.

Dawson PE. *Evaluation, Diagnosis, and Treatment of Occlusal Problems*. 2nd ed. St. Louis: Mosby; 1989.

Drake RL. *Gray's Anatomy*. 2nd ed. Philadelphia: Churchill Livingstone; 2015.

Drake RL. *Gray's Anatomy for Students*. 3rd ed. Philadelphia: Churchill Livingstone; 2015.

DuBrul EL. *Sicher's Oral Anatomy*. 8th ed. St. Louis: Ishiyaku EuroAmerica, Inc; 1988.

Farman AG, Escobar V. Duplication of oral and maxillofacial structures. *Quintessence Int*. 1986;17(11):731.

Fehrenbach M. *Illustrated Anatomy of the Head and Neck*. 5th ed. St. Louis: Elsevier; 2017.

Fehrenbach M. *Illustrated Dental Embryology, Histology and Anatomy*. 5th ed. St. Louis: Elsevier; 2020.

Fuller JL, Denehy GE. *Concise Dental Anatomy and Morphology*. 3rd ed. Chicago: Year Book Medical Publications; 1999.

Grahnen H, Granath LE. Numerical variations in primary dentition and their correlation with permanent dentition. *Odontol Rev*. 1961;12:348.

Johnson DR, Moore WJ. *Anatomy for Dental Students*. 3rd ed. Oxford, UK: Oxford University Press; 1997.

Kessler HP, Kraut RA. Dentigerous cyst associated with an impacted mesiodens. *Gen Dent*. 1989;48:47.

King NM, Wei SH. Developmental defects of enamel: A study of 12 year olds in Hong Kong. *J Am Dent Assoc*. 1986;112:835.

Kraus BS, Jordan E, Abrams L. *Dental Anatomy and Occlusion*. 2nd ed. St. Louis: Mosby; 1992.

Liebgoot B. *The Anatomic Basis of Dentistry*. 3rd ed. St. Louis: Mosby; 2011.

Logan BM. *Head and Neck Anatomy*. 4th ed. Philadelphia: Elsevier; 2010.

Logothetis DD. *Local Anesthesia for the Dental Hygienist*. 2nd ed. St. Louis: Elsevier; 2017.

Mangold WG, Pol L, Abercrombie CL, Berl R. New community residents' preferences for dental service information. *J Am Dent Assoc*. 1986;112:840.

Massler M, Schour I. *Atlas of the Mouth in Health and Disease*. 2nd ed. Chicago: American Dental Association; 1975.

Mohl ND. *A Textbook of Occlusion*. Lombard, IL: Quintessence; 1988.

Mourino AP, Camm JH. Multiple anomalies of a newborn: report of a case. *J Am Dent Assoc*. 1987;114:335.

Nanci A. *Ten Cate's Oral Histology*. 8th ed. St. Louis: Mosby; 2013.

Nelson S. *Wheeler's Dental Anatomy, Physiology and Occlusion*. 11th ed. St. Louis: Elsevier Inc; 2020.

Proffit WR, Fields HW, Nixon WL. Occlusal forces in normal and long-face adults. *J Dent Res*. 1983;62:566.

Ramfjord S, Ash MM. *Occlusion*. 3rd ed. Philadelphia: WB Saunders Co.; 1983.

Ramfjord S, Ash MM. Significance of occlusion in the etiology and treatment of early, moderate, and advanced periodontitis. *J Periodontol*. 1981;52:511.

Rankine-Wilson RW, Henry P. The bifurcated root canal in lower anterior teeth. *J Am Dent Assoc*. 1965;70:1162–1165.

Renner RP. *An Introduction to Dental Anatomy and Esthetics*. Lombard, IL: Quintessence; 1985.

Ruhenstein L, Byrne BE. Supraosseous extracanal invasive resorption. *Gen Dent*. 1993;41:430–433.

Vertucci FJ. Root canal anatomy of the human permanent teeth. *Oral Surg Oral Med Oral Pathol*. 1984;58:589–599.

Woelfel JB. *Dental Anatomy: Its Relevance to Dentistry*. 5th ed. Philadelphia: Lea & Febiger; 1997.

Zeisz R. *Dental Anatomy*. St. Louis: Mosby; 1949.

Oral Histology and Embryology

17

Basic Tissues

This chapter on the basic tissues of the body is in no way meant to be a complete discussion, but rather, an introduction to the basic concepts and structure of the body's tissues. The body is composed of four basic tissues: **epithelium**, **connective tissue**, **muscle**, and **nervous tissue**. A tissue is an accumulation of cells, fibers, crystals, or fluids; any one or all might compose a tissue. The basic description of a **cell** should be the starting point for discussing basic tissues (see Fig. 17.1A.)

Cell Structure

A cell can be thought of as a bag of fluid, generally varying in size from 0.01 to 0.05 mm in diameter. The wall of this bag is called the **cell membrane**, and its function is to keep the cellular fluid inside and unnecessary foreign materials outside. The cell membrane has the potential to allow molecules of different sizes to pass through it, and it can incorporate other membranes into it or add to it by itself. Fig. 17.1A, shows the area inside the cell membrane, a fluid medium known as **cytoplasm**. Within the cytoplasm are other components of the cell, but by looking through a light microscope, you can probably distinguish only one structure—the **nucleus**. The nucleus is the master control of the cell. It contains **deoxyribonucleic acid (DNA)** and **ribonucleic acid (RNA)**, which control the operation of the cell. DNA is found in chromosomes and most of RNA is found within the **nucleolus**; both of these are located within the nucleus. The function of RNA is to carry genetic information or instructions from DNA to the manufacturing parts of the cell.

Organelles

Looking through an electron microscope, which further enlarges cellular structures, you can see other parts of the cell. Most cell parts are called **organelles**, which are small functioning parts. They allow the cell to remain alive and carry out its particular function.

Small, usually oblong organelles known as **mitochondria** are responsible for energy production and for the rate at which the cell uses energy—commonly referred to as the **metabolism** of the cell. If the mitochondria are injured, the cell will not be able to function and may die. The number and location of the mitochondria are an indication of cellular activity and where the majority of activity is located within the cell. The mitochondria in Fig. 17.1B show the infoldings of the inner membrane of the mitochondria that form leaf-like projections called **cristae**. The cristae have **enzymes** on their surface that aid in cell metabolism. Just as an increased number of mitochondria indicates increased cellular activity, an increase in cristae also indicates a more active cell.

Another organelle, called the **endoplasmic reticulum**, is a sort of network within the fluid of the cell. The endoplasmic reticulum is a series of interconnecting tubules that are responsible for the manufacture of various products to be used inside or outside the cell. This function is controlled by several types of RNA from the nucleus and from the cytoplasm itself. Some of the endoplasmic reticulum have small granules of RNA known as **ribosomes** on their surface and are referred to as **rough endoplasmic reticulum**. In other instances, the endoplasmic reticulum has a smooth surface and no ribosomes and is known as **smooth endoplasmic reticulum**. The rough endoplasmic reticulum is responsible for the production of **proteins**.

Once the protein material is produced, it is often necessary to "package" it, as one would do in the shipping room of a factory. The organelle in the cell that takes care of this packaging is known as the **Golgi apparatus** or **Golgi complex**. The Golgi apparatus is a series of flattened saccules that produce a thin membrane to surround the material produced by the endoplasmic reticulum so that it can be moved around the cell and later outside of the cell without mixing with the cell's cytoplasm. To accomplish this type of cell secretion, known as **merocrine secretion**, the protein that has been surrounded by a membrane produced by the Golgi apparatus moves to the inner surface of the cell membrane and fuses to it. At the point of fusion, a rupture occurs in the cell membrane and in the membrane produced by the Golgi, and the contents are released without any loss of cytoplasm. The Golgi membrane is then incorporated into the cell membrane.

Another organelle found in many cells is called a **lysosome**, a structure that acts as a scavenger for the cell. If any other organelles of the cell die, or if the cell takes in some kind of foreign material, the lysosome will digest the substances. This organelle

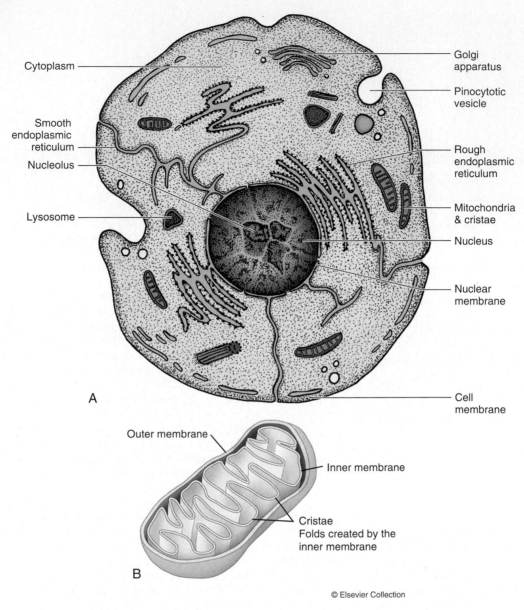

Cytoplasm

Golgi apparatus

Pinocytotic vesicle

Smooth endoplasmic reticulum

Nucleolus

Rough endoplasmic reticulum

Lysosome

Mitochondria & cristae

Nucleus

Nuclear membrane

A

Cell membrane

Outer membrane

Inner membrane

Cristae Folds created by the inner membrane

B

© Elsevier Collection

• **Figure 17.1** A cell showing all basic components, except for lipid or glycogen inclusions **(A)**. Mitochondria structure showing the cristae created by the folding of the inner membrane **(B)**. This folding of the inner membrane increases the functional surface area of the cristae.

contains very powerful digestive enzymes to perform its job, and if it is injured, the enzymes will leak out and consume the cell.

Along with the presence or absence of pressure from cells around it, most cells maintain their shape because of the existence of organelles known as **microtubules** or **microfilaments**. These structures are ultrastructural—that is, they are so small that they can only be seen with an electron microscope. The microtubules are hollow rods of proteins and are often associated with the cell's motile parts, called *cilia* or *flagella.* Microfilaments are solid protein rods and are found in all cells except mature **erythrocytes**, or red blood cells. They run in many directions throughout the cell and often bind to the cell membrane or to other microfilaments. **Centrioles** are found as a pair of multitubular rods that function in mitosis, aiding in alignment of the poles of the dividing cell.

Cellular Inclusions

Organelles are intermixed in many cells with what are called **cellular inclusions**. This term indicates that the contents of the inclusions are not produced by the cell, but rather are stored in the cell to be used at a later time and possibly another place. These inclusions may be little spheres of fat, known as **lipid droplets**, or multiple units of the sugar glucose, known as **glycogen**. Both lipid droplets and glycogen are storage forms of energy. When the body requires energy, they are released from the cell that stores them to travel to other parts of the body to be used as needed (Fig. 17.2). Many of these inclusions enter the cell by a process known as **pinocytosis**, which means *drinking in.* The product pushes into the cell membrane from outside, and the membrane caves inward, finally pinching itself off and surrounding the inclusion without any loss of cytoplasm.

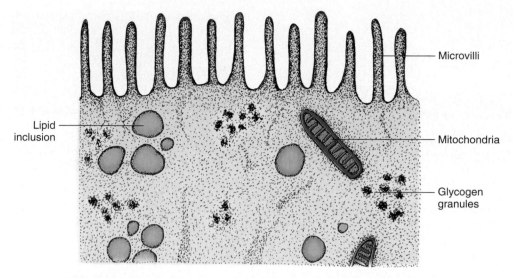

• **Figure 17.2** A portion of an absorptive cell showing glycogen and lipid inclusions.

Although this is only a brief discussion of cells and their components, a number of different types of cells have different functions. This chapter further explores the similarities and differences of these cells and their functions within the four basic tissues of the body.

Epithelial Tissue

Epithelium is a group of cells that makes up skin and lines the inside of the tubes and cavities of the body. Examples of these lining layers include the inside of blood vessels or the digestive tract and the lining of the walls of the thoracic (chest) and abdominal cavities. Glands, such as salivary glands, sweat glands, pancreas, and liver, also originate from epithelium. The shapes of epithelial cells differ, and they are in a variety of relationships. Because of these differences, each type of epithelium has a different classification according to its number of cell layers—simple epithelium is single layered and stratified epithelium has multiple layers.

Simple Epithelium

Simple Squamous Epithelium

The word *squamous* means *flat* or *platelike*. If you looked at the surface of **simple squamous epithelium**, it would look like a collection of fried eggs side by side in a big pan. If you looked at

the cross section of this epithelium, it would look like an overdone fried egg cut right through the yolk (Fig. 17.3). When looking at it from the side view, you can imagine that such a thin layer would not be an extremely protective type of structure but might be thin enough for some materials to pass through between the cells. This type of epithelium is of the following two types:

Endothelial cells: found lining blood vessels, **lymphatic vessels**, and lining the heart.

Mesothelial cells: found lining cavities in the body such as **pleural, peritoneal**, and **pericardial cavities.**

Simple Cuboidal Epithelium

Simple cuboidal epithelial cells are cubelike in shape and only one layer thick; however, that one layer is much thicker than the squamous layer. These cells are located in a number of areas in the body, such as the kidneys, the glands, and the respiratory passages (Fig. 17.4A). There may be cilia on some of these cells, which are movable and can trap contaminants and help move them out of the organ or tract.

Simple Columnar Epithelium

Columnar cells are tall, rectangular-shaped cells that line the digestive tract from the stomach to the anal region (see Fig. 17.4B). In this location, the main function of the epithelium is absorption of the breakdown products within the digestive tract. To do a more thorough job in this process, the end of the cell facing

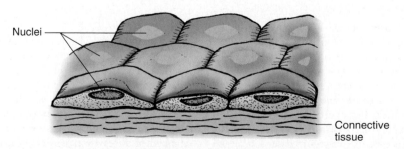

• **Figure 17.3** Simple squamous epithelium. In the cross-sectional picture at the front, the cells and nuclei are flat. On the upper surface, the nuclei are slightly raised, like the yolk of an egg.

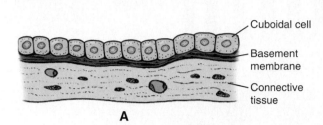

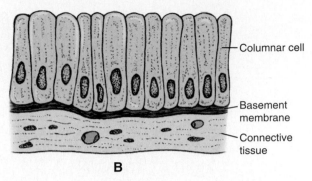

© Elsevier Collection

• **Figure 17.4 (A)** Simple cuboidal epithelium is similar to simple columnar epithelium as you can see, but its cells are shorter and cuboidal in shape. **(B)** Simple columnar epithelium. The cells are tall and all the same height. They rest on a basement of connective tissue.

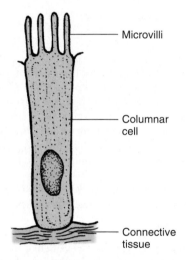

• **Figure 17.5** Simple columnar cell with microvilli. Microvilli are exaggerated in length and width so that you can see how they would increase the surface area of the cell membrane.

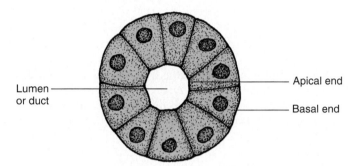

• **Figure 17.6** Columnar cells forming a tube or duct pushed into a pyramidal pattern. Apical ends are narrower than basal ends. Secretions come from the apical ends.

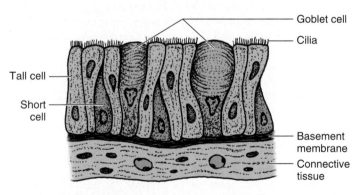

• **Figure 17.7** Representation of pseudostratified columnar epithelium from the trachea. Note that goblet cells are intermixed. More than one row of cells appears to be evident, but in actuality only one is, because all cells rest on the basement membrane. Also note cilia at the cells' surface.

toward the lumen has small ultrastructural projections known as **microvilli**. These microvilli increase the surface area of the cell end by many times its original surface, thereby increasing the amount of nutrients that can be absorbed in the digestive tract (Fig. 17.5). The cells are also found in the ducts of various glands. When these columnar cells are packed together to form small ducts, they tend to form a pyramid shape (Fig. 17.6) and are often referred to as **pyramidal cells**. These cells often have microvilli for the same purpose as cuboidal cells.

Pseudostratified Columnar Epithelium

The term **pseudostratified columnar epithelium** means *falsely layered epithelium* or epithelium that looks like more than one layer. Viewed under a microscope, it appears that several rows of nuclei are present, which would suggest more than one row of cells. However, on closer examination, it is evident that all the cells reach down to the underlying tissue, the **basement membrane**. Some of the cells are very short, but others begin on the basement membrane with a very narrow stem and then expand once they reach the upper part of the cell layer. This type of epithelium is seen in several areas of the body, but most prominently in the respiratory passages. In the respiratory tract and in other places, epithelium has many

small, single-celled glands called **goblet cells** intermixed with epithelium (Fig. 17.7). These glands secrete a mucous substance and lubricate the surface of the epithelium for a number of functions. Along with goblet cells, this epithelium also has small, hairlike projections known as **cilia**, which perform a waving, beating motion. These cilia are coated with mucus from goblet cells and then trap the contaminants passing through the duct or tract. These trapped particles are passed along from cilium to cilium by means of the beating motion until they reach an opening out of the body. Some simple columnar epithelia also have cilia.

Stratified Epithelium

Of the three varieties of multiple-layered, or stratified, epithelia, only two are commonly found in the body.

Stratified Cuboidal or Stratified Columnar Epithelium

A type of epithelium not commonly found is **stratified cuboidal** or **stratified columnar epithelium**. It consists of two or possibly more rows of cuboidal or columnar cells on top of one another and is generally only found forming large ducts of glands.

Transitional Epithelium

The term *transitional* indicates change, and that appropriately describes **transitional epithelium**. It changes in thickness and appearance as the need arises. Composed of multiple layers of cells and varying in thickness, it is found in the urinary system, with the primary concentration in the urinary bladder and the ureter. Relaxing and stretching of the tissue can make it appear that the number of layers is varying (Fig. 17.8A, B). This change in appearance accounts for the name "transitional" and represents a very functional arrangement of cells.

Stratified Squamous Epithelium

The most common type of epithelium is **stratified squamous epithelium**. As skin, it covers the body and also makes up the mucosa of the oral cavity, pharynx, esophagus, and anal region. In a discussion of this type of epithelium, it seems appropriate to consider the changes seen in the cells at different layers of the stratified squamous epithelium.

Stratum Basale

A single layer of cuboidal cells that rests on the underlying connective tissue of the basement membrane is known as **stratum basale**. It is in this layer that the cells divide and form more cells to maintain the supply and replace the cells that are lost.

Stratum Spinosum

As more cells form in the **basal layer**, they become displaced because of the crowding; thus they are pushed out of the basal layer into the layers above them toward the surface. The **stratum spinosum** varies in its number of cell rows from 2 to 3 to 10 or more. Like the basal layer, some cell division can still be seen in this layer. These cells are no longer cuboidal but seem to be star shaped or have many small points, hence the adjective "spinosum." The reason for the star-shaped appearance is that the cells are attached at points of intracellular modifications, called **desmosomes**, on the walls of adjacent cells. During preparation of tissue for study under a microscope, the cells dehydrate and shrink away from each other but are held together at the points of desmosomal attachments and thus appear star shaped. The cells continue to be pushed toward the surface by the newly forming basal cells and eventually reach the next layer.

Stratum Granulosum

Not clearly seen in many areas of the mucosa of the oral cavity, **stratum granulosum** is particularly evident in thick skin. When seen, it appears as two or three layers of flattened cells that contain granules or spots within their cytoplasm. These granules are made up of a material called **keratohyalin** and eventually cause the cell to die when the amount of **keratin** becomes great enough.

Stratum Corneum

The term *corneum* has the same meaning as the term *keratinized*; it means *hornlike*. **Stratum corneum** resembles the tissue of the fingernail but is less dense and therefore softer. In many instances, stratum corneum is misnamed because the top layers of cells are not always cornified or keratinized. Three different situations can be seen in this layer:

1. The cells may be alive, and epithelium is then referred to as **nonkeratinized** stratified squamous epithelium. In this type, no stratum granulosum is present.
2. The cells on the surface, although still showing signs of nuclei, may be in the process of dying and are referred to as partly keratinized, or **parakeratinized**, stratified squamous epithelium. Here the stratum granulosum is very thin.
3. The cells on the surface may be dead, and epithelium is then referred to as **keratinized stratified squamous epithelium**. Here the upper layer has no nuclei, and the cells appear somewhat opaque when they are not stained with dyes for microscopic study (Fig. 17.9; see also Fig. 23.1).

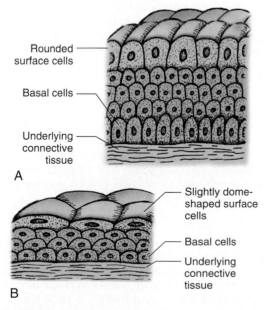

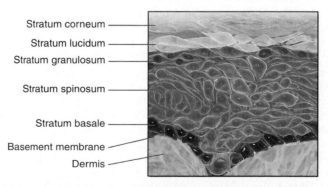

• **Figure 17.8 (A)** Relaxed transitional epithelium of bladder. About five rows of cells are present. **(B)** Stretched transitional epithelium. Fewer rows are evident, and the surface cells and their nuclei are more flattened.

• **Figure 17.9** Stratified squamous epithelium. The stratum spinosum and stratum corneum would be thicker. Because this is thick skin, a stratum lucidum can be seen. (From: Figures 17-9 Blausen.com staff (2014). "Medical gallery of Blausen Medical 2014". WikiJournal of Medicine 1 (2). DOI:10.15347/wjm/2014.010. ISSN 2002-4436. - Own work.)

TABLE 17.1	Classification of Epithelia			
Cell Type	**Cell Shape**	**Cell Modifications**	**Characteristics**	**Location**
Simple				
1. Squamous				
a. Endothelial	Spindle			Lines heart, blood, and lymph vessels
b. Mesothelial	Oval to polygonal			Lines pleural, pericardial, and peritoneal cavities
2. Cuboidal	Cube		Cilia may appear	Kidney, glands, respiratory passages
3. Columnar	Rodlike		Microvilli, cilia may appear	Most glands, small intestines, respiratory passages
4. Pseudostratified	Rodlike with thin section		Cilia, stereocilia	Respiratory passages, male reproductive organs
Stratified				
1. Squamous	Polyhedral		Intercellular bridges	Covering of the body, mouth, pharynx, vagina
2. Columnar	Columnar cells on cuboidal or columnar on columnar			Oropharynx, larynx
3. Transitional	Cube to pear		Distension causes cell flattening	Urinary passages, bladder

From Gartner L. & Hiatt J. *Color Textbook of Histology*. 3rd ed. Publisher location is Edinburgh: Saunders; 2007.

The thickness of this dead upper layer varies, depending on the amount of trauma or rubbing to which the tissue is subjected. As you know, working with a shovel or rake will eventually cause a callus to form in the hand—a result of a thickening of the stratum corneum and stratum spinosum. In thick skin, such as the palms of hands or the soles of feet, a clear layer known as the **stratum lucidum** can be seen between the stratum granulosum and the stratum corneum. The cells are continually produced in the basal layer of the epithelium and move up through the other layers until they reach the surface, where they are shed. Our bodies possess a mechanism that regulates the cells produced and lost, adjusting to meet any needed changes. Without this control, we would have either skin as thick as an elephant's or no skin at all (Table 17.1).

Another important mechanism relating to cell replacement in skin has to do with pigment in skin and changes in that pigment level. Skin normally has a yellowish color because it contains the pigment **carotene**. Some pink color is also imparted to it by the underlying blood vessels. Immediately beneath the basal layer of cells in all humans except albinos are cells called **melanocytes**, which produce a pigment called **melanin** (Fig. 17.10). These cells, when stimulated by **ultraviolet rays**, produce more pigment, which becomes incorporated into epithelial cells and is carried to the surface. As this happens, skin darkens. When the person is no longer subjected to these ultraviolet rays, the pigment level is reduced, the cells containing it are eventually lost, and skin lightens in color. Ethnic groups with typically darker-colored skin have more melanocytes present. These cells are constantly producing more melanin, thus maintaining the darker color of their skin. In the absence of melanocytes, or with a limited number of them, a more pinkish color is imparted to skin.

Glands

Most of the glands of the body are developed from epithelium. As epithelium develops, some of the basal cells begin to grow downward into the connective tissue beneath epithelium. As the basal cells grow downward, they form a cord of epithelial cells that later hollow out to form a tube. When these tubes have reached a certain depth, they form a number of bulblike or tubelike processes on their ends, which are generally referred to as **acini** or tubules, respectively. Glands can be classified in a number of ways.

Distributive Mechanisms

The term *distributive mechanism* refers to the manner in which the secretory products are carried away from the gland. **Exocrine** glands contain products that are carried away by ducts leading from the gland. **Endocrine** glands have ducts that are lost after the gland develops and has products that are carried away from the gland in the bloodstream. Salivary glands are an example of exocrine glands, and the thyroid gland is an endocrine gland example.

Secretory Mechanisms

The secretory mechanism is the manner in which the product is secreted from the gland. In **holocrine** glands, the entire cell dies, and the secretion is expelled when the cell membrane breaks up. This sort of process is seen in the sebaceous glands of the hair follicles. The oil of the hair is a result of the death of the cells of the gland. The secretory products of **merocrine** glands pass through the cell wall without allowing any cell cytoplasm to escape. This is how the salivary glands secrete, without any loss of cytoplasm.

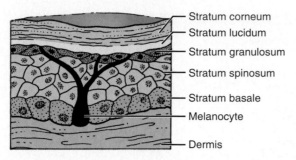

- **Figure 17.10** The body of the melanocyte cell lies beneath the basal layer of epithelium, and melanin granules are secreted into the layers above.

Merocrine secretion was described earlier in the discussion on the Golgi apparatus.

Arrangement of Components

Exocrine glands have secretory and excretory portions. The secretory portion is composed of cells that actually secrete and modify the substance being produced by the gland. The excretory portion is that part of the duct system that carries the product to the surface epithelium without changing the makeup of the secretory substance. The arrangement of these components varies, depending on whether the gland is a simple tubular gland, which is just a straight tube, or a **compound tubuloalveolar** gland (e.g., salivary glands). A compound gland has numerous levels of branching within its duct system, similar in appearance to a bunch of grapes—that is, tubelike secretory parts with a rounded alveolus or acinus at the end of each tube (Fig. 17.11).

Products

Salivary glands produce the following types of secretions:
1. **Serous** secretion—a thin, watery substance containing most of the digestive enzymes found in saliva

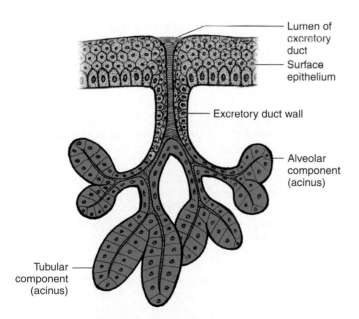

- **Figure 17.11** Representation of compound tubuloalveolar glands. Branchings of ducts have rounded alveolar end pieces and elongated tubular end pieces.

2. **Mucous** secretion—a thicker, more viscous substance containing mucins for lubrication and protection
3. **Seromucous or mucoserous** secretion—a substance produced by many of the glands that have both serous and mucous cells and in varying quantities within the same gland

Embryonic Origin

An individual, and in-turn all basic tissues, develops from a single cell, the fertilized ovum. From this one cell the following occurs: the fertilized ovum divides into two cells, the two into four, and so on. This multiplication forms a ball of cells, which becomes hollow with a thickened inner layer on one side. This hollow ball is called a **blastocyst** (Fig. 17.12). The outer layer of cells of this blastocyst is called the **trophoblast layer,** and the thickened inner layer is called the **embryoblast layer**. The trophoblast layer becomes part of the membranes surrounding the developing embryo and the placenta. The embryoblast layer forms the actual embryo itself, one of the membrane layers, and a sac called the *amnion*. At first, the embryoblast is an elongated flat structure made up of two layers of epithelial cell layers. The outer layer of epithelial cells is called the **ectoderm**. The inner layer of epithelial cells will be replaced eventually by cells from the ectoderm and become the **endoderm**. Later, more cells of the ectoderm layer work their way between these two layers and become the **mesoderm**, or middle layers. The downward migration of the cells in the middle of the embryo is called the **primitive streak**. This downward growth is caused by an increase in proliferation of cells into the middle of the embryo. Eventually the embryo will be divided into a right half and a left half. Each half mirrors the other in growth. As the ectoderm migrates, it forms a mesodermal layer and an endodermal layer.

Lastly, a group of ectodermal cells within the neural plate differentiate and form the **neural crest**. All the other cells of the body develop from these four layers. Different kinds of epithelium may come from three of these basic embryonic layers: (1) The ectoderm develops into the epidermis of skin and into the central nervous system; (2) the endoderm forms the epithelium of the digestive tract, the respiratory system, and some glands; and (3) the mesoderm gives rise to the connective tissue dermis, bone and cartilage, the squamous lining of the abdominal and thoracic cavities, and the inner lining of blood vessels (Fig. 17.13). Glands generally arise from either the ectoderm or the endoderm. Most dental connective tissues are derived from the neural crest—including pulp, dentin, cementum, alveolar process, and the periodontal ligament.

Connective Tissue

The term *connective tissue* refers to tissues that connect and support other tissues and parts of the body. All the various types of connective tissues originate from the mesoderm. Connective tissues can be divided into connective tissue proper and more specialized connective tissues, such as cartilage, bone, and blood.

Connective Tissue

Connective tissue is composed of cells, fibers, the fluidlike material referred to as **ground substance**, and a filtrate of blood plasma called *extracellular fluid*. Connective tissue is subdivided into connective tissue proper and dense connective tissue.

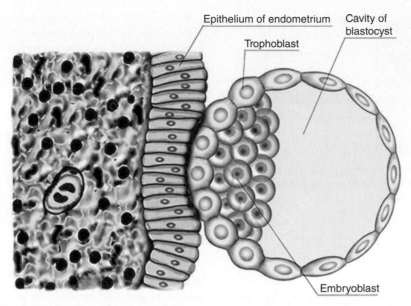

• **Figure 17.12** The embryoblast layer of the blastocyst will later become the embryo, and the trophoblast layer will help form the placenta. (From: Asklepios Medical Atlas/Science Photo Library.)

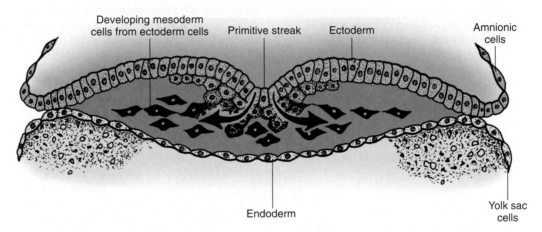

• **Figure 17.13** Cross section through a flat plate of cells of a 16-day embryo. The primitive streak divides the embryo into right and left halves. All germ layers originate from the downgrowth of the primitive streak.

Connective Tissue Proper

Loose connective tissue, which is found in superficial and deep fasciae, supports the internal frameworks of all organs. It is made up of collagen, elastic fibers, fibroblasts, macrophages, and mast cells.

Dense Connective Tissue

Regular Connective Tissue

The term *regular connective tissue* simply means that collagen fibers run parallel to one another, with fibroblasts squeezed between them. Dense regular connective tissues are found as tendons, which attach muscle to bone, and ligaments, which attach bone to bone. Collagen fibers are arranged in parallel rows, with fibroblasts aligned between the rows. The presence of fibroblasts indicates the ability of tendons or ligaments to repair themselves most of the time. If tendons or ligaments are completely torn, then surgery is required.

Dense Irregular Connective Tissue

When some epithelia, such as the epithelium of the skin on the arm, are examined, they are found to be quite movable. Epithelium has no blood vessels, and yet its cells are active and therefore must have a nutrient source somewhere. The dense irregular connective tissue immediately below skin serves as this source. Besides cells, fibers, and ground substance, irregular connective tissue also contains nerves and blood vessels that supply the area (Fig. 17.14). Many different types of connective tissue cells are evident. One of the most important cells is the **fibroblast**. The suffix *blast* means *to sprout*. Therefore the word *fibroblast* refers to one of the cells that sprouts or forms fibers. These are known as **collagen** fibers. They are nonelastic and function by holding epithelium to the underlying muscle or bone, thus holding bones together or attaching muscles to bone. The collagen fiber is also the fiber that attaches the tooth to its socket. This chapter later discusses how collagen fibers can be formed by cells that produce

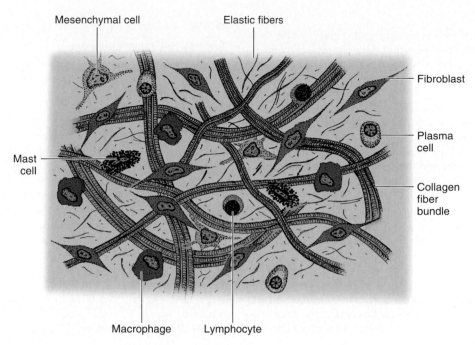

Mesenchymal cell   Elastic fibers

Fibroblast

Plasma cell

Mast cell

Collagen fiber bundle

Macrophage   Lymphocyte

• **Figure 17.14** Irregular connective tissue with fibroblasts, collagen fibers, and other cells and fibers of connective tissue. Invisible ground substance holds it all together.

bone, cartilage, dentin, and cementum. Numerous varieties of collagen fibers are found, each with a Roman numeral designation. The most common one in irregular connective tissue is designated **type I collagen**.

Another type of cell found in connective tissue is a primitive cell of mesodermal origin and is called the **mesenchymal cell**. This is the first cell seen when the mesoderm develops in the early embryo. This cell has the potential to change into a number of other cell types that produce bone, cartilage, muscle, and fibroblasts. The presence of mesenchymal cells in tissue allows for the replacement of some components of connective tissue that are lost through injury.

Cells present in connective tissue produce antibodies to fight off or resist certain microorganisms or foreign substances entering the body. The most common of these is the tissue lymphocyte, which is virtually the same as the lymphocyte that travels in circulating blood. These lymphocytes are designated as either **B-lymphocytes** or **T-lymphocytes**. B-lymphocytes originate from bone marrow and then move to many lymphoid organs, such as the spleen, lymph nodes, and others, where they multiply. When stimulated antigenically by foreign substances, they duplicate and enlarge to form **plasma cells**, which secrete antibodies. T-lymphocytes also originate from bone marrow and then migrate to the thymus gland and multiply there to form cells that have numerous functions. The most common of these functions is to combat virus-infected cells, various tumors, and grafted tissues and organs. In transplantation, these cells therefore have to be destroyed or have their function suppressed by chemotherapeutic agents before tissues or organs can be transplanted. If they are not destroyed, T-lymphocytes attack the newly transplanted tissues and cause them to be rejected.

Some cells called **macrophages** act as scavengers and devour dying cells and microorganisms. Because of their function, macrophages contain *lysosomes,* the scavenger organelle found in many cells (refer to the beginning of this chapter). Macrophages may be fixed in certain areas or may be capable of wandering freely throughout connective tissue.

Another type of cell that is found in varying quantities within connective tissue is the **fat cell**, or **adipocyte**. Adipocytes can be found in large quantities in the bottom layers of connective tissue. Fat cells can accumulate in large quantities in some areas of the body, such as the abdomen, gluteal region, and thighs.

In addition to these cells, fibers are also present within connective tissue. One, the **reticular fiber**, primarily functions as a framework for a number of organs. This reticular fiber is formed by a cell that looks virtually identical to a fibroblast. Another fiber is the **elastic fiber**, which stretches and then returns to its original length. Elastic fibers found beneath skin are depleted with aging, and the results of this process can readily be seen in bags under the eyes and wrinkles in the face because they are most apparent in areas of thin skin, such as the face.

Irregular connective tissue is so named because its fibers run in all directions. It is further subdivided into *loose irregular connective tissue* and *dense irregular connective tissue.* The former primarily contains reticular fibers, elastic fibers, lymphocytes, and plasma cells, as well as the cells already discussed. Dense irregular tissue, however, replaces most other types of fibers with coarse bundles of collagen fibers.

The third major component of connective tissue, the ground substance, is a gluelike substance that holds the cells and fibers together. This is supplemented with varying amounts of gel-like water found as intercellular fluid, which is a filtrate of blood plasma. The gel consistency results from several groups of combinations of proteins and carbohydrates called **proteoglycans** and **glycoproteins**.

Loose Connective Tissue With Special Properties
Mucous Connective Tissue
This type of tissue is primarily made up of fibroblasts and collagen and is found in the umbilical cord as well as the vocal cords.

Elastic Tissue

This tissue is made up of fibroblasts and yellow elastic fibers. It is found in the vocal cords, as supporting tissue in general connective tissue, and in the ligaments connecting the spinous processes of the vertebrae.

Reticular Tissue

This type of tissue is a fine series of fibers that helps form the structural framework of several organs. The tissue comprises **reticular fibers** and cells. These form the stroma, or framework, of lymphoid organs, such as lymph nodes and the spleen. The functioning cells of these organs surround the supporting reticular tissue.

Adipose Tissue

Better known as "fatty tissue," it is composed of fat cells, or adipocytes. It is found in loose connective tissue and in larger deposits throughout the body.

Pigment Tissue

As mentioned earlier, melanocytes, or better called **melanoblasts**, are found below and within the bottom layers of skin. They produce melanin granules that increase the pigmentation of skin.

Cartilage

Cartilage is a noncalcified supporting component of the body; however, cartilage does calcify in some areas, such as the larynx. It is composed of cells called **chondroblasts** or **chondrocytes**, fibers of either collagen or **elastin**, and a ground substance. The three types of cartilage are **hyaline cartilage, fibrocartilage**, and **elastic cartilage**.

Hyaline Cartilage

Hyaline cartilage is firmer than the other two types of cartilage and contains fine collagen fibers, chondrocytes, and chondroblasts. It can be seen in an adult in such areas as the larynx, trachea, bronchi, nasal cartilages, and certain parts of bones. During a person's development from the embryonic stage into adulthood, many of the areas that originate as hyaline cartilage later change into bone. It is also this hyaline cartilage that allows the bones of arms and legs to lengthen.

Elastic Cartilage

Elastic cartilage contains elastic fibers, chondrocytes, and chondroblasts, and it is very flexible. It is found in the firm but flexible part of the ear, in the epiglottis over the larynx, and in the eustachian tube.

Fibro Cartilage

Fibrocartilage contains a great deal of collagen fibers and functions as a cushioning substance. It is found in such areas as intervertebral disks between the vertebrae of the spinal column and, in the adult, the temporomandibular joint (TMJ) of the jaw.

One significant characteristic about cartilage is that it grows in two ways. First, it grows by adding to its surface, which is known as **apposition** or **appositional growth**. Cartilage is surrounded by a double layer of tissue known as **perichondrium** (meaning *around the cartilage*). The outer layer is composed of collagen fibers, and the inner layer contains cells that become chondroblasts and form cartilage. This is the layer that causes appositional growth. Second, the chondrocytes found inside the cartilage undergo cell division and enlargement and cause growth from within. This is known as **interstitial growth**. If it were not for this process of interstitial growth, it would not be possible for the long bones of the body to grow in length.

Bone

Spongy or Cancellous Bone

This is the bone tissue that is found in the middle of bone. It is usually referred to as *bone marrow*. Small bridges of bone have space in between, and these spaces function as either blood-producing or fat-storing tissue.

Compact or Dense Bone

This is the hard outer layer of bone. What makes bone hard? Bone is made up of cells called **osteoblasts** (meaning *bone formers*) or **osteocytes** (meaning *bone cells*), collagen fibers, and ground substance. Bone also has microscopic crystals of a substance called **hydroxyapatite**. These crystals of calcium and phosphate are found packed into the ground substance and fibers between cells, giving bone its hardness. If a bone is placed in an acidic substance, the crystals dissolve, and only the other three components are left. Consider the following experiment in which a chicken bone is placed in vinegar. After a few days, the chicken bone can be bent into a pretzel shape. Vinegar, which is acetic acid, dissolves the crystals, which makes the bone flexible.

Intramembranous Ossification

Similar to cartilage, bone forms in more than one way. One way is by **intramembranous ossification**, or formation within tissue. Bone forms in regular connective tissue when some of the primitive mesenchymal cells differentiate into osteoblast cells. These osteoblast cells are soon surrounded by a double-layered structure called **periosteum**. The outer layer is made up of collagen, and the inner layer is made up of osteogenic cells that become osteoblasts and form more bone. These cells secrete ground substance, collagen fibers, and then hydroxyapatite crystals. The crystals grow and pack tightly together, and the forming bone hardens. Osteoblasts that get entrapped within their own matrix stop forming more bone and become known as *osteocytes*. These cells play a role in the nutrition of bone. Most of the bone growth in the head area is of the intramembranous type (Fig. 17.15).

Endochondral Ossification

The second way in which bone forms is called **endochondral ossification**. With this type of bone formation, cartilage is first formed, covered by perichondrium; the inner layer of the perichondrium contains cells that become chondroblasts, which produce a cartilage model of the future bone shape. The cartilage is then invaded by bone cells, which replace the cartilage with bone (Fig. 17.16). As bone replaces cartilage, it does so in two end sections called the **epiphyses** and a center section called the **diaphysis**. Between each epiphysis and diaphysis is a block of cartilage known as the **epiphyseal plate**. Within this plate is an interstitial growth of cartilage that causes the plate to lengthen; then some of either side of the plate is converted to bone, and the bone thus grows in length. Without that block of cartilage, the bone would be unable to have a directional growth. Perichondrium is eventually replaced by periosteum. When the pituitary gland stops producing growth hormone, the epiphyseal plate disappears, and the bone is no longer in three sections but unites as one. In addition to this type of growth in long bones and vertebrae, certain important areas of the bones in the bottom of the skull also grow endochondrally, which allows for lengthening of the bones from within and at the bone surface.

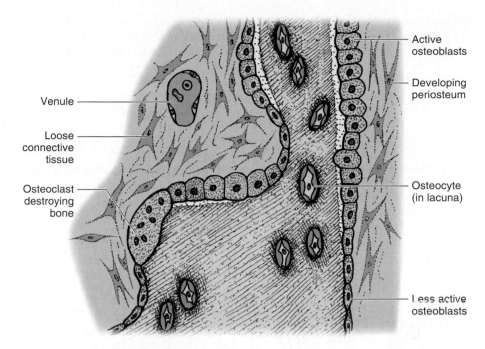

• **Figure 17.15** Intramembranous ossification. Osteoblasts secrete components and become trapped in the mix. They are then referred to as *osteocytes*. Space occupied by these osteocytes is referred to as *lacuna*. To the left, a multinucleate osteoclast can be seen destroying bone.

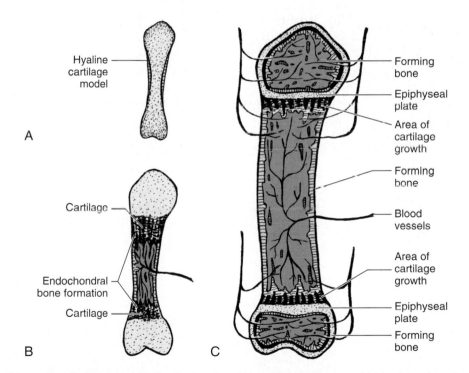

• **Figure 17.16** Endochondral ossification in a long bone. **(A)** A cartilage model of a future long bone. **(B)** Center of the model is now converted to a bony shell, and areas toward the ends are where cartilage is changing to bone and elongating. **(C)** Here bone is at either end and in the middle, with a cartilage epiphyseal plate between them. This is where elongation of the bone takes place.

Bone Structure

Once bone has developed, it appears the same microscopically. Without studying the bone while it is developing, you would not be able to determine from the final microscopic appearance whether it developed by intramembranous or endochondral ossification. Bone is about 65% hydroxyapatite crystals with the rest made up of collagen, ground substance, and water. It is covered on the outside with a double layer of periosteum. As was indicated earlier, the outer layer of the periosteum is fibrous, and the inner layer is composed of cells that become osteoblasts and can form bone. In the center of bone is a cavity, generally referred to as the **marrow cavity**. This space serves as a site of blood cell production. Later in the person's life, the marrow cavity in many bones changes into storehouses for fat. The inner wall of the marrow cavity is lined by an **endosteum**, which forms modified bone on the inside during remodeling of bone-in-bone growth.

The hard structure between the periosteum and the marrow cavity, known as *cortical bone* or *plate,* has numerous blood vessels running through it to keep it vital. Around these blood vessels are gathered many trapped bone cells, referred to in their trapped state as *osteocytes.* This arrangement of blood vessels and osteocytes is called a **Haversian system** (see Fig. 17.17A, B), a series of blood vessels running parallel to one another along the length of the bone. As bone grows, these blood vessels lying on the surface go through a series of changes whereby bone surrounds blood vessels, resulting in a hollow tube in the bone with a blood vessel in the middle. The osteoblasts lining this tube begin to secrete bony layers and eventually entrap themselves as osteocytes. These layers continue building and fill in the tube until the blood vessel is completely surrounded. Figs. 17.17A and B show the openings of

these Haversian systems as circular structures known as **Haversian lamellae**. The longitudinal blood vessels of the Haversian systems are connected with other blood vessels running perpendicular to them and traveling through tubes called **Volkmann's canals,** or *nutrient arteries.* These arteries interconnect with one another, bringing blood inside the bone. Within the Haversian system, nutrients are passed on to the entrapped osteocytes closest to the blood vessel, and they, in turn, pass the nutrients on to the cells farther from the blood vessels. Blood is also carried into the **marrow spaces**, where more blood cells are manufactured and passed out of bone. Before the arteries reach the marrow cavity, they actually go through a capillary bed and enter the marrow cavity as **venules**. Therefore the endosteal lining of the marrow cavity is similar to an endothelial lining of a vein. Then veins carry the blood and new cells produced by the marrow cavity back out of the bone and into the venous circulation of the body and back to the heart.

The area between Haversian systems also has entrapped bone cells and layers known as **interstitial lamellae**. These are parts of older Haversian systems that have been partly destroyed and replaced by newer systems. This bone resorption and apposition is known as *bone remodeling.* Bone is also deposited on its own surface by periosteum. These layers formed by periosteum and lying immediately adjacent to it are known as **circumferential lamellae**. On the inside, adjacent to the marrow spaces, are layers produced known as **endosteal lamellae**.

Haversian systems are best seen in a cross section of long bones of the arms or legs (see Fig. 17.17A, B). These same systems exist in flat bones and in some irregular-shaped bones of the skull. In flat bones the marrow cavities are very narrow and are known as **diploë**.

It is important that bone be nourished with blood because it is a constantly changing structure. A perfect example is orthodontic treatment (Fig. 17.18). The tooth movement is only possible because bone is able to change and remodel itself as the tooth moves. Cells called **osteoclasts** are involved in this remodeling process. The suffix *clast* means *something that destroys,* and the

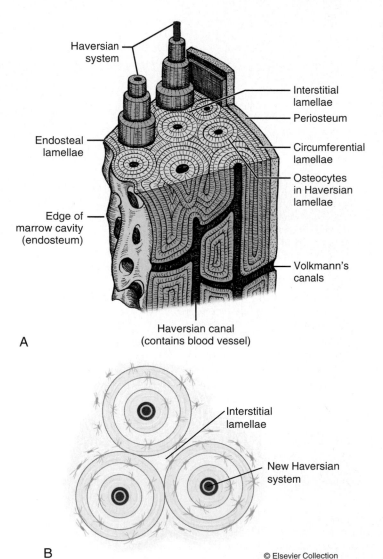

A

B

© Elsevier Collection

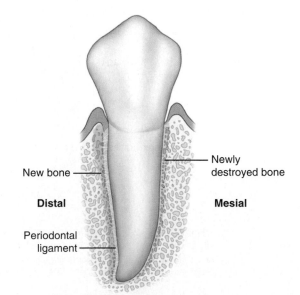

Mandibular Right Second Premolar
Buccal view

© Elsevier Collection

• **Figure 17.17** **(A)** Section through a portion of a long bone of an extremity. To the left side would be the inner marrow cavity lined with endosteum. Arteries are entering bone through Volkmann's canals and feeding into the Haversian system. Around the Haversian artery is the Haversian bone containing osteocytes. You can also see circumferential lamellae around the outside and interstitial lamellae representing old Haversian systems that are being replaced. **(B)** Interstitial lamellae are the old layers of bone cells trapped between the Haversian systems. Bone more recently formed replaces old bone in the Haversian system.

• **Figure 17.18** Bone on the side to which the tooth moves is destroyed. This is done to allow room for the tooth to move into this area. This bone is destroyed by cells known as *osteoclasts.* On the other side of the tooth, osteoblasts form bone to fill in the space vacated by the tooth.

prefix *osteo* means *bone;* thus osteoclasts are bone-destroying cells. Osteoblasts and osteoclasts work together to change bone constantly as stresses are placed on it (Table 17.2).

Blood

Blood is another type of special connective tissue. Arteries, veins, and capillaries, which carry blood, and the heart, which pumps it, are part of the organ system known as the *cardiovascular system.* Blood is made up of two components—the fluid part and the cellular part. The fluid part is called **plasma** and is similar in composition to the fluid found between the cells of the body. The cellular part is divided into erythrocytes (**red blood cells**), leukocytes (**white blood cells**), and **platelets**.

Erythrocytes

Every cubic millimeter (mm^3) of blood contains 4 to 6 million red blood cells. Red blood cells are unusual in that they have no nucleus in their mature state. They are described as **biconcave disks** and are very thin in the middle and thick at the edges. Red blood cells have an iron-containing element called **hemoglobin**. Hemoglobin has the ability to attach oxygen molecules to its structure and carry them from the lungs to the cells where oxygen is needed. It can also carry carbon dioxide, which is the waste product, from cells to the lungs for elimination. Red blood cells have a life span of about 4 months and are eliminated by the spleen, located in the upper left abdominal area, when they are worn out.

Clinical Considerations

Any significant decrease in the number of red blood cells or their ability to carry oxygen causes a condition known as **anemia**. Of the several types of anemia, one of them is brought on by a deficiency of vitamin B_{12} and another by a lack of iron in the body. Both of these are **acquired deficiencies**. One **inherited anemia** is found primarily in people of African descent, in which red blood cells change shape irreversibly when exposed to low oxygen conditions. This is known as **sickle cell anemia** because of the C shape of the red blood cell. These sickle-shaped cells do not carry oxygen well. This results in a condition called **anoxia**. Anoxia causes severe damage, even death, to the cells.

Leukocytes

Far fewer white blood cells are present than red blood cells, numbering only 4,500 to 11,000 per cubic millimeter (mm^3) of blood. White blood cells are divided into two groups by the presence or absence of granules in their cytoplasm. Those with granules are referred to as **granulocytes** and those without are **agranulocytes**.

Granulocytes

There are three types of granulocytes based on the staining properties of their granules.

Neutrophils

Of white blood cells, 40% to 60% have granules that do not stain readily and are therefore referred to as **neutrophils**. They

---

TABLE 17.2 Classification of Connective Tissue

Tissue Type	Associated Cells	Fibers		Location and Function
I. Connective Tissue Proper				
A. Loose connective tissue	Fibroblasts, macrophages, mast cells	Yellow elastic White collagen		Fascia, superficial and deep; organ framework support
B. Dense connective tissue				
1. Dense regular	Fibroblasts, macrophages	White fibrous		Tendons, ligaments; muscle to bone attachment
2. Dense irregular	Fibroblasts, macrophages	Mostly white fibrous, elastic, and reticular fibers		Sheets, dermis, some sternum, capsules; support of organs
C. Loose connective tissue with special properties				
1. Mucous connective tissue	Stellate fibroblasts	Collagenous		Umbilical and vocal cords; support
2. Elastic tissue	Fibroblasts	Yellow elastic		Ligamenta nuchae, vocal cords; support
3. Reticular tissue	Reticular cells	Fine reticular		Framework of lymph node and spleen

Continued

TABLE 17.2   Classification of Connective Tissue—cont'd

Tissue Type	Associated Cells	Fibers		Location and Function
4. Adipose tissue	Fat cells	None		Scattered in all loose connective tissue and in deposits
5. Pigment tissue	Melanoblasts	None		Corium of dark skin Choroid and iris of eye
II. Cartilage A. Hyaline cartilage	Chondrocytes	Fine collagenous		Articular and nasal cartilages, trachea, bronchi; support
B. Elastic cartilage	Chondrocytes	Elastic, collagenous		External ear, eustachian tube, epiglottis; support
C. Fibrous cartilage	Chondrocytes	Collagenous (dense)		Intervertebral disks; support
III. Bone A. Spongy or cancellous	Osteocytes, osteoblasts, osteoclasts	Collagenous		Center of long bones
B. Compact or dense	Osteocytes, osteoclasts, osteoblasts	Collagenous		Outer shaft of bones
IV. Blood and Lymph	Erythrocytes, leukocytes			Blood vascular and lymphatic systems

From Chiego D. *Essentials of Oral Histology and Embryology: A Clinical Approach.* 5th ed. St. Louis: Elsevier; 2018.

live for only about 2 days. During that time, they function as **phagocytes**, killing and devouring microorganisms. When microorganisms enter the body where they are not normally found, they trigger an **inflammatory reaction**. The four signs of inflammation are redness, warmth, swelling, and pain. The redness and warmth are attributable to more blood being sent to that region; the swelling and pain are caused by an increase in **extracellular fluid**. This increase in fluid between the cells is caused by blood plasma that leaks from the smallest of blood vessels—the capillaries and venules—of the area. As the fluid leaks out of the blood vessels, so, too, do neutrophils. Neutrophils are the first white blood cells to arrive at the site of cellular injury. They move to the area of the invading microorganisms and begin devouring them.

Eosinophils

Of white blood cells, 1% to 4% stain red with a dye known as eosin. These **eosinophils** function to help combat **allergic reactions** and inflammatory reactions. Eosinophils are involved in fighting parasitic infections.

Basophils

Of white blood cells, 0.5% to 1% stain blue with a basic stain and are known as **basophils**. These cells, along with connective tissue cells known as **mast cells**, contain a substance known as **histamine**, which is released in reaction to an **allergenic** substance. Histamine causes fluid to leak from blood vessels and the local tissues to swell. To decrease this swelling, a drug that combats this histamine reaction is used and is therefore known as an **antihistamine**. This combats the action of the histamines, which stops the leakage of the vessels, and the swelling decreases.

Agranulocytes

Two types of white blood cells have no granules and are therefore referred to as *agranulocytes*. They are the **lymphocytes** and **monocytes**.

Lymphocytes

Of white blood cells, 20% to 40% are lymphocytes. They are found in circulating blood and in **lymphoid tissues**, such as lymph nodes, spleen, and tonsils. Two different types of lymphocytes provide **immunity**. One of these lymphocytes produces a cell known as a *plasma cell,* also associated with immune responses and seen readily in tissue where long-lasting infections have occurred. There are two types of lymphocytes—B-type lymphocytes and T-type lymphocytes.

Monocytes

Of white blood cells, 2% to 8% are monocytes. Monocytes become macrophages in acute inflammation. In such cases, neutrophils, lymphocytes, and monocytic macrophages can all be found within the inflamed tissues. Monocytes fuse together in mitotic multiplication and are believed to form osteoclasts, which are large, multinucleated cells that destroy bone and other hard tissues of the body, such as dentin, cementum, and possibly enamel.

During the disease process, the number of white blood cells increases, particularly neutrophils and lymphocytes. In **leukemia**, a disease of white blood cells, one type of white blood cell starts multiplying rapidly, choking out the production of red blood cells. Most blood cells are produced in bone marrow, spleen, thymus, lymph nodes, and tonsils, where lymphocytes are formed. People who have received bone-marrow transplants, as discussed previously, are first treated with drugs that kill their own defective marrow and then receive new marrow, which should produce a normal blood cell population.

Platelets

In each cubic millimeter of blood, 150,000 to 400,00 platelets can be found. Platelets are a membrane-bound particle of a larger cell called a **megakaryocyte**, which is found in bone marrow. These platelets play an important role in the clotting of blood. When platelets reach a broken blood vessel, they may break and release a substance called **serotonin**, which causes blood vessels to contract, similar to other **vasoconstrictors**, such as **epinephrine**, which are used as dental anesthetic agents. Other platelets simply stack up in the leakage area and begin forming what will eventually be a blood clot.

Muscle Tissue

The third basic tissue, muscle, is found throughout the body. The three types of muscle tissue are skeletal, cardiac, and smooth muscles. All muscle tissues, through contraction, or shortening, in length, accomplish their work.

Skeletal Muscle

The most widely studied muscle is skeletal muscle, also known as striated **voluntary muscle**. The term *striated* refers to the striped appearance of the muscle fibers under a microscope. The word *voluntary* means that the contraction, or shortening, of muscles is under the willful control of the person or animal. A skeletal muscle, such as the biceps in the upper arm, is made up of thousands of individual muscle fibers, or muscle cells. Each of these skeletal muscle cells has not just one but hundreds of nuclei. This cell is referred to as a **myofiber**. The myofiber runs the full length of the muscle. (To avoid confusion, various muscle shapes should be noted, including how some muscles have tendons positioned throughout their length. Therefore a muscle fiber may run into a tendon and not really run the full length of the apparent muscle; in some instances, it may be 1 inch long, whereas in other muscles it may be several feet long.) Each fiber is made up of many smaller cell components called **myofibrils**. Between myofibrils are the usual components of cells, such as mitochondria and the endoplasmic reticulum. These myofibrils also have the striated appearance indicative of skeletal muscle. Myofibrils are made up of two smaller **myofilaments** called **actin** and **myosin**. The thinner actin filaments slightly overlap the thicker myosin filaments, and a chemical reaction causes the two filaments to slide over one another. The overall fiber shortening takes place by this sliding mechanism. This whole process is repeated hundreds of times in a single myofibril. Hundreds of light and dark staining bands are present in a fibril. The light band is called the **I band,** and the dark band is called the **A band**. Halfway through the I band is a thin, dark line called the **Z line**. The distance between two Z lines is called a **sarcomere**, and within one sarcomere are all the components necessary for this sliding filament mechanism of skeletal muscle. Therefore the sarcomere is the functional unit of skeletal muscle (Fig. 17.19).

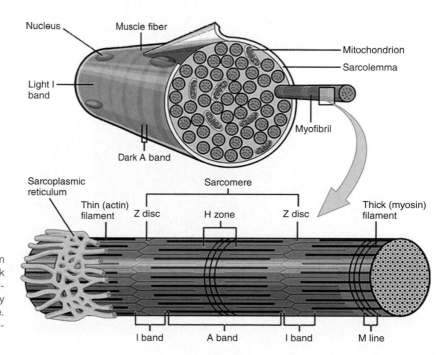

• **Figure 17.19** Entire realm of skeletal muscle tissue, from whole muscle to components of sarcomere. Thin and thick filaments slide over one another in contraction. (From Vladimirsky, S. (2020, September 7). What is muscle hypertrophy and how does it work? Kinesis Magazine. kinesismagazine.com/2020/09/07/what-is-muscle-hypertrophy-and-how-does-it-work/.)

Cardiac Muscle

Heart muscle, or cardiac muscle, is referred to as striated **involuntary muscle**; that is, it has striping similar to the skeletal muscle. The term *involuntary* means that control of the heart is not under the willful control of the individual but rather is regulated automatically by the body. Cardiac muscle differs from skeletal muscle in that it has only one or two nuclei per cell, and the muscle cells or fibers branch as they meet one another. Similar to skeletal muscle, cardiac muscle has banding, and the sarcomere is the smallest functioning unit. The heart muscle is also unusual in that it has specialized muscle cells, called **Purkinje's fibers**, that act like nerves in the heart and conduct messages through the heart to help it contract or beat properly.

Smooth Muscle

Smooth muscle is the third kind of muscle tissue and is nonstriated involuntary muscle. This means that it does not have stripes and cannot be willfully controlled. These muscle fibers are found lining such areas as the digestive tract (where they move the food through the tract), in blood vessels (where they regulate the flow of blood to different parts of the body), in the lungs (where they contract the air passages and alveolar sac areas), and in many other organs. Smooth muscle has actin and myosin components as is found in the other two kinds of muscle; however, these components are not regularly arranged, and as a consequence, the muscle fibers do not appear striped (Fig. 17.20).

Nervous Tissue

Nervous tissue serves as the communicating system of the body. Sensory or **afferent** messages are carried from the outer parts of the body toward the brain. They provide information for the brain, and it reacts accordingly. The messages leaving the brain for distant parts of the body are referred to as motor or **efferent** messages; they usually cause some kind of action to take place.

The cell of the nervous system is called the **neuron**. The three parts of the neuron are the **cell body**, the **axon**, and the **dendrite**. A neuron functions to carry a message by sodium and potassium ions passing in and out through the cell membrane. This sets up a small electrical charge that passes along the cell wall. These changes in the polarity of the neuronal cell membrane are referred to as *depolarization* and *repolarization*. This current does not have a message in it, but only a wave of electricity. It is the brain itself that converts the current to information based on the type of neuron carrying the message, where it is from, and, at times, the relationship to a past experience. Neurons carry messages generally in only one direction. The wave of electricity passes from the dendrite to the cell body and out along the axon. When it reaches the end of the axon, it contacts the dendrite or cell body of the next neuron and passes the message or impulse to the adjacent neuron through small vesicles or droplets that are made up of **acetylcholine** or **epinephrine**. The wave of depolarization travels along that neuron until it reaches its destination. Thus neurons carry messages to the brain, and other neurons carry messages away from the brain (Fig. 17.21).

Characteristic	Skeletal	Cardiac	Smooth
Body location	Attached to bones or, for some facial muscles, to skin 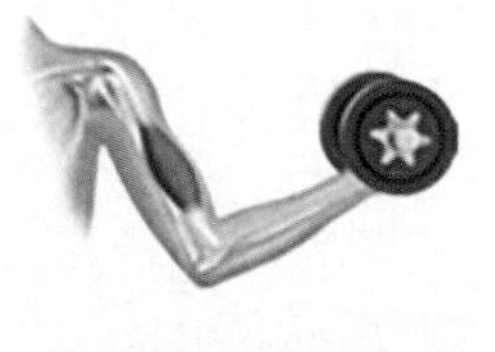	Walls of the heart 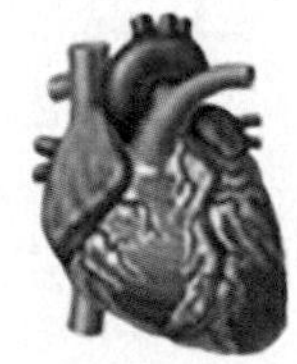	Mostly in walls of hollow visceral organs (other than the heart) 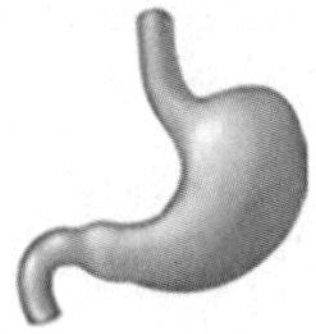
Cell shape and appearance	Single, very long, cylindrical, multinucleate cells with very obvious striations 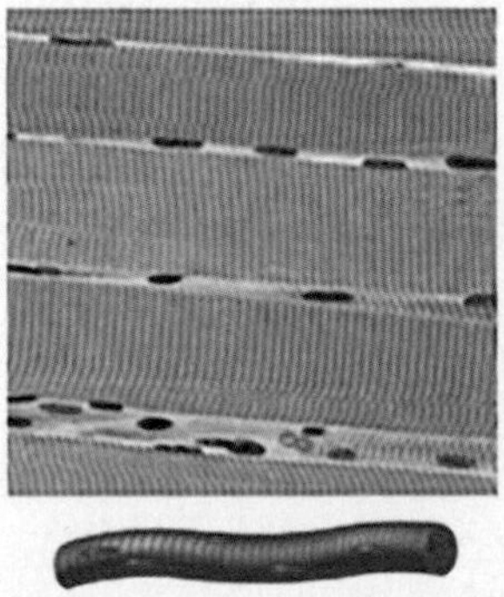	Branching chains of cells; uninucleate, striations; intercalated discs 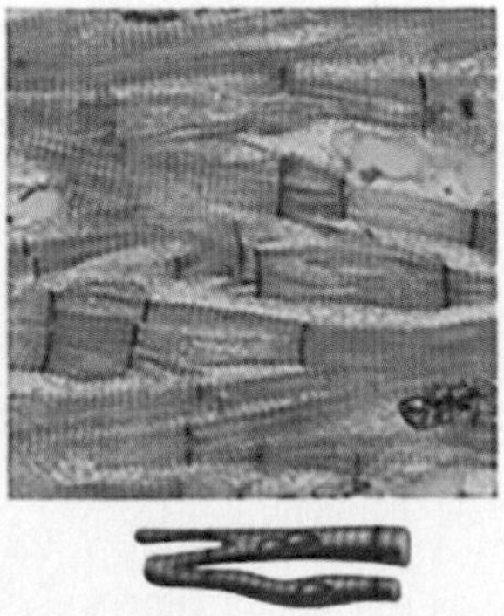	Single, fusiform, uninculeate; no striations 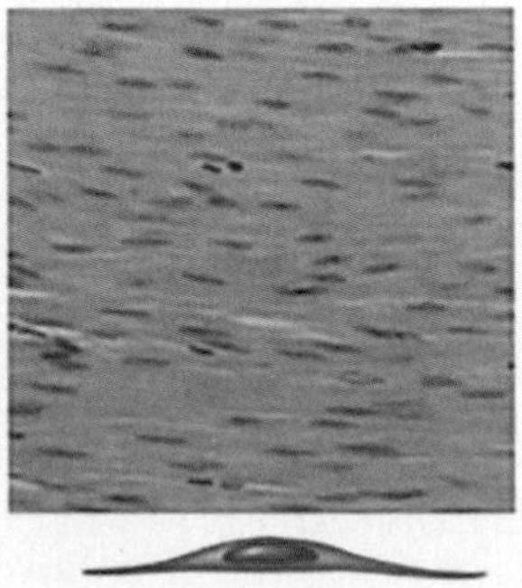

• **Figure 17.20** Comparison of skeletal, cardiac, and smooth muscles. (From Comparison of skeletal, cardiac, and smooth muscles found in Marieb, E. (2014). Essentials of human anatomy & physiology (11th ed.). Pearson.)

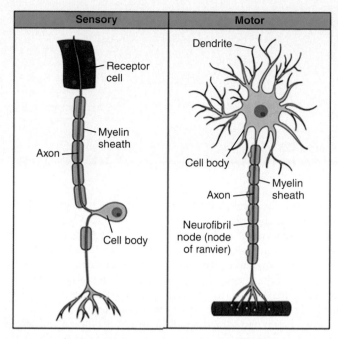

Sensory

- Receptor cell
- Myelin sheath
- Axon
- Cell body

Motor

- Dendrite
- Cell body
- Myelin sheath
- Axon
- Neurofibril node (node of ranvier)

• **Figure 17.21** Some different types of neurons—sensory and motor. The impulse passes from dendrites and the cell body down along the axon to meet with another neuron. (Modified from https://valentinapernarcic.cumbresblogs.com/category/ingles/biology/ and https://www.tutor2u.net/psychology/reference/biopsychology-sensory-relay-and-motor-neurons.)

Many of these nerve cells, or neurons, have a protective covering around their axons called a **myelin sheath**; therefore some nerves are referred to as **myelinated** nerves. This myelin sheath plays a very important role in some nerves. The size of the axon and degree of myelinization controls the speed at which the message travels along the nerve. Another role it plays is in regeneration of damaged nerves. For example, consider a lower tooth extraction in which the lip and jaw in that area remain numb after surgery. In most instances, the numbness disappears after a period. A simplified explanation of what may occur is as follows: the dendrite is injured, and part of it may die. When it dies, it breaks down but may leave portions of the protective myelin sheath cells in place. The nerve, or more accurately the dendrite or axon, regrows down this reforming tube until it reaches the point where it once supplied sensation; then the numbness disappears. If the myelin sheath is damaged, when the dendrite starts to regenerate, it may be unable to locate the old area, which will remain numb.

Neurons are found in the nerves that run out into the body and in the spinal cord and brain. Most nerves have neurons carrying messages both ways. It often takes two or three neurons in a chain to relay the message to the brain and another two or three to transfer it from the brain back to the various parts of the body. See Chapter 34 for additional discussion on the nervous system.

Review Questions

1. Name the organelles of the cell and their general functions.
2. What is pinocytosis?
3. What is the difference between cell organelles and cell inclusions?
4. What is the function of the cell membrane?
5. Define *epithelium*.
6. Which is the most common type of epithelium?
7. How do the epithelial cells arise in skin, and what happens to them?
8. What are desmosomes?
9. Where do glands come from?
10. How are glands classified?
11. Name the embryonic germ layers. Which layer or layers does epithelium come from?
12. What forms from the outer cell mass and inner cell mass of the blastocyst?
13. Name the components of irregular connective tissue.
14. How do cartilage and bone differ?
15. What makes bone hard?
16. What is a Haversian system?
17. What are the components of endochondral ossification?
18. What are the divisions of blood cells?
19. What are the functions of each of the white blood cells and platelets?
20. Where do we find hemoglobin, and what is its function?
21. Name the three types of muscle tissue, and give examples of their locations.
22. Define or describe the following:
    a. myofiber
    b. myofibril
    c. myofilament
23. What is a sarcomere?
24. How does skeletal muscle contract?
25. What are the parts of a neuron?
26. Define *afferent* and *efferent*.
27. What is a myelin sheath?
28. What is the role of the myelin sheath in nerve regrowth?
29. In what direction does a current or message travel in a neuron?

18
Development of Orofacial Complex

OBJECTIVES

- To be aware of the developmental stages of the human from fertilization to birth
- To list the embryonic structures that form the face and discuss the approximate age of formation
- To discuss the mechanism involved in the development of the maxillary lip
- To name the structures involved in the formation of the palate and the timing of its development
- To describe the mechanism involved in the development of the palate
- To describe the other structures arising from the pharyngeal arches
- To discuss the embryonic structures involved in the development of the cleft lip and palate

Embryologic Stages

From the time of fertilization of the ovum until full-term development is reached, the developing human goes through the following stages:

1. Preembryonic period—from the time of fertilization through week 2 of gestation
2. Embryonic period—from week 3 through 8 of gestation
3. Fetal period—from week 9 through 36 of gestation

During the preembryonic period, cells are differentiating into tissues that will form the three germ layers of the body—ectoderm, mesoderm, and endoderm—as well as the surrounding membranes that protect and nourish the human as they develop. The ectoderm forms teeth, skin, fingernails, eye tissues, and so on. The mesoderm gives rise to muscle, blood vessels, lymphatics, connective tissue, bone, and cartilage. The endoderm develops into the respiratory epithelium, digestive system, liver, pancreatic, and other glands.

Prefacial Embryology

The early features of the face can be seen developing by the embryonic age of 3 weeks. By the time the embryo is about 3 weeks old, its length measures approximately 3 to 4 mm from the top of the head to the tail area. Even at that small size, the forerunners of the structures that will become the face can be seen. Fig. 18.1 is a lateral view of the embryo, and several important features can be seen. The umbilical cord (shown cut here) attaches the embryo to the placenta embedded in the wall of the uterus. The heart bulge appears as it does because it develops in an extremely anterior position and pushes out on the upper body wall, which will later become the thorax. As the

thorax and ribs develop, the heart will assume a position inside the thoracic cage and will no longer bulge outward. Finally, ridges of tissue, the **pharyngeal arches**, can be seen bulging out laterally. The pharyngeal arches seen in Fig. 18.1 are actually "U"-shaped bars of tissue. The open end of the "U" faces posteriorly and surrounds the upper end of the foregut and part of the primitive oral cavity. Eventually six of these arches will develop; the ones closest to the head are the largest, and those farther down are smaller in size.

For a better understanding of the structure of these pharyngeal arches, it is necessary to look at a longitudinal section through the embryo, which is divided into halves (Fig. 18.2). The body is relatively hollow, with the exception of a tube closed at its upper and lower ends and running through the middle of the body cavity, the lining of which developed from the endoderm. This tube is the developing digestive tract and is divided into three parts. The upper part is the **foregut**, which forms the digestive tube from the throat region to the duodenum. The middle portion is the **midgut**, which forms the rest of the small intestine as well as the cecum, ascending colon, and most of the transverse colon. The lower portion is the **hindgut**, which forms the descending colon, sigmoid colon, and rectum of the large intestine.

In Fig. 18.2, you can see the foregut with the tube still closed at the top and the hindgut at the bottom as well. During the latter part of week 4, the membrane closing off the top of the foregut disintegrates. This connects the tube with the primitive oral cavity, which is a depression known as the **stomodeum**, and forms the oral cavity and the oral pharynx. At about week 7, the bottom end of the tube fuses and disintegrates and becomes the anal and urethral openings. The point in Fig. 18.2 where the foregut region and the stomodeum share a common wall is known as the **oropharyngeal membrane**. This membrane is found in the location that will become the region between the palatine tonsils and an area about two-thirds of the way back from the tip of the tongue. When the oropharyngeal membrane breaks down at the beginning of week 4, the connection between the oral cavity and the digestive tract is established.

Facial Development

Facial development can be visualized using five facial processes/prominences that surround the oral cavity. They include the paired mandibular processes, paired maxillary processes, and frontonasal prominence. The lower face is derived from the mandibular processes, the maxillary processes develop the midface, and the frontonasal prominence gives rise to the upper face.

The upper two pharyngeal arches, numbered with Roman numerals I and II, are also known respectively as the **mandibular arch** and the **hyoid arch**. First, the mandibular arch begins to show growth from the upper surface of the posterior end of the arch and will become the maxillary process. When that begins to happen, it can be subdivided into **mandibular processes** below and **maxillary processes** above (Fig. 18.3). The mandibular processes will form the mandible, and the maxillary processes will form the maxillae, the zygomatic bones of the cheek, and the palatine bones, which form the hard palate in the roof of the mouth. The maxillae also comprise the upper jaw.

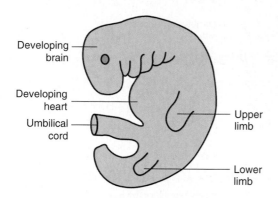

• **Figure 18.1** Lateral view of a week 3 embryo showing cardiac bulge, three pharyngeal arches, and a developing eye and ear.

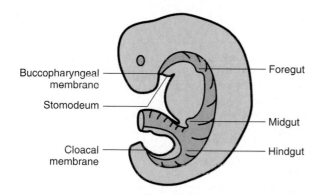

• **Figure 18.2** Longitudinal section through a week 3 embryo. Note the relationship between the stomodeum; the oropharyngeal membrane; and the foregut, midgut, and hindgut. The gut tube is closed at either end until the latter part of week 4.

In the anterior (frontal) view of a 3-week embryo, note the forehead area, known as the **frontonasal prominence**, the stomodeum (primitive oral cavity), and the mandibular processes of the mandibular arch (Fig. 18.4). During week 4, some changes can be seen. First, two small depressions form low on the frontonasal prominence; these are the **nasal pits**, the beginning of the nasal cavities. The areas on either side of these nasal pits begin to form a ridge and become the **medial nasal process** and the **lateral nasal process** (Fig. 18.5). From the side of the head, note that the maxillary processes are starting to enlarge slightly and seem to be growing toward the midline. By week six, the two medial nasal processes have fused to each other and to the two maxillary processes to form the upper lip (Fig. 18.6). The lateral nasal process takes no part in forming the upper lip; it gets pushed up and out of the way. Around the same time, the nasal pits deepen until they open into the primitive oral cavity at about week 6. The **mandibular symphysis** is formed by the fusion of the mandibular processes at about week 7.

The medial nasal and maxillary processes begin to fuse at their lower end, and that connection then starts to form perforations in it. Connective tissue flows into this groove and begins to fill in the area that lies between these perforations. There is an increase in the connective tissue of the upper lip around the groove, and the groove fills in and slowly disappears (Fig. 18.7). This process is known as **migration**. If this migration fails, the tissues will lack the ability to stretch as development continues; the resulting breakage will lead to a separation between the medial nasal process and maxillary process. A separation can also be the result of ectoderm (outer layer of tissue covering the processes) becoming trapped between the fusing medial nasal and maxillary processes; thereby preventing the fusion from occurring. This is known as a **cleft lip**. If this occurs, it takes place by week 6 of embryonic development.

Palatal Development

The formation of the palate, or roof of the mouth, involves the same processes—both maxillary processes and the medial nasal processes and begins during week 5. The medial nasal processes form a block of tissue that includes the area of the maxillary central and lateral incisors as well as a small "V"-shaped wedge of tissue lingual to these teeth back to the **incisive foramen** (see Fig. 26.12). This is known as the **primary palate** (Fig. 18.8A

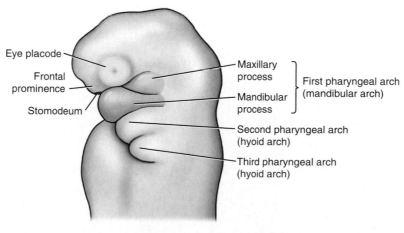

© Elsevier Collection

• **Figure 18.3** Lateral view of a week 3 embryo. Note the frontonasal prominence of the forehead region and the first three pharyngeal arches. Also, observe that the mandibular arch is now divided into maxillary and mandibular processes. The eye placode is starting to develop.

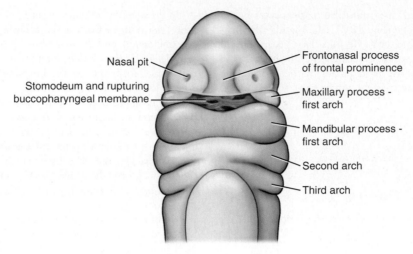

Nasal pit

Stomodeum and rupturing buccopharyngeal membrane

Frontonasal process of frontal prominence

Maxillary process - first arch

Mandibular process - first arch

Second arch

Third arch

• **Figure 18.4** Frontal view of a week 3 embryo. Note that the maxillary process is barely visible. The nasal pits are beginning to develop.

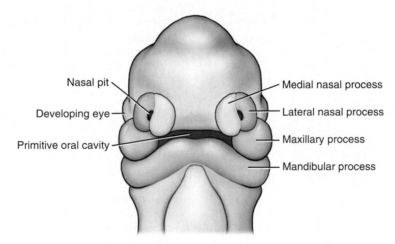

Nasal pit

Developing eye

Primitive oral cavity

Medial nasal process

Lateral nasal process

Maxillary process

Mandibular process

• **Figure 18.5** Embryo at week 4. The lower end of the frontal prominence has divided into medial and lateral nasal processes. Forward growth of the maxillary process has also occurred.

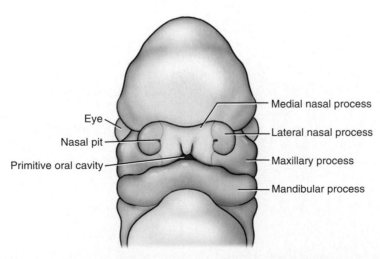

Eye

Nasal pit

Primitive oral cavity

Medial nasal process

Lateral nasal process

Maxillary process

Mandibular process

• **Figure 18.6** Embryo at week 6. Medial nasal processes and maxillary processes are filling in the groove to form the upper lip. The primitive oral cavity is the slit between the maxillary and mandibular processes.

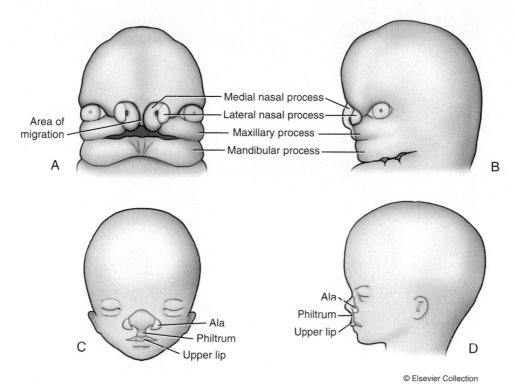

© Elsevier Collection

• **Figure 18.7** The medial nasal processes fuse to form the philtrum of the upper lip and beginning of the nasal septum and lip of the nose. The lateral nasal processes form the alae of the nose (wing of nose). **(A)** and **(B)** show the embryo before fusion is complete, while **(C)** and **(D)** show the process already fused in the infant.

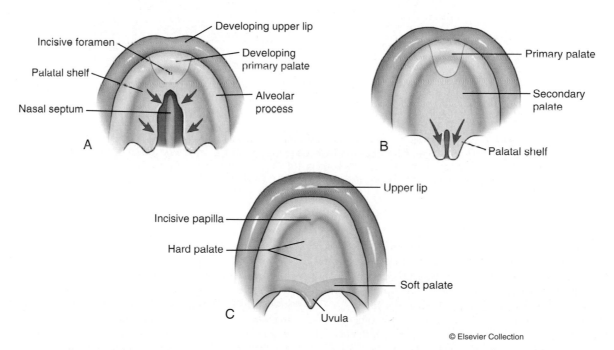

© Elsevier Collection

• **Figure 18.8** **(A)** Inferior view. The developing palate closes from the anterior to posterior. **(B)** The last parts of the palate to close are the palatal shelves. **(C)** Complete closure of the palate.

and B). The medial nasal processes also help form the nasal septum, the wall that divides the nasal cavity into right and left halves.

The remainder of the hard and soft palates (**secondary palate**) also develops from the maxillary processes. This action begins during week 6, with the growth of the medial nasal processes into the primary palate. Small ledges of epithelial-covered tissue start to grow inward from the maxillary processes and form the **palatal shelves** (Fig. 18.8B). As they grow in, they tend to become trapped beneath the developing tongue (Fig. 18.9A). However, at this time, the face is growing in a downward and forward

**Frontal section
through the head**

**Ventral view of the
palatine shelves**

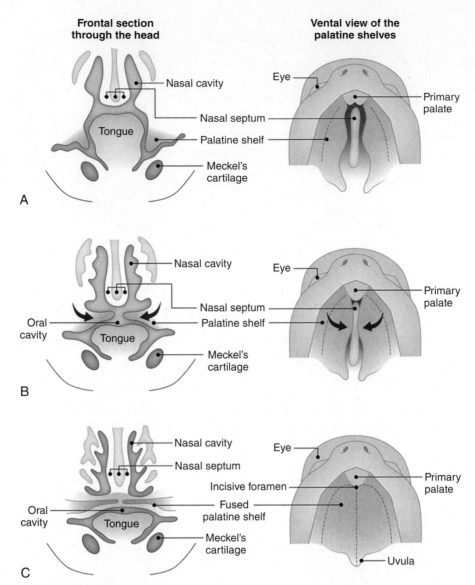

• **Figure 18.9** Frontal and ventral views. **(A)** Week 8 embryo. The palatal shelves are trapped beneath the tongue. **(B)** Week 9 embryo; the tongue has flattened to the floor of the mouth and allows for the palatal shelves to move upward and in a horizontal position. **(C)** Week 11 embryo; the palatal shelves have fused with each other and are fusing with the nasal septum. (From DeSesso, J, & Scialli, A. (2018). Bone development in laboratory mammals used in developmental toxicity studies. Birth Defects Research, 110, 1157–1187. https://doi.org/10.1002/bdr2.1350 Figure 9.)

direction, and the tongue moves down, pulling out from between the palatal shelves. The palatal shelves move into a horizontal position and come into contact first with the primary palate and then, more posteriorly, with each other, and fuse dorsally with the downward-growing nasal septum (Fig. 18.9B and C).

What occurs next is the breakdown of the contacting epithelial layers of the palatal shelves because of the influence of chemicals produced by the epithelial cells. When this happens, the connective tissue beneath the epithelium on either palatal shelf flows together and fuses. This process is referred to as **fusion**. However, if this area is viewed microscopically, one can see that not all of the epithelial cells break down; rather, a few of them remain embedded in connective tissue. These cells are referred to as **epithelial rests**. It is possible that at a later time these clumps of epithelial cells will begin to multiply and form a sac of cells known as a **cyst**, which is generally filled with fluid.

If the cyst develops along the fusion line of the two palatal shelves, it is in the midline of the palate and is known as a **median palatine cyst**. If it develops along the lines of fusion between the primary palate and the palatal shelves, it tends to be known as a **globulomaxillary cyst**. This cyst lies between the maxillary lateral incisor and canine. It may grow and distort the tissues around it, possibly causing teeth to be pushed out of alignment, and it generally should be removed.

In summary, the two maxillary processes fuse with the primary palate during weeks 7 to 8 and then fuse with one another, first in the anterior region and then moving posteriorly. This process is completed by week 12. If a **cleft palate** were to develop, it will occur between weeks 7 and 12. Depending on when it occurs during development, earlier vs. later, the defect may involve the entire palate, just the soft palate, or only the uvula (Fig. 18.10).

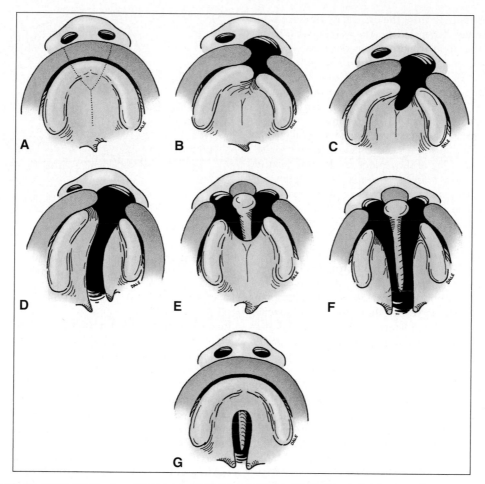

• **Figure 18.10** Inferior view. **(A)** Normal. **(B)** Unilateral cleft lip. **(C)** Unilateral cleft lip and primary palate. **(D)** Unilateral cleft lip and palate. **(E)** Bilateral cleft lip and primary palate. **(F)** Bilateral cleft lip and palate. **(G)** Late palatal cleft.

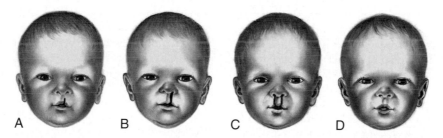

• **Figure 18.11 (A)** Unilateral cleft lip. **(B)** Unilateral cleft lip and primary palate. **(C)** Bilateral cleft lip. **(D)** Palatal cleft not involving the lip.

Cleft Lips and Palates

Clinical Considerations

A combined cleft lip and palate occurs in about 1 in 700 births among Caucasians in the United States. For African Americans in the United States, the rate is about 1 in 2000. It is more frequent in Asians, at about 3 in 2000. It is interesting to note that in clefts involving only the palate, and not the lip, the ratio is about the same for all races—1 in 2500. Males tend to have a higher incidence of cleft lip, or cleft lip with cleft palate, whereas females have more isolated incidence of cleft palate.

The two most common types of cleft lip are unilateral and bilateral cleft lips. Unilateral cleft lip involves lack of connective tissue migration between one maxillary process and the fused medial nasal processes. Bilateral cleft lip involves lack of connective tissue migration between both maxillary processes and the fused medial nasal processes. This usually includes an outward protrusion of the midline of the lip and the primary palate, including bone (see Fig. 18.10E and F, and Fig. 18.11C). Cleft lip can occur with or without a cleft palate.

The cleft palate has similar terms. Unilateral cleft palate occurs when only one of the two palatal processes fuses with the nasal septum, resulting in an opening from the oral cavity into one side of the nasal cavity. Bilateral cleft palate occurs when neither palatal process fuses with the opposing process or the nasal septum. This leaves an opening from the oral cavity into both sides of the nasal cavity (see Fig. 18.10E and F, and Fig 18.11C). The unilateral cleft lip tends to be a parallel cleft, whereas the bilateral cleft palate tends to be a "V"-shaped cleft, widening at the posterior end. Cleft palate can occur with or without cleft lip.

Cleft lip and cleft palate can usually be treated surgically with good results. Currently, cleft lip surgery is encouraged as early as the first few months after birth. One of the reasons for this is if done at an early age, there is no negative recollection of the surgical treatment, and the patient is not usually traumatized by the surgery. The other is, if done later, the increased chance of the child interacting socially with other children or adults and being teased about their appearance. People can be cruel at times and may make fun of the individual, which can lead to psychosocial problems that can psychologically scar the affected individual for a long time. Performing a corrective operation at an early stage in life can help reduce these problems.

Even after all surgical options have been attempted, there may still be a need for replacement of lost function, and a maxillofacial prosthodontist may fabricate an appliance to fill in any remaining gaps in the roof of the mouth. A speech therapist can then work with the person to regain proper speech patterns.

Clinical Considerations

The surgical correction of cleft lip and cleft palate is performed not just for aesthetic reasons. Functional problems created by cleft lip and cleft palate can be very serious and even life threatening. When the patient with cleft palate eats, food is pushed into the nasal cavity and can cause airway obstruction and food aspiration. The openings may also lead to the inability to latch and suckle while nursing; this may contribute to malnutrition in infants. This opening into the nasal cavity also causes extreme speech difficulties. Speech impediment creates psychological problems and opens the door to harassment by other children. The speech therapist records the child's speech before surgery and then records speech after surgery. The children are so amazed that they ask if the previous recording is really their speech. Such a response can be very rewarding!

One final thing to consider in studying cleft lip and cleft palate is the relationship between the timing of the occurrences and their potential causes. Earlier in the chapter, we noted that cleft lip develops at week 6 after fertilization of the ovum, and cleft palate can occur between weeks 7 and 12 after fertilization. Hereditary factors are involved in the development of clefts, and if there is any family history of clefts, they will occur with greater frequency in that family than in a family without that history. The other main factor is environmental; if a pregnant woman uses specific types of drugs, smokes, drinks alcohol, or is in an environment that has potentially damaging pollutants in the air or water, her child may have a greater risk of suffering birth defects, such as clefts. It is also possible for a woman to expose herself to potentially harmful situations at a time when she is not yet aware that she is pregnant. Because cleft deformities develop so early, it is important that women of child-bearing age be cognizant of the harmful factors that might affect fetuses.

Other Structural Development Inside the Pharyngeal Arches

A number of important structures develop from the pharyngeal arches. To understand these structures better, it is helpful to

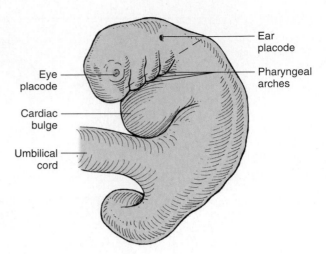

• **Figure 18.12** Duplicate of Fig. 18.1, with a dotted line marking a cut made from left to right through the pharyngeal arches.

imagine a cut from left to right, down through the head and the pharyngeal arches (Fig. 18.12). If you remove the front half of the head and neck along the dotted line, and view it from behind, you see a series of bulges with depressions between them (Fig. 18.13). The external bulges in the future neck region are known as **pharyngeal arches**. The depressions on the neck surface are known as **pharyngeal grooves**, and the areas between the grooves are known as **pharyngeal pouches**. In Fig. 18.13, you can see each of the arches numbered. In each arch is a bar of cartilage, an artery, a cranial nerve, and mesenchymal tissue. Additionally, specific bone, cartilage, and muscle structures will develop from each one of these arches. For example, the cranial nerve of the first arch is the fifth cranial nerve, or **trigeminal nerve**, and the cranial nerve of the second arch is the seventh cranial nerve, or **facial nerve**. In later chapters on the muscles of the head and neck, you will learn that the muscles of mastication are innervated by the fifth cranial nerve and the muscles of facial expression by the seventh cranial nerve. This tells you that the muscles of mastication arose from the first arch and the muscles of facial expression arose from the second arch. Table 18.1 lists the pharyngeal arches, the cranial nerves involved in each arch, and the muscles, bones, and cartilages that arise from these arches.

Fig. 18.14 is a view of one side of the cut seen in Fig. 18.13. The upper internal groove forms the external auditory meatus and one layer of the eardrum, whereas the upper pouch forms the inner layer of the eardrum, the primitive tympanic cavity (also known as *middle ear*) and the **eustachian tube**, or **auditory tube**, which leads into the posterior nose region or nasal pharynx. At this point, let us look at the pharyngeal grooves below the first and the lower grooves. A fold of tissue grows down externally from the second arch and covers over the grooves below. That gives a smooth contour to the area that will become the neck. The second pouch forms the palatine tonsils, and the pouches below the palatine tonsils form some of the **endocrine glands**, such as the **parathyroid** and **thymus** glands. In the middle portion of Fig. 18.15, you can see the region where the tongue and the **thyroid gland** develop. In this view, you can see a number of structures that go into making up the tongue, the basic ones being the **lateral lingual swellings**, the **tuberculum impar**, and the **copula**. You can also see a small depression, known as the **foramen**

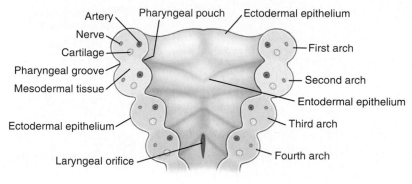

• **Figure 18.13** Drawing of pharyngeal arches removed with the cut shown in Fig. 18.12 and viewed from behind showing four of the six arches. Note the external grooves and internal pouches. The *dotted line* separates the ectodermal epithelium above from the endodermal epithelium below.

TABLE 18.1	Pharyngeal Arch Innervation and Arch Derivatives		
Arch	**Cranial Nerves**	**Muscles**	**Cartilages/Bones**
I	V	Muscles of mastication Mylohyoid Anterior digastric Tensor tympani (in ear) Tensor veli palatini	Malleus and incus bones
II	VII	Muscles of facial expression Posterior digastric Stylohyoid Stapedius (in ear) Greater cornu of hyoid	Stapes Styloid process Lesser cornu of hyoid Upper body of hyoid Lower body of hyoid
III	IX	Stylopharyngeus	Greater cornu of hyoid Lower body of hyoid
IV and VI*	X (XI)	Muscles of larynx Muscles of pharynx Most muscles of soft palate	Cartilages of larynx

*Fifth pharyngeal arch is only rudimentary in humans.

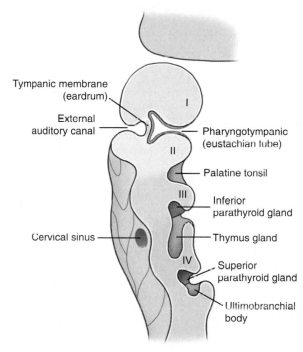

• **Figure 18.14** Later view of one side of Fig. 18.13. All but the first external groove has been covered over. Note the other structures arising from the pouches.

cecum, in the middle of the posterior tongue. This is the point where the thyroid gland begins to develop and then migrates downward, eventually lying in the lower front neck region. The thyroid gland is an endocrine gland, and so eventually, after reaching its location in the neck, it will lose its duct and become an endocrine gland. Sometimes it does not lose its duct system, and a thyroglossal duct remains as a source of cysts developing in the neck along the course of the duct. The timing for these structures varies somewhat, but their development takes place over several months.

Clinical Considerations

In the development of the tongue, a few things can go wrong.

1. If the tongue is too small for the mouth it results in a condition known as *microglossia*—the size of the tongue can cause eating and speech problems.
2. If the tongue is too large, it results in a condition known as *macroglosssia*—it can cause difficulties with speech, eating, and breathing and may require surgery and speech therapy.
3. Another condition that can cause speech problems of the tongue is *ankyloglossia* (being tongue tied). This condition is associated with constrictive movements of the tongue. This is caused by too short a lingual frenum, which limits the movement of the tongue.

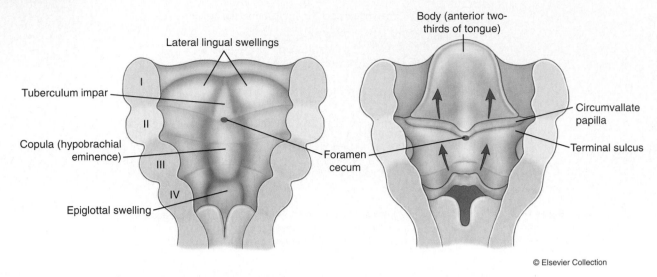

Lateral lingual swellings

Body (anterior two-thirds of tongue)

Tuberculum impar

Copula (hypobrachial eminence)

Epiglottal swelling

I
II
III
IV

Foramen cecum

Circumvallate papilla

Terminal sulcus

© Elsevier Collection

• **Figure 18.15** Various structures that go into the formation of the tongue and the epiglottis.

Review Questions

1. What are the three stages of human development and when do they occur?
2. During which developmental weeks do lips form?
3. What is the oropharyngeal membrane and when does it rupture?
4. Which processes form the upper lip?
5. Which processes form the hard and soft palates and when do they form?
6. What are epithelial rests and what might they do in later life?
7. What is a cyst, and if located in the bone of the jaw, what might it do?
8. What are unilateral and bilateral cleft lips and cleft palates?
9. When does a cleft lip or a cleft palate form?
10. Which muscles arise from the first pharyngeal arch? Which bones?
11. What pharyngeal arch does the muscles of facial expression arise from, and what is their innervation?
12. What groups of muscles form from the IV and VI pharyngeal arches?
13. What are the differences in the mechanism between the development of the upper lip and the palate?
14. What structures fuse together to form the upper lip?
15. Which of the following in the first trimester could cause facial deformity?
    a. alcohol
    b. airborne contaminants
    c. recreational drugs
    d. certain prescription drugs
    e. all of the above
16. Which of the following clefts begin later in development?
    a. cleft lip
    b. bilateral cleft and primary palate
    c. unilateral cleft and secondary palate
    d. cleft soft palate and uvula

19
Dental Lamina and Enamel Organ

OBJECTIVES

- To define the dental lamina and indicate in what embryonic week it is first seen
- To describe the bud, cap, and bell stages of the enamel organ and the various layers found in each
- To define successional and vestibular laminae
- To describe the dental papilla, the dental sac, and their functions

Dental Lamina

The first signs of tooth development are seen during week six of the embryonic period. At that time, embryonic **oral** (stratified squamous) **epithelium** begins thickening. As epithelium thickens, it grows downward into the underlying connective tissue and does not create a visible ridge in the oral cavity at the time. This thickened oral epithelium is known as the **dental lamina**. It is a U-shaped thickening of the epithelium of the primitive oral cavity and is found in a position corresponding to the future arch-shaped arrangement of maxillary and mandibular teeth (dental arch). This thickening does not begin all at once throughout the mouth, but is first seen in the anterior midline and slowly spreads posteriorly toward the molar region (Fig. 19.1). It takes several weeks for this thickening to extend to the future position of primary molars.

During week eight of the embryonic period, starting at the midline and spreading posteriorly, there is a continued thickening in the dental lamina in 10 areas of the maxillary arch and 10 areas of the mandibular arch. These 20 localized thickenings correspond to the position of the future primary dentition and will form the enamel of future teeth. However, enamel could be affected by a condition called **ectodermal dysplasia**, in which there is poor development of structures arising from the ectoderm, such as the sweat, salivary, and sebaceous glands; skin; hair; and tooth enamel. It can also involve the white sclera of the eye, causing discoloration.

Enamel Organ

Bud Stage

The initial budding from the dental lamina at the 10 thickened areas in each arch is referred to as the **bud stage** (Fig. 19.2); the first stage in the development of the **enamel organ** that forms the tooth enamel. At first, the buds look like blobs of cells from the dental lamina projecting deeper into the underlying connective tissue. The cells in the middle of the buds come from the outer or superficial layers of the oral epithelium, whereas the cells in the periphery of the bud come from the deep or basal layers of the oral epithelium. The buds seem to stretch out from the dental lamina as they grow. As development continues, the deepest parts of the buds become slightly concave. It is at this point that the developing enamel organ goes from the bud stage to the **cap stage**.

Cap Stage

As the enamel organ moves into the cap stage, it consists of the following three components: outer enamel epithelium (OEE), inner enamel epithelium (IEE), and stellate reticulum.

Outer Enamel Epithelium

The outermost part of the structure of the cap stage is the **outer enamel epithelium**. It is a direct continuation of the basal layer of oral epithelium. These are low columnar or cuboidal cells.

Inner Enamel Epithelium

The cells that outline the concavity in the deepest part of the cap stage compose the **inner enamel epithelium**. These cells are continuous with the OEE cells and also come from the basal layer of the oral epithelium.

Stellate Reticulum

The cells between the IEE and the OEE include the **stellate reticulum**. These cells originate from the superficial layers of the oral epithelium. Although they may resemble embryonic mesenchymal cells, they are actually ectodermal cells, as are other parts of the enamel organ (Fig. 19.3). As the concavity of the cap grows more pronounced, the enamel organ reaches the **bell stage**.

Bell Stage

The differentiation between the cap stage and the bell stage is made when a fourth layer of epithelium, the **stratum intermedium**, appears in addition to the three previously mentioned. The stratum intermedium is composed of several layers of flattened squamous cells lying between the IEE and the stellate reticulum (Fig. 19.4).

As the development continues in the bell stage, two processes occur. First, the future outline or form of the crown of the tooth is determined by the way in which the cell layers expand as the enamel organ grows. Second, there are changes in various cells, particularly the IEE cells, and these changes will lead to the production of enamel (see also Chapter 20).

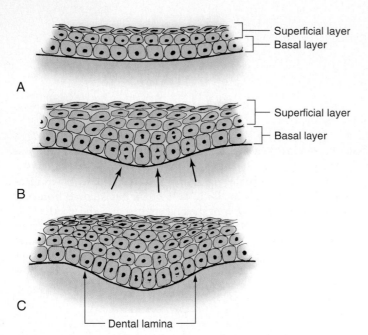

• **Figure 19.1** **(A)** Embryonic oral epithelium before development of dental lamina. Note the thickness of the superficial and basal layers of cells. Embryonic connective tissue lies beneath embryonic oral epithelium. **(B)** Thickening of the superficial layer and multiplication of cells *(arrows)* in the basal layer. **(C)** Further advancement in completed thickening of dental lamina.

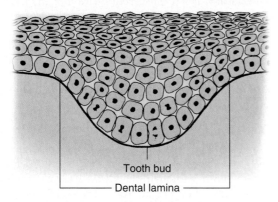

• **Figure 19.2** Bud stage. Note the further downward extension of the cells of the oral epithelium to form the bud. The stretching out of cells is still considered part of the dental lamina.

Functions of the Four Layers of the Enamel Organ

1. The OEE is considered a protective layer for the entire enamel organ. Later, it will play a role in attaching the gingiva to the tooth (see Fig. 19.4).
2. The cells of the IEE elongate and change internally to become **ameloblasts**, which are responsible for actual enamel formation (see also Chapter 20).
3. The stellate reticulum functions as a cushioned protection for IEE cells and has a role in nourishment of the stratum intermedium by allowing vascular fluids to move between the loosely packed cells.

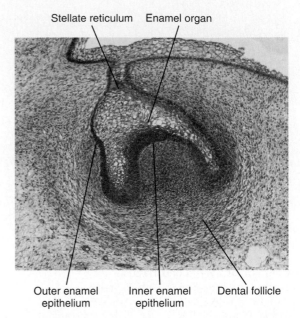

• **Figure 19.3** Cap stage. Basal layer of the cells of the oral epithelium is continuous with the inner and outer enamel epithelium. Stellate reticulum can be seen as a continuation of the superficial layers of the oral epithelium. (From Nanci A. *Ten Cate's Oral Histology.* 8th ed. St. Louis, MO: Mosby; 2013.)

4. The cells of the stratum intermedium help provide nourishment for IEE cells. They are also producers of protein and may receive products from and provide products for the ameloblasts.

Successional Lamina

In the developing primary teeth, the dental lamina develops an extension to the lingual side of each tooth (see Fig. 19.4). This extension is known as the **successional lamina**. Successional lamina goes through bud, cap, and bell stages, just like primary teeth, and forms permanent incisors, canines, and premolars. Permanent molars develop from a posterior growth of the dental, or general, lamina and are nonsuccessional. The rate of formation will vary from tooth to tooth, with the permanent teeth developing at a much slower rate than the primary teeth.

As each developing tooth reaches the bell stage, the laminar attachment begins to break down. This happens first in the anterior region and spreads posteriorly. The original laminar attachment begins to break down as the bell stage is reached. This primary tooth lamina is now known as the *lateral lamina* because that is its relationship to the successional lamina (Figs. 19.5 and 19.6).

Vestibular Lamina

The vestibular lamina is a thickening of the oral epithelium in a facial or buccal direction from the dental lamina. This epithelium thickens, and then a clefting or splitting can be seen in the thickened area (Fig. 19.7). Eventually this cleft forms a groove that becomes the area of the mucobuccal or mucolabial fold in the future vestibule. If this vestibular lamina did not form, the vestibule would end at the level of the alveolar ridge, and denture construction would be very difficult or impossible.

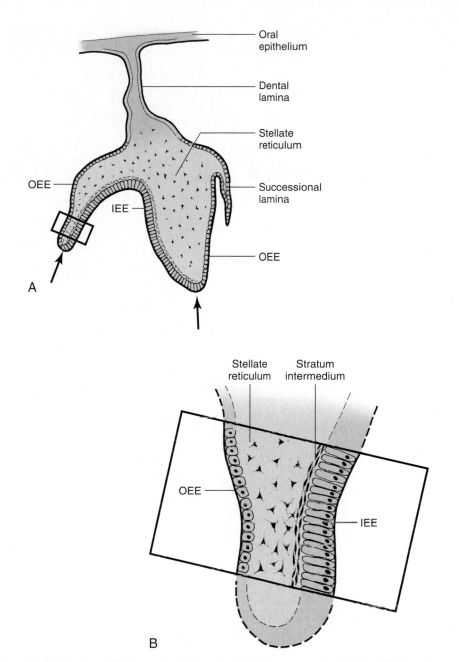

- **Figure 19.4** Bell stage. **(A)** Concavity of the cells of the inner enamel epithelium (IEE) has increased in the bell stage. Successional lamina can be seen developing to the lingual side of the primary tooth. **(B)** Enlargement of the boxed section of (A). There are several layers of flattened cells, that are stratum intermedium, as well as IEE, OEE, and stellate reticulum.

Dental Papilla and Dental Sac

The **dental papilla** is a small area of condensed cells arising from mesenchyme and located next to or deep to the IEE. It is first seen in the late bud stage and grows and becomes more pronounced as it goes through the bell stage. This structure forms the dentin and pulp of the tooth. As the development progresses from bud to bell stage, the cells of the dental papilla become more compact, and the area enlarges. It sits within the conical shape of the IEE cells and becomes very pronounced, bulging out from the enamel organ. The basement membrane between the dental papilla and enamel organ will later give rise to the dentoenamel junction.

The nerves and blood vessels of the pulp formed by the dental papilla are first seen in the early stages of development of the dental papilla. They invade the early pulpal tissue, and as the rest of the tooth forms, the neural and vascular components of the pulp are already present.

The **dental sac**, also known as the **dental follicle**, is composed of several rows of flattened cells; they surround that part of the dental papilla not in contact with the IEE cells and also surround part of the enamel organ. Like the dental papilla, the dental sac also arises from mesenchyme, and it forms the periodontium (cementum, periodontal ligament, and alveolar bone) of the tooth (Fig. 19.8).

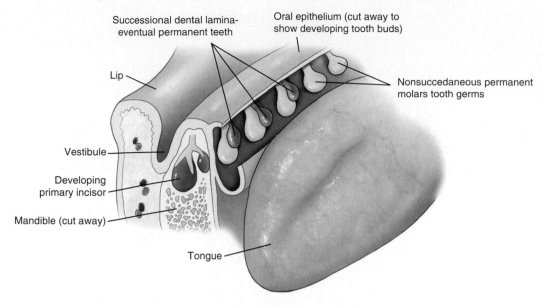

• **Figure 19.5** Development of tooth buds in alveolar process. Anterior teeth are more advanced than posterior teeth. The anterior lamina has begun to degenerate as the posterior lamina forms. When tooth buds have differentiated, the lamina is no longer needed.

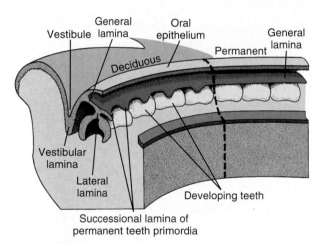

• **Figure 19.6** Dental lamina system is shown in relation to general lamina. From successional lamina come permanent teeth, which replace primary teeth except in the posterior arch area. (From Chiego D. *Essentials of Oral Histology and Embryology*. 4th ed. St. Louis, MO: Mosby; 2014.)

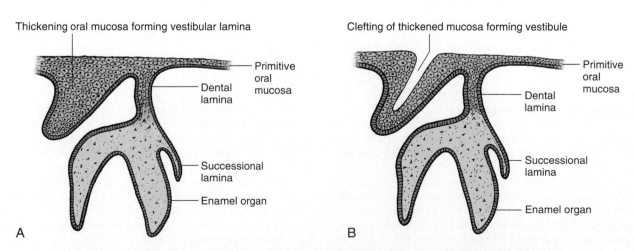

• **Figure 19.7** **(A)** Thickened epithelium of future vestibule forming facial to the dental lamina. **(B)** A cleft has developed in the vestibular lamina and a vestibular fold has formed.

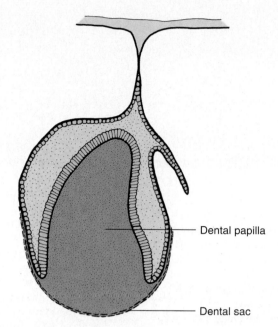

Dental papilla

Dental sac

• **Figure 19.8** Condensed mesenchymal cells, which make up the dental papilla, and flattened layers of the dental sac, which surrounds part of the dental papilla and part of the enamel organ.

Review Questions

1. What is the first sign of tooth development and when is it seen?
2. Oral epithelium is an example of what type of epithelial arrangement?
3. The enamel organ comes from which germ layer?
4. What are the stages of the enamel organ and what general changes are taking place?
5. What is ectodermal dysplasia and what is the significance of the origin of the enamel organ in relation to this pathologic condition? Besides enamel, what other structures develop abnormally from this condition?

6. What are the four layers of the enamel organ as seen in the bell stage and what is their function?
7. Define and describe the roles of the following:
   successional lamina
   vestibular lamina
   dental papilla
   dental sac

20
Enamel, Dentin, and Pulp

A close relationship exists in the formation of enamel, dentin, and pulp. Enamel develops from the enamel organ, which is derived from the ectoderm, whereas dentin and pulp develop from the dental papilla, which is derived from the mesoderm. The mesoderm of the dental papilla determines the shape of the developing crown of the tooth. Animal experiments have shown that if the dental papilla is transplanted from an anterior tooth beneath the enamel organ of a posterior tooth, the posterior tooth will assume the shape of the anterior tooth from which the dental papilla came. Although there is an interrelationship between enamel and dentin, it is the dental papilla that seems to have genetic control over tooth shape.

Dental Papilla

During the bud stage, the *mesenchymal cells* of the embryonic connective tissue deep to the bud are large and multipointed. As the enamel organ goes into the cap stage, the mesenchymal cells adjacent to the cap become more rounded and condensed and are then called *dental papilla cells*. The enamel organ is also enlarging at this time (Fig. 20.1). This condensation continues into the bell stage, during which further changes occur. At this time, the relationship

between enamel formation (**odontogenesis**) and dentin formation (**dentinogenesis**) becomes more obvious. The following is a list of events that occur during the formation of enamel and dentin:

1. During the bell stage, cells of the IEE become taller and differentiate into **preameloblasts**. They line up along the basement membrane, and the nucleus of each cell moves away from the basement membrane. This repolarization is important to their change from IEE cells to preameloblasts.
2. Next, the preameloblasts induce the peripheral cells of the dental papilla, causing them to become low columnar or cuboidal cells and differentiate into **odontoblasts**. Just like it does with the preameloblasts, the odontoblasts nuclei migrate away from the basement membrane and they become a mirror image with the preameloblasts.
3. After repolarization of both cells, the basement membrane between them disintegrates.
4. Next, the odontoblasts begin laying down dentin, which is known as dentinogenesis. The predentin is set down adjacent to the preameloblasts, where the basement membrane used to be.
5. The preameloblasts come in contact with the predentin, and this induces them to differentiate into ameloblasts. After that happens, amelogenesis begins. Amelogenesis is the laying down of enamel matrix. The enamel matrix is secreted from the Tomes's process of the ameloblasts adjacent to the dentin, where the basement membrane used to be.
6. The deposition of the enamel matrix up next to the dentin matrix creates the future **dentinoenamel junction (DEJ)** (Fig. 20.2).
7. Dentin begins to lay down hydroxyapatite crystals, and they calcify (crystals begin growing).
8. Enamel begins to lay down hydroxyapatite crystals, and they calcify (crystals begin growing).

This process is identical for all developing teeth. It is seen first in developing anterior teeth and later in posterior teeth. It tends to be seen first in the mandibular arch slightly before it is seen in the maxillary arch. Within any single tooth, this type of interrelationship is first seen at the tip of the cusp of a tooth and later spreads toward the cervical line.

Whether permanent or primary, this development takes place in each tooth. Permanent molars develop as a budding off of a posterior extension of the dental lamina, whereas anterior permanent teeth and permanent premolars develop from a lingual budding off of the dental lamina of primary teeth. If, for any reason, the primary tooth bud does not form, then a permanent tooth bud cannot develop from it. If this happens, then primary and permanent teeth are both congenitally missing.

Enamel Composition

Enamel is the hardest calcified tissue in the body. It is generally white but at times appears yellowish because of the reflection of

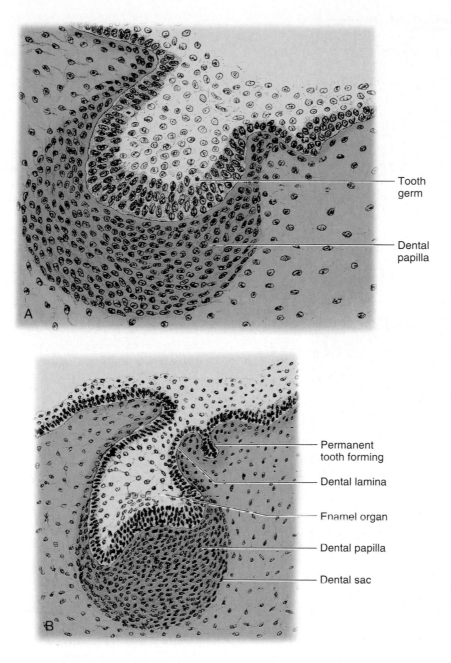

• **Figure 20.1** **(A)** General condensation of dental papilla. **(B)** Later stage. Condensation of the cells in dental papilla is more pronounced. Note the permanent tooth bud developing lingual to the primary tooth dental papilla. (Modified from Bevelander G. *Outline of Histology*. 8th ed. St. Louis: Mosby; 1979.)

the color of the underlying dentin. Enamel is 96% inorganic in composition. This inorganic structure is composed of many millions of crystals of hydroxyapatite, the chemical formula of which is Ca_{10} $(PO_4)_6$ $(OH)_2$. The other 4% of enamel is composed of water (3%) and a fibrous organic material (1%).

The enamel structure comprises two parts—the **rod sheath** and the **enamel rod**. The rod sheath outlines the rod and contains most of the fibrous organic substance. However, the rod, which is made up of hydroxyapatite crystals, is the primary unit of the structure of enamel. The rod is a column of enamel that runs all the way from the DEJ to the surface of the tooth. It is perpendicular to the DEJ and to the surface of the crown (Fig. 20.3).

At least three or four ameloblasts act together to form one enamel rod by laying down fibers and a matrix composed of a gluelike material called *ground substance* and depositing millions of hydroxyapatite crystals into the matrix.

Enamel rods fit together tightly because of a cementing substance called *interrod substance*. Most enamel rods appear with the keyhole shapes (Fig. 20.4A) that have a wide upper end and a narrowed bottom end. The reason for the different appearances of the upper and lower parts of the keyhole is that the crystals in those parts are oriented in different directions. When ameloblasts produce the matrix and then deposit the crystals into the matrix, the secreting ends of ameloblasts bulge outward in the direction of the

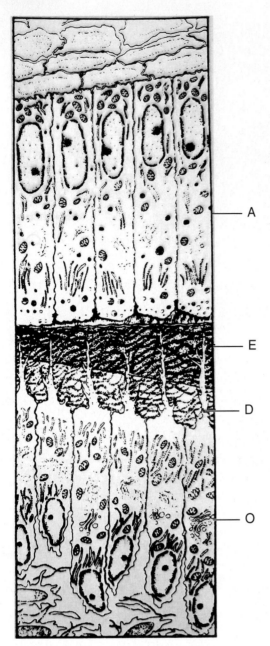

• **Figure 20.2** Diagram of enamel and dentin apposition. (A) Ameloblasts with the nuclei moved away from the disintegrated basement membrane. *E*, Enamel matrix being laid down toward the future dentinoenamel junction (DEJ). *D*, Dentin matrix being laid down toward the future DEJ. *O*, Odontoblasts with the nuclei moved away from the disintegrated basement membrane. (From Avery, J. (2000). *Essentials of oral histology and embryology. A clinical approach* (2nd ed.). Mosby. Page 59.)

DEJ. This asymmetric bulge is called the *Tomes's process* of an ameloblast. Each ameloblast does not lie parallel to the long axis of the enamel rod but is canted at an angle. As the crystals are secreted, they emerge from the pointed part of the ameloblast in an arrangement perpendicular to the cell membrane. The result is that the crystals in the upper part of the keyhole are arranged in a pattern longitudinal to the long axis of the rod, whereas the crystals in the lower end are angled almost 60 degrees off the long axis.

A cross-sectional view of the rod shows the upper-end crystals cut vertically and the lower-end crystals cut at an angle, giving each area a distinct appearance. It was only the advent of new

microscopes and techniques that allowed study of individual crystals and better understanding of the differing descriptions of enamel. The appearances of the enamel rods cut at different angles (see Fig. 20.4B) help visualize the different enamel rod shapes. There is a slight curving of the rods, and this changes the rods' appearance from lighter to darker. These are referred to as *Hunter-Schreger bands*. The rods develop at a rate of 4 μm per day.

Development of Enamel

As previously discussed, ameloblasts begin to lay down a matrix and in a few days deposit millions of hydroxyapatite crystals into a small area of the matrix. This is seen first at the tip of a cusp and then further toward the cervical line. It is important to remember that all the crystals that will ever be in that particular area of rod are laid down initially. This is referred to as the **mineralization stage** of enamel rod calcification (Fig. 20.5A).

The second stage of calcification is called the **maturation stage** (see Fig. 20.5B). During this stage, the crystals grow in size until they are tightly packed together. The ameloblast produces the matrix and enamel at a rate of 4 mm per day. Every fourth day, there seems to be a change in the development of the rod, and a brownish line develops in the enamel. These lines are called the **striae of Retzius** and curve outwardly and occlusally from the DEJ (Fig. 20.6). They can be seen in the longitudinal section of a tooth and can also be seen in a tooth and on the surface of a number of teeth. On the surface of an anterior tooth, horizontal lines can be seen on the crown. These are known as **imbrication lines** and are surface manifestations of the striae of Retzius. Unfavorable metabolic activities or nutritional deficiencies affect the formation of these lines. Such a nutritional disturbance occurs on the day of birth. The resulting imbrication lines display what are called **neonatal lines**, which can be seen on the surface of primary teeth.

Fate of Enamel Organ

As the ameloblast moves away from the DEJ toward the OEE, it begins to compress the two layers in the middle—the stratum intermedium and the stellate reticulum. These two middle layers eventually lose their identity, and the ameloblasts contact the OEE (Fig. 20.7). This is the signal for ameloblasts to cease formation of enamel. The final job of the ameloblast is to lay down a protective layer over enamel, called the **primary enamel cuticle**, or **Nasmyth's membrane**. This membrane covers the crown and remains there for many months after eruption until worn away by tooth brushing and other abrasion. It is this membrane that is stained green or yellow in the newly erupted teeth of young children, particularly in the cervical one-third of the crown. The stained membrane can be removed by polishing and by the action of other instruments.

After the ameloblast produces the primary cuticle, it begins flattening out and blending with the OEE cells in what is called the **reduced enamel epithelium (REE)**. This REE produces an adhesive-like secretion called the **secondary enamel cuticle**, or **epithelial attachment**, which functions to hold the gingiva to the tooth. This epithelium adheres to the tooth and is known as the **attachment epithelium**. It is found at the base of the gingival sulcus (see Chapter 22).

Abnormalities of Enamel

A number of enamel abnormalities exist. Some are readily seen with clinical examination, others are confirmed with radiographic

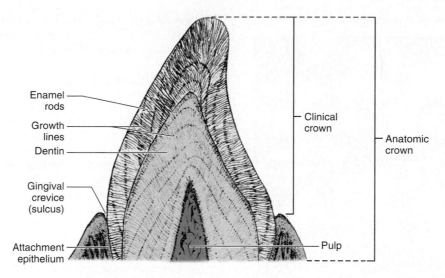

• **Figure 20.3** Note the slight curvature of enamel rods and that the ends of the rods are perpendicular to the dentinoenamel junction (DEJ) and outer surface of the tooth. (Modified from Ham AW, Cormack D. *Histology*. 8th ed. Philadelphia: JB Lippincott Co.; 1979.)

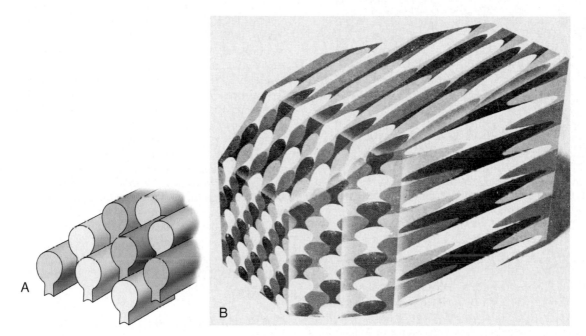

• **Figure 20.4** **(A)** Key shaped enamel rods. **(B)** Groups of rods and their relation to one another. Note how different cutting angles change appearance of the key-shaped rods. (Neal RJ. Structure of mature human dental enamel as observed by electron microscopy. *Arch Oral Biol* 1965;10:775.)

examination, and still others are seen only through histologic examination of the sectioned tooth.

Enamel Dysplasia

Both enamel hypocalcification and enamel hypoplasia are types of enamel dysplasia. With **hypocalcified enamel**, spots or entire areas of the exposed tooth surface appear white to whitish yellow in color. It is the result of insufficient growth of the enamel crystals or an insufficient number of crystals originally deposited in the matrix. If the crystals do not grow to full size during the maturation stage, they are not packed together tightly, and enamel is less than 96% inorganic, causing hypocalcification. Because enamel is less dense than normal, it may decay more rapidly.

The density of **hypoplastic enamel** is generally normal, but the enamel is thin. Enamel will have a yellow to gray hue and may be seen radiographically as a thinner than normal layer.

Enamel Lamellae

Cracks in enamel caused by developmental problems or **trauma** are called **enamel lamellae**. The most common types are those caused by trauma, which includes rapid changes in temperature applied to teeth, such as may come from different types of food

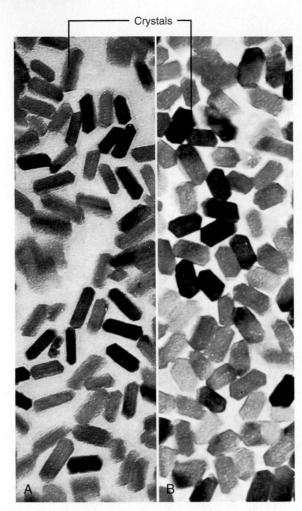

• **Figure 20.5** **(A)** Mineralization stage of calcification. Note the spaces between crystals. **(B)** Same magnification as (A) but showing maturation stage with crystal growth and increased density. (From Bhaskar SN. *Orban's Oral Histology and Embryology*. 8th ed. St. Louis: Mosby; 1976.)

and drinks. Clinically they appear as hairline cracks in enamel and may extend all the way through enamel and even into dentin. The less common type of lamella is a developmental defect and is the result of one or more ameloblasts ceasing enamel production and thus leaving a space between other enamel rods and providing a potential pathway through enamel for bacteria to enter. These are usually seen histologically and not clinically.

Enamel Tuft

A small area of hypocalcified enamel seen at the DEJ and extending about one-fourth to one-third of the way through enamel is an **enamel tuft**. It is only seen in a histologic section of tooth, and it has no clinical significance. It is the result of early enamel formation at the DEJ not being complete and therefore hypomineralized.

Enamel Spindle

An **enamel spindle** is an **odontoblastic process**, a cellular extension of the odontoblast, which becomes trapped between ameloblasts in early development and thus ends up in the enamel (Fig. 20.8). It is seen only histologically, and its clinical implications are not known.

Dentin Composition

Dentin is a hard yellowish substance. It is 70% inorganic hydroxyapatite crystal; 20% organic, composed of collagen, mucopolysaccharide ground substance; and 10% water. Clinically, dentin appears to be solid. Microscopically, dentin comprises the following three distinct areas (Fig. 20.9).
1. **Dentinal tubule**—a long tube, running from the DEJ, or dentinocemental junction (DCJ), to the outer pulp wall. Each dentinal tubule contains an **odontoblastic process, dentinal fluid,** and possibly a **sensory axon**.
2. **Peritubular dentin**—an area of higher crystalline content immediately surrounding the dentinal tubules.
3. **Intertubular dentin**—the bulk of the dentinal material, found between the tubules.

Formation of Regular Dentin (Primary Dentin)

As the odontoblast begins to secrete dentin matrix at the future DEJ or DCJ, the cell begins to move toward the pulp. The odontoblast differs from the ameloblast in that it leaves part of the cell behind and secretes matrix around it. Through this process, the cell wall stretches or lengthens so that part of the odontoblast stretches all the way from the DEJ or DCJ inward to the periphery of the pulp (Fig. 20.10). The secreted matrix from an odontoblast spreads peripherally until it meets with other dentin matrices and eventually calcifies and forms intertubular dentin. Later, the odontoblastic process contained within the intertubular dentin shrinks in diameter, and the space that it formerly occupied is filled with a highly calcified dentin known as *peritubular dentin* (see Fig. 20.9). When the tooth erupts into the oral cavity, the dentin that has formed by that time is known as **primary dentin**, or regular dentin. Dentin continues to be formed as either secondary or reparative dentin.

Formation of Secondary and Reparative Dentin

Secondary Dentin

The layer formed inside the regular dentin and positioned closest to the pulp is **secondary dentin**. It starts forming when the tooth erupts and comes into contact with the opposing tooth. It is formed by the same odontoblasts that form the regular dentin. As the secondary dentin forms, it causes the overall size of the pulp chamber to decrease. This is most noticeable when comparing radiographs of newly erupted permanent maxillary central incisors with radiographs of much older permanent maxillary central incisors (Fig. 20.11). Newly erupted teeth have large pulp chambers and prominent pulp horns. As secondary dentin formation proceeds, a decrease in the size of the pulp canals, chambers, and pulp horns occurs. It is this process of secondary dentin formation that allows metal crowns to be constructed on teeth after they had erupted a few years earlier. If this formation did not take place, cutting tooth structure for the placement of crowns would tend to injure the large prominent pulp horns and pulp chambers of teeth.

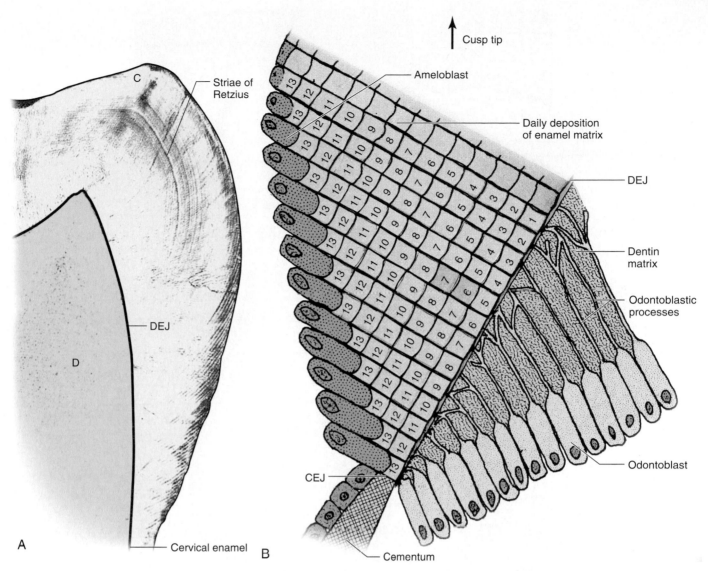

↑ Cusp tip

• **Figure 20.6 (A)** Heavy black lines represent striae of Retzius. Note their curving direction. *C*, Cusp; *DEJ*, dentinoenamel junction; *D*, dentin. **(B)** Enlarged representation of several enamel rods. Segments are labeled according to the day of formation. Enamel formation is most advanced at the cusp tip. (*CEJ*, cementoenamel junction.) (A, Modified from Provenza DV. *Fundamentals of Oral Histology and Embryology*. 2nd ed. Philadelphia: JB Lippincott Co.; 1972.)

Reparative Dentin

Reparative dentin is formed in response to local trauma and is located immediately beneath the area of trauma. The trauma may be one of several varieties—occlusal, mechanical, or chemical trauma.

Occlusal trauma is the condition that exists when one tooth or part of a tooth is subjected to more occlusal stress than normal. This usually relates to the cusp area of the tooth. The odontoblast layer beneath the cusp responds to the trauma by quickly producing dentin. This dentin has very few, if any, dentinal tubules and, under the microscope, looks very dense and unorganized.

Mechanical trauma is usually the result of cavity preparations in the tooth. Cavity preparations generally extend through enamel and into dentin. When dentin is cut, odontoblastic processes are

damaged. Most of this damage leads to the death of the odontoblasts in that area. These odontoblasts are replaced by reserve mesenchymal cells from the adjacent pulpal tissue, which change into odontoblasts and produce reparative dentin.

Chemical trauma is usually brought about by the acids produced by the bacteria that cause dental caries. Chemical trauma is also sometimes produced by substances used in filling teeth if the cavity preparation has not been lined in some manner. Lining the cavity preparation protects the pulp from the chemicals used in restorations, and some of them also help soothe the pulpal tissue that has been damaged by the preparatory process.

It is possible to radiographically determine the type of trauma. Occlusal trauma results in reparative dentin being produced beneath the involved area, usually a cusp tip. Mechanical and chemical traumas occur in areas where there has been decay or

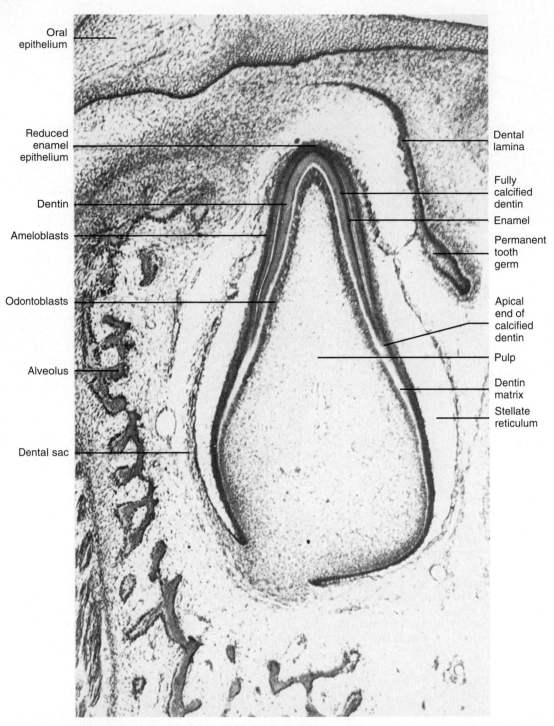

Oral epithelium

Reduced enamel epithelium

Dentin

Ameloblasts

Odontoblasts

Alveolus

Dental sac

Dental lamina

Fully calcified dentin

Enamel

Permanent tooth germ

Apical end of calcified dentin

Pulp

Dentin matrix

Stellate reticulum

• **Figure 20.7** Enlargement of dental papilla area. Ameloblasts at the tip of cusps have met the outer enamel epithelium (OEE), forming reduced enamel epithelium (REE). (From Bevelander G. *Atlas of Oral Histology and Embryology.* Philadelphia: Lea & Febiger; 1967.)

cavity preparations, such as occlusal grooves or cervical or interproximal areas (Fig. 20.12).

Abnormalities in Dentin

Several abnormalities can be found in dentin. Because dentin lies beneath either enamel or cementum, most of the more common abnormalities cannot be seen without sectioning the tooth and studying it under a hand lens or microscope.

Interglobular Dentin

During the process of calcification, some areas of poorly calcified dentin become entrapped. These poorly calcified areas are the

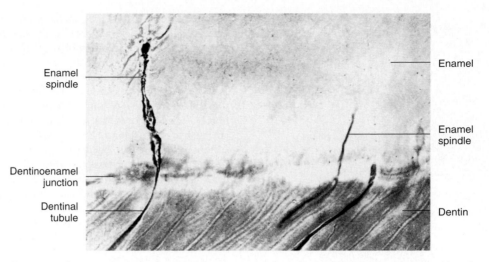

• **Figure 20.8** An enamel spindle or odontoblastic process extension crossing the dentinoenamel junction (DEJ) and lying in enamel. (From Bhaskar SN. *Orban's Oral Histology and Embryology*. 8th ed. St. Louis: Mosby; 1976.)

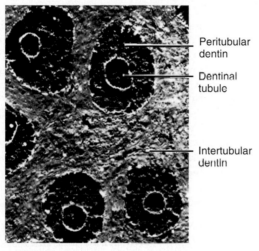

• **Figure 20.9** Cross-sectional view of dentin. (From Bhaskar SN. *Orban's Oral Histology and Embryology*. 8th ed. St. Louis: Mosby; 1976.)

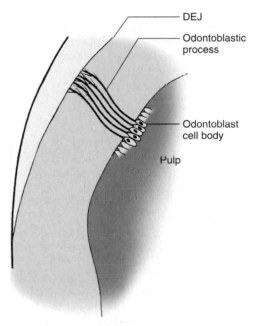

• **Figure 20.10** Cell body of an odontoblast with an elongated odontoblastic process stretching from the dentinoenamel junction (DEJ) to the pulp.

interglobular dentin. They are found next to the DEJ in the crown and the DCJ in the root. The root interglobular dentin has no clinical significance and is generally called the **granular layer of Tomes**.

Dead Tracts

Dentinal tubules that are empty because of the death of the odontoblasts that originally occupied them are known as **dead tracts**. These are not seen clinically, but only microscopically. Because the tubules are empty, they provide decay-causing bacteria with a pathway to the pulp. This means more rapid penetration of decay once it has reached the DEJ, and there is insufficient time for reparative dentin to be formed.

Sclerotic Dentin

A condition in which the dentinal tubules are filled with dentin material, due to occlusal trauma or decay, is called **sclerotic**

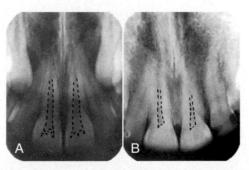

• **Figure 20.11** Radiographs of maxillary central incisors. **(A)** Radiograph of an 8-year-old. **(B)** Radiograph of a 43-year-old. Note the prominence of the pulp horns and chamber size of pulp in the 8-year-old compared with that in the 43-year-old.

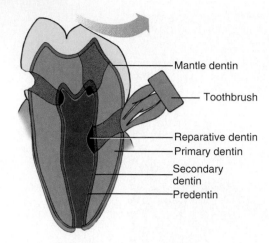

- **Figure 20.12** Primary, secondary, and reparative dentin. Note how the secondary dentin has decreased the size of the entire pulp chamber, whereas reparative dentin is formed only beneath traumatic areas, such as carious regions or areas of occlusal wear. (From Nanci A. *Ten Cate's Oral Histology*. 8th ed. St. Louis: Mosby; 2013.)

dentin. The odontoblastic processes in the area of the trauma retract and begin secreting matrix substance, filling in the empty tubule. The odontoblasts may also degenerate, and the tubules of the degenerating odontoblasts are filled. This has also been referred to as **transparent dentin**.

Pulp

The pulp develops from the mesenchymal tissue of the dental papilla. It will eventually consist of blood and lymph vessels, nerves, fibroblasts, and collagen fibers, as well as other cells of connective tissue. As dentin grows inward, it compresses the inner tissue of the dental papilla. At this point, blood vessels, lymphatic channels, nerves, and connective tissue cells are very evident. Many of the mesenchymal cells become fibroblasts and begin forming collagen fibers (Fig. 20.13). The nerves of the pulp are primarily sensory and transmit only one type of sensation—pain. Some autonomic sympathetic nerves innervate the smooth muscle cells in the walls of the blood vessels and cause them to constrict. This kind of reaction is important in the vascular changes in the pulp caused by irritation to the tooth.

Young pulpal tissue is considered primarily cellular with a lesser concentration of fibers compared with older pulp. A number of cell types are present. Besides fibroblasts, there are macrophages, which will protect the pulp, and a large number of reserve mesenchymal cells. These mesenchymal cells are the kind seen in the dental papilla as the tooth starts to develop. They are undifferentiated and have the ability to change into differing types of cells, including fibroblasts and odontoblasts. As the pulp ages, some of these cells are used to form odontoblasts to replace those that are damaged. (Although odontoblasts are an integral part of dentin, they are also the peripheral cells of the pulp [Fig. 20.14].) Some of them will change to fibroblasts and produce more collagen. With aging of the tooth, the pulp becomes smaller because of the production of secondary and reparative dentin and is less able to resist trauma because it loses its reserve cells; this explains why, compared with adults, young people are less susceptible to permanent pulpal damage.

Abnormalities in Pulp

Pulp stones are the primary abnormality seen in the pulp. They are small, circular, calcified areas found in the pulps of about 80% of persons 70 to 80 years of age. With such a high rate of occurrence, identifying them as abnormalities may be questionable, but they are considered a pathologic condition. There are several classifications of stones based on their origin and density. True pulp stones originate from odontoblasts and are very rare. False stones are the most common type and probably originate from dead cells with concentric layers of calcium phosphate around them. When studied under the microscope, a false stone resembles an onion cut in cross section. Another classification of stones refers to them as *diffuse calcifications*; they are tiny, calcified structures found in groups.

Pulp stones are also classified according to their locations. Free pulp stones are found in the middle of the pulp. Attached pulp stones are those that have become attached to the dentin in the periphery of the pulp. Embedded stones are those that are attached to the dentin and become surrounded by secondary dentin (Fig. 20.15).

Clinical Considerations

Pulp stones do not usually affect the health of the pulp. The pulp can have a number of stones and still be vital. They may be seen as small globular **radiopacities** on radiographs. The only problem that may occur would be in the endodontic treatment of a tooth with numerous pulp stones. The stones could make it difficult to remove pulpal tissue.

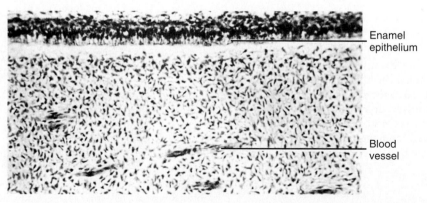

- **Figure 20.13** Young pulp with mesenchymal cells and developing blood vessels. (From Bhaskar SN. *Orban's Oral Histology and Embryology*. 8th ed. St. Louis: Mosby; 1976.)

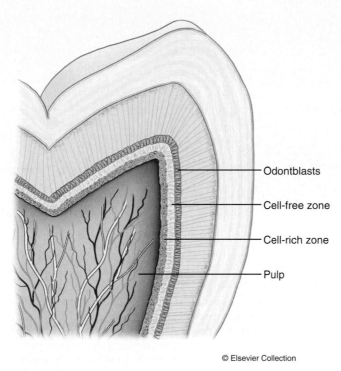

© Elsevier Collection

• **Figure 20.14** Odontoblasts surrounding pulp as the outer layer.

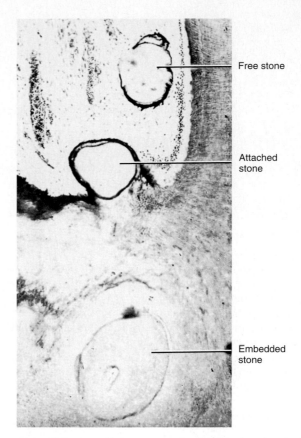

• **Figure 20.15** Pulp stones in three stages: free, attached, and embedded. (From Bhaskar SN. *Orban's Oral Histology and Embryology*. 8th ed. St. Louis: Mosby; 1976.)

Review Questions

1. How do the cells of the inner enamel epithelium (IEE) change to become preameloblasts?
2. How do preameloblasts change to become ameloblasts?
3. What is the reciprocal relationship between enamel and dentin during formation?
4. What happens if enamel crystals do not grow to full size?
5. What is the orientation of crystals in the upper and lower parts of the keyhole-shaped enamel rod?
6. What is Nasmyth's membrane?
7. What are enamel lamellae?
8. What are the three distinct areas of primary dentin?
9. What is the difference between secondary dentin and reparative dentin in terms of composition?
10. What are dead tracts?
11. What is sclerotic (or transparent) dentin?
12. What happens to the pulp as it ages?
13. What are pulp stones?
14. How are pulp stones classified by their location?
15. How do pulp stones affect the health of the pulp?

21

Root Formation and Attachment Apparatus

OBJECTIVES

- To discuss the role of the epithelial root sheath in root formation and dentin formation
- To describe the fate of the epithelial root sheath
- To describe the beginning of cementum formation, the two varieties, and where they are found
- To define and diagram alveolar bone and its components
- To define periodontal ligament and list its various groups and subgroups of fibers
- To briefly describe bone's reaction to pressure and tension and how this affects tooth movement

This chapter deals with the formation of the root—how its form is determined and developed—and the development of cementum, the periodontal ligament (PDL), and alveolar bone, collectively referred to as the attachment apparatus.

Root Formation

Root formation begins after the outline of the crown has been established but before the full crown is calcified. If you refer to Figs. 19.4, 20.2, and 20.3 (bell stage), you will see that the point where the outer enamel epithelium (OEE) meets the inner enamel epithelium (IEE) is located at the deepest part of the enamel organ and is known as the **cervical loop**. There are no interposing layers of stellate reticulum or stratum intermedium here, which one would see more coronally in the crown. These layers of OEE and IEE, which make up the **epithelial root sheath** (**Hertwig's epithelial root sheath**), begin to undergo rapid **mitotic division** and grow deep into the underlying connective tissue—the beginning of root formation. It is important to keep in mind the relationship of the dental papilla and the dental sac to this growing epithelial root sheath. The dental papilla is on the inside, and the dental sac is on the outside (Fig. 21.1). As the apical growth continues, the tip of the epithelial root sheath turns horizontally inward; this turned-in portion is known as the **epithelial diaphragm** of the root sheath. The epithelial root sheath and epithelial diaphragm guide the shape and the number of roots.

Figs. 21.1 and 21.2 are two-dimensional representations of three-dimensional objects. To help you understand this better, visualize a paper cup in three dimensions. The rim of the cup

represents the cervical line of the tooth, and the side of the cup is the epithelial root sheath. If you cut a round hole in the bottom of the cup about two-thirds the diameter of the cup and made a vertical cut through the middle, the horizontal bottom of the cup that remained would represent the epithelial diaphragm. The way in which this epithelial diaphragm continues to grow inward determines whether the tooth will have one, two, or three roots.

Changes continue to occur at the deep surface of the epithelial diaphragm. As the vertical epithelial root sheath grows longer, forming the root length, the horizontal epithelial diaphragm continues to grow in toward the middle of the tooth. If the entire circumference of the diaphragm grows evenly, it will eventually form a single-rooted tooth. If two areas opposite one another grow inward more rapidly and meet, it will then separate into two columns of root formation to form a birooted tooth. If three areas grow inward to meet, a tri-rooted tooth will be formed (Fig. 21.3). In multirooted teeth, the point where the epithelial diaphragm meets is the bifurcation or trifurcation of the tooth.

Attachment Apparatus

Dentinocemental Junction

Fig. 21.1 shows the relationship of the epithelial root sheath to the dental papilla and dental sac. As the root sheath grows from the cervical line deeper into connective tissue, it influences the peripheral cells of the dental papilla to change into odontoblasts, similar to what happens in the crown of the tooth. Odontoblasts begin to secrete matrix and calcify. Once dentin begins to form next to the epithelial root sheath, cellular influence causes the root sheath to begin to break up. There is still some debate as to which cells cause this breakup. It may be the odontoblasts inside, or it may be the cells of the dental sac on the outside.

To envision this deterioration of the epithelial root sheath, imagine that the sheath is originally a solid wall of cells surrounding the developing tooth root. Later it becomes riddled with holes, like a piece of Swiss cheese. With the appearance of these holes, there is no longer any barrier separating the odontoblasts and dentin on the inside from the cells of the dental sac on the outside. Some of the undifferentiated dental sac cells contact dentin are induced to change into cementoblasts, move through the holes, and begin to form cementum. This cementum is laid down against the previously formed dentin and establishes the dentinocemental junction (DCJ) (Fig. 21.4). Remember that the epithelial root sheath is perforated; therefore, the cementoblasts that contact dentin are able to accomplish the transformation only in the areas where the sheath

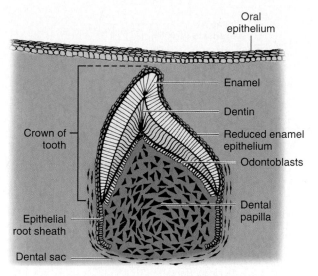

• **Figure 21.1** Beginning root development. The epithelial root sheath interposed between the dental papilla and the dental sac.

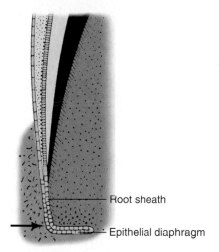

• **Figure 21.2** The epithelial diaphragm is the horizontal component of the epithelial root sheath. Mitosis and growth of the root sheath take place at the point of the arrow. (Modified from Bhaskar SN. *Orban's Oral Histology and Embryology*. 8th ed. St. Louis: Mosby; 1976.)

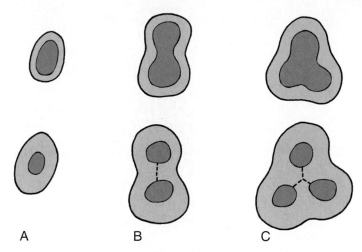

• **Figure 21.3** Inferior view of an epithelial diaphragm. **(A)** The entire circumference of the epithelial diaphragm grows inward, and a single-rooted tooth will be formed. **(B)** The epithelial diaphragm grows inward at two opposite areas and meets in the middle, forming a double-rooted tooth. **(C)** The epithelial diaphragm grows inward at three areas and meets, forming a tri-rooted tooth.

cells later begin dividing, they may lead to the formation of periodontal cysts in the jaws, similar in origin to the palatal cysts mentioned in Chapter 18.

Cementum

Cementum is a hard, yellowish substance covering the root of the tooth. It is composed of about 50% to 60% inorganic hydroxyapatite crystals, and the remaining 40% to 50% is made up of organic components and water. As in most hard substances in teeth, except for enamel, the organic component is primarily collagen fibers and mucopolysaccharide ground substance.

As cementum formation begins, it is first seen at the cervical line of the tooth, also called the *cementoenamel junction (CEJ)*. As cementum is laid down, it may assume three different relationships with the enamel of the crown. In about 15% of the cases, cementum overlaps enamel, in 55% cementum meets enamel at a sharp junction, and in the remaining 30% of the cases, cementum and enamel do not meet, thus leaving dentin exposed at the cervical line. Exposed dentin may make the tooth very sensitive in that area if the patient develops gingival recession (Fig. 21.5).

As the cementoblast begins laying down cementum, it moves away from the DCJ and secretes matrix behind it. This type of deposition results in **acellular cementum**, in which all of the cementoblasts remain on the surface rather than becoming trapped within cementum. These surface cementoblasts not only initially build cementum, but also aid in rebuilding cementum when it is damaged. This type of cellular arrangement is noted in the cervical two-thirds of the root but not usually to any extent in the apical one-third.

As root formation and, thus, cementum formation proceed from the cervical line to the apex of the root, cementoblasts surround themselves and become entrapped as they are secreting matrix, similar to osteoblasts in bone formation becoming osteocytes. A histologic examination of the tissue reveals numerous entrapped cells, which are referred to as **cementocytes**. Because of these cells, the tissue is described as **cellular cementum**. In the middle and apical thirds of the root, cellular cementum can be

has broken up. While this occurs, the remaining root sheath cells pull away from dentin, and the cementoblasts contact the entire dentin and establish the rest of the DCJ. Occasionally some epithelial root sheath cells do not pull away and may differentiate into ameloblasts, forming small globs of enamel on the surface of dentin. These are referred to as **enamel pearls** and are usually found in root furcations. Enamel pearls may interfere with attachment and cause periodontal problems. Accessory root canals are another defect that may occur during this time. When the root sheath fails to continue apically or encounters a blood vessel, it may produce a horizontal pathway to the periodontium from the tooth. These canals may make it difficult for a dentist to remove all pulpal tissue completely if the tooth has to be treated endodontically.

After the cells of the epithelial root sheath have disintegrated and moved away from dentin, the remaining root sheath cells are found in the periodontal space next to the tooth and are called **epithelial rests of Malassez** or simply *epithelial rest cells*. If these

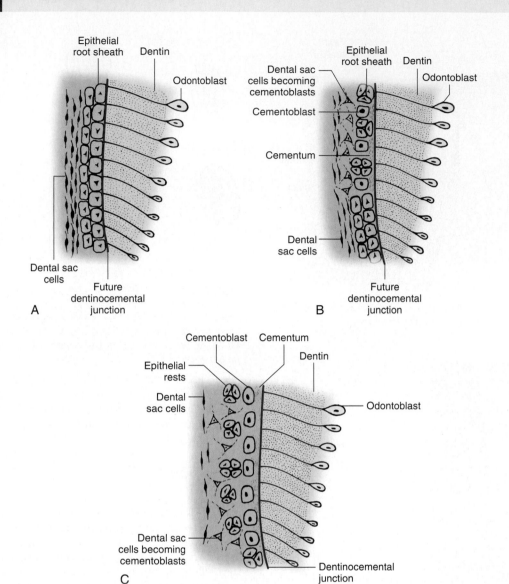

• **Figure 21.4** **(A)** The epithelial root sheath separates dentin from the dental sac cells. **(B)** The epithelial root sheath breaks up, and the dental sac cells become cementoblasts. **(C)** The epithelial root sheath moves away from dentin, and the dentinocemental junction (DCJ) is formed.

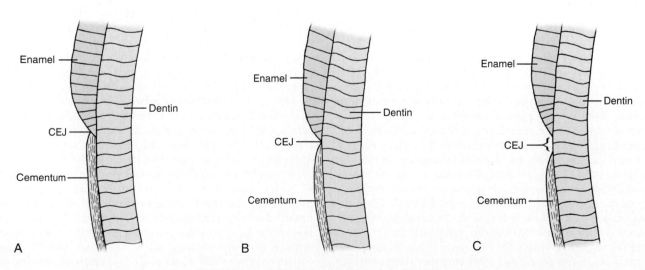

• **Figure 21.5** Variations in cementoenamel junction (CEJ). **(A)** Cementum overlaps enamel. **(B)** Cementum and enamel meet in a sharp junction. **(C)** Cementum and enamel do not meet, and dentin is exposed.

seen overlapping acellular cementum (Fig. 21.6). Because of the presence of the cementocytes, cellular cementum is more vital than acellular cementum and therefore more responsive to remodeling itself, albeit a slow process. However, to remain vital, the entrapped cells within cellular cementum must be maintained. Therefore, cementocytes have long cellular processes that point toward the surface of the tooth, where they gain nourishment from the blood vessels of the periodontium.

The cellular cementum at the apex of the root tends to increase in thickness with the passage of time and other considerations. Potential factors may include occlusal trauma, pathologic conditions (apical inflammation), systemic conditions, or attrition. This thickening is called **hypercementosis** and in general causes no great problem to the tooth unless it becomes necessary to

extract it. A bulbous apex due to hypercementosis might make extraction more difficult, and it may be necessary to remove the adjacent bone as well (Fig. 21.7A–B).

The outer layer of cementum is lined with cementoblasts, which are capable of cementum formation throughout a person's life. As the **periodontal membrane** or **ligament** (PDL) forms from the middle of the layer of cells in the old dental sac, the ends of the periodontal fibers become surrounded by cementoblasts, whose secretion hardens around the ends of the fibers, attaching them to cementum. The parts of the PDL embedded in cementum are known as **Sharpey's fibers**. The periodontal fibers surrounded by alveolar bone on the other side of the tooth socket are also known as *Sharpey's fibers* (Fig. 21.8).

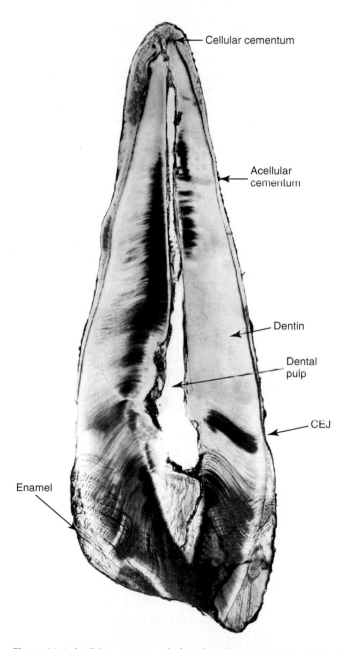

• **Figure 21.6** Acellular cementum is found on the cervical two-thirds of the root. Cellular cementum covers the apical one-third of the root, overlapping the acellular cementum near the middle. (From Nanci A. *Ten Cate's Oral Histology.* 8th ed. St. Louis: Mosby; 2013.)

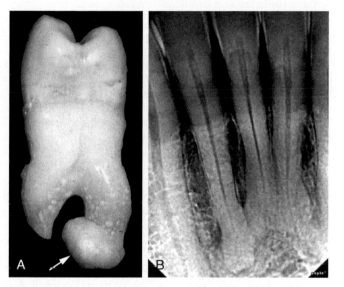

• **Figure 21.7** Hypercementosis. **(A)** The apex of the root has become quite bulbous and can make extraction very difficult because the cementum overgrowth traps the root within the socket. **(B)** Radiograph of hypercementosis on mandibular anterior teeth. (A, From: Vijah, R. & Chandan, S. (2015). Hypercementosis: Review of literature and report of a case of mammoth, dumbbell-shaped hypercementosis. Journal of Indian Academy of Oral Medicine and Radiology, 27 (1), 160-163. https://doi.org/10.4103/0972-1363.167154 Figure #4.)

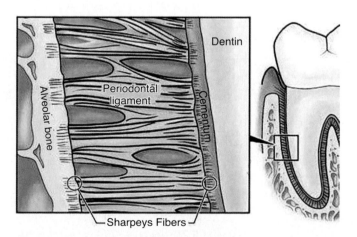

• **Figure 21.8** The ends of the periodontal ligament entrapped in bone and cementum; these entrapped fibers are called *Sharpey's fibers.* (From: Gehrig, J. & Willmann, D. (2016). Foundations of periodontics for the dental hygienist (4th ed.) Wolters Kluwer. Page 38, figure 2-16.)

Cementum Repair

When cementum experiences trauma, the cementum is resorbed by odontoclasts. Also known as osteoclasts, the same cell that destroys bone and dentin, the odontoclasts remove the damaged cementum at the site of trauma. Once this is completed, the cementoblasts lined up along the PDL begin to secrete cementoid and repair the lesion. Cementum repair is not continuous and only occurs due to severe trauma. Typical trauma that may damage cementum can be from occlusal forces, orthodontic movement, the eruption of permanent teeth, and the exfoliation of primary teeth. Later in the chapter, we will discuss bone repair, which is the same type of reaction seen in cementum. However, the process is slower in cementum because of a lower metabolic rate. Therefore cementum is not affected by trauma as quickly as bone is; this is an important consideration in orthodontic tooth movement.

Alveolar Bone

By definition, **alveolar bone** or **alveolar process** is the bone of the maxillary or mandibular jaw that comprises the sockets for teeth. The composition of dried bone varies, depending on whether it is young bone or adult bone. Adult bone is about 60% inorganic crystal; the remaining 40% organic composition is about 89% collagen and 11% noncollagenous material. Alveolar bone originates by intramembranous development (as discussed in Chapter 17) and is mesodermal in origin, as are all types of connective tissue.

Alveolar bone is composed of three layers, as seen in cross section (Fig. 21.9A). The layer of compact bone on the buccal or lingual surface is referred to as the **cortical plate** of bone. It is typical bone with a normal periosteum. The bone that forms the socket for the tooth is also a compact bone but does not have a normal periosteum. Although this is a compact layer, it contains numerous holes that allow for the passage of blood vessels, connecting the deeper part of the bone with the vessels of the periodontal space. This layer is called the **cribriform plate** or **alveolar bone proper**. Radiographically it is referred to as the **lamina dura**. The cribriform plate originates from the outer layer of the dental sac.

The tooth socket is constantly being remodeled, and additional bone, called **bundle bone**, is laid down on the cribriform plate (see Fig. 21.9B).

Finally, in between the cortical plate and the cribriform plate is a layer of **spongy** or **cancellous bone**. This spongy bone is bone marrow (Chapter 17).

Radiographically, the cortical plate can only be seen on occlusal radiographs when the beam is aimed perpendicular to the occlusal plane. It cannot be seen on other intraoral radiographs because it is only on the buccal and lingual sides of the socket. Intraoral radiographs will only show the cribriform plate, the spongy bone, and the crest of bone that joins two sockets, called the interdental septum. The contours of the interdental septum are a good indicator of periodontal health and are frequently utilized to provide a visual representation of bone loss to patients (Fig. 21.10).

Like cementum, alveolar bone can repair itself. Although the processes are similar, the higher metabolic rate and superior blood supply of alveolar bone make it a more effective and efficient remodeler.

Periodontal Ligament

The PDL also develops from the middle layer of mesodermal cells of the dental sac. This happens after cementum has begun forming. As the dental sac cells begin to change, they first become fibroblasts, and the fibroblasts form collagen fibers. At first, these fibers are arranged around the tooth and parallel with the root surface in the middle of the periodontal space. The fibers that are forming adjacent to cementum and alveolar bone are initially more obliquely oriented. Later, they will band into groups of fibers that span the periodontal space.

About the same time the fibers are forming, the other components of the PDL are also starting to appear, including blood

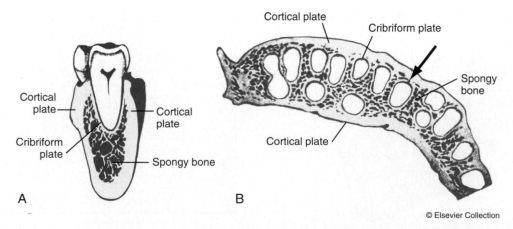

© Elsevier Collection

• **Figure 21.9** Alveolar bone. **(A)** A cross-section view through a mandible. The cortical plate is on the buccal and lingual sides with the cribriform plate in the socket. Spongy bone is present in between. **(B)** A longitudinal horizontal section through a mandible. Note the thickened lamina dura *(arrow)*. This is caused by bundle bone being deposited on the cribriform plate. (From Bhaskar SN. *Orban's Oral Histology and Embryology.* 8th ed. St. Louis: Mosby; 1976.)

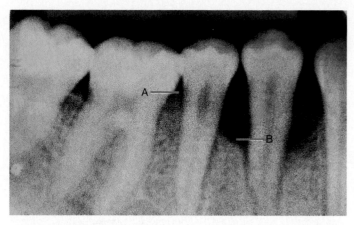

• **Figure 21.10** The arrows point to the alveolar bone crest. Healthy **(A)** and blunted **(B)** alveolar crest indicative of periodontal disease. (From: Bergantin, B., Rios, D., Oliveira, D., Júnior, E., Hanemann, J., & Honório, H. (2018). Localized bone loss resulted from an unlikely cause in an 11-year-old child. Case Reports in Dentistry, article ID 3484513. https://doi.org/10.1155/2018/3484513.)

vessels, lymphatic vessels, nerves, and various types of connective tissue cells. Unlike the nerves of the pulp, which can transmit only impulses of pain, the nerves of the periodontal space also have fibers that allow one to feel light touch and pressure, as well as heat and cold. When biting down on something hard produces a sharp pain, it is the nerves of the PDL that are stimulated, not the pulp of the tooth. After root canal treatment, it is still possible to feel pain at times; however, this is not from the pulpal area but from the PDL. The blood vessels of the ligament space are branches of the same vessels that go to the pulp, but they also have branches that penetrate the holes in the wall of the cribriform plate and join with the vascular channels in the spongy part of alveolar bone, and still others come from the gingival blood supply and interconnect with these other vessels.

As the fibers of the ligament form, they begin to arrange themselves in a definite pattern. When the fibers reach their final arrangement, they are known as the principal fiber groups and descriptively arranged into three groups: alveolodental fibers, transeptal fibers, and **gingival fibers**.

1. Alveolodental fibers—main principal fiber group that orient from the tooth neck to the apex and attach cementum to alveolar bone (Fig. 21.12)
   a. Alveolar crest group—runs from cementum, slightly below the CEJ into alveolar bone; helps resist horizontal movements
   b. Horizontal group—runs from cementum, inferior to the alveolar crest; helps resist horizontal movements
   c. Oblique group—most numerous, runs from cementum coronally into alveolar bone; main fiber group for resisting occlusal stresses
   d. Apical group—runs from cementum at the apex of the tooth into adjacent alveolar bone; resists forces trying to pull the tooth from its socket
   e. Interradicular group—found only on multirooted teeth; runs from cementum of one root to the cementum of another and has no bony attachment; resists the forces trying to remove the tooth (Fig. 21.11)
2. Transeptal ligament fibers—also called interdental ligament fibers; connects interdentally, runs from the cervical cementum of one tooth to the cervical cementum of an adjacent tooth and has no bony attachment; function is to hold the teeth in interproximal contact (Fig. 21.12).

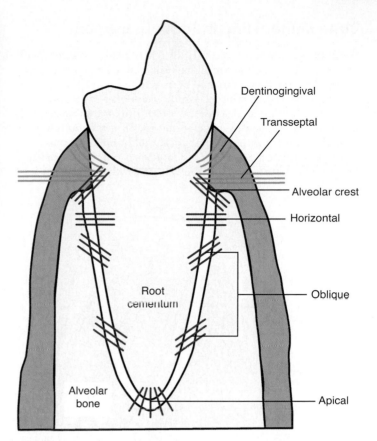

• **Figure 21.11** Diagram showing the five groups of alveolodental fibers. Interradicular fibers are only present in multirooted teeth. (From: de Jong, T., Bakker, A., Everts, V., & Smit, T. (2017). The intricate anatomy of the periodontal ligament and its development: Lessons for periodontal regeneration. Journal of Periodontal Research, 52(6), 965-974. https://doi.org/10.1111/jre.12477.)

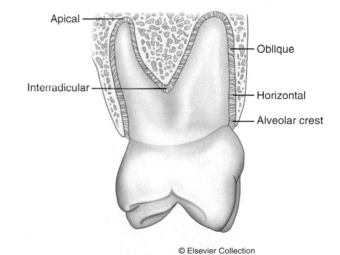

© Elsevier Collection

• **Figure 21.12** Gingival and transseptal fibers. The transseptal fibers go from the cementum of one tooth to the cementum of an adjacent tooth. The gingival fibers extend from cementum up into the gingiva.

3. Gingival fibers—found in the lamina propria of marginal gingiva and not with the PDL. They do not resist tooth movement forces but help support the relationship between marginal gingiva and the tooth. Not considered a principal fiber group by some.

Bone Remodeling in Tooth Movement

What happens when a tooth is lost? Many times the tooth adjacent to the missing tooth will tilt toward the unoccupied space. This phenomenon has been referred to as *mesial drift*. The same type of movement can be accomplished in orthodontic tooth movement. Because each tooth fits into a socket, it is necessary to change the shape of that socket if the tooth is to be moved. In most tooth movement, the tooth does not move as a whole but tilts on an axis. This rotational point on a tooth is located about two-thirds of the way down the root. If a tooth

tilts mesially (Fig. 21.13A; also see Fig. 21.14), bone is resorbed on the cervical two-thirds of the mesial side and on the apical one-third of the distal side. This resorption is a result of the tooth putting pressure on alveolar bone in these areas, causing reduced blood flow, which results in the formation of osteoclasts, cells that destroy bone. As the tooth moves, there is tension on the periodontal fibers in the apical one-third of the mesial side and the cervical two-thirds of the distal side. This tension causes osteoblasts to build new bone, and the socket fills in at the area once occupied by the tooth's root (Fig. 21.13B; also see Fig. 21.14).

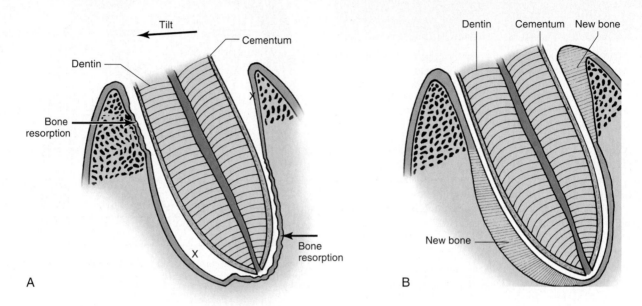

• **Figure 21.13** **(A)** Mesial drift. The tooth is tilted mesially, and bone is destroyed at the areas marked *X,* which were once occupied by teeth. **(B)** Remodeled bone. Hash marks indicate new bone formation after tooth movement and new bone apposition.

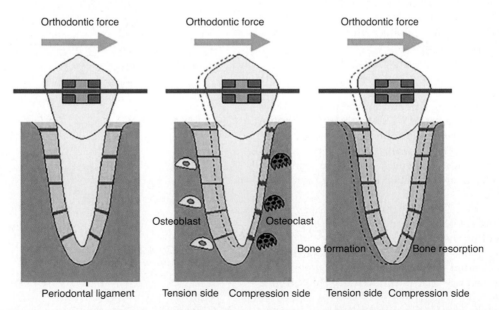

• **Figure 21.14** Orthodontic tooth movement and the actions of osteoblasts and osteoclasts in response to tension and compression. (From: Kitaura, H., Kimura, K., Ishida, M., Sugisawa, H., Kohara, H., Yoshimatsu, M., & Takano-Yamamoto, T. (2014). Effect of cytokines on osteoclast formation and bone resorption during mechanical force loading of the periodontal membrane. The Scientific World Journal, Article ID 617032. https://doi.org/10.1155/2014/617032 Figure #2.)

Review Questions

1. What early structures develop into the epithelial root sheath?
2. What happens to the epithelial root sheath after root dentin starts to form?
3. What are epithelial rests? What might happen to them later in life?
4. Cells of the dental sac form three structures. What are they?
5. What are the two types of cementum? Where are they found on the root?
6. What are Sharpey's fibers? What is their function?
7. What are the layers of alveolar bone?
8. What is the lamina dura? What clinical implications can be made if the lamina dura is thickened?
9. What are the various periodontal ligament principal fiber groups and the functions of each?
10. How would mesial drift occur?
11. What causes bone resorption and apposition (remodeling)?

22
Eruption and Shedding of Teeth

OBJECTIVES

- To name the three stages of active tooth eruption and the points at which each stage begins
- To discuss the fate of the epithelial layers covering the crown of the tooth
- To discuss briefly what causes the shedding of primary teeth
- To diagram or describe the origin and position of permanent teeth compared with deciduous teeth
- To list and describe the factors that lead to a retained primary tooth

Active Tooth Eruption

The term *active tooth eruption* implies the emergence of a crown into the oral cavity. In general, however, the term refers to the total life span of the tooth, from the beginning of crown development until the tooth is lost or the individual dies. This eruptive process is usually divided into three stages, and although there may be some difference in the terminology, they refer to the same mechanism.

Preeruptive Stage

The **preeruptive stage** begins as the crown starts to develop. Recall that dental lamina formation—bud, cap, and bell stages, as well as the calcification of the crown—takes place in the connective tissue beneath the oral epithelium. During this time the bone of the maxilla or mandible surrounds the developing primary tooth in a U-shaped crypt or beginning socket (Fig. 22.1).

The eruptive movement associated with the preeruptive stage is of two varieties—spatial and eccentric. In spatial movement, the crown develops while the bottom of the socket fills in with bone, pushing the crown toward the surface. A similar facial movement accompanies jaw growth. In eccentric, or off-center, growth, the crown of a tooth does not grow in a perfectly symmetric pattern. As the crown enlarges, it grows more in one area than in another, and so the tooth seems to be moving because the center of the tooth is shifting. It appears to have moved because the center point of the developing crown has shifted. This is the activity of the preeruptive stage. It involves crown growth and some movement toward the surface while the crypt is developing.

Eruptive Stage

The **eruptive stage** or **prefunctional eruptive stage** begins with the development of the root. While the root continues to lengthen, the tooth begins to move toward the surface of the oral cavity. As it approaches the oral cavity, alveolar bone is growing to keep pace with it. However, in time, the tooth moves faster than the growing alveolar bone and approaches the surface of the oral epithelium and breaks into the oral cavity.

The crown of the tooth is surrounded by reduced enamel epithelium. Around the reduced enamel epithelium, there are cells of the dental sac, or follicle, that covers the crown. Cells of the dental follicle form a cord of connective tissue epithelium. This fibrous cord is known as the **gubernacular cord** and forms a **gubernacular canal** that leads the way and, with the help of macrophages and osteoclasts, breaks down the bone between the tooth and the surface oral epithelium for the primary tooth to erupt (Fig. 22.2). As the tooth moves to the surface, the reduced enamel epithelium moves with it until it compresses connective tissue and causes it to disintegrate. The reduced enamel epithelium then contacts the oral epithelium, and these two layers fuse into one layer—the **united oral epithelium**. Lastly, an enzyme is released that facilitates the tooth breaking through the oral epithelium and emerging into the oral cavity. This stage continues until the erupting teeth meet the opposing teeth.

For both primary and secondary dentition, tooth movement in the eruptive stage tends to be occlusal and facial, more facial in anterior teeth than in posterior teeth. When we think about the pathway for secondary teeth, we have to consider that they develop. Permanent anterior teeth develop slightly lingual to their primary predecessors and permanent posterior teeth develop below their primary counterparts (Fig. 22.3).

Posteruptive Stage

The **posteruptive stage** begins when teeth come into occlusion and continues until they are lost or death occurs. This posteruptive stage functions in several ways. First, as the mandible continues to grow and the space between the maxilla and the mandible increases, teeth will continue to erupt to maintain a balance in the arches. Second, as teeth wear occlusally because of prolonged masticatory stress and wear, they will continue to erupt to maintain tooth contact. Third, because there is slight interproximal wear, a slight mesial eruptive force will keep teeth in contact. There is a physiologic mesial drift inherent to teeth by virtue of their inclination in the jaws; this is referred to as *mesial drift* (Fig. 22.4). Finally, if an opposing tooth is lost, the tooth may continue to erupt in what is generally referred to as **supraeruption** or **hypereruption**. Supraeruption can cause serious problems in the replacement of a missing tooth because it makes it difficult to reestablish the normal occlusal plane.

Shedding of Primary Dentition

As mentioned before, the 20 permanent teeth that follow primary teeth develop as offshoots of the primary dental lamina. Recall that anterior permanent teeth develop apically and lingually to

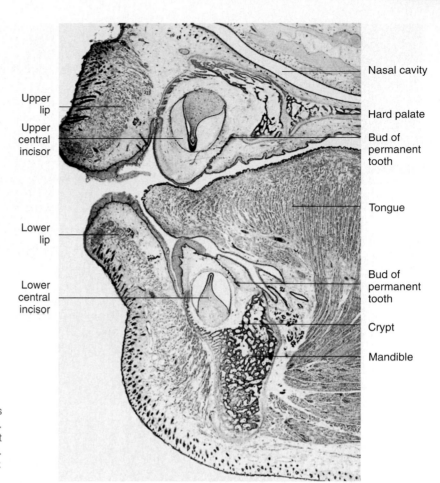

• **Figure 22.1** Primary mandibular and maxillary incisors developing in the recess or crypt of bone, forming a socket. The depth of the crypt builds up from osteoclastic activity at its base and increases in height to form future alveolar bone. (From Bhaskar SN. *Orban's Oral Histology and Embryology.* 8th ed. St. Louis: Mosby; 1976.)

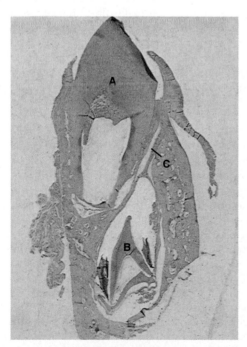

• **Figure 22.2** Buccolingual section through an erupted deciduous canine **(A)** and its erupting successor **(B)**. Note the position of the gubernacular canal **(C)**, the pathway that leads the permanent tooth to the surface oral epithelium.

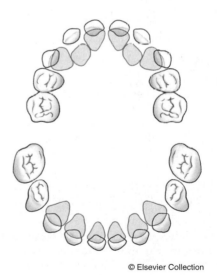

© Elsevier Collection

• **Figure 22.3** Permanent anterior teeth *(red)* develop lingual to their deciduous predecessors *(black)*.

primary teeth (Fig. 22.5), whereas permanent premolars develop between the roots of primary molars (Fig. 22.6). Regardless of its position, the fact that the permanent tooth is present and is in the eruptive stage means that the permanent tooth is moving toward the surface and putting pressure on the root of the primary tooth.

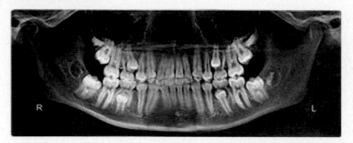

• **Figure 22.4** Teeth are inclined toward the mesial. Note that premolars are tilted toward the midline even before they erupt.

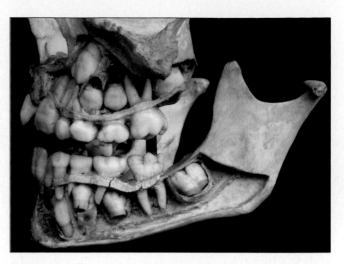

• **Figure 22.6** Dried skull of an 8-year-old with the outer cortical plate cut away. Permanent premolars lie apical to and between the roots of their deciduous molar predecessors. (From Retained deciduous root fragment. https://oralradiology.wordpress.com/radiographic-interpretation/pulpalapical-findings/apical-findings-other/retained-deciduous-root-fragment/.)

Retained Primary Teeth

There are several reasons why primary teeth are retained beyond their normal time for **exfoliation**. This discussion does not consider a general delayed eruption that you may see in some patients because of varying growth patterns but, rather, the cases in which one or two teeth are retained well beyond the expected period for them to be lost.

The reasons for this are several. First, there may be no permanent successor, and the tooth remains. Second, there may be **ankylosis** of the primary tooth, a condition in which the alveolar crest of bone fuses in the cervical area with the cementum of a resorbing root. Although virtually all of the root may have been resorbed, the tooth remains firmly in place, preventing the permanent tooth below from erupting. This may remain that way for years, and yet when the ankylosed tooth is removed, the permanent tooth will generally begin to erupt. The last reason for a retained primary tooth is that the permanent tooth does not erupt in its normal position and therefore does not cause resorption of the primary tooth root or roots, and the tooth remains. This is frequently seen in the anterior mandibular area when the permanent teeth erupt too far lingually. In this case permanent teeth erupt completely lingual to their deciduous predecessors so that two sets of anterior teeth will be seen, one behind the other.

Another problem associated with shedding of primary teeth is unresorbed root fragments. This condition is usually, but not always, associated with a misaligned primary or permanent tooth. If the root tip of a primary tooth is not in the path of eruption of a permanent tooth, the cervical portion of the root may be resorbed, leaving the apical part still embedded in the jaw (Fig. 22.7). The fragments may eventually work their way to the surface and be removed. These retained roots are seen in radiographs from time to time.

The schedule of eruption and shedding is varied. In general, posterior teeth go through a slower process compared with anterior teeth. Not only does the length of time for eruption vary, but its beginning or ending time also varies from one person to another. There is a range for normal eruption time, and only when this period is exceeded is there cause for concern (see Chapter 5).

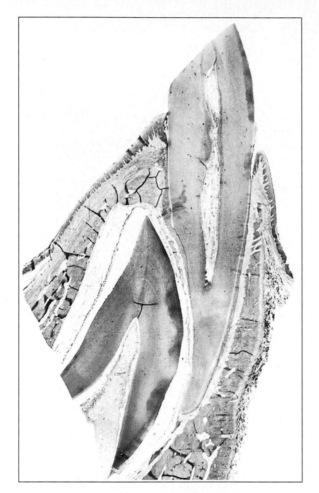

• **Figure 22.5** A permanent mandibular anterior tooth lying lingual and apical to its deciduous predecessor, causing resorption of that tooth. (From Nanci A. *Ten Cate's Oral Histology*. 8th ed. St. Louis: Mosby; 2013.)

It is believed that this pressure causes osteoclasts to form and begin resorbing the primary tooth root. This resorption is intermittent and not constant. This is the usual manner in which resorption occurs, but other factors may be involved. Although most primary teeth would be retained if a permanent tooth did not develop, it is still possible to see a primary tooth undergo root resorption in the absence of a permanent tooth and a primary tooth retained in the presence of a permanent tooth. Therefore although the pressure of a developing tooth is a major factor in resorption of primary teeth, it is not the only factor; there is a focus on the role of the enamel organ of the erupting tooth in the whole process.

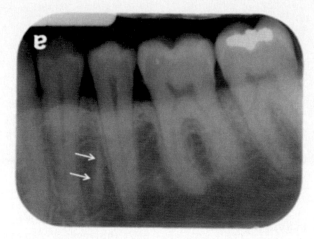

• **Figure 22.7**   Arrows point to remnants of the roots of a deciduous molar still embedded in bone because of a lack of resorption.

Review Questions

1. What is active eruption, and how long does it last?
2. What are the three stages of active tooth eruption? When do they begin and end?
3. What is supraeruption?
4. What causes the breakdown of the oral epithelium as the tooth breaks through and erupts?

5. What is the position of permanent teeth in relation to their deciduous predecessors?
6. What is ankylosis? What problems could it cause? How is it treated?
7. Give three causes of retained primary teeth.

23

Oral Mucosa

OBJECTIVES

- To name the three categories of oral mucosa and discuss where they are found
- To name the three stages of keratinization of oral mucosa and discuss where these different types are found
- To discuss the factors that affect the mobility of various types of the mucosa
- To understand what the submucosa is and where it is found
- To describe the four stages of passive eruption
- To describe the typical clinical picture of the normal gingiva
- To describe some of the changes seen in diseased gingiva

Divisions of Oral Mucosa

The lining of the oral cavity is referred to as the *oral mucosa* or *oral mucous membrane.* It is a stratified squamous epithelial arrangement that runs from the margins of the lips posteriorly to the area of the tonsils. Although this same epithelium is found posterior to this point, it is part of the oral pharynx and not of the oral cavity. Behind the tonsils and in the posterior throat wall it would be referred to as the *pharyngeal mucosa.* Oral mucosa is divided into three categories:

1. **Specialized mucosa**—mucosa on the dorsal and lateral surfaces of the tongue.
2. **Masticatory mucosa**—comprises the gingiva and hard palatal tissue; undergoes trauma or compression during mastication (see Chapter 8).
3. **Lining mucosa**—all other areas of oral mucosa (see Table 8.1).
   Oral mucosa is composed of stratified squamous epithelium and connective tissue. Stratified squamous epithelium can have various characteristics on its surface (Fig. 23.1) depending on whether it is keratinized, parakeratinized, or nonkeratinized.
1. **Keratinized**—on its surface are layers of dead cells without nuclei. This layer is generally called the *stratum corneum.* The stratum granulosum layer beneath the corneum is relatively evident at this stage of keratinization. As keratinization increases, there tends to be an increase in the thickness of the stratum spinosum.
2. **Parakeratinized**—on its surface are some dead cells without nuclei and some apparently dying cells with slightly shriveled nuclei. The stratum granulosum is not quite as evident as in the keratinized mucosa.
3. **Nonkeratinized**—cells on the surface all tend to have nuclei that appear fairly healthy and normal. The stratum granulosum is missing in this type of mucosa.

The lining mucosa is nonkeratinized to parakeratinized under most circumstances. The basal layer of cells rests on the underlying connective tissue with a basement membrane between these two components. Although this underlying connective tissue contains some well-developed collagen fibers, it is still loose enough to allow the overlying epithelium to be fairly movable. Also, allowing for this mobility is the way in which the epithelium and the connective tissue interdigitate with one another.

As seen in Fig. 23.2, there is a definite interdigitating between the epithelium and connective tissue. In this illustration, the ridges appear to interdigitate between the two; however, a three-dimensional representation (Fig. 23.3) shows that there are not only ridges of connective tissue but also pegs of connective tissue projecting up into the epithelium. The length of these ridges and connective tissue pegs determines how tightly the epithelium attaches to the underlying connective tissue and therefore how movable the epithelium is. The connective tissue is attached to underlying bone in some areas or to fatty or muscle tissue in other areas.

Specialized Mucosa

Within the oral cavity, specialized mucosa presents as lingual papillae on the dorsal and ventral surfaces of the tongue. The epithelium is parakeratinized and a lamina propria is present. This mucosa will be discussed in detail in Chapter 24.

Masticatory Mucosa

Masticatory mucosa (free and attached gingivae) is the mucosa of the gingiva and hard palate. It is firm, thick, and immovable with a rubbery, resilient texture.

The gingiva is divided into two regions, the **free gingiva (marginal gingiva)** and the **attached gingiva**. These two regions combine to form the peak of gingiva that extends coronally between the teeth, which is known as the **interdental papilla** (Fig. 23.4). The function of the interdental papilla is to prevent food from collecting interproximally and causing an irritation.

The **col** is the part of the interdental papilla that is apical to the contact area and connects the facial and lingual interdental papillae. The col is nonkeratinized and not subjected to as much trauma during mastication as the rest of the attached gingiva. If there is drifting of teeth, or if interproximal restorations are done with improper contact area margins, then the col will become irritated. At first, the trauma may cause swelling and bleeding of the col, but later the col may become keratinized. If the proper contact areas are regained and/or restored, there will be a slow return to nonkeratinized epithelium.

By observing teeth and gingiva, you will find that there is a very shallow groove or sulcus around the tooth. The average depth

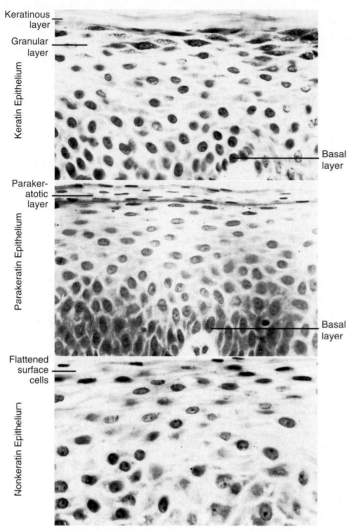

Keratinous layer
Granular layer

Keratin Epithelium

Basal layer

Parakeratotic layer

Parakeratin Epithelium

Basal layer

Flattened surface cells

Nonkeratin Epithelium

• **Figure 23.1** (A) Keratinized epithelium. Note the thick layer at the top without any sign of nuclei. These are dead cells. (B) Parakeratinized epithelium. Although nuclei are present even at the top, there are fewer than in nonkeratinized epithelium, and they appear flattened and shriveled. (C) Nonkeratinized epithelium. Nuclei are obvious even at the top. (From Bhaskar SN. *Orban's Oral Histology and Embryology.* 8th ed. St. Louis: Mosby; 1976.)

of this sulcus measured with a periodontal probe is about 2 mm (see Figs. 23.4 and 23.5). The stratified squamous epithelium that lines this sulcus is nonkeratinized, and at the bottom of the sulcus, the epithelium is continuous with the cells that attach to the tooth, known as the **attachment epithelium (junctional epithelium)**. In cases of periodontal disease, the sulcus deepens either as a result of the free gingiva swelling or the attachment epithelium breaking down or moving farther apically on the tooth. The extent of the free gingiva is usually readily seen because there may be a shallow groove on the gingival surface that corresponds to its depth. This is called the **free gingival groove**.

The interdental papilla is an extremely important part of the gingiva. In a healthy state, it fills the area between teeth up to their contact areas and prevents food from becoming lodged or impacted between teeth during mastication. It is also one of the first areas involved in periodontal disease, becoming swollen and blunted. As this happens, the lack of original contour causes it to

be further irritated during mastication, and the problem becomes more complicated. For this reason, it is an important area to study and check for swelling, blunting, or redness as disease indicators.

The remainder of the gingiva is called the *attached gingiva*. Its name is derived from the fact that it is tightly attached to the underlying connective tissue and bone (see Figs. 23.4 and 23.5). In a healthy state, the gingiva usually has a stippled or dimpled appearance. This is caused by the connective tissue fibers attaching the epithelium to the underlying bone. In periodontal disease, one of the first signs of gingival problems is a loss of stippling. This is initially caused by swelling, or **edema**, of gingival tissues. The normal color of this gingiva is pink, but in the diseased state, it might become reddish, whitish, or have ulcerations or outgrowths of the mucosa.

Where the attached gingiva meets the **alveolar mucosa**, there is change in color and loss of stippling because the epithelium is not attached tightly to bone. The alveolar mucosa is more reddened by the underlying blood vessels and thinness of the epithelium of the mucosa.

In the maxillary arch, the lingual attached gingiva does not meet up against alveolar mucosa but is directly continuous with the masticatory mucosa of the hard palate. This palatal mucosa is generally the area of thickest mucosa in the oral cavity and the most likely to be keratinized.

In this area of masticatory mucosa, the interconnection between connective tissue and the epithelium are long and narrow and therefore help make the epithelium very adherent and relatively immovable (Fig. 23.6). It is within this connective tissue that blood vessels, nerves, small salivary glands, and some fatty deposits are found. Also helping to provide a firm base for the hard palate tissue is the absence of a submucosa in the medial portion. Although the lateral borders of the hard palate contain a submucosa and are palpable, most of the hard palate has no submucosa; instead, it has a **mucoperiosteum** (Fig. 23.7). The mucoperiosteum is made of a mucous membrane directly connected to the periosteum of the underlying bone. This provides an unmovable surface on the palate.

Lining Mucosa

Lining mucosa is found in six different areas of the mouth: the **buccal mucosa, labial mucosa, alveolar mucosa, ventral surface of the tongue, floor of the mouth, and soft palate.**

The lining mucosa is stretchable, loose, flexible, easily compressed, and unattached. Lining mucosa tends to have poorly developed epithelial–connective tissue interdigitating, and this allows it to move freely on the underlying tissue. This degree of mobility is also influenced by the attachment of the connective tissue to the type of tissue lying beneath it.

Lining mucosa do not undergo the same trauma to which the attached gingiva is exposed. Their epithelium is thinner and nonkeratinized, and the lamina propria exhibits connective tissue, elastic fibers, and extensive vascularity. The deeper submucosa may contain connective tissue, adipose tissue, elastic fibers, and minor salivary glands. It is loosely attached to muscle and bone.

1. *Buccal mucosa*—if the buccal mucosa, the mucosa of the cheek, is constantly traumatized by chewing, it will become thickened and keratinized in a line corresponding to the occlusal plane of teeth. Sebaceous glands are frequently found in the buccal mucosa.

2. *Labial mucosa*—trauma to mucosa of the lip may cause some thickening as in the cheek, but more frequently it will cause

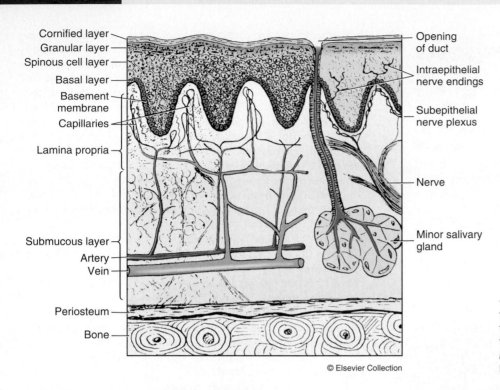

Cornified layer
Granular layer
Spinous cell layer
Basal layer
Basement membrane
Capillaries
Lamina propria
Submucous layer
Artery
Vein
Periosteum
Bone

Opening of duct
Intraepithelial nerve endings
Subepithelial nerve plexus
Nerve
Minor salivary gland

© Elsevier Collection

• **Figure 23.2** Epithelium–connective tissue junction in a two-dimensional representation. Note the interdigitation of the ridges or pegs of each tissue layer. (From Bhaskar SN. *Orban's Oral Histology and Embryology.* 8th ed. St. Louis: Mosby; 1976.)

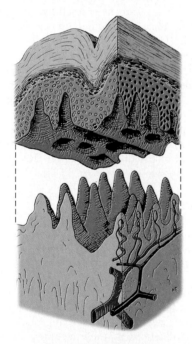

• **Figure 23.3** In a three-dimensional representation, connective tissue pegs can be seen projecting up from ridges into the epithelium. (Modified from Elias H, et al. *Human Microanatomy.* 4th ed. Philadelphia: FA Davis Co.; 1978.)

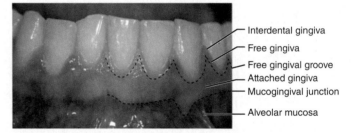

Interdental gingiva
Free gingiva
Free gingival groove
Attached gingiva
Mucogingival junction
Alveolar mucosa

• **Figure 23.4** Free gingiva and the free gingival groove, which divides the free gingiva from attached gingiva. Note the stippled appearance of the gingiva compared with the alveolar mucosa. (From Modified by Marcos Gridi-Papp (https://cnx.org/contents/Mw1rkOh8@32.1:6lOQ91t1@1/ The-Anatomy-of-the-Gum) from original by Mohamed Hamze (https:// commons.wikimedia.org/w/index.php?curid=3304239)).

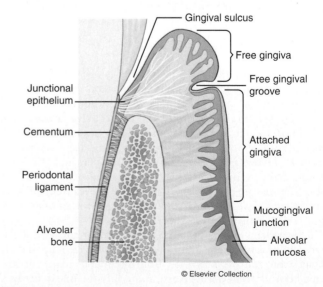

Gingival sulcus
Free gingiva
Free gingival groove
Junctional epithelium
Cementum
Attached gingiva
Periodontal ligament
Mucogingival junction
Alveolar bone
Alveolar mucosa

© Elsevier Collection

• **Figure 23.5** Attached gingiva and alveolar mucosa meet at the mucogingival junction.

trauma to a minor salivary gland and cause a blister-like lesion known as a **mucocele**.

3. *Alveolar mucosa*—elastic fibers, loose connective tissue, and minor salivary glands keep tissue flexible and moist.

4. *Mucosa of the soft palate*—mucosa of about the same thickness as the buccal and labial mucosae, although not as easily traumatized because of its location.

5. *Floor of the mouth and ventral surface of tongue*—these areas are moderately protected from trauma. However, the epithelium

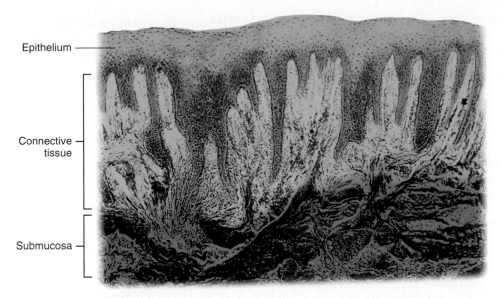

Epithelium

Connective
tissue

Submucosa

• **Figure 23.6** Long interdigitations between the epithelium and connective tissue. These make masticatory mucosa immovable. (Modified from Bhaskar SN. Orban's *Oral Histology and Embryology*. 8th ed. St. Louis: Mosby; 1976.)

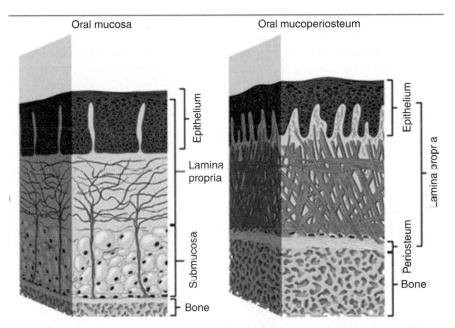

Oral mucosa

Oral mucoperiosteum

Epithelium

Lamina
propria

Submucosa

Bone

Epithelium

Lamina propria

Periosteum

Bone

• **Figure 23.7** Unlike most areas of oral mucosa, the lateral border of the hard palate lacks a submucosa and is attached directly to the periosteum of underlying bone. This firm, inelastic attachment is called a mucoperiosteum. (Adapted from figure 12-6 on https://pocketdentistry.com/12-oral-mucosa/.)

is very thin and a laceration or irritation to the mucosa may occur if it is traumatized by something sharp.

Submucosa

The **submucosa** is the connective tissue beneath the mucosa and contains blood vessels, nerves, and connective tissue. This connective tissue helps determine the mobility of the mucosa by the length of its ridges and pegs. It is not present in all areas of the oral cavity, but when it is, it tends to increase the mobility of the mucosa on top of it. If a submucosa is present, it tends to contain fatty tissue, minor salivary glands, or both. There is very little, if any, submucosa in the gingiva and anteromedial hard palate. In these areas, the mucosa is tightly attached to the periosteum of the underlying bone.

Passive Eruption

Chapter 22 detailed active eruption and how the tooth breaks through the mucosa and into the oral cavity. There is also a process known as **passive eruption**, in which the attachment epithelium moves from the crown of the tooth apically. Remember that as the tooth breaks through into the oral cavity, the attachment epithelium is formed from the reduced enamel epithelium. This is frequently referred to as the **primary attachment epithelium**. Later, the primary attachment epithelium is replaced by a **secondary attachment epithelium**, which arises from the basal layer of the epithelium in the free gingiva. Passive eruption is generally divided into the following four stages (Fig. 23.8).

Stage I—the attachment epithelium at the base of the gingival sulcus rests entirely on enamel. The more recent the eruption, the more incisally or occlusally it may be located.

Stage II—the attachment epithelium is primarily on enamel with a bit on cementum. This may be a relatively long stage.

Stage III—the attachment epithelium extends from the cementoenamel junction (CEJ) onto cementum. This may also be a relatively long stage.

Stage IV—the attachment epithelium is entirely on cementum apical to the CEJ.

There is no specific timing for the process of passive eruption, and it may never reach stage IV, which is considered pathologic and is referred to as *gingival recession.*

The attaching of the epithelium to tooth is an extremely active process. The cells that provide for this attachment are replaced every 4 to 6 days, and this rapid turnover aids in the repair of early gingival or periodontal disease. With proper dental hygiene therapies, there can be significant improvements in attachment epithelium in a week or slightly longer.

Changes in Oral Mucosa

Sometimes the tissue of the oral cavity deviates from its normal color; it may appear quite reddish or whitish. Epithelial cells have no color themselves, but they may take up pigments produced by the body and carry them to the surface. It is this carried pigment that gives differential colors to the skin. The redness of the mucosa comes from the oxygen-carrying pigment in blood, known as *hemoglobin.* These blood vessels are located immediately beneath the mucosa in connective tissue, and the reflection of blood through the epithelium imparts the red color to the mucosa. When the mucosa is excessively red, this is the result of inflammation—the blood vessels beneath the mucosa expand and bring more blood to the area to fight the causative irritation. In a pathologic condition, you will find that redness is one of the primary signs of inflammation. How then can the epithelium appear whitish? Is it because there is less blood beneath the epithelium? It generally is the result of irritation of the mucosa, which causes the cells to multiply faster and the epithelium to become thicker, a condition similar to the development of a callus. When it becomes thicker, the tissue becomes more **opaque**, and the blood does not show through easily; therefore the tissue is whiter than normal. When examining the thickened, whitish mucosa histologically, you can see that the thickened layers are the stratum spinosum and the stratum corneum. This, of course, is a keratinizing epithelium.

It cannot be stressed enough that the oral mucosa is a very important indicator for both the oral and general health of the person. The color, tone, and contours of the tissue are extremely important health indicators. These tissues must be studied carefully because they provide important information.

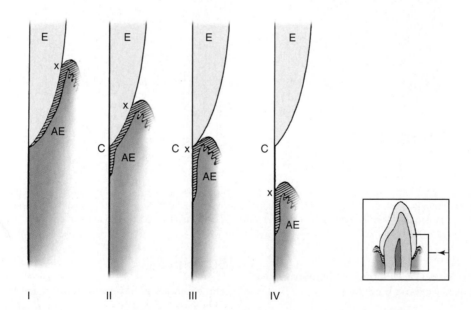

• **Figure 23.8** Four stages of passive eruption. *X,* Base of sulcus; *AE,* attachment epithelium; *C,* cementum; *E,* enamel.

Review Questions

1. What are the three divisions of the oral mucosa, and where are they located?
2. What are the three variations of stratified squamous epithelium?
3. What are the changes in layers evident in these variations?
4. What factors determine the mobility of the mucosa?
5. What are the general causes of change in mucosal color? What is indicated by mucosa that appears red in color? What is indicated by mucosa that appears white in color?
6. What structures can be found in the submucosa?
7. What is the average depth of the gingival sulcus?
8. What is the function of the interdental papilla?
9. What is the col?
10. What is the descriptive term used for normal gingival appearance?
11. Describe the relationship of the attachment epithelium to the tooth in the four stages of eruption.

24

The Tongue

OBJECTIVES

- To describe the formation of the tongue as it relates to the embryonic germ layers and pharyngeal arches
- To discuss the difference between the extrinsic and intrinsic muscles of the tongue
- To describe briefly how tongue movement is accomplished
- To describe the papillae of the tongue and their function
- To describe the kinds of changes seen on the tongue that indicate health problems

Development of the Tongue

As discussed in Chapter 18, bars of tissue are found on the anterior surface of the developing embryo, which are referred to as *pharyngeal arches*. The first pharyngeal arch is the mandibular arch, the second is the hyoid arch, and the remainder are numbered III, IV, V, and VI. Just above the first arch and extending down behind all the arches is a hollow tube, the digestive tract. Before the end of the fourth embryonic week, this tube is closed off at the upper end by the oropharyngeal membrane, which separates the foregut from the stomodeum. The epithelium anterior to the oropharyngeal membrane develops from the outer germ layer, or *ectoderm*. The tube behind the buccopharyngeal membrane develops from the inner germ layer, or endoderm. At the beginning of week four, the oropharyngeal membrane disintegrates, but the epithelium in that area still comes from two distinct germ layers. It is at this point that the tongue starts to develop as a swelling that arises out of the back part of the pharyngeal arches (Fig. 24.1). This swelling develops from the future floor of the mouth. The epithelial covering of the tongue develops from the ectoderm and the endoderm—the anterior two-thirds from the ectoderm and the posterior one-third from the endoderm. The tongue is basically a sac of epithelium filled with muscles. These muscles arise from the middle germ layer of the embryo, the *mesoderm*.

If you refer back to Chapter 18, you will find that the anterior two-thirds of the tongue develops from two lateral lingual swellings and a midline tuberculum impar (see Fig. 18.19). These are both from the first pharyngeal arch. The posterior one-third of the tongue develops from the copula and the third pharyngeal arch. The root of the tongue and epiglottis develop from the epiglottal swelling of the fourth pharyngeal arch.

Tongue Muscles

As mentioned before, the tongue is an epithelial sac filled with muscles and connective tissue. These muscles can be controlled willfully and are generally referred to as *skeletal muscle* or *voluntary striated muscle*. They are divided into two groupings: **intrinsic** and **extrinsic** muscles. Those that start and end wholly within the tongue are referred to as *intrinsic muscles*. These muscles do not have a fixed end or movable end, but their function depends upon where each muscle is more stabilized, and the less stabilized end will move toward the more stabilized end. There are four pairs of intrinsic muscles. They are:

1. *Superior longitudinal group*—runs anterior to posterior and lies near the dorsum of the tongue. This moves the superior surface of the tongue anteriorly or posteriorly.
2. *Inferior longitudinal group*—also runs anterior to posterior but lies near the ventrum of the tongue.
3. *Transverse group*—runs from side to side and narrows the tongue.
4. *Vertical group*—runs from dorsal to ventral and flattens the tongue.

These muscles are located within the tongue tissue and do not have a specific origin or insertion; they are named for their location. What happens when the muscles in these groups contract? If the longitudinal group of fibers contracts, the tongue is shortened. Shortening the tongue makes it thicker and wider. If you contract the group that runs transversely, the tongue may get a little thicker and longer. Contract the vertical group, and the tongue may get wider and longer.

Along with the intrinsic muscles in the tongue are a group of muscles that originate outside the tongue and run into it; these are the *extrinsic muscles*. These muscles are named after their origin and insertion. The origin of a muscle is the immovable attachment of the muscle, and the insertion is the movable attachment of the muscle. The muscle moves the insertion toward the origin. There are four pairs of muscles, left and right. The **hyoglossus** runs from the lateral sides of the **hyoid** bone up into the lateral borders of the tongue and pulls the lateral edges or borders of the tongue down onto the floor of the mouth (Fig. 24.2). The **styloglossus** runs from the styloid process down and forward into the lateral borders of the tongue and blends with the hyoglossus. The styloglossus pulls the tongue backward and slightly upward. The **palatoglossus** runs from the anterior soft palate down and slightly forward into the lateral borders of the tongue. It elevates the posterior part of the tongue and pulls it slightly backward. The **genioglossus** originates from the superior **genial tubercles** on the midline of the mandible and inserts into the midline of the tongue from the tip to the base. It aids in protrusion, retrusion, or depression of the tongue (Table 24.1).

Papillae

The tongue is covered with stratified squamous epithelium. The ventral surface of the tongue has very thin epithelium, but the

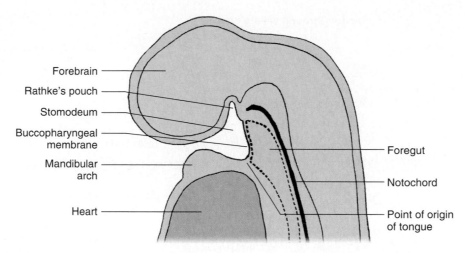

• **Figure 24.1** An anteroposterior section through an embryo. The mandibular or first pharyngeal arch is marked, and others are below it partially covered by the heart. The tongue arises from an area at the lower end of the buccopharyngeal membrane. (Modified from Bhaskar SN. *Orban's Oral Histology and Embryology.* 8th ed. St. Louis: Mosby; 1976.)

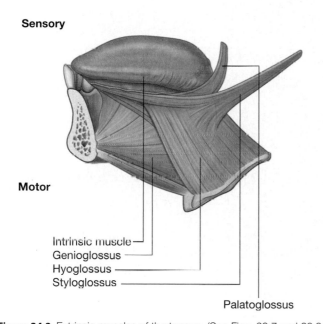

• **Figure 24.2** Extrinsic muscles of the tongue. (See Figs. 28.7 and 28.8.)

dorsal surface has thick parakeratinized to keratinized epithelium. Scattered throughout this epithelium on the uppermost surface are four types of elevated structures known as *papillae.*

Circumvallate Papillae

One type of papilla is the **circumvallate papilla**, a V-shaped row of circular raised papillae. There are 7 to 15 elevations in the V, which is located about two-thirds of the way back on the tongue with the point of the V facing posteriorly. This row anatomically divides the anterior two-thirds of the tongue from the posterior one-third and marks the area that develops from different pharyngeal arches with different nerve supplies (see also Chapter 34). Under a microscope, the circumvallate papillae appear to rest in troughs, and they have many tiny **taste buds** all around their lateral surfaces (Fig. 24.3). These taste buds are made up of many cells that support several small hairlike nerve endings that perceive taste (Fig. 24.4). Small salivary glands are located at the bottom of the trough, and they serve to wash the papillae clean, making them ready to perceive new tastes. These salivary glands are known as the **glands of von Ebner.**

<table>
<tr><td colspan="2">TABLE 24.1</td><td colspan="3">Extrinsic Muscles of the Tongue</td></tr>
</table>

Muscle	Origin	Insertion	Action
Hyoglossus	Hyoid bone	Lateral of tongue	Pulls lateral of tongue down
Styloglossus	Styloid bone	Lateral of tongue	Pulls tongue back and upward
Palatoglossus	Soft palate	Lateral of tongue	Elevates back of tongue and pulls it backward
Genioglossus	Genial tubercles of mandible	Midline of tongue	Aids in protrusion, retrusion, depression of tongue

Section through vallate papilla

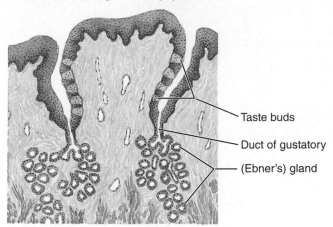

Taste buds

Duct of gustatory

(Ebner's) gland

• **Figure 24.3** Large circumvallate papilla in a trough, with light-colored taste buds along its sides. The von Ebner gland duct can be seen emptying into the trough around the papillae. (From Netter illustration used with permission of Elsevier Inc. All rights reserved. www.netterimages.com).

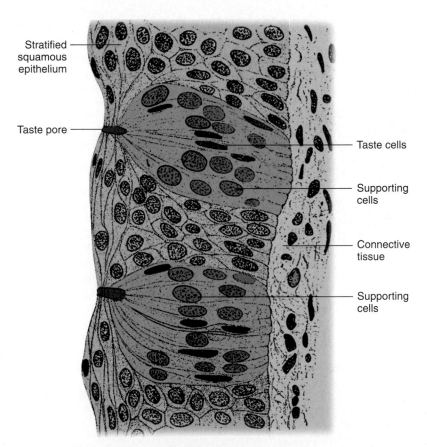

Stratified squamous epithelium

Taste pore

Taste cells

Supporting cells

Connective tissue

Supporting cells

• **Figure 24.4** The hairlike receptors of taste buds are located in taste pores. (Modified from Bhaskar SN. *Orban's Oral Histology and Embryology*. 8th ed. St. Louis: Mosby; 1976.)

Fungiform Papillae

The anterior two-thirds of the tongue's dorsal surface has tiny, round, raised spots. In younger persons, these spots frequently appear redder than the area around them. These are the **fungiform papillae**. The fungiform papillae have taste buds that are located on the top of the papillae (Fig. 24.5).

Filiform Papillae

The remainder of the anterior two-thirds of the tongue is covered with tiny, pointed projections of parakeratinized to keratinized epithelium known as **filiform papillae**. They are the most abundant lingual papilla and have no taste function; they provide tactile sensation on the tongue.

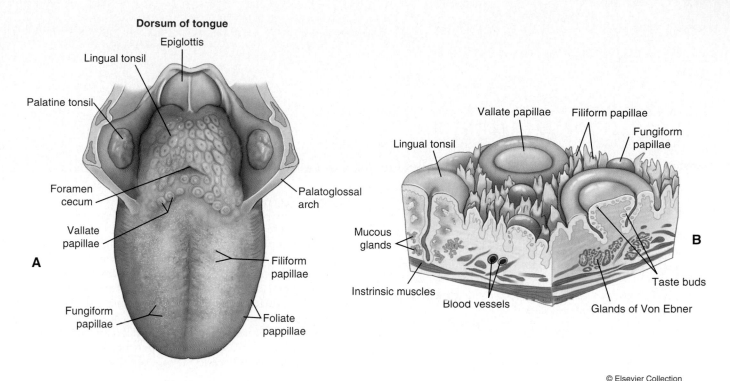

• **Figure 24.5.** **(A)** Dorsal view of tongue showing the roughened large lingual tonsils on the posterior of the tongue and the foliate papillae on the side. **(B)** Section of dorsal of the tongue showing a cutaway through lingual papillae and showing von Ebner's glands at the base of the vallate papillae.

Clinical Considerations

Sometimes the epithelia on papillae grow very long and trap food and pigments originating from oral bacteria and food. When papillae are very long, the condition is called hairy tongue. Other times the epithelia of papillae are lost and the surface in that area becomes very smooth. This is referred to as glossitis, and it occurs in several conditions, one of which is vitamin deficiencies.

Foliate Papillae

If you grasp the tip of the tongue with a piece of gauze and pull it out and to the side, you will see a roughened lateral surface back toward the base of the tongue. The **foliate papillae** are 4 to 11 leaf shaped, vertical ridges that contain few taste buds.

Clinical Considerations

The posterior lateral border of the tongue where the foliate papillae are located is an area that can become irritated and reddened. It is also an area where oral cancer can begin but be obscured because of the location and folds of tissue. It is therefore an important area to check in oral examinations.

Review Questions

1. How many embryonic germ layers form the entire tongue?
2. What is the difference between extrinsic and intrinsic muscles?
3. How are various tongue movements and shapes accomplished?
4. Name the papillae of the tongue, their locations, and their functions.

5. What two functions do taste buds perform?
6. What kinds of changes relating to a person's health can you see on the tongue?

25

Histology of the Salivary Glands

In this chapter, we will attempt to describe only the histology of salivary glands. For the description of size, location, and function of these glands, refer to Chapter 33.

Components of a Salivary Gland

As discussed in Chapter 17, salivary glands arise from a cord of epithelium growing into the underlying connective tissue, and the cord later forms a tube. At the end of this tube, clusters of secretory cells form, and these clusters, which look like bunches of grapes, will have end pieces that are either round or tubelike. The secretion of these glands involves protein production.

Acini

The secretory end pieces are known as **acini**. The secretions of these glands are proteins. There are two kinds of acinar cells, **mucous acini** and **serous acini**. Although these cells form grapelike or tubular end pieces, in cross section, they are described as **pyramidal cells** (Fig. 25.1). The outer edge or base of the cells rests on a basement membrane between the cells and the connective tissue. Within this connective tissue are the nerves and blood vessels necessary for the various aspects of cellular activity. The apex of the cells faces the center of the tube or grapelike structure. The base of the cells is surrounded by connective tissue, and partially surrounding each secretory acinus is a **myoepithelial cell** (Fig. 25.2). This cell has long cellular projections, resembling a squid, and it can contract like a muscle. Hence the prefix *myo*, meaning muscle. These projections surround a portion of the acinus, and when the myoepithelial cell contracts, it squeezes the acinus and aids in the secretion of saliva that has accumulated in the hollow center of the acinus, thus helping to move it out the duct system (Fig. 25.3). There are also some indications that these myoepithelial cells may play a role in suppressing the growth of epithelial-involved tumors. All types of acini—mucous, serous, and seromucous—secrete their products through this process known as *merocrine secretion*.

Serous Acini

(See Fig. 25.1A.)

The makeup of serous acinus secretions is similar to that of mucous acini, only without the mucins; a **serous** secretion is a thinner, more watery secretion. A **serous acinus** is the *primary* source of a protein known as *amylase*. Amylase is found in saliva as well as in pancreatic fluid and converts starch and glycogen into simple sugars. The secretory granules stain deeply, the lumen is very small and difficult to see, and the adjacent cell membranes are not easily seen. A serous cell is pyramidal in shape with a round nucleus that is close to the base of the cell.

Seromucous Acini

(See Fig. 25.1B, seromucous demilune.)

In glands that have both mucous and serous components, you can see the separate types of acini, and you can also see them joined together as mixed or **seromucous acini**. In a seromucous acinus, the mucous cells form a tubelike structure, and on the end of the tube a group of serous cells forms into a half-moon cluster. These are referred to as **serous demilunes**. The serous demilune cells secrete their product between the cell walls of the underlying mucous cells, and their secretion enters the lumen of the gland. As the term **seromucous** suggests, these acini produce both mucous and serous secretions (see Fig. 25.1).

Mucous Acini

(See Fig. 25.1C.)

A **mucous** secretion is slightly viscous because of the production of several **mucins**. Although its product is 99% water, it does have a number of inorganic ions, such as sodium, potassium, and chloride. A mucous acinus is more tubular and has a larger **lumen** compared with a serous acinus, and the cell membranes can more easily be seen at adjacent sides of the cells. The nucleus of a mucous cell is usually very flat and lies against the basal end of the cell, and the cell itself is pyramidal in shape. The apical end of these cells appears frothy under the light microscope. Under the electron microscope, one can see a great number of mucous droplets that stain very poorly and so give an empty, frothy appearance to the apical end.

Connective Tissue Capsule

A salivary gland is surrounded by a connective tissue capsule. The connective tissue not only surrounds the gland but also sends partitions, called septums, into the gland carrying nerves and blood vessels with it and dividing the gland into lobes and smaller units called **lobules** (Fig. 25.4).

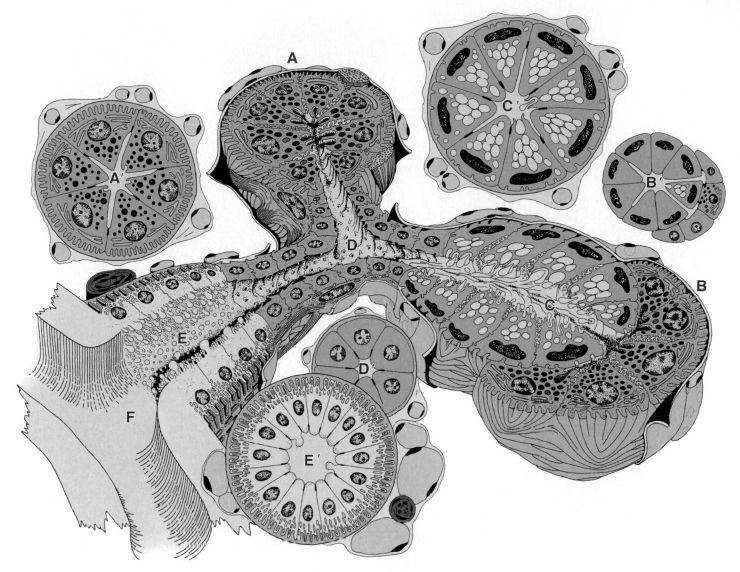

• **Figure 25.1** Schematic diagram of typical salivary gland. **(A)** Serous end piece in cross section. **(B)** Seromucous demilune in cross section. **(C)** Mucous end piece in cross section. **(D)** Intercalated duct in cross section. **(E)** Striated duct in cross section. **(F)** Terminal excretory duct. (Modified from Ten Cate AR. *Oral Histology.* 2nd ed. St. Louis, MO: Mosby; 1985.)

Duct System

Salivary glands have varying numbers of lobules, depending on their sizes, and each lobule is surrounded by connective tissue. There are a series of different kinds of ducts that may be located within the lobule, between the lobule, outside of the gland, or in the surrounding connective tissue that leads to the surface of the oral cavity.

Intralobular Ducts

Within the lobule are two kinds of ducts that by location are classified as **intralobular ducts**, meaning "within the lobule." There are two types of intralobular ducts: intercalated ducts and striated ducts (Fig. 25.5). In addition, there are interlobular ducts located between lobules.

Intercalated Ducts

Intercalated ducts are very small intralobular ducts that directly drain the acini. The cells in these ducts are single cuboidal and not much taller than their nuclei. In some glands, the ducts are long and easily seen, whereas in others, they are short and rarely seen. These intercalated ducts transport the secretions and add lactoferrin (an antimicrobial component of the immune system) and lysozyme (an antibacterial) to the secretions.

Striated Ducts

Intralobular **striated ducts** are so named because the bases of the columnar cells within these ducts appear to be striped. The basal cell membrane has infoldings in which mitochondria become trapped and aligned between the infoldings. These mitochondria

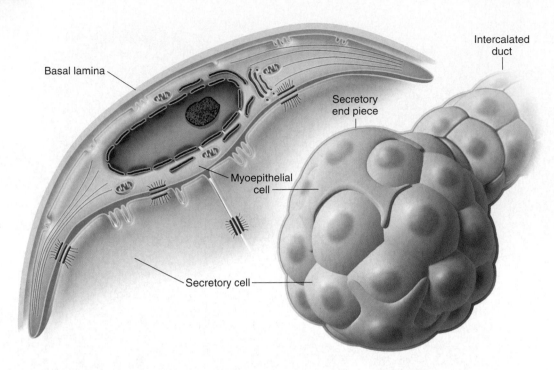

• **Figure 25.2** A myoepithelial cell can be seen with its processes surrounding an acinus. (From Nanci A. *Ten Cate's Oral Histology.* 8th ed. St. Louis, MO: Mosby; 2013.)

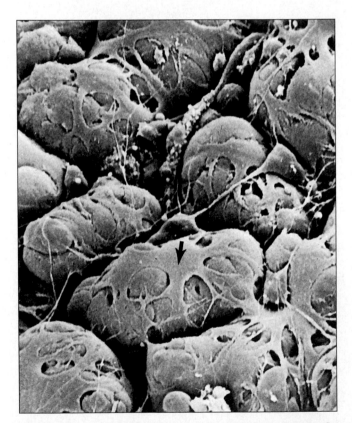

• **Figure 25.3** Scanning electron micrograph of myoepithelial cells. Contraction of the myoepithelial cells helps in active secretion of saliva by expelling the saliva from the acini into the duct system and out of the gland.

can be stained, causing a striped appearance. Water and various substances, such as sodium, potassium, chloride, and other ions, are reabsorbed by being secreted out of the basal end of the cell where they are picked up again by the capillaries and lymphatic vessels. This function is important because it conserves water and electrolytes (see Fig. 25.1). Both the intercalated and the striated ducts are also called *secretory* because as the salivary fluid passes through them, their content is modified.

Interlobular Ducts

Interlobular ducts lie within the connective tissue between lobules of the gland. These ducts contain pseudostratified columnar cells that transition to stratified cuboidal or squamous cells as they get closer to the oral mucosa. They are generally referred to as **excretory ducts**. These ducts do not modify the salivary secretions but simply carry them out of the gland and to the surface tissues of the oral cavity (Fig. 25.6).

Control of Secretions

Secretory control comes from the **autonomic nervous system**, particularly the parasympathetic nervous system (see Chapter 34). The control of secretions is associated with chewing, taste, and smell. Each of these is capable of modifying the amount and consistency of the salivary secretions.

Formation of Saliva

Saliva is formed within the endoplasmic reticulum of individual cells. The future saliva is packaged by a membrane within the

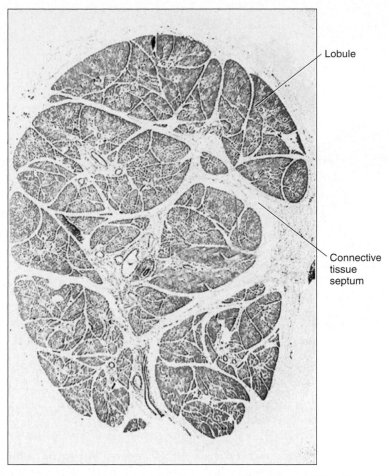

Lobule

Connective
tissue
septum

• **Figure 25.4** Connective tissue surrounds this salivary gland and further subdivides it into lobules. (From Nanci A. *Ten Cate's Oral Histology.* 8th ed. St. Louis, MO: Mosby; 2013.)

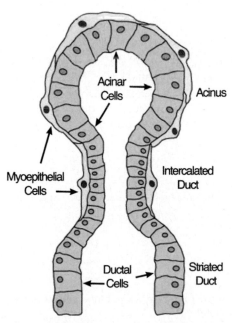

Acinar
Cells

Acinus

Myoepithelial
Cells

Intercalated
Duct

Ductal
Cells

Striated
Duct

• **Figure 25.5** Illustration of the cells found within and around a salivary gland acini and secretory salivary ducts. (From: Sakr, M. (2021). Diagnostic techniques and therapeutic strategies for parotid gland disorders. IGI Global. http://doi:10.4018/978-1-7998-5603-0 page 9).

Golgi apparatus and moves out into the cytoplasm of the mucous or serous acini. The apical end of the cell accumulates these granules of future saliva, and when the gland is stimulated by the parasympathetic nervous system, the granules move to the apical cell membrane, fuse with it, and release their substance into the center lumen of the acini. From there, the secretion moves through the intercalated, striated, and excretory ducts until it reaches the duct opening, leading into the oral cavity.

As it passes through the striated ducts, the fluid content actively changes. Water is pulled out of the lumen of the duct, through the striated duct, and into the capillaries lying at the base of the cells of the duct. At the same time, conservation of electrolytes and secretion of potassium and bicarbonate occurs. The fluid within the duct becomes more concentrated. Depending on the type of secretion, the amount of amylase will vary and be available to begin the breakdown of starches before further breakdown in the stomach and the duodenum. There are also immunoglobulins, which are antibodies in the saliva, as well as antibacterial lysozymes that protect the body from bacteria. The saliva also acts as a pH buffer, which plays a role in resistance to decay.

Function of Saliva

Basically, saliva functions to help prepare the bolus of food so that it can be swallowed more easily. It helps keep the mucous

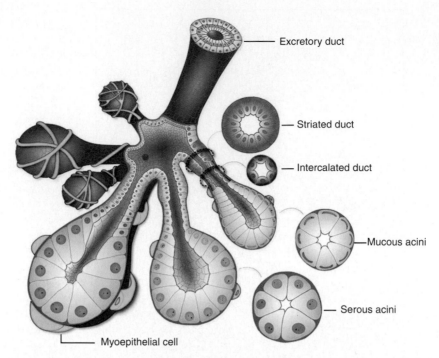

• **Figure 25.6** The intercalated duct can be seen directly connected to the acini, followed by striated ducts, and lastly the excretory duct, which is responsible for carrying the final secretion to the oral cavity. (From: de Paula, F., Teshima, T.H.N., Hsieh, R., Souza, M.M., Nico, M.M.S., and Lourenco, S.V. (2017). Overview of human salivary glands: Highlights of morphology and developing processes. The Anatomical Record, 300(7), 1180-1188. https://doi.org/10.1002/ar.23569).

membranes lubricated to protect them from drying out. As mentioned, saliva also acts as a pH buffer, and the immunoglobulins and lysozymes within saliva play a role in protecting the body. Saliva helps cleanse the surfaces of teeth, and by neutralizing the acids produced by bacteria and bathing the teeth in fluoride rich saliva, it helps prevent tooth decay. Not all of saliva's functions are beneficial; it also helps create biofilm and provides minerals for supragingival calculus formation.

Review Questions

1. What are acini and what are the three types? Describe their appearances.
2. What is a myoepithelial cell and what is its function?
3. Define the following and their functions:
    a. Intercalated duct
    b. Striated duct
    c. Secretory duct
    d. Excretory duct
    e. Intralobular duct
    f. Interlobular duct
4. What are serous demilunes?
5. What controls the secretion of salivary glands?
6. What enzyme is found in saliva, and what does it do?
7. What are the functions of saliva?

Unit III Test

1. Which of the following is *not* a cell organelle?
    a. nucleus
    b. glycogen
    c. endoplasmic reticulum
    d. Golgi apparatus
2. The skin and oral mucosa are examples of _____ epithelium.
    a. simple squamous
    b. simple columnar
    c. transitional
    d. stratified squamous
    e. pseudostratified squamous
3. Which of the following would *not* be classed as connective tissue?
    a. bone
    b. cartilage
    c. collagen
    d. tendon
    e. ligament
    f. none of the above
4. Which of the following white blood cells is *not* a granulocyte?
    a. neutrophil
    b. lymphocyte
    c. basophil
    d. eosinophil
    e. none of the above

5. Which of the following muscle tissues is classified as striated voluntary muscle?
   a. cardiac
   b. skeletal
   c. smooth
   d. all of the above
   e. none of the above
6. The smallest functioning unit of skeletal muscle is the
   a. myofibril
   b. sarcomere
   c. Z line
   d. myofiber
   e. intercalated disk
7. The protective covering around a nerve cell is known as a(n)
   a. dendrite
   b. axon
   c. myelin sheath
   d. Schwann cell
   e. node of Ranvier
8. In the development of the embryonic germ layers, where does the mesoderm come from?
   a. ectoderm
   b. endoderm
   c. ectoderm or endoderm
   d. the membranes surrounding the embryo
   e. none of the above
9. What type of epithelium is found in the urinary bladder and urethra?
   a. simple columnar
   b. stratified squamous
   c. pseudostratified columnar
   d. stratified columnar
   e. transitional
10. One of the most important and abundant cells in irregular connective tissue is the
    a. reticulocyte
    b. fibroblast
    c. elastocyte
    d. macrophage
    e. basal cell
11. What is the developmental period of the embryo?
    a. 0 to 2 weeks
    b. 3 to 8 weeks
    c. 8 to 12 weeks
    d. 12 to 36 weeks
12. The maxillary lip develops from the
    a. medial nasal process
    b. lateral nasal process
    c. maxillary process
    d. mandibular process
    e. a and b
    f. b and c
    g. a and c
    h. none of the above
13. The maxillary lip forms by a process of _____, whereas the palate forms by a process of _____.
    a. elongation, migration
    b. migration, fusion
    c. fusion, elongation
    d. none of the above

14. The premaxilla comes from the
    a. lateral nasal processes
    b. medial nasal processes
    c. mandibular process
    d. maxillary processes
    e. none of the above
15. The oropharyngeal membrane disintegrates at the beginning of the _____ embryonic week.
    a. second
    b. third
    c. fourth
    d. sixth
16. The critical time for development of the upper lip is weeks
    a. 2 to 5
    b. 3 to 6
    c. 5 to 9
    d. 7 to 10
17. The critical time for palatal development is weeks
    a. 2 to 6
    b. 3 to 7
    c. 5 to 9
    d. 7 to 12
18. There are _____ pharyngeal arches, not counting the rudimentary fifth pharyngeal arch.
    a. 2
    b. 3
    c. 4
    d. 5
19. A combined cleft lip and palate occurs about once in every _____ live births among Caucasians in the United States.
    a. 300
    b. 700
    c. 1500
    d. 7000
    e. 10,000
20. Which of the following is *not* part of an early pharyngeal arch?
    a. cartilage
    b. bone
    c. nerve
    d. blood vessel
    e. mesodermal tissue
21. The first signs of tooth development are seen in the _____ week.
    a. 4th
    b. 6th
    c. 10th
    d. 12th
22. The first stage of the enamel organ is the _____ stage.
    a. cap
    b. bell
    c. bud
    d. incisive
23. The beginning of the bell stage occurs with the appearance of the
    a. outer enamel epithelium
    b. stellate reticulum
    c. stratum intermedium
    d. inner enamel epithelium

24. Which of the following does *not* arise from the dental sac?
    a. dentin
    b. cementum
    c. periodontal ligament
    d. none of the above

25. The ameloblast arises from the
    a. dental papilla
    b. inner enamel epithelium
    c. outer enamel epithelium
    d. stellate reticulum

26. Enamel is _____ inorganic hydroxyapatite crystals.
    a. 5%
    b. 30%
    c. 70%
    d. 96%

27. What is the *last* thing produced by the ameloblast?
    a. primary enamel cuticle
    b. Nasmyth's membrane
    c. reduced enamel epithelium
    d. secondary enamel cuticle
    e. a and b

28. What is the shape of an enamel rod?
    a. round
    b. hexagonal
    c. keyhole shaped
    d. flat
    e. both a and b

29. Cracks in the enamel are known as
    a. enamel spindles
    b. enamel tufts
    c. imbrication lines
    d. enamel lamellae
    e. none of the above

30. Dentin is _____ inorganic hydroxyapatite crystals.
    a. 10%
    b. 30%
    c. 50%
    d. 70%
    e. none of the above

31. Dentin that has formed under an area of decay is known as _____ dentin.
    a. primary
    b. reparative
    c. secondary
    d. none of the above

32. Pulp develops from
    a. the dental papilla
    b. mesenchyme
    c. pulp stones
    d. the dental sac
    e. a and b

33. When odontoblasts die they are replaced by
    a. other odontoblasts
    b. fibroblasts
    c. mesenchymal cells
    d. cementoblasts
    e. a and c

34. Cementum is _____ inorganic hydroxyapatite crystals.
    a. 10–20%
    b. 30–40%

c. 50–60%
d. 70–80%
e. 90–100%

35. Hertwig's epithelial root sheath develops from the
    a. enamel organ (outer and inner enamel epithelium)
    b. dental papilla
    c. dentin
    d. dental sac

36. What cells lay down cellular and acellular cementum?
    a. osteoblasts
    b. odontoblasts
    c. cementoblasts
    d. fibroblasts
    e. none of the above

37. At the cementoenamel junction (CEJ), cementum overlaps enamel about _____ of the time.
    a. 15%
    b. 20%
    c. 30%
    d. 55%
    e. 95%

38. Which of the following is *not* a true statement concerning Sharpey's fibers?
    a. They are found in cementum.
    b. They are found in dentin.
    c. They are found in alveolar bone.
    d. They are the embedded portion of the periodontal ligament.
    e. None of the above.

39. Cellular cementum is usually found
    a. at the cementoenamel junction
    b. in the cervical third of the root
    c. in the middle third of the root
    d. in the apical third of the root

40. Which of the following is *not* originally found as alveolar bone is forming?
    a. bundle bone
    b. cribriform plate
    c. spongy bone
    d. cortical plate
    e. none of the above

41. Which of the following alveolodental fiber groups would resist occlusal forces?
    a. apical
    b. horizontal
    c. oblique
    d. alveolar crest
    e. none of the above

42. In active tooth eruption, the "eruptive" stage begins when
    a. crown formation begins
    b. root formation begins
    c. tooth erupts into the oral cavity
    d. root formation is completed
    e. none of the above

43. In tooth eruption, the normal path of eruption is
    a. occlusal and facial
    b. occlusal and lingual
    c. apical and facial
    d. apical and lingual
    e. straight occlusally

44. What is the most probable cause of tooth eruption?
    a. growth of pulpal tissue
    b. root growth

  c. bone growth in socket
  d. changes within the periodontal ligament
  e. b, c, and d
45. The permanent molars develop
  a. between the roots of the primary molars
  b. between the roots of the premolars
  c. independent of the primary molars
  d. lingual to primary molars
46. Attached gingiva is an example of
  a. specialized mucosa
  b. lining mucosa
  c. masticatory mucosa
  d. b and c
47. Specialized mucosa is found
  a. on the hard palate
  b. on the soft palate
  c. on the dorsum of the tongue
  d. on the mucosa of the cheek
48. What kind of epithelium is found in the gingival sulcus?
  a. simple squamous
  b. simple cuboidal
  c. stratified squamous
  d. pseudostratified columnar
49. The height of the free gingiva is generally the same height as the
  a. attached gingiva
  b. alveolar mucosa
  c. gingival sulcus
  d. interdental papilla
50. Which of the following papillae of the tongue do *not* have taste buds?
  a. filiform
  b. fungiform
  c. circumvallate
  d. foliate
51. The intrinsic muscles of the tongue run
  a. anterior to posterior
  b. ventral to dorsal
  c. from one lateral side to the other lateral side
  d. All of the above.
52. Which of the following muscles functions to pull the lateral borders of the tongue downward?
  a. styloglossus

  b. genioglossus
  c. geniohyoid
  d. palatoglossus
  e. none of the above
53. Hairy tongue is an elongation of the
  a. fungiform papillae
  b. filiform papillae
  c. circumvallate papillae
  d. foliate papillae
54. The salivary gland ducts that carry secretions directly out of the acini are _____ ducts.
  a. interlobular
  b. excretory
  c. striated
  d. intercalated
  e. none of the above
55. What salivary enzyme splits starches into long-chain sugars?
  a. peptidase
  b. sucrase
  c. amylase
  d. protease
56. Secretory function of the salivary glands is controlled by the
  a. autonomic nervous system
  b. parasympathetic nervous system
  c. sympathetic nervous system
  d. a and b
  e. none of the above
57. Which of the following is a function of striated salivary ducts?
  a. They aid in conserving water.
  b. They aid in conserving electrolytes.
  c. They modify the saliva.
  d. All of the above.
  e. none of the above
58. Which of the following statements is *not* true about intercalated ducts?
  a. Their nucleus is almost as high as the cell.
  b. They are interposed between acini and striated ducts.
  c. They modify the salivary content as it passes through.
  d. They may be short or long ducts.
  e. All of the above.

Unit III Suggested Readings

Berkovitz BK, Holland GR, Moxham BJ. *Color Atlas and Textbook of Oral Anatomy, Histology, and Embryology.* 5th ed. London: Mosby; 2017.

Berkovitz S. *The Cleft Palate Story.* Carol Stream, IL: Quintessence; 2021.

Bevelander G. *Outline of Histology.* 8th ed. St. Louis: Mosby; 1979.

Bhaskar SN. *Orban's Oral Histology and Embryology.* 14th ed. St. Louis: Mosby; 2018.

Carlson BM. *Human Embryology and Developmental Biology.* 6th ed. St. Louis: Mosby; 2018.

Chiego D. *Essentials of Oral Histology and Embryology: A Clinical Approach.* 5th ed. St. Louis: Elsevier; 2018

Fehrenbach M. *Illustrated Anatomy of the Head and Neck.* 6th ed. St. Louis: Elsevier; 2020.

Nanci A. *Ten Cate's Oral Histology, Development, Structure and Function.* 9th ed. St. Louis: Elsevier; 2017.

Sadler TW. *Langman's Medical Embryology.* 14th ed. Philadelphia: Lippincott, Williams & Wilkins; 2018.

Schoenwolf G., Bleyl S., Brauer P., & Francis-West, P. (2014). *Larsen's human embryology.* St. Louis: Elsevier.

UNIT IV

Head and Neck Anatomy

26

Osteology of the Skull

The bones of the skull play several roles. They surround the brain and protect it from injury, form the facial skeleton, and participate in the growth process of the jaws, which, in turn, controls whether a patient has malocclusion (improper relationship of teeth and jaws) and whether there is balance between the midface and the lower face.

This chapter presents a description of the more important bones of the skull and their landmarks. However, the discussion is certainly not all inclusive.

Excluding the three small **ossicles** (the malleus, incus, and stapes in each ear, which aid in hearing), the skull is composed of 22 bones. Some of these are single bones, and some are paired bones. They are grouped into two categories—one group surrounds the brain and one forms the face.

The following eight bones make up the **neurocranium**, the bones surrounding the brain:

- frontal bone (single)
- sphenoid bone (single)
- ethmoid bone (single)
- occipital bone (single)
- temporal bones (paired)
- parietal bones (paired)

Of these eight bones, sphenoid and ethmoid bones are difficult to visualize because they cannot be seen in their entirety on the surface of the skull. The ethmoid bone is primarily located in the facial area of the nose, but because a small part of it surrounds the brain, it is classified as part of the **neurocranium**.

The 14 bones that make up the **viscerocranium** of the face include the following:

- **mandible** (single)
- **vomer** (single)
- **nasal bones** (paired)
- **lacrimal bones** (paired)
- **zygomatic bones** (paired)
- **inferior nasal conchae** (paired)
- **palatine bones** (paired)
- **maxillae** (paired)

Instead of considering the bones around the brain and of the face as two completely separate groups, this chapter will present various views of the skull and study the relationships of the bones to one another. Refer back to these lists, as necessary.

Several terms are used in the following chapters and should be introduced. One of the first terms you will come across is **suture**, which is a joining together of two or more bones. Two other key terms are **foramen** and **canal**. A foramen is a hole or opening through bone, and a canal is a tubelike opening through bone.

Views of the Skull

Fig. 26.1 is an exploded view of all the bones in the skull. Those of you who enjoy jigsaw puzzles should be able to get a pretty good sense of which bones are part of the neurocranium and which are part of the viscerocranium in the anterior or frontal view of an adult skull. A close study of the area (see Fig. 26.1) should make it easier to put the pieces together. Fig. 26.2 is a small accomplishment of that task. Each of the views is presented in color. Use Fig. 26.1 and Fig. 26.2 as a guide to determine position and identity.

Anterior View of the Skull

Fig. 26.3 is an enlargement of the anterior view and is a similar enlargement of the views that follow. If you use the list of bones of the neurocranium and the viscerocranium, you should be able to see that the frontal bone is located from the eyes up to the top of the skull. In the frontal bone, you can see the **supraorbital notch** or **foramen**. This carries the **supraorbital nerve** and **artery** to the skin of the forehead. The area below the eyes down to the occlusal plane between the upper and lower teeth is made up of paired **zygomatic bones**, or cheekbones, and paired maxillae. The **infraorbital canal** and **foramen** carry the infraorbital artery and nerve to the cheek region. The paired nasal bones form the bridge of the nose, and the lower jaw is formed by the single mandible. The inner or medial corner of the eye cavity (**orbit**) contains a small lacrimal bone. Within the nasal cavity the vertical **nasal**

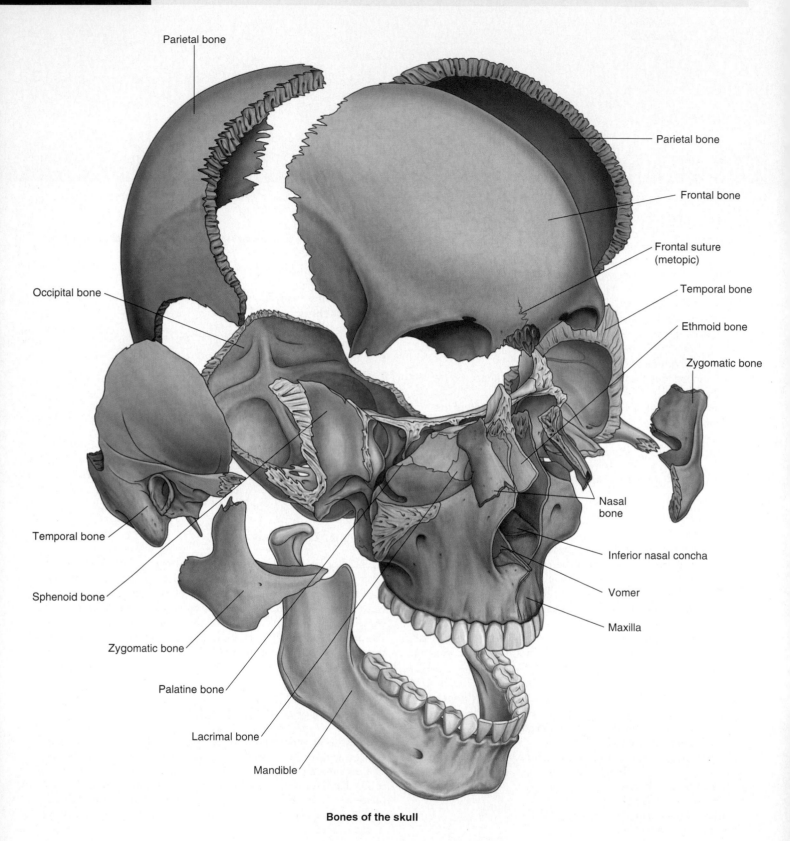

Parietal bone

Parietal bone

Frontal bone

Frontal suture
(metopic)

Occipital bone

Temporal bone

Ethmoid bone

Zygomatic bone

Nasal
bone

Temporal bone

Inferior nasal concha

Sphenoid bone

Vomer

Zygomatic bone

Maxilla

Palatine bone

Lacrimal bone

Mandible

Bones of the skull

• **Figure 26.1** Bones of the skull, exploded view.

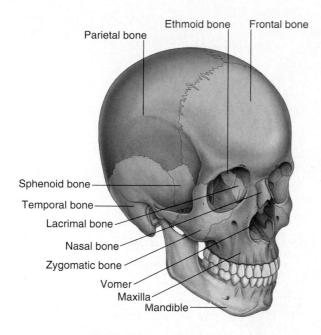

Parietal bone
Ethmoid bone
Frontal bone
Sphenoid bone
Temporal bone
Lacrimal bone
Nasal bone
Zygomatic bone
Vomer
Maxilla
Mandible

• **Figure 26.2** Bones of the skull by color.

septum is composed of the **septal cartilage**, vomer, and the **perpendicular plate** of the ethmoid bone. The inferior nasal conchae are found in the lower, lateral portions of the nasal cavity. More details of the bones of the nasal cavity are discussed in Chapter 27.

If you look at the diagram of the orbit, in the medial wall you can see the **orbital portion of the lesser and greater wings of the sphenoid**, forming the **superior orbital fissure** in the posterolateral part of the orbit. The lesser wing is above the fissure, and the greater wing is below the fissure. The roof of the orbit is formed primarily by the **orbital plate of the frontal bone**. The lateral wall of the orbit is primarily zygomatic bone, and the floor of the orbit is primarily the maxillae and some of the zygomatic bone. Note that the **rim of the orbit** is formed from equal parts of frontal, zygomatic, and maxillary bones.

Study each of the lines to make sure you can see each of the lines to the structure identified. Eventually, make sure you know the function of the identified structure. Use the colored version of the diagram of the structure.

Lateral View of the Skull

At the lateral edges of the skull, some parts of the parietal and temporal bones are visible, as well as the greater wing of the sphenoid bone. From a lateral view (Fig. 26.4), parts of the bones that can be seen are: the frontal, zygomatic, maxillary, mandibular, nasal, and lacrimal bones; a small bit of the ethmoid bone in the medial wall of the orbit; the greater wing of the sphenoid (seen only in the colored view of Fig. 26.4); the parietal, occipital, temporal, and frontal bones; and their accompanying sutures. The view of the skull in Fig. 26.4 shows jagged suture lines separating one bone from another. It may be difficult to see some of them, but it is important to study them well. The most difficult identifications of the skull for the novice student of anatomy are the numerous points or landmarks. It is difficult to see the suture lines between the bones in many instances.

You can see the **coronal**, or **frontal-parietal suture,** as well as the **lambdoid suture** or the **parieto-occipital suture**. The

lambdoid suture forms an inverted V, only half of which can be seen from the lateral view. The area outlined by the dotted line is the **temporal fossa**, which is made up of areas of the frontal, parietal, sphenoid, and temporal bones. Within the temporal fossa, between the squamous part of the temporal bone and parietal bone, is the **squamosal suture**.

Clinical Considerations

The squamosal suture is an interesting suture in that most suture joints butt up against one another. An overlapping suture results in slippage of the suture. Some believe that some temporomandibular joint (TMJ) problems are caused by slippage of the overlapping suture, and an attempt is made to manually manipulate the suture to relieve the resulting TMJ pain.

The **mastoid process** is the projection on the temporal bone just behind the **external auditory meatus**, or outer ear canal. The mastoid process serves as the insertion for the sternocleidomastoid muscle. Projecting forward from the temporal bone and joining with the zygomatic bone is the zygomatic arch. This arch is made up of the **zygomatic process** of the temporal bone and the **temporal process** of the zygomatic bone. The **mandibular fossa**, which articulates with the **mandibular condyle**, is found in this area. Just anterior to the mandibular fossa is the **articular eminence** of the temporal bone. These two structures are possibly better seen in an inferior view of the skull. Below and medial to the ear is a small projection, the **styloid process**, for the attachment of some muscles and ligaments of the neck region.

Inferior View of the Skull

Another view of the skull to be considered is the view of the bottom of the skull. The most difficult view is that of the inferior portion of the skull; in the palatal region, you can see the **incisive foramen, median palatine suture**, and **transverse palatine** or **palatomaxillary suture**, just anterior to the **hard palate** of the palatine bone (Fig. 26.5). In the palatal region is the posterolateral portion of the hard palate; you can also see the **greater palatine foramen**. **Lesser palatine foramen** are found just posterior to the greater palatine foramen. Just behind that are the **pterygoid hamuli** or **hamular processes** of the **medial pterygoid plate**. The medial and **lateral pterygoid plates** join anteriorly to form the **pterygoid fossa** between them. Just lateral to that area, in the sphenoid bone, is the **foramen ovale**, which transmits the fifth cranial nerve to the lower jaw. Posterior to the foramen ovale is the **foramen spinosum**, which transmits the middle meningeal artery, the major blood supply, to the coverings of the brain and is frequently a source of severe headaches. Posterior to these structures are the openings for the internal carotid arteries, the **carotid canals**. Medial to the foramen ovale and foramen spinosum is the **foramen lacerum**, an opening in the floor of the carotid canal, which is filled with cartilage during the person's life.

In Fig. 26.6A, you see a jagged red line which is the junction of the sphenoid bone and the occipital bone. This is the **spheno-occipital synchondrosis**. This is a major area of endochondral bone growth involving the longitudinal growth of the base of the skull, which is an important factor in the development of facial profiles and types of malocclusions. Grouped together are the styloid processes, mastoid processes, and **stylomastoid foramina**, from which exits the facial nerve to the muscles of facial expression. The mandibular fossae of the TMJ and the articular eminence just anterior to it can also be seen from an inferior view, as

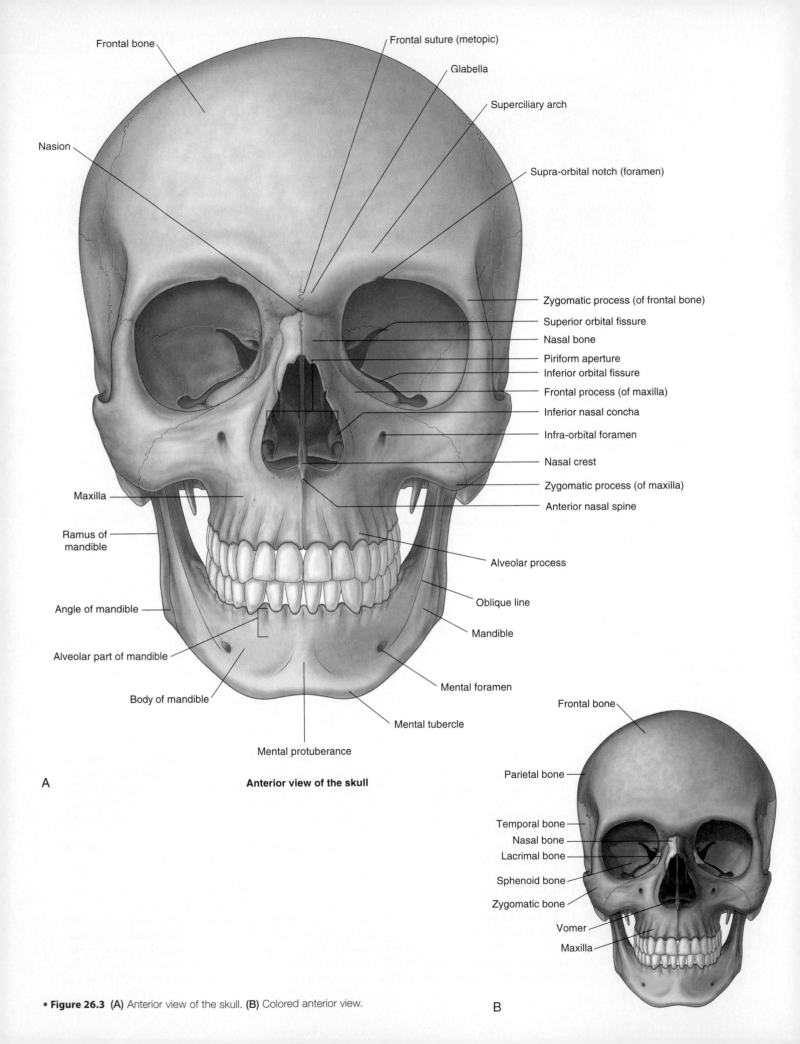

Frontal bone

Frontal suture (metopic)

Glabella

Superciliary arch

Nasion

Supra-orbital notch (foramen)

Zygomatic process (of frontal bone)

Superior orbital fissure

Nasal bone

Piriform aperture

Inferior orbital fissure

Frontal process (of maxilla)

Inferior nasal concha

Infra-orbital foramen

Nasal crest

Zygomatic process (of maxilla)

Anterior nasal spine

Maxilla

Ramus of mandible

Angle of mandible

Alveolar part of mandible

Body of mandible

Mental protuberance

Alveolar process

Oblique line

Mandible

Mental foramen

Mental tubercle

Anterior view of the skull

A

Frontal bone

Parietal bone

Temporal bone

Nasal bone

Lacrimal bone

Sphenoid bone

Zygomatic bone

Vomer

Maxilla

B

• **Figure 26.3** **(A)** Anterior view of the skull. **(B)** Colored anterior view.

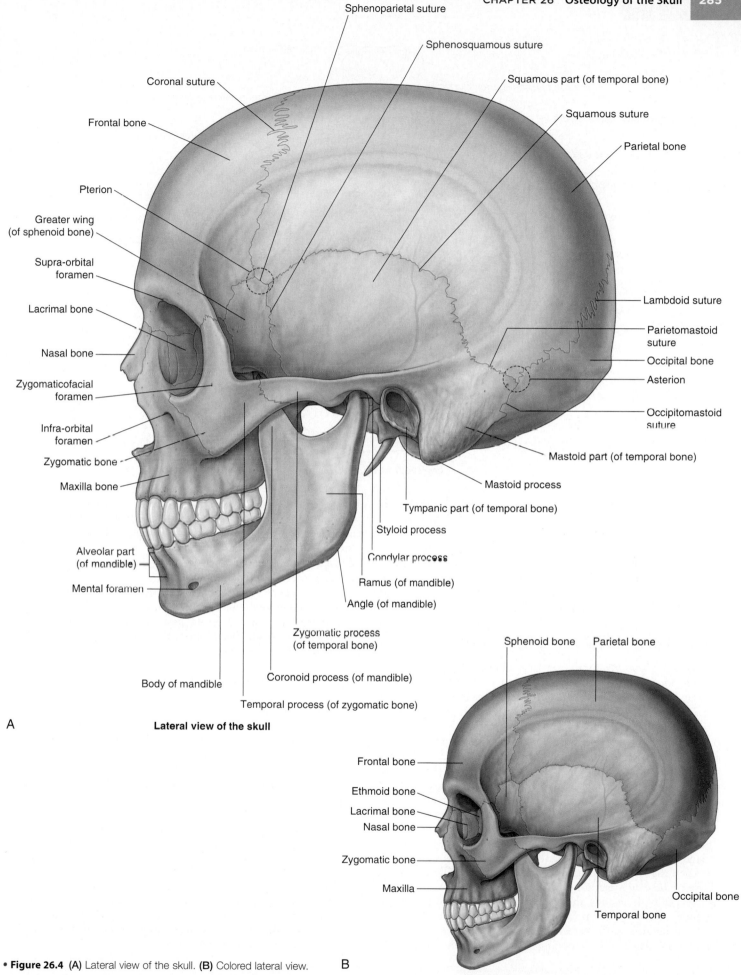

A

Lateral view of the skull

B

• **Figure 26.4** **(A)** Lateral view of the skull. **(B)** Colored lateral view.

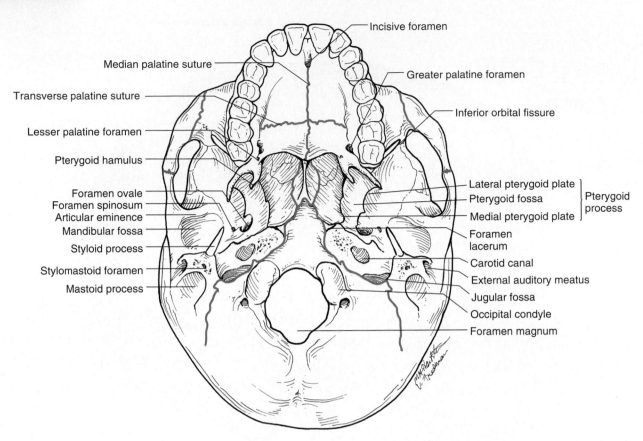

- **Figure 26.5** Inferior view of the skull.

well as the **jugular fossae** or **foramina** and the **occipital condyles**. The individual bones are separately colored so they can easily be identified in Fig. 26.6B.

Although there are many more points of study in this view, it is probably sufficient to be familiar to those mentioned previously. (Only the lead lines you should be familiar with at this point in your education have been mentioned here. The remaining lead lines will be of value in your radiographic studies.)

Floor of the Cranial Cavity (Fig. 26.7)

In Fig. 26.7B, you can see the red jagged line as the spheno-occipital synchondrosis mentioned in the inferior view of the skull. Internally, you can see the **crista galli**, serving as an attachment for the **falx cerebri**, which is part of the dura mater that superiorly separates the left and right cerebral hemispheres down to the corpus callosum (the crossing brain fibers from one side to the other), and the **cribriform plate**, which is the passageway for the olfactory nerve or nerves of smell from the nasal cavity to the brain. Both are parts of the ethmoid bone. Just behind this are the greater and lesser wings of the sphenoid bone extending from the body of the sphenoid. From the lesser wing of the sphenoid bone, anterior to the frontal bone, is the **anterior cranial fossa**, which houses the frontal lobe of the brain. **Sella turcica** is a boney projection on the sphenoid bone. It is elevated and shaped like a Turkish saddle, raised on the front and back, and the **hypophyseal fossa** rests in between these two elevations. Within this fossa lies the master control gland of the body, the pituitary gland. Also in the sphenoid are the foramen ovale and **foramen rotundum**, where the nerves to the lower and upper teeth leave the skull. You can also see the foramen spinosum and, by looking down through the anterior end

of the carotid canal, the foramen lacerum. The large opening toward the posterior of the skull is the **foramen magnum** of the occipital bone. Just lateral to this the **jugular foramen** and the **internal acoustic meatus** can be seen in Fig. 26.7. Above the internal acoustic meatus is the crest of the petrous **temporal bone**, which houses the middle and inner ear. From this crest forward to the lesser wing of the sphenoid is the **middle cranial fossa**, which houses the temporal lobe of the brain. From the crest of the petrous temporal bone back to the posterior of the skull is the **posterior cranial fossa**, which houses the brainstem (pons and medulla) and the cerebellum.

Posterior View of the Skull

Fig. 26.8 presents the sutures and bones in the posterior view of the skull. The **sagittal suture** runs from the **frontal suture** on the anterior skull, posteriorly to the lambdoid suture on the posterior of the skull. It is shaped like an upside-down U. That suture encompasses the occipital bone on the posterior and laterally to the **parietal sutures**. The temporal bone is in the ear region.

Roof of the Cranial Cavity of the Skull

Fig. 26.9A shows the superior view of the skull. The three main sutures seen are the sagittal or interparietal suture, the coronal suture, and the lambdoid suture. You can also see parts of the frontal, temporal, parietal, and occipital bones. Fig. 26.9B is an internal view of the roof of the skull; the sutures are hard to identify from this view, but notice the grooves for the superior sagittal sinus and the middle meningeal arteries.

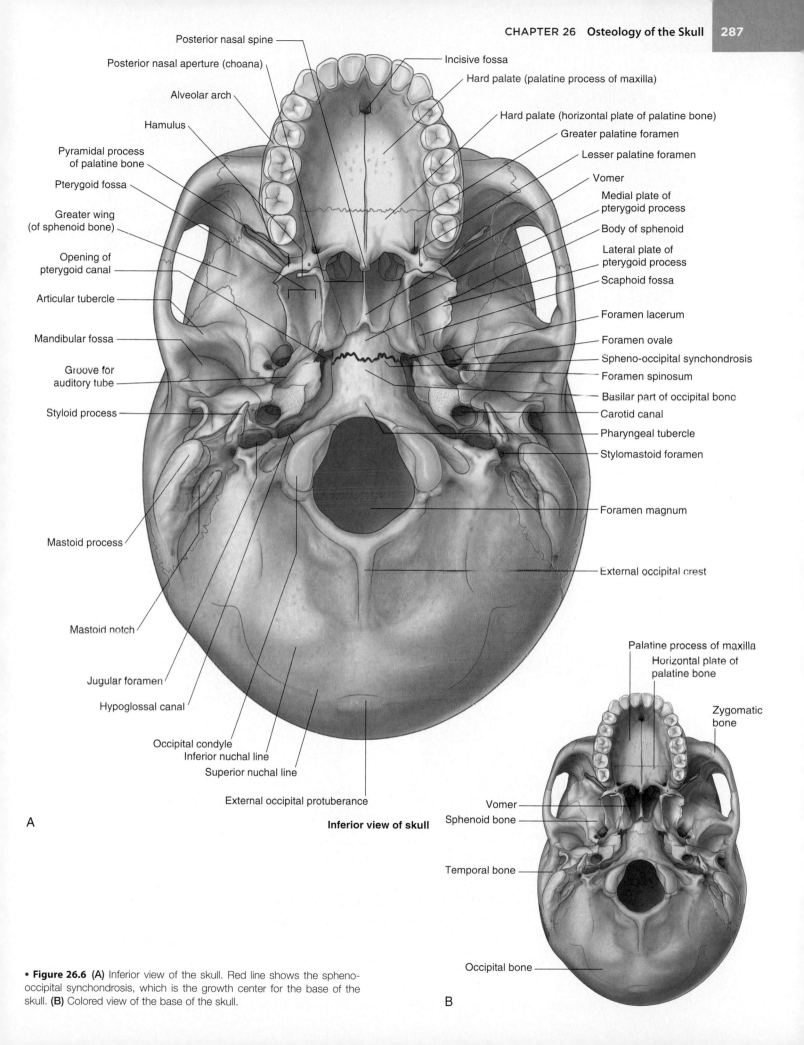

Posterior nasal spine
Posterior nasal aperture (choana)
Alveolar arch
Hamulus
Pyramidal process of palatine bone
Pterygoid fossa
Greater wing (of sphenoid bone)
Opening of pterygoid canal
Articular tubercle
Mandibular fossa
Groove for auditory tube
Styloid process
Mastoid process
Mastoid notch
Jugular foramen
Hypoglossal canal
Occipital condyle
Inferior nuchal line
Superior nuchal line
External occipital protuberance

Incisive fossa
Hard palate (palatine process of maxilla)
Hard palate (horizontal plate of palatine bone)
Greater palatine foramen
Lesser palatine foramen
Vomer
Medial plate of pterygoid process
Body of sphenoid
Lateral plate of pterygoid process
Scaphoid fossa
Foramen lacerum
Foramen ovale
Spheno-occipital synchondrosis
Foramen spinosum
Basilar part of occipital bone
Carotid canal
Pharyngeal tubercle
Stylomastoid foramen
Foramen magnum
External occipital crest

Inferior view of skull

A

Palatine process of maxilla
Horizontal plate of palatine bone
Zygomatic bone
Vomer
Sphenoid bone
Temporal bone
Occipital bone

B

• **Figure 26.6 (A)** Inferior view of the skull. Red line shows the spheno-occipital synchondrosis, which is the growth center for the base of the skull. **(B)** Colored view of the base of the skull.

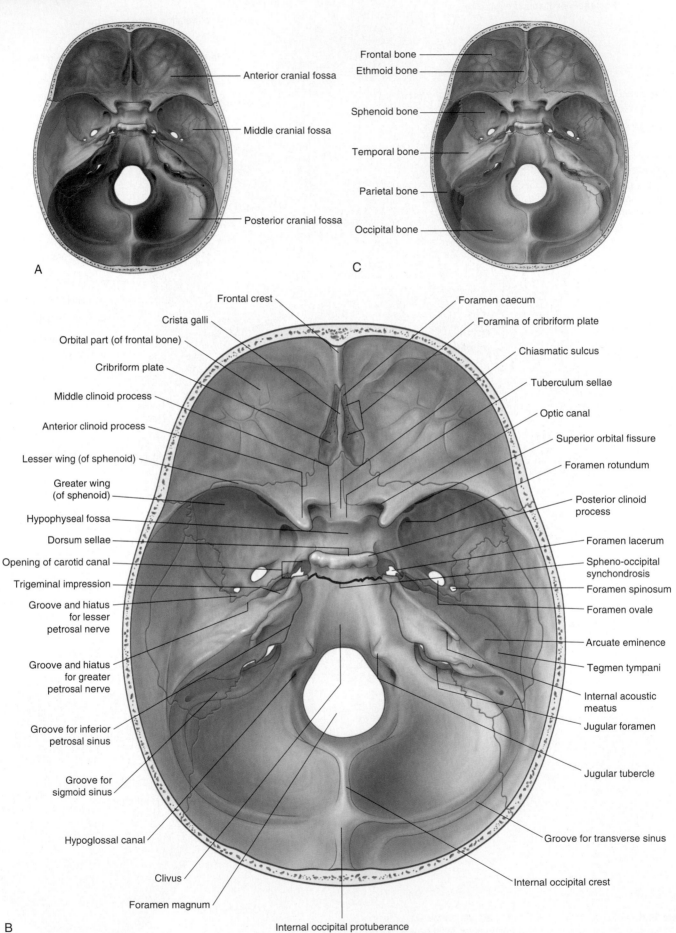

A

C

Anterior cranial fossa

Middle cranial fossa

Posterior cranial fossa

Frontal bone
Ethmoid bone
Sphenoid bone
Temporal bone
Parietal bone
Occipital bone

Frontal crest
Crista galli
Orbital part (of frontal bone)
Cribriform plate
Middle clinoid process
Anterior clinoid process
Lesser wing (of sphenoid)
Greater wing (of sphenoid)
Hypophyseal fossa
Dorsum sellae
Opening of carotid canal
Trigeminal impression
Groove and hiatus for lesser petrosal nerve
Groove and hiatus for greater petrosal nerve
Groove for inferior petrosal sinus
Groove for sigmoid sinus
Hypoglossal canal
Clivus
Foramen magnum

Foramen caecum
Foramina of cribriform plate
Chiasmatic sulcus
Tuberculum sellae
Optic canal
Superior orbital fissure
Foramen rotundum
Posterior clinoid process
Foramen lacerum
Spheno-occipital synchondrosis
Foramen spinosum
Foramen ovale
Arcuate eminence
Tegmen tympani
Internal acoustic meatus
Jugular foramen
Jugular tubercle
Groove for transverse sinus
Internal occipital crest

B

Internal occipital protuberance

• **Figure 26.7** **(A)** Colored view of the floor of the cranial cavity. **(B)** Floor of the cranial cavity.

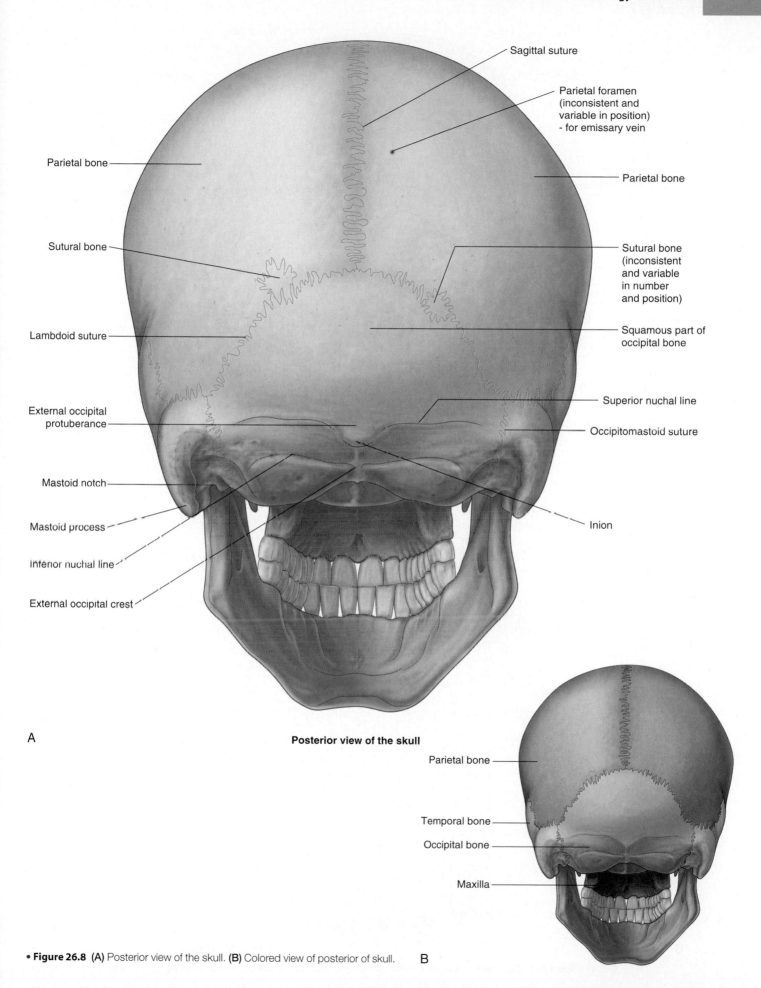

Sagittal suture

Parietal foramen (inconsistent and variable in position) - for emissary vein

Parietal bone

Parietal bone

Sutural bone

Sutural bone (inconsistent and variable in number and position)

Squamous part of occipital bone

Lambdoid suture

Superior nuchal line

External occipital protuberance

Occipitomastoid suture

Mastoid notch

Mastoid process

Inion

Inferior nuchal line

External occipital crest

A

Posterior view of the skull

Parietal bone

Temporal bone

Occipital bone

Maxilla

B

• **Figure 26.8** (A) Posterior view of the skull. (B) Colored view of posterior of skull.

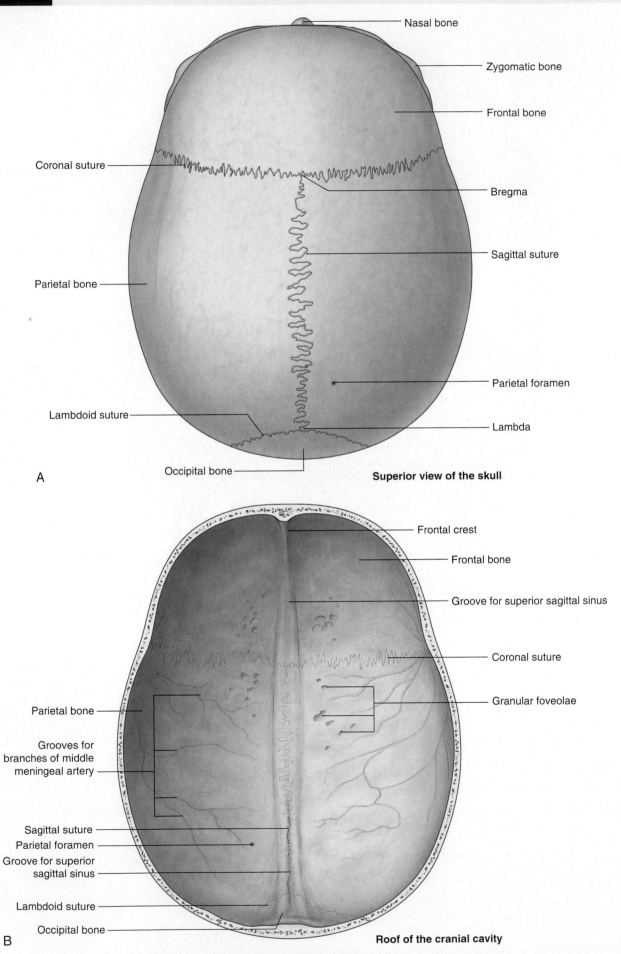

Nasal bone

Zygomatic bone

Frontal bone

Coronal suture

Bregma

Sagittal suture

Parietal bone

Parietal foramen

Lambdoid suture

Lambda

Occipital bone

Superior view of the skull

A

Frontal crest

Frontal bone

Groove for superior sagittal sinus

Coronal suture

Granular foveolae

Parietal bone

Grooves for branches of middle meningeal artery

Sagittal suture

Parietal foramen

Groove for superior sagittal sinus

Lambdoid suture

Occipital bone

Roof of the cranial cavity

B

• **Figure 26.9** **(A)** Superior view of the skull. **(B)** Internal view of the roof of the cranial cavity.

Major Bones of the Skull

The bones of the skull are divided into two groups: ones that surround the brain, called the *neurocranium*, and the ones that do not surround the brain, but have to do with the respiratory and digestive functions of the body, called the *viscerocranium*. The neurocranium is composed of four single and two paired bones. The following eight bones make up the **neurocranium,** the bones surrounding the brain:

frontal bone (single)
sphenoid bone (single)
ethmoid bone (single)
occipital bone (single)
temporal bones (paired)
parietal bones (paired)

The 14 bones that make up the **viscerocranium** bones of the face include the following:

mandible (single)
vomer (single)
nasal bones (paired)
lacrimal bones (paired)
zygomatic bones (paired)
inferior nasal conchae (paired)
palatine bones (paired)
maxillae (paired)

Neurocranium

Four of these bones—frontal, parietal, temporal, and occipital—cover the outside of the brain. They afford major protection to the front, back, top, and sides of the brain. The inferior portion of the brain is protected by parts of the ethnoid and sphenoid bones.

The sphenoid bone is composed of a body, greater and lesser wings, and paired **pterygoid processes.** Within the body is one of the pairs of paranasal sinuses—the sphenoid sinuses. The areas of greatest interest are the pterygoid processes, which project down

from the body of the sphenoid, just behind the maxillae. Each process has two thin walls of bone that project backward—the medial and lateral pterygoid plates. Projecting down from the medial pterygoid plate is the hamulus or hamular process, which plays a role in the function of a muscle of the anterior soft palate. The area between these plates is a depression known as a pterygoid fossa. From the fossae and the lateral pterygoid plates originate two pairs of muscles of mastication that move the jaw (Fig. 26.10). Between the maxillae and the pterygoid processes is an opening into an area behind and below the eye known as the **pterygopalatine fossa** (Fig. 26.11). Major nerves and blood vessels to the oral and nasal cavities and midface branch into this area.

Viscerocranium

The nasal bones, vomer, lacrimal bones, and zygomatic and inferior nasal conchae afford support to the respiratory opening and also support the eye socket. This will be covered in Chapter 27.

The maxillae, palatine bones, and mandible afford support to the masticatory system, which houses teeth, gingivae, palates, and the tongue.

Maxillae

Processes

The maxillae consist of a body and four processes in each bone. The **frontal process** and the zygomatic process are the projections of the maxilla that meet the frontal and zygomatic bones, respectively; between these processes, bone forms about one-third of the rim of the orbit. The third process is the **alveolar process** of the maxilla, which forms the sockets for upper teeth. The fourth is the **horizontal palatine process** of the maxilla, which, together with its counterparts, forms most of the hard palate.

There are two separate maxilla bones that fuse to form the maxillae.

Maxillary Sinuses

Within the bodies of the maxillae are **maxillary sinuses**, the largest and possibly most troublesome of the paranasal sinuses. As you

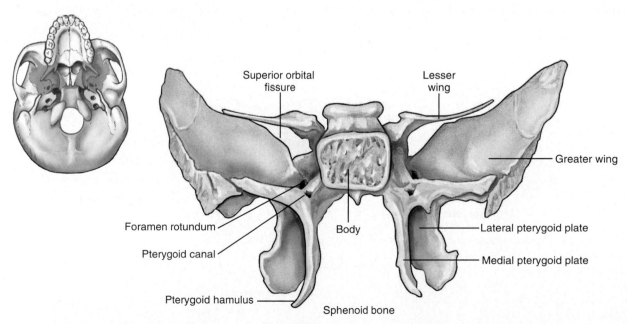

• **Figure 26.10** Posterior view of the sphenoid bone. Note the pterygoid processes and their components. (From Patton KT, Thibodeau GA. *Anatomy & Physiology.* 8th ed. St. Louis, MO: Mosby; 2013.)

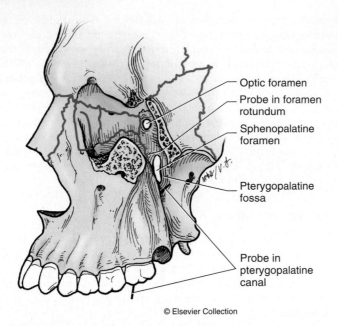

Optic foramen
Probe in foramen rotundum
Sphenopalatine foramen

Pterygopalatine fossa

Probe in pterygopalatine canal

© Elsevier Collection

• **Figure 26.11** In this lateral view, zygomatic bone has been removed to better show the opening between the maxilla and the pterygoid process (pterygomaxillary fissure), which leads into the pterygopalatine fossa.

will study in radiology, maxillary sinuses are quite large, forming a very thin wall of bone between the roots of maxillary posterior teeth and the sinus spaces themselves. Infections in the sinuses may affect teeth, and, conversely, infections in teeth may affect the sinuses (see Chapter 27).

Lateral View

Fig. 26.12 presents the lateral view of the maxilla. Here you can see the body as well as the alveolar, zygomatic, and frontal processes. You can also see how the maxilla forms half of the opening of the nasal cavity. At the lower end of the nasal cavity, in front, is the **anterior nasal spine**. This is a radiographic landmark frequently used in lateral head films for orthodontics. In the alveolar

process, you can see how anterior teeth and sometimes premolars cause bulgings in bone, known as **alveolar eminences**. Above the canine, the **canine fossa** can be seen, and in the upper end of that fossa area is the **infraorbital foramen**. If you look behind the third molar region, you see the posterior bulging of bone; this is known as the **maxillary tuberosity**. In this area, blood vessels and nerves enter bone to supply posterior teeth and part of the maxillary sinus. It is also the area where much of the growth of maxillae takes place. This growth causes the maxillary bones to become longer in an anteroposterior direction. Insufficient growth usually means inadequate room for third molars to erupt and an upper jaw that may be shorter than it should be, possibly causing the mandible to appear to be more forward than it is, thus causing an apparent class III occlusion. Growth of these bones, and therefore of the upper face, takes place not only at that point but also between the palatine processes, between the frontal bone and the maxillae, and between the zygomatic bones and the maxillae.

Inferior View

Fig. 26.13 is an inferior or palatal view of the maxillae. Note the median palatine suture line, which accounts for lateral palatal growth, and also the incisive foramen in the anterior region. Also visible are the palatine bones that form the posterior part of the soft palate. Between the maxilla and the palatine bone is the **transverse palatine suture**.

Medial View

A medial view of the maxilla from the nasal cavity shows several landmarks, as already mentioned, but it primarily shows the opening into the nasal cavity of the maxillary sinus (Fig. 26.14). The opening is known as the **hiatus** or the **ostium of the maxillary sinus** and varies considerably in size. The smaller this opening, the more likely the sinus will become clogged from nasal

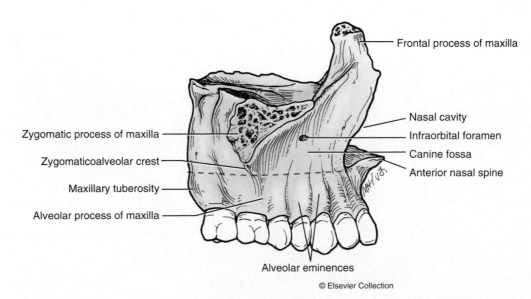

Frontal process of maxilla
Nasal cavity
Infraorbital foramen
Canine fossa
Anterior nasal spine
Zygomatic process of maxilla
Zygomaticoalveolar crest
Maxillary tuberosity
Alveolar process of maxilla
Alveolar eminences

© Elsevier Collection

• **Figure 26.12** Lateral view of the maxilla. Little room is available for the third molar to erupt at this point. Division between the body of the maxilla and the alveolar process (*broken line*).

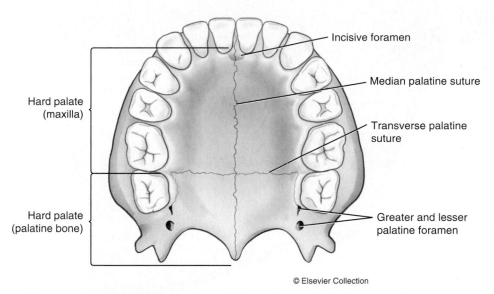

© Elsevier Collection

• **Figure 26.13** Inferior or palatal view of the maxillae and part of the palatine bone. The hard palate covers the maxillary palate with attached papillary gingiva, and the soft palate covers the palatal bones with a more movable palatal mucosa.

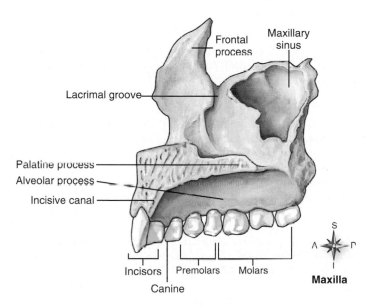

• **Figure 26.14** Medial view of the maxilla. Note the thickness of the hard palate separating the oral cavity from the nasal cavity. (From Patton KT, Thibodeau GA. *Anatomy & Physiology.* 8th ed. St. Louis, MO: Mosby; 2013.)

congestion and edema. This opening (not shown in the figure) is underneath the middle concha of the three conchae. In this view, you can see the **lacrimal groove**, which runs down from the inner corner of the eye. This is the source from which tears flow into the nose, accounting for the runny nose that occurs when a person is crying. You can also see a cutaway view of the sinus, which continues down to the area surrounding the apices of the maxillary teeth roots.

Mandible

The mandible is a single bone made up of three parts: the **horizontal body**, with the alveolar process on top of it, and the vertical portion of bone known as the **ramus**. Generally, they are considered

to be one body and one alveolar process but two rami in a mandible (Fig. 26.15).

The **mental protuberance** forms the chin portion of the mandible. The area above the dotted line is the **alveolar process,** which is the bone that forms the sockets for the teeth.

Lateral View

In Fig. 26.16, you can see other landmarks of the mandible. Just posterior from the mental protuberance is the **mental foramen**, from which the mental blood vessels and nerves for the lower lip and chin emerge. These nerves and blood vessels are branches of the inferior alveolar arteries and nerves. This foramen is just about

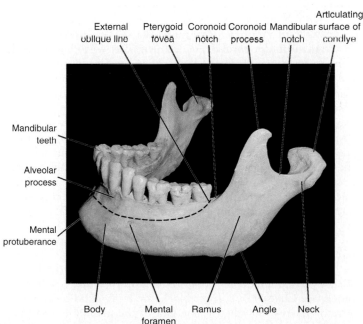

• **Figure 26.15** Lateral view of the mandible. The alveolar process begins above the dotted line. (From Fehrenbach MJ, Herring SW. *Illustrated Anatomy of the Head and Neck.* 4th ed. St. Louis, MO: Saunders; 2012.)

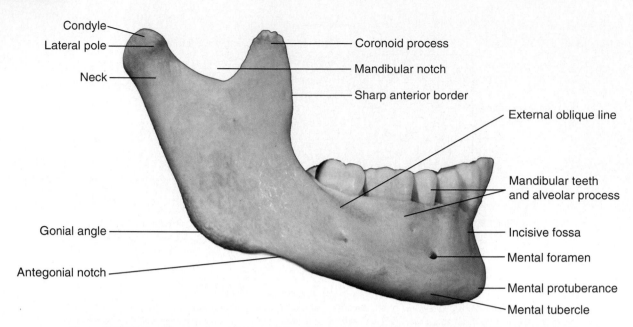

Condyle
Lateral pole
Neck
Coronoid process
Mandibular notch
Sharp anterior border
External oblique line
Mandibular teeth and alveolar process
Gonial angle
Antegonial notch
Incisive fossa
Mental foramen
Mental protuberance
Mental tubercle

• **Figure 26.16** Lateral landmarks of the mandible. (From Liebgott B. *The Anatomic Basis of Dentistry.* 3rd ed. St. Louis, MO: Mosby; 2011.)

at a position that divides the body of the mandible below from the alveolar process above it. The point where the **inferior border of the mandible** turns upward is the **mandibular angle,** also called the **gonial angle.** This is the dividing line between the body and the ramus.

Clinical Considerations

On the inferior border of the body of the mandible, just anterior to the gonial angle, you can see or feel an indentation, the antegonial notch. This is where the facial artery and vein cross the mandible. This is a pressure point to slow bleeding in cuts of the face (see Chapter 32).

Moving up along the posterior border of the ramus, we come to the **mandibular condyle,** which articulates with the temporal bone to form the TMJ. The slightly narrowed area just beneath the condyle is known as the **condylar neck.** The *mandibular condyle* and the *neck of the condyle* together form the **condylar process.** In front of the condyle, the depression in the ramus is called the **mandibular notch.** Just anterior to this notch is the **coronoid process,** which is the attachment for one of the muscles of mastication, the temporalis. The anterior border of the ramus ends in the **external oblique line,** which shows up as a radiopacity on posterior periapical or panographic radiographs. There is a notch in the anterior of the ramus just inferior to the coronoid process and posterior and superior to the external oblique line. This notch is called the **coronoid notch.**

The *coronoid notch* is used as a landmark in the administration of an inferior alveolar block.

The anterior border of the neck of the mandibular condyle is used as a landmark in the administration of the Gow-Gates block (see Chapter 36). These blocks are local mandibular nerve anesthetics that anesthetize one half of the mandible with one injection.

Growth of the mandible takes place in several areas. First, the alveolar process and body increase in width and height. The lengthening of the mandibular arch takes place by bone being added to the posterior border of the ramus and taken away from the anterior border. If there is insufficient growth, there may be no room for the normal eruption of mandibular third molars.

Medial View

In Fig. 26.17, about midway up the ramus, is the **mandibular foramen,** where the nerves and blood vessels for the lower teeth and lip enter the mandible. Just in front of the foramen and running forward and down is the **mylohyoid line,** the attachment for the mylohyoid muscle. Below the mandibular foramen is the **mylohyoid groove** for the passage of the mylohyoid nerve and vessels to the mylohyoid and anterior digastric muscles. Toward the anterior part of that line are two depressions in the bone, one above the line and one below it. These are the **sublingual** and **submandibular fossae.** The sublingual and submandibular salivary glands lie in these depressions. The area immediately behind the third molars is referred to as the **retromolar triangle.** The lateral margin of this triangle is the external oblique line or ridge, and the medial margin of this triangle is the **internal oblique line** or **ridge.**

Posterior View

In Fig. 26.18, directly at the midline, are two small, grouped projections, one above and one below. These are the **superior and inferior genial tubercles,** or **mental spines.** They are attachments for muscles that aid in tongue movement and swallowing—the genioglossus and geniohyoid muscles. Just below these projections at the inferior border of the mandible are the **digastric fossae,** which are also points of attachment for the anterior digastric muscle. The last landmark is the **lingula,** which means "little tongue." The lingula is a projection of bone that partially covers the opening of the mandibular foramen. This is a point of attachment for the **sphenomandibular ligament.** Variation in size and location of the lingula may, at times, affect the effectiveness of anesthesia in this area.

There is a ridge that runs vertically down the midline of the mandible. This ridge, the **mandibular symphysis,** is evidence of

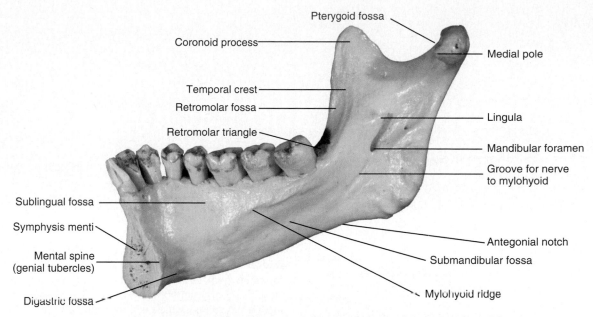

• **Figure 26.17** Medial landmarks of the mandible. (From Liebgott B. *The Anatomic Basis of Dentistry*. 3rd ed. St. Louis, MO: Mosby; 2011.)

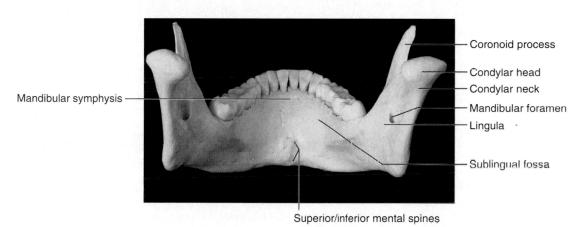

• **Figure 26.18** Posterior view of the mandible. Note the genial tubercles, digastric fossae, and lingulae, which could not be easily seen on the medial view of the mandible. (From Abrahams PH, Spratt JD, Loukas M, et al. *McMinn and Abraham's Clinical Atlas of Human Anatomy*. 7th ed. London, UK: Elsevier; 2013.)

the fusion of the two mandibular processes during embryonic development. A right and a left mandibular process join at this symphysis at about the seventh embryonic week (Fig. 26.18). Further inferiorly we see two pairs of small spines projecting lingually; these form the attachment site for muscles of the tongue and hyoid bone.

From time to time, review this chapter on the osteology of the skull. You will find a great deal of correlation between this material and your radiology, clinical, and anesthesia studies. A thorough knowledge of osteology will make you a better practitioner of radiologic and anesthetic techniques and will benefit the patient you are treating.

Review Questions

1. How many bones form the skull?
2. How are the bones subdivided?
3. Define the following:
   a. suture
   b. foramen
   c. canal
   d. fossa
4. Which bones form the hard palate?
5. What would be another name for each of the following sutures?
   a. coronal
   b. sagittal
   c. lambdoid

6. Where is the largest of the paranasal sinuses?
7. Name the bony area immediately behind maxillary third molars.
8. What are the divisions of the mandible?
9. Name the major bone landmarks of the maxillae and the mandible.
10. Discuss the growth of mandibular and maxillary arches.
11. What are the parts of the sphenoid bone?
12. What bones make up the rim of the orbit?
13. What part of what bone divides the anterior and middle cranial fossae, and which one divides the middle and posterior cranial fossae?

27

Nose, Nasal Cavity, and Paranasal Sinuses

Nose and Nasal Cavity

External View

The nose and the nasal cavity are a complex arrangement of hard and soft tissues. The nose is that portion of the nasal complex that protrudes outward from the skeletal component. The nose, or more properly, the external nose, is attached superiorly to nasal bones and inferiorly to the anterior nasal spine. Each protruding lateral margin is known individually as a wing of the nose, or an **ala**. The external nose is divided in half by the cartilaginous part of the **nasal septum**, which is the wall that divides the nasal complex into right and left halves (Fig. 27.1). If you look at a skull, you will see that the nasal aperture, the anterior most portion of the nasal cavity, is somewhat pear shaped.

Internal View

Peering inside the nasal cavity, you can see the *nasal septum*. The lateral walls of the nasal cavity have three shelves, called *nasal conchae*, which project into the septum. The superior portion of the bony nasal cavity has small holes that open into the anterior cranial fossa through the **cribriform plate** of the ethmoid bone to transmit olfactory nerves from the nose up to the brain.

The septum is formed from the vomer bone and a portion of the ethmoid bone as well as the fibrocartilaginous part of the septum (Fig. 27.2). The inferior portion or floor of the cavity is formed from the bones of the hard palate, which are the palatal processes of the maxillae and the horizontal portion of the palatine bones. The most complex portion of the nasal cavity is its lateral walls. The upper half to two-thirds of the lateral wall of the cavity is formed from parts of the ethmoid bone. It consists of the

wall and two shelflike structures, known as the **superior** and **middle nasal conchae**. The lower part of the lateral walls is formed by portions of the maxillae. At the point where the maxillae and the ethmoid bone meet in the lateral wall, there is a third medial projection, which is a separate bone itself, known as the **inferior nasal concha** (Fig. 27.3). The soft tissue part of the middle nasal concha is referred to as the uncinate process.

The openings between the nasal cavities and the nasopharynx begin at the posterior of the nasal septum. These two oval-shaped openings are known as the **choanae**, or **posterior nasal apertures**. Posterior to this is the nasal pharynx. The posterosuperior part of the nasal cavity is composed of a portion of the body of the sphenoid bone where it meets the ethmoid bone and is known as the **sphenoethmoidal recess**.

Clinical Considerations

With the advent of fiberoptics and microscopic instruments, surgery on tumors of the pituitary gland can be performed by going through the nasal cavity, into the sphenoid sinus, and cutting away the roof of that sinus, thereby gaining access to the pituitary gland from below and operating on it without having to go through the skull.

The pituitary fossa is used as a cephalometric landmark in orthodontics. The deepest part of this fossa is called *sella turcica* (see Fig. 27.3). The pituitary fossa houses the pituitary gland.

Epithelial Lining

Recall from Chapter 17 on epithelial tissues that there is one type of epithelium known as *pseudostratified columnar epithelium with goblet cells*. This epithelial tissue is usually called **respiratory epithelium,** because it is primarily found in the respiratory tract. (You should be aware by now that the nasal cavity is the beginning of the respiratory tract or system.) The epithelium has many hairlike projections, known as *cilia*, which move in a synchronized beating pattern toward the anterior portion of the nasal cavity. The tiny goblet cells secrete a sticky mucous substance onto the cilia, trapping contaminants as they enter the nasal cavity and moving them toward the front where they are removed by blowing the nose; during sleep, this mucus may flow backward as postnasal drip. For this mechanism to be successful, it is important to have as much surface area as possible in the nasal cavity. The conchae help accomplish that.

The epithelium in the roof of the nasal cavity and coming down onto the upper surface of the superior concha and upper

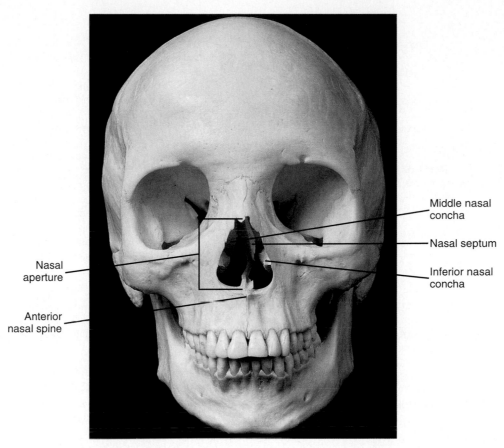

Middle nasal concha

Nasal septum

Inferior nasal concha

Nasal aperture

Anterior nasal spine

• **Figure 27.1.** Anterior view of a skull showing the nasal aperture, nasal septum, and nasal conchae. (From Abrahams PH, Spratt JD, Loukas M, et al. *McMinn and Abraham's Clinical Atlas of Human Anatomy.* 7th ed. London, UK: Elsevier; 2013.)

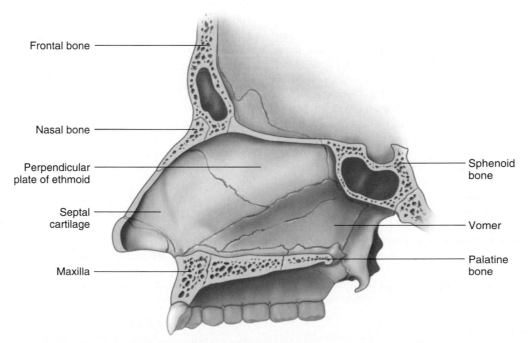

Frontal bone

Nasal bone

Perpendicular plate of ethmoid

Septal cartilage

Maxilla

Sphenoid bone

Vomer

Palatine bone

• **Figure 27.2.** Sagittal section showing the nasal septum and its components. (From Fonseca RJ, Barber HD, Powers M, et al. *Oral and Maxillofacial Trauma.* St. Louis, MO: Saunders; 2013.)

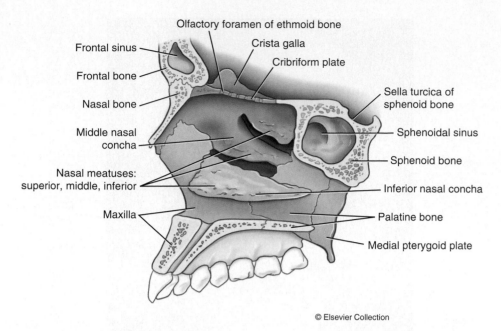

Olfactory foramen of ethmoid bone
Crista galla
Cribriform plate
Frontal sinus
Frontal bone
Nasal bone
Sella turcica of
sphenoid bone
Sphenoidal sinus
Sphenoid bone
Middle nasal
concha
Inferior nasal concha
Nasal meatuses:
superior, middle, inferior
Maxilla
Palatine bone
Medial pterygoid plate

© Elsevier Collection

• **Figure 27.3.** Sagittal section of right nasal cavity, with the septum removed, showing the lateral nasal wall and bony conchae.

nasal septum is modified and has nerve fibers that perceive odors. This is called the **olfactory epithelium.**

Paranasal Sinuses

Location

You now should have a clearer picture in your mind of the nasal cavity. To visualize it even better, it would be helpful to study a skull that has been specially prepared by being split along the midline. This would give you a greater appreciation of the complexity of the structure. Studying this area more closely, you would see that there are numerous openings into the nasal cavity from other areas. Most of these openings are from compartments or cavities of various sizes known as the **paranasal sinuses.** There are four pairs of these sinuses—two ethmoids, two frontals, two maxillaries, and two sphenoids. These sinuses are not easily seen at first; the nasal conchae must first be located. These conchae on either side of the nasal cavity are there for several reasons, one of them being to increase the surface area for the respiratory epithelium, which, as mentioned earlier, acts as a filter of incoming air.

The area of the lateral nasal wall sheltered underneath each concha is known as the **meatus** of each concha. The **inferior meatus** is beneath the inferior nasal concha and has one small opening, which is the opening of the nasolacrimal duct. This duct carries tears from the corner of the eye into the nasal cavity. The middle meatus lies beneath the middle nasal concha, where there is a crescent-shaped opening called the **hiatus semilunaris**, which means a half-moon-shaped opening. In this area are a number of other openings, which will be discussed shortly. The bulbous ridge above the hiatus semilunar is called the **ethmoid bulla.** The **superior meatus** lies beneath the superior concha and is the smallest meatus (Fig. 27.4).

Frontal Sinuses

The paired **frontal sinuses** are located in the frontal bone just above the orbital cavity; these vary in size from person to person.

They frequently cross the midline and may be partially located on the opposite side. These sinuses drain into the very anterior end of the hiatus semilunaris. Infections in these sinuses cause pressure and pain just above the eye.

Sphenoid Sinuses

The paired **sphenoid sinuses** are located in the body of the sphenoid bone just underneath the pituitary fossa, which is located in the middle cranial fossa (Fig. 27.5). These sinuses also cross the midline. They open into the highest and most posterior part of the nasal cavity—the *sphenoethmoidal recess.* Infections in the sphenoid sinuses cause pressure and a congested feeling that is hard to localize but is deep in the midline of the head.

Ethmoid Sinuses

The **ethmoid sinuses** are frequently called **ethmoid air cells,** because they are not single-paired sinuses like the other paranasal sinuses but are subdivided into numerous small compartments (Fig. 27.5). Infections in the ethmoid sinuses are difficult to treat because of the small compartments. When infected, they cause a feeling of congestion and aching within the nasal cavity area.

These clusters of air cells are further divided into anterior, middle, and posterior ethmoid air cells.

Anterior Ethmoid Air Cells

The anterior ethmoid air cells are located in the lateral wall of the nasal cavity at the base of the middle nasal concha. These air cells open into the hiatus semilunaris just posteroinferior to the opening for the frontal sinus.

Middle Ethmoid Air Cells

The middle ethmoid air cells are also located in the base of the middle nasal concha, just behind the anterior air cells. They are also located within the ethmoid bulla. These may have a couple of

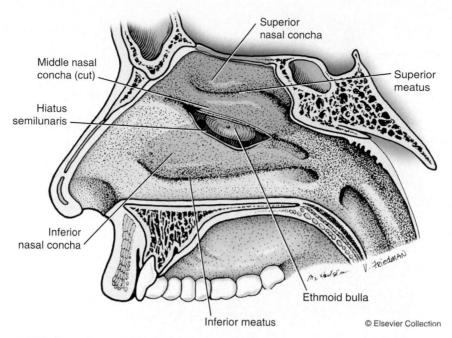

• **Figure 27.4.** Same view as in Fig. 27.3, but covered with nasal mucosa. The middle concha has been partially removed to show the hiatus semilunaris and the ethmoid bulla in the middle meatus.

Sagittal section

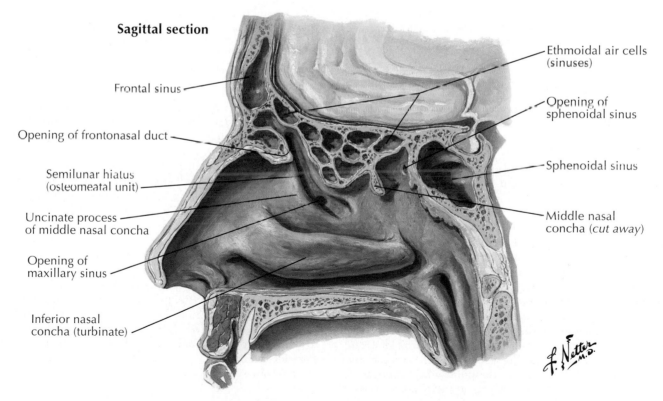

• **Figure 27.5.** A cutaway of the lateral wall of the nasal cavity. This is a view as seen from the medial toward the lateral. This view shows the relationship of the semilunar hiatus to the opening of the maxillary sinus. (From Netter F. *Atlas of Human Anatomy.* 2nd ed. East Hanover, NJ: Novartis; 1997.)

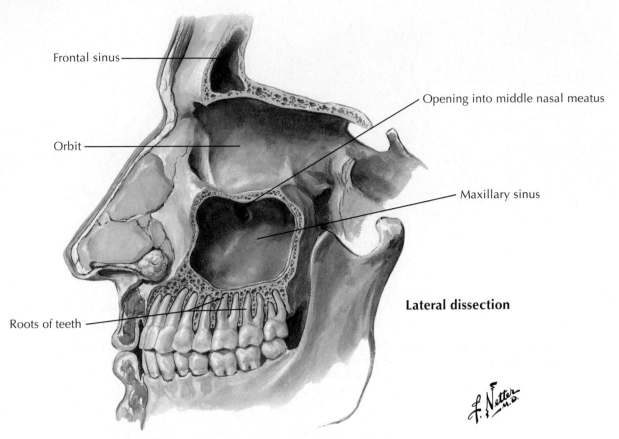

Frontal sinus

Orbit

Roots of teeth

Opening into middle nasal meatus

Maxillary sinus

Lateral dissection

• **Figure 27.6** A cutaway view of the maxillary sinus exposing the maxillary sinus and its proximity to the roots of the maxillary teeth. The opening from the maxillary sinus into middle nasal meatus can also be seen. (From Netter F. *Atlas of Human Anatomy.* 2nd ed. East Hanover, NJ: Novartis; 1997.)

openings, one on the ethmoid bulla and another possibly in the hiatus semilunaris.

Posterior Ethmoid Air Cells

The posterior ethmoid air cells are located in the base of the superior nasal concha and open into the superior meatus.

Maxillary Sinuses

Maxillary sinuses are the largest of the paranasal sinuses and open into the posterior end of the hiatus semilunaris through one or more openings. At birth, the maxillary sinus in each maxilla is the size of a small pea. As growth takes place, each sinus continues to expand and occupy a greater portion of the body of the maxilla. In a young adult, the maxillary sinus occupies an area from just posterior to the maxillary canine back to the area of the third molar in an anteroposterior direction. In a superoinferior direction, it would extend from the floor of the orbital cavity inferiorly to the point where it might extend down around the root tips of the maxillary posterior teeth (Fig. 27.6). The maxillary sinus may develop compartmental walls, but generally all of them are connected by large openings. If you look at the location of the opening for the maxillary sinus in the middle meatus region and compare it with its location on the medial wall of the sinus, you will find that this opening is almost two-thirds of the way up the medial wall (see Fig. 27.6). You can appreciate the significance of trying to drain

a cavity through an opening that is near the top of the space. Several things come into play here, the first being that every individual's maxillary sinus is different. Sometimes there is more than one opening in each sinus, sometimes the opening or openings are very small, and sometimes they are very big. During a nasal infection, swelling occurs in the nasal mucosa. If the maxillary sinus has a very small opening or openings, it may swell shut as a result of the mucosal edema. Preexisting infection in the sinus continues to increase, and the fact that the sinus is now a warm, closed space causes it to act like an incubator for the microorganisms causing the infection. As the infection increases in severity, pressure increases in the maxillae. Tilting the head forward causes the pressure to increase because the fluid produced by the infection flows forward against the anterior wall of the sinus. The use of nasal sprays frequently gives some temporary relief, but then the cavity eventually clogs again. If there is some opening of the sinus, tilting the head to one side while lying down may allow for some drainage from the opposite side or the high-side sinus.

Clinical Considerations

When this clogging happens repeatedly, an ear, nose, and throat (ENT) specialist sometimes punches a hole from the inferior meatus into the medial wall of the maxillary sinus near its base and enlarges it to achieve good drainage and a decrease in maxillary sinus infections.

Function of Sinuses

Historically, several functions have been discussed regarding the sinuses. Probably the most popular was that the sinuses warm the air as it passes into the respiratory system. Later studies showed that the flow of air into and out of these sinuses is actually very minimal. The general belief now is that the hollow cavities of the nasal sinuses function to lighten the overall bone weight.

Clinical Problems

Besides the problems mentioned regarding the maxillary sinus, there are also dental considerations relating to this structure. The same nerves that supply maxillary posterior teeth also supply maxillary sinuses. These are sensory nerves that carry different types of messages to the brain. In everyday life, these nerves are constantly sending messages to the brain from maxillary teeth. Biting down on a piece of bone or a seed, for example, results in a painful stimulus being sent to the brain. The same nerves to teeth also have fibers from maxillary sinuses, but sinuses seldom send messages to the brain. As a result, the brain gets used to interpreting everything that travels along those nerves as messages from teeth. However, during a maxillary sinus infection, sinuses also send messages along the same nerves. The brain correctly interprets these messages as pain; however, it incorrectly interprets the pain as coming from the tooth because that is where all the messages came from in the past.

When this occurs, the individual usually contacts the family dentist and complains about a rather severe toothache. When that patient is examined, no apparent signs of any caries are found, there are no periodontal pockets, and the tooth is only mildly sensitive to percussion. A **periapical** radiograph shows no periapical lesion and no interproximal caries, although at times there may be a cloudiness appearing in the maxillary sinus. This is usually a sign of fluid buildup. Testing of the pulp yields normal results.

Where do we go from here? There could be problems that are often undetectable, such as a cracked tooth, but we need to explore one other option before proceeding with any other tests or treatment. We need to go back to the medical and dental history form and check for a history of sinus infections. If the history form in your office does not have that category, then question the patient concerning sinus infections, especially recent sinus problems. If the patient confirms a problem with sinus infections, then refer him or her to a physician for treatment. This will usually take care of the problem unless it recurs after medical treatment. Under such circumstances, further evaluation must be done.

Another area of concern is the relationship of the floor of the sinus to teeth. In a number of instances, the floor of the sinus dips down around the tip of one or more roots of posterior teeth. Under some circumstances, it is possible that a periapical infection of a tooth may involve the sinus. It is also possible that the sinus may dip between the roots of a maxillary molar. If that molar has roots that are **dilacerated** (curved because of disturbances in development) and it needs to be extracted for any reason, use reliable radiographs to assess the situation. It would be embarrassing and considered negligent treatment if, without radiographs of the region, you proceeded to extract a molar tooth and found that a part of the maxillary sinus floor was also extracted in addition to the extracted tooth. Generally, a tooth with dilacerated roots needs to have the roots sectioned and removed one at a time to minimize the possibility of a fracture of the sinus floor.

When maxillary teeth are extracted and healing has occurred, the maxillary sinus tends to enlarge into the area formerly occupied by posterior maxillary roots and impacted third maxillary molars. This means that the thickness of bone in the maxillary tuberosity and alveolar ridge up to and sometimes including the canine region may be very thin and has to be evaluated when deciding what type of treatment to use to replace teeth when a **prosthetic appliance** is present.

Evaluation and treatment need to go beyond teeth and involve other areas or systems of the body. This is just one more reason why the members of the dental team need to know more about total evaluation of the patient.

Review Questions

1. Which bones or structures form the nasal septum?
2. What bones would you find in the lateral wall of the nasal cavity?
3. What is a meatus?
4. What is the function of respiratory epithelium?
5. What opens into the following?
   a. inferior meatus
   b. middle meatus
   c. superior meatus
   d. sphenoethmoidal recess
6. Where specifically is the olfactory epithelium found?
7. Anatomically, why might maxillary sinuses create problems with sinus infections and with extractions of maxillary posterior teeth?
8. Why might a maxillary sinus infection seem to be coming from teeth?

28

Muscles of Mastication, Hyoid Muscles, and Sternocleidomastoid and Trapezius Muscles

OBJECTIVES

- To describe the origin, insertion, action, and nerve and blood supply of the muscles of mastication
- To categorize the muscles according to their roles in elevation, depression, protrusion, retrusion, and lateral excursion of the mandible
- To describe the functions of the sternocleidomastoid and trapezius muscles and their roles in referred pain to various areas, including the temporomandibular joint
- To name the suprahyoid and infrahyoid muscles and their roles in mandibular movement, swallowing, and phonation

Because this is the first of three chapters dealing with muscles and their functions, it seems appropriate to mention briefly some terms relevant to this subject. In general, a person reading about muscles constantly sees five terms: *origin, insertion, action, nerve supply,* and *blood supply.* Because nerve supply and blood supply are self-explanatory, we will be primarily concerned with the first three. The **origin** of a muscle is generally considered to be the end of the muscle that is attached to the least movable structure. The **insertion** of a muscle is the other end of the muscle, which is attached to the more movable structure. In some muscles, there could be movement at either end, and so the terminology is a bit confusing. The **action** is the work that is accomplished when the muscle fibers contract. If you are familiar with the action of a muscle but are not sure which end is the origin or the insertion, keep in mind that, in general, the insertion moves toward the origin when the muscle is contracted. Likewise, if you know the direction of the muscle fibers, you can usually deduce the action by imagining the insertion moving toward the origin and picturing what happens. Keep in mind that there may at times be more than one function to a particular muscle because either end of a muscle can function as an insertion if the other end is fixed or because different fiber directions within the muscles and different groups of fibers may be called into function, thereby creating different actions.

Muscles of Mastication

The muscles of **mastication** are four pairs of muscles attached to the mandible and primarily responsible for elevating, protruding,

retruding, or causing the mandible to move laterally. They develop from the first (mandibular) pharyngeal arch, which is also responsible for the development of some of the bony facial structures. Because they develop from this arch, they are innervated by the nerve of the first arch, the fifth cranial nerve (trigeminal nerve). More specifically, the muscles are innervated by the third part of the fifth nerve, which is called the *mandibular division,* or V_3. The blood supply to these muscles comes from the maxillary artery, which is a branch of the external carotid artery. Blood vessels and nerves are further discussed in Chapters 32 and 34 (see Table 28.1).

Masseter Muscle

The **masseter muscle** is probably the most powerful of the muscles of mastication. It takes its origin from two areas on the zygomatic arch. The superficial head originates from the inferior border of the anterior two-thirds of the zygomatic arch. The deep head arises from the inferior border of the posterior third of the zygomatic arch and the entire medial side of the zygomatic arch. The fibers of the superficial head run down and slightly back to be inserted into the angle of the mandible on the lateral side. The deep head has vertically oriented fibers. When the masseter muscle contracts, it elevates the mandible, closing the mouth (Fig. 28.1).

Temporal Muscle

The **temporal muscle**, frequently called the **temporalis muscle**, has a very wide origin from the entire temporal fossa and the fascia covering the muscle. The anterior fibers run almost vertically, but the posterior fibers run in a more horizontal direction over the ear. All these fibers insert into the coronoid process of the mandible and sometimes run down the anterior border of the ramus of the mandible as far as the third molar (Fig. 28.2). If the entire muscle contracts, the overall action pulls up on the coronoid process and elevates the mandible, closing the mouth. If only the posterior fibers are contracted, the result is a horizontal pulling of the coronoid process in a posterior direction. This pulls the mandible backward, which is referred to as *retruding the mandible.*

Medial Pterygoid Muscle

In studying the origin of the **medial pterygoid muscle**, it is probably best to examine a model of the skull while reading the

TABLE 28.1	Muscles of Mastication				
Muscle	Origin	Insertion	Action	Nerve Innervation	Arterial Supply
Masseter	Inferior border of zygomatic arch	Lateral side of the angle of mandible	Elevates mandible	Cranial nerve V, division 3	Maxillary artery
Temporal muscle	Temporal fossa	Coronoid process	Elevates mandible and retrusion of mandible	Cranial nerve V, division 3	Maxillary artery
Medial pterygoid muscle	Pterygoid plate and fossa and maxillary tuberosity	Medial side of angle of mandible	Elevates mandible	Cranial nerve V, division 3	Maxillary artery
Lateral pterygoid muscle	Infratemporal crest and lateral pterygoid plate	Anterior border of temporomandibular joint (TMJ) and neck of condyle	Protrudes and depresses mandible, lateral excursion of mandible	Cranial nerve V, division 3	Maxillary artery

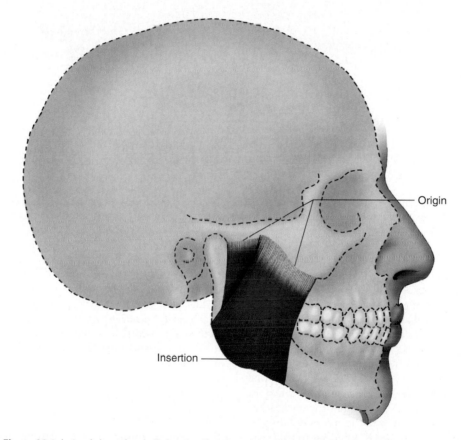

• **Figure 28.1** Lateral view of a skull showing that the origin of the masseter muscle is from the zygomatic arch. Fibers run down and slightly back to insert into the angle of the mandible.

description. The muscle has two origins. The larger and major origin is from the medial side of the lateral pterygoid plate and the pterygoid fossa as well as a tiny area of the palatine bone at the lower end of the medial and lateral pterygoid plates. This area is called the *pyramidal process* of the palatine bone. The smaller origin is just anterior to that area, coming from the maxillary tuberosity just behind the third molar. All the fibers run down and slightly posteriorly and laterally to be inserted into the angle of the mandible on the medial side. This is just opposite the masseter insertion on the lateral side. When the muscle contracts, the resulting action is elevation of the mandible and closing of the mouth (Fig. 28.3).

Lateral Pterygoid Muscle

The **lateral pterygoid muscle** also has two separate origins. The smaller, superior origin or head arises from the area called the *infratemporal crest* of the greater wing of the sphenoid bone. The larger, inferior origin or head arises from the lateral side of the lateral pterygoid plate. This is just opposite the origin of the medial pterygoid muscle. The fibers from both origins of the lateral pterygoid muscle run horizontally in a posterior direction. Some fibers from the superior head penetrate the capsule of the temporomandibular joint (TMJ) and insert into the anterior border

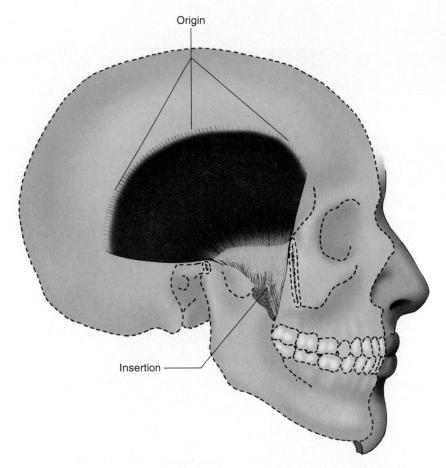

Origin

Insertion

• **Figure 28.2** The temporal muscle has a wide origin from the temporal fossa. Note the vertical, inclined, and horizontal muscle fibers, which insert primarily on the medial side and the tip of the coronoid process.

of the disk of the joint. The remainder of the fibers from that origin and the fibers of the inferior head insert into the neck of the condyle on the anterior and medial side (see Fig. 28.3).

The lateral pterygoid muscle has several actions. The inferior head pulls the condyle forward and helps protrude and depress the mandible. The disk is also brought forward because of its attachment to the condyle. When both left and right inferior heads function, the mandible is protruded and depressed. If only one lateral pterygoid is contracted, there will be lateral excursion to the opposite side of the contracted muscle. The superior head of the lateral pterygoid functions primarily in the action of biting or what is sometimes called the *power stroke*. It functions to guide the posterior movement of the disk and condyle as it goes back to a centric position. In other words, as other muscles are pulling posteriorly, the upper head of the lateral pterygoid is relaxing and controlling that movement (see Fig. 28.3).

Hyoid Muscles

We have just discussed the muscles that accomplish virtually all jaw movements except strong depression of the mandible or opening of the mouth and some retrusion of the mandible. These actions are accomplished by muscles in the neck, called the **hyoid muscles** (see Table 28.2).

Hyoid muscles are so named because they attach to or are associated with the hyoid bone in the neck. The hyoid is a

horseshoe-shaped bone suspended beneath the mandible, with the open end of the horseshoe pointed posteriorly (Fig. 28.4). It is unusual in that it articulates with no other bone; its only connection with other bones is by muscles and ligaments. These muscles are divided into two groups—those above the hyoid are called **suprahyoid muscles**, and those below are called **infrahyoid muscles**.

Suprahyoid Group

Digastric Muscle

The **digastric muscle** has a relatively unusual arrangement of fibers, with muscle fibers at either end of the muscle and a collagenous tendon in the middle. Classically, it has been described as having two bellies: an *anterior* and a *posterior*. The digastric muscle is a V-shaped muscle that has its origin on the digastric notch of the temporal bone and has its insertion at the digastric fossa of the mandible on the inferior surface of the midline. Along the way, this muscle has two bellies with an intermediate tendon. The **posterior digastric belly** of this muscle begins from its origin on the digastric notch of the temporal bone to this intermediate tendon. A sling of fascia forms a loop that allows the intermediate tendon to slide through it. The **anterior digastric belly** of the digastric muscle continues from this intermediate tendon and then to its origin and inserts on the inferior midline of the mandible. For clearer understanding, it might be best to say that its origin is at the digastric

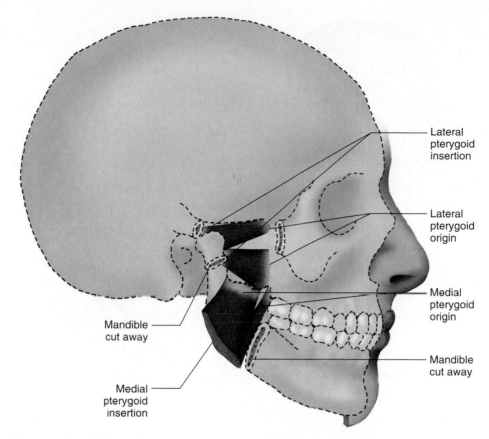

• **Figure 28.3** Lateral view of a skull showing the origins of the lateral pterygoid muscle from the infratemporal crest and pterygoid plate, with fibers inserting into the disc and neck of the condyle. Note the medial pterygoid muscle originating from the pterygoid area, as well as a small origin from the maxillary tuberosity. Insertion onto the medial side of the angle of the mandible is also visible.

TABLE 28.2   Muscles of the Hyoid

Muscle	Origin	Insertion	Action	Nerve Innervation	Arterial Supply
Digastric muscle	Digastric notch	Digastric fossa	Retrudes mandible and elevates hyoid	Cranial nerve V, division 3 and cranial nerve VII	Maxillary artery
Mylohyoid muscle	Mylohyoid line	Hyoid bone	Depresses mandible and elevates hyoid	Cranial nerve V, division 3	Lingual artery
Geniohyoid muscle	Inferior genial tubercle	Hyoid bone	Depresses mandible and elevates hyoid	Cervical nerve I	Lingual artery
Stylohyoid muscle	Styloid process	Hyoid bone	Pulls hyoid up and back	Cranial nerve VII	Facial and occipital arteries
Omohyoid muscle	Scapula and hyoid bone	Sternocleidomastoid muscle	Pulls hyoid down	Cervical nerves II and III	Lingual artery and superior thyroid artery
Sternohyoid muscle	Manubrium of sternum	Hyoid bone	Pulls hyoid down	Cervical nerves II and III	Lingual artery and superior thyroid artery
Sternothyroid muscle	Sternum	Thyroid cartilage of larynx	Pulls larynx down	Cervical nerves II and III	Superior thyroid artery
Thyrohyoid muscle	Thyroid cartilage	Hyoid bone	Lifts larynx or depresses hyoid	Cervical nerve I	Superior thyroid artery

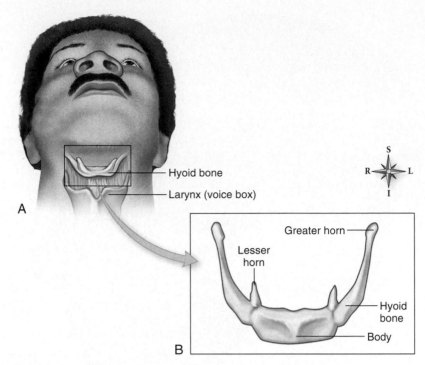

• **Figure 28.4** Hyoid bone. **(A)** Anterior view. **(B)** Superior view. This bone articulates with no other bone but is attached to other bones entirely by muscles. (From Patton KT, Thibodeau GA. *Anatomy & Physiology.* 8th ed. St. Louis, MO: Mosby; 2013.)

notch just medial to the mastoid process behind the ear. The fibers run forward and down to the area of the intermediate tendon, which attaches to the hyoid bone by a tendinous loop through which it can slide. From here the muscle fibers extend forward and slightly up to be inserted into the digastric fossa on the inferior surface of the mandible at the midline (Figs. 28.5 and 28.6).

The action of this muscle is twofold. By contracting, it can create a backward pull on the mandible, thus retruding it. If the jaw is clenched, contraction of the muscle elevates the hyoid bone and lifts up on the larynx or voice box. It can also aid in pulling the mandible down if the infrahyoid muscles pull the hyoid bone down.

The digastric muscle is also unusual in that it has two nerves supplying it. The anterior part of the muscle is supplied by the third part of the trigeminal nerve (V_3), and the posterior part is supplied by the facial nerve (VII). What does that tell you about the pharyngeal arch origin of these muscles?

Mylohyoid Muscle

The **mylohyoid muscle** forms what is called the *floor of the mouth.* The muscle originates from the mylohyoid line on the medial surface of each side of the mandible, running down and inserting into the hyoid bone. The left and right muscles also fuse together in the midline of the neck. This type of fusion is known as the **raphe**. The action is related to the depression of the mandible or the elevation of the hyoid bone. The nerve supply is the mylohyoid branch of V_3 (trigeminal). The blood supply is a branch of the inferior alveolar artery (see Figs. 28.5 and 28.6).

Geniohyoid Muscle

The **geniohyoid muscle** originates from the inferior genial tubercle or mental spine on the lingual surface of the mandible at the midline. It lies deep to the mylohyoid muscle, running down

and back to insert into the hyoid bone by the midline. It also acts as a depressor of the mandible or elevator of the hyoid bone. Its nerve supply comes from the first cervical nerve in the neck. The blood supply is a branch of the lingual artery (Fig. 28.7).

Stylohyoid Muscle

The **stylohyoid muscle** takes its origin from the styloid process of the base of the skull. The muscle runs down and forward to insert into the posterior part of the hyoid bone. At its insertion on the hyoid bone, the muscle splits and part of the posterior portion of the digastric muscle passes through it. The action of the muscle is to pull the hyoid bone back and up. The nerve supply is a branch of the facial nerve (VII), which also supplies the posterior belly of the digastric muscle. The facial and occipital arteries provide its blood supply (see Figs. 28.5 and 28.6).

Infrahyoid Group

Omohyoid Muscle

The two muscular bellies of the **omohyoid muscle** are separated by an intermediate tendon. One of the bellies arises from the upper border of the scapula (shoulder blade), and the other arises from the hyoid bone. The two bellies are joined by an intermediate tendon deep to the **sternomastoid (sternocleidomastoid) muscle** in the side of the neck. When the muscle contracts, it pulls the hyoid bone down. The nerve supply comes from the second and third cervical nerves, and the blood supply from the lingual and superior thyroid arteries (see Figs. 28.5 and 28.6).

Sternohyoid Muscle

The **sternohyoid muscle** takes its origin from the upper border of the manubrium of the sternum. It runs up to be inserted into the

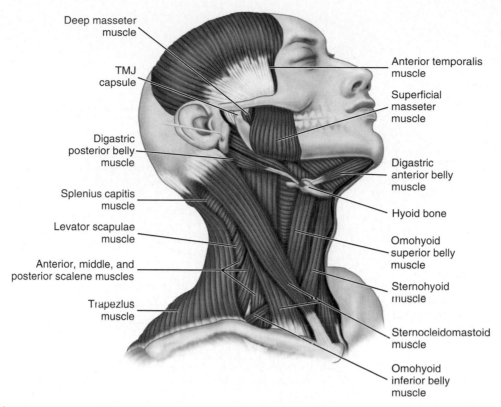

• **Figure 28.5** Lateral view of the neck showing the digastric muscle suspended above the hyoid bone and attaching to it by a ligamentous loop. Mylohyoid and stylohyoid muscles are also visible above the hyoid bone, and omohyoid, thyrohyoid, and sternohyoid muscles are visible below the hyoid bone. Also, the large sternocleidomastoid muscle covers a large area on the side of the neck. (From Nelson SJ, Ash M. *Wheeler's Dental Anatomy.* 9th ed. St. Louis, MO: Saunders; 2010.)

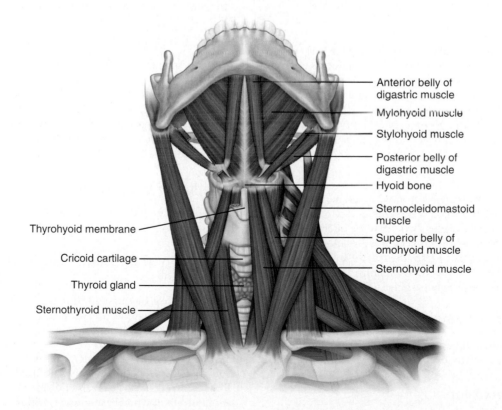

• **Figure 28.6** Anterior/inferior view of the mylohyoid muscle. Left and right muscles fuse in the midline and form a slinglike arrangement that forms the mouth floor. You can also see the anterior view of digastric, stylohyoid, sternohyoid, sternothyroid, and sternocleidomastoid muscles. (From Fonseca RJ, Barber HD, Powers M, et al. *Oral and Maxillofacial Trauma.* St. Louis, MO: Saunders; 2013.)

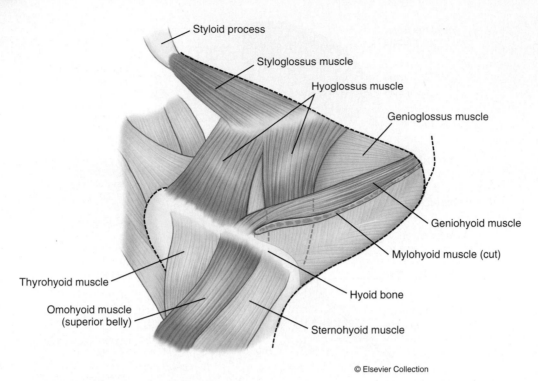

Styloid process

Styloglossus muscle

Hyoglossus muscle

Genioglossus muscle

Geniohyoid muscle

Mylohyoid muscle (cut)

Hyoid bone

Sternohyoid muscle

Thyrohyoid muscle

Omohyoid muscle
(superior belly)

© Elsevier Collection

• **Figure 28.7** With the mylohyoid muscle cut away, the geniohyoid muscle extends from the genial tubercles of the mandible down to the hyoid bone.

front part of the body of the hyoid bone. When the muscle contracts, it pulls the hyoid bone down. Its nerve supply is from the second and third cervical nerves. Its blood supply is the lingual and superior thyroid arteries (see Figs. 28.5 and 28.6).

Sternothyroid Muscle

The **sternothyroid muscle** arises from the upper part of the sternum, running up to be inserted onto an oblique line on the side of the thyroid cartilage of the larynx. It is not easily seen because the sternohyoid muscle tends to lie superior to it. When the muscle contracts, it pulls the larynx down. The nerve supply comes from the second and third cervical nerves. The blood supply is from the superior thyroid artery (Fig. 28.8; also see Fig. 28.6.)

Thyrohyoid Muscle

The **thyrohyoid muscle** originates from the oblique line on the lateral side of the thyroid cartilage, which serves as the insertion of the sternothyroid muscle. The fibers run up to be inserted into the hyoid bone. When the muscle contracts, it either lifts the thyroid cartilage and raises the **larynx** or helps depress the hyoid bone. The first cervical nerve provides the nerve supply, and the superior thyroid artery is the blood supply (see Figs. 28.5 and 28.8).

Movements of the Jaw and Larynx

The following is a brief description of the movements accomplished by the muscles of mastication and the hyoid muscles.

Mandibular Protrusion

Lateral pterygoid muscles acting together produce mandibular **protrusion**.

Mandibular Retrusion

The posterior or horizontal fibers of the temporal muscle, as well as the digastric muscle, accomplish **retrusion** of the mandible.

Lateral Excursion of the Mandible

One of the lateral pterygoid muscles acting by itself accomplishes **lateral excursion**. If the left lateral pterygoid muscle contracts, the left condyle is pulled forward, and the mandible will move to the right. Contraction of the right lateral pterygoid muscle accomplishes the opposite movement. While the one lateral pterygoid is contracting, the opposite elevators of the mandible hold the other condyle in place (Fig. 28.9).

Elevation of the Mandible

The medial pterygoid, masseter, and temporal muscles accomplish **elevation**.

Depression of the Mandible, Opening of the Mouth

The **depression** of the mandible is accomplished by the inferior head of the lateral pterygoid muscle plus hyoid muscles. Remember that this includes suprahyoid and infrahyoid muscles. If the mandible is to be depressed, it is important that infrahyoid muscles contract and pull down on the hyoid bone. Once the hyoid bone is stabilized or held down from below, contraction of suprahyoid muscles can aid in pulling the mandible down. These muscles influence the inferior head of the lateral pterygoid muscle to accomplish depression of the mandible.

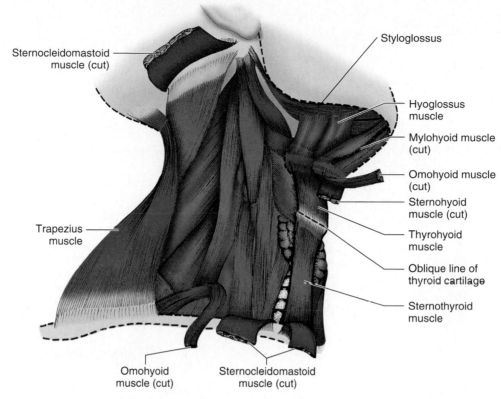

• **Figure 28.8** Lateral view of the neck, with several muscles cut and turned back (reflected). Note the extent of sternothyroid and thyrohyoid muscles.

Laryngeal Movements

The larynx moves up and down in swallowing and phonation. For this to be accomplished, certain muscles must contract. Before continuing, try this demonstration. Place your fingers lightly on the larynx and swallow. What happens? The larynx moves up and under the shelter of the **epiglottis**, which moves back over the laryngeal opening so that anything being swallowed would pass over the laryngeal opening and enter the esophagus. Actually, most of this action is accomplished by the tongue moving the food to the back of the mouth and pushing back on the epiglottis. If this action did not take place, you could choke when trying to swallow food. The hyoid bone is pulled slightly up by the contraction of suprahyoid muscles. The thyrohyoid muscle then contracts, elevating the thyroid cartilage of the larynx and, along with the contraction of the muscles attached to the epiglottis and the backward movement of the tongue, moves the epiglottis over the opening of the larynx, allowing the swallowed material to enter the esophagus (Fig. 28.10).

This, by no means, covers all the muscles in the neck area, but it does include those most closely involved in mandibular and laryngeal movements, providing a better understanding of some of the controls of mastication and swallowing (**deglutition**).

Sternocleidomastoid Muscle

In an extraoral examination of a patient, it is necessary to press or palpate beneath the posterior border of the sternocleidomastoid muscle to check for enlargement of the lymph nodes lying against the internal jugular vein in the neck. This muscle is also involved in referred pain.

The sternocleidomastoid muscle has its origin in the upper border of the sternum and the medial one-third of the clavicle or collarbone. The muscle runs up and back on the side of the neck to insert into the mastoid process of the temporal bone. The action of the muscle is involved in tilting and rotating the head. It is innervated by the eleventh (XI) cranial nerve (accessory nerve), and its blood supply is a branch of the external carotid artery (see Figs. 28.5 and 28.6; see Table 28.3).

Trapezius Muscle

The **trapezius muscle** takes its origin from the external occipital protuberance on the occipital bone and from the bony ridges on the vertebrae by means of the ligamentum nuchae. The superior nuchal lines run lateral from the vertebrae to the trapezius muscle. It also originates from the spinous processes of cervical and thoracic vertebrae. Its insertion is into the spine of the scapula, the acromial process of the scapula, and the lateral one-third of the clavicle. Its function is to **adduct** and elevate the scapula and to slightly rotate it (see Figs. 28.5 and 28.8). Shrugging of shoulders is a major function of the trapezius muscle. Some work, such as typing at an improper height, can cause pain in the trapezius as a result of holding the arms in a raised position while doing the work. The superficial branch of the transverse cervical artery is the principal blood supply of the trapezius muscle.

Sternomastoid and trapezius muscles can involuntarily contract under tension or in conjunction with migraine headaches. Some malocclusions can also cause such spasms. Because these muscles have some of their sensory nerve supply from the second, third, and fourth cervical nerves, they are in close approximation

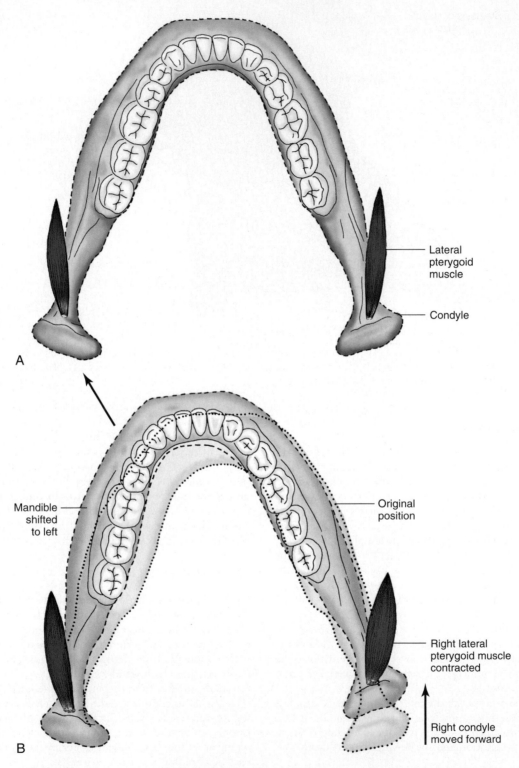

Lateral pterygoid muscle

Condyle

A

Mandible shifted to left

Original position

Right lateral pterygoid muscle contracted

Right condyle moved forward

B

• **Figure 28.9** (A) Superior view of the mandible in rest position showing the condyles and lateral pterygoid muscles. (B) The right lateral pterygoid muscle has contracted, pulling the condyle on that side forward. The mandible swings to the opposite side, as shown by the *dashed line* and *arrow*.

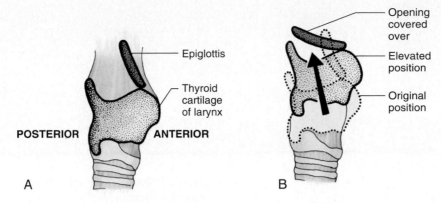

• **Figure 28.10** (A) Thyroid cartilage of the larynx and epiglottis is suspended in part from the hyoid bone. (B) As the suprahyoid muscles are contracted along with the thyrohyoid muscle, the larynx is elevated, and the epiglottis moves back and down to cover the laryngeal opening.

TABLE 28.3 Muscles of the Neck

Muscle	Origin	Insertion	Action	Nerve Innervation	Arterial Supply
Sternocleidomastoid muscle	Upper border of sternum and medial third of clavicle	Mastoid process	Tilts and rotates head	Cranial nerve XI	External carotid artery
Trapezius muscle	External occipital protuberance of occipital bone and spinous processed of cervical and thoracic vertebrae	Scapula and clavicle	Adducts and elevates scapula, slightly rotates scapula	Cranial nerves II, III, and IV	Superficial transverse cervical artery

to the lower part of the trigeminal nerve nucleus in the upper spinal cord. This can at times cause pain to emanate from the area of the TMJ. Many people come to dental offices complaining of TMJ pain. When nothing wrong can be found within the joint or associated muscles, one might try to anesthetize the sternomastoid and/or trapezius muscle. If the pain in the joint disappears, this would confirm that the anesthetized muscle is the offending culprit. This illustrates the importance of considering all muscles, even the muscles of mastication, when diagnosing problems in the area of the TMJ.

Review Questions

1. How can you distinguish the origin of a muscle from its insertion?
2. Describe the action of a muscle.
3. Define or describe the following terms in relation to mandibular movements:
   a. elevation
   b. protrusion
   c. retrusion
   d. depression
   e. lateral excursion of the mandible
4. Name the muscles involved in creating the actions mentioned in question 3.
5. What does the fact that the anterior belly of the digastric muscle is innervated by the trigeminal nerve, and the posterior belly is innervated by the facial nerve, tell you about the embryologic origin of the muscle?
6. Which groups of muscles affect the movements of the larynx?
7. Of the hyoid muscles, which group is found below the hyoid bone?
8. What is referred pain? What muscles can refer pain to the TMJ?
9. Which suprahyoid and infrahyoid muscles are innervated by cervical nerves as opposed to cranial nerves?

29

Temporomandibular Joint

OBJECTIVES

- To diagram and label a sagittal section of the temporomandibular joint (TMJ)
- To define the role of a synovial cavity
- To describe the two movements of the TMJ as the mouth opens and know where these movements take place
- To describe the role of the superior posterior elastic lamina, the inferior posterior collagenous lamina, and the superior and inferior heads of the lateral pterygoid muscle as the jaw goes through its various functional movements
- To define disc derangement, subluxation, bruxism, and TMJ sounds
- To discuss probable causes of TMJ pain

Structure

As the name indicates, the **temporomandibular joint** (TMJ) is the articulation between the temporal bone and the mandible. A joint is a joining together of two bones, and there are a number of joint types. A suture of the skull is one type of joint that we have already studied (see Chapter 26), and the TMJ is another type because it is a joint where the surface of one bone moves over the surface of another.

Actually, the TMJ comprises two joints that move and function as one. It is also a bilateral, or two-sided, joint in that the mandible is fused at the midline so that the left and right joints are interrelated in their movements. In Chapter 26, you learned the osteology or the system of bony parts of the TMJ. Fig. 29.1 shows the mandibular fossa, posterior tubercle, and articular eminence of the temporal bone, as well as the condyle of the mandible. Between these two bones, you can see a small fibrous pad of dense collagen tissue called the **articular disc**. The upper surface of the disc is concave and convex to match the contours of the **mandibular fossa** and the articular eminence, whereas the lower surface of the disc is concave to match the contour of the condyle. Fig. 29.1 shows that the articular disc is thickest at its posterior end, it is thinnest at its middle, and there is a slight increase in thickness at its anterior end. The thick posterior area is called the *posterior band,* the thin middle area is called the *intermediate zone,* and the slightly thicker anterior area is called the *anterior band.* Above and below this disc are small, saclike compartments called **synovial cavities**. Part of the tissue lining these cavities is an epithelium that secretes a few drops of lubricating liquid called **synovial fluid**, which allows the surfaces to rub over one another without irritation. The **synovium** is the covering that lines the synovial cavity.

The entire TMJ is surrounded by a thick fibrous capsule. The lateral side of this capsule is thickened between the articular tubercle and the lateral pole of the condyle. This thickened area is the **temporomandibular ligament**. This ligament prevents the condyle from being displaced too far inferiorly and posteriorly and provides some resistance to lateral displacement (Fig. 29.2). On the medial side are two other ligaments that help to control the movement of the TMJ. They are the **stylomandibular ligament** and the **sphenomandibular ligament**.

The articular disc is attached both medially and laterally to the poles of the condyle (Fig. 29.3). Anteriorly it is attached to some fibers of the superior head of the lateral pterygoid muscle. These fibers penetrate the capsule and insert into the disc. The area posterior to the disc is the **retrodiscal pad**. This is an area composed of relatively loose connective tissue in which much of the blood and nerve supply to the joint is located. The blood supply comes from the **ascending pharyngeal**, **superficial temporal**, **deep auricular**, and **anterior tympanic arteries**. All these arteries branch directly or indirectly off of the *external carotid artery*. The nerve supply to the joint comes from the following three branches of the third division of the *trigeminal nerve*: **auriculotemporal**, **deep temporal**, and **masseteric nerves**. Running from the upper posterior part of the disc is an elastic lamina or tissue layer that lies above the retrodiscal pad. Posteriorly, it attaches to the tympanic plate of the temporal bone. Running from the lower posterior border of the disc is a collagenous lamina that lies below the retrodiscal pad and attaches to the posterior neck of the condyle, where the capsule attaches to it (see Fig. 29.1).

Movement

The TMJ has two distinct types of movement—a rotational movement and a gliding movement along an inclined plane. This is frequently called a *hinge and sliding joint* or a *gliding joint*. As teeth begin to separate (the first few millimeters), there is a rotational movement in the lower synovial cavity between the disc and the condyle below. The reason for the rotational movement is the posterior elastic lamina. As the condyle begins rotating, the disc wants to move anteriorly with it because it is attached to the poles of the condyle. However, the elastic lamina pulls posteriorly on the disc, and the disc and condyle rotate on one another. As the jaw opens farther, the rotational movement continues, but an additional anterior gliding movement along the posterior slope of the articular eminence also occurs. This gliding movement takes place between the disc and the temporal bone above. The forward movement is caused by contraction of the inferior head of the lateral pterygoid muscle (see Chapter 28). The condyle and the disc move forward until they reach a point just slightly anterior to the crest of the articular eminence.

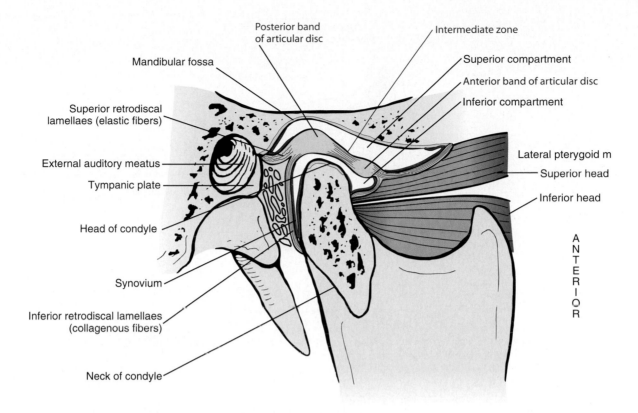

Posterior band of articular disc

Intermediate zone

Mandibular fossa

Superior compartment

Anterior band of articular disc

Inferior compartment

Superior retrodiscal lamellaes (elastic fibers)

External auditory meatus

Tympanic plate

Lateral pterygoid m

Superior head

Inferior head

Head of condyle

Synovium

Inferior retrodiscal lamellaes (collagenous fibers)

Neck of condyle

ANTERIOR

• **Figure 29.1** Longitudinal section through the temporomandibular joint (TMJ). Synovium is marked in red; the inferior retrodiscal lamellae, disc, and attachments are gray. (From Liebgott B. *The Anatomical Basis of Dentistry*. 3rd ed. St. Louis: Mosby; 2011.)

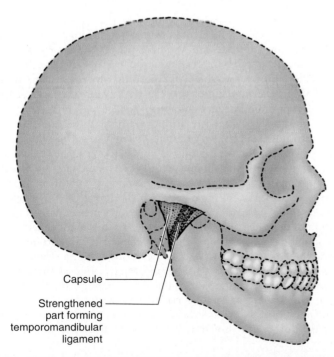

Capsule

Strengthened part forming temporomandibular ligament

• **Figure 29.2** The capsule surrounding the entire temporomandibular joint (TMJ). The capsule is strengthened on the deep side of the lateral surface by the temporomandibular ligament, which helps prevent lateral, posterior, and inferior movements of the condyle out of the fossa.

When the jaw moves back into a centric relation, the superior head of the lateral pterygoid controls the posterior movement of the disc by controlling the release of its contraction and balancing the posterior pull exerted by the elastic lamina. The lower posterior collagenous lamina prevents the elastic lamina and disc from being pulled too far forward, thereby preventing injury.

During chewing, the mandible is depressed by the hyoid muscles, and the lateral pterygoid muscle pulls forward and down. As this depression takes place, the lateral pterygoid muscle opposite the chewing side pulls forward even more, causing the mandible to move into a lateral excursion to the chewing side. As you begin the power stroke and elevate the mandible and begin to bite down on a thick piece of food placed between the teeth on the chewing side, the condyle on that side will be in a position where the condyle, disc, and temporal bone are in contact with one another. However, on the nonchewing side, as you continue to bite down, the condyle, disc, and temporal surfaces will be pulled slightly apart. This makes the nonchewing side of the joint somewhat unstable, which could cause the surfaces to bounce against one another and possibly injure the structures. However, this does not happen because the superior head of the lateral pterygoid muscle contracts, pulling the disc forward. In doing so, it moves the thicker posterior part of the disc forward, which fills the space created by the surfaces moving slightly apart and so it balances and stabilizes the joint on that side. With continued contraction, the posterior fibers of the temporalis muscle on the nonchewing side contract, pulling back on the coronoid process

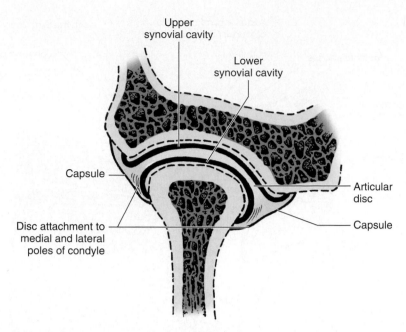

• **Figure 29.3** From left to right, a frontal section through the condyle, disc capsule, and fossa. The disc fibers curve down to insert into the poles of the condyle.

and thus pulling the condyle posteriorly, causing the occlusal surface of mandibular teeth to grind the food as the mandible moves from lateral excursion back into a more centric position. By slowly relaxing its contracted fibers, the upper head of the lateral pterygoid muscle controls the posterior movement of the disc with a posterior pull from the superior elastic lamina, and a smooth closing movement takes place.

Problems Associated With the TMJ

There is a myriad of problems associated with the TMJ, and in many cases, there is disagreement over how these problems should be treated. The following discussion presents some of these problems and their possible causes. It is quite likely that you will see many of these cases in the office, where they will be either treated or referred elsewhere for treatment.

Pain in the TMJ Area

Many patients complain of pain in the region of the TMJ. If radiographic studies show a normal TMJ and there does not seem to be any pain upon palpation of the area, the possibility of referred pain should be considered (see Chapter 28). Referred pain is a condition in which sensory messages, seemingly coming from the area of the TMJ, are actually traveling to the brain from other regions of the body. Often such pain comes from spasms in neck muscles and from the muscles of mastication. Muscle relaxants or physical therapy allow these muscles to relax and subsequently relieve the pain. In Chapter 34, you will study the cranial nerves. Four of these nerves—the cranial nerves V, VII, IX, and X—supply the sensory areas around the ear. Involvement of these nerves may cause pain that seems to come from the TMJ. Pain in the TMJ may also come from malocclusion, caused by shifting, wear, or loss of teeth. (It should be pointed out here, in reference to pain originating in the disc, that the central portion of the disc has no nerve supply, which is why a hole can be worn through the

disc and not be recognized. The medial and lateral attachments of the disc to the condyle and anterior and posterior attachments are in areas that have nerve supply, and injury to those areas will cause significant pain.) Many of these problems are referred to as **myofascial pain dysfunction (MPD)**, which involves a myriad of possible factors.

Internal Problems of the TMJ

TMJ Sounds

Many patients complain of a popping, clicking, or grinding *(crepitus)* in the TMJ and yet have no other symptoms, such as pain. The popping or clicking noise may occur when the disc is pulled too far forward in the opening movement. The thick posterior band of the disc gets caught between the head of the condyle and the articular eminence. It then pops forward and is displaced too far anteriorly. It may also pop posteriorly from its trapped position. This closing sound would be called a *reciprocal* pop or click. Often the dentist is not able to hear the clicking or popping without the aid of a stethoscope. Sometimes by palpating the joint as popping occurs, a jumping movement of the condyle can be felt as the disc pops forward. If this only happens on one side, you can frequently see the movement by standing in front of the patient and observing whether the mandible moves in a straight downward movement or whether it shifts to one side and then moves back to the midline during opening. These problems can be treated with ultrasonography, physical therapy, or application of a plastic splint similar to a night guard. The grinding sound (crepitus) may be caused by adhesions in the synovial membranes of the joint, arthritic changes, or possibly perforations of the disc. It can also be treated by ultrasonography, although it may recur.

Disc Derangement

The cause of TMJ sounds may also be the result of a type of disc derangement. In constant anterior displacement of the disc,

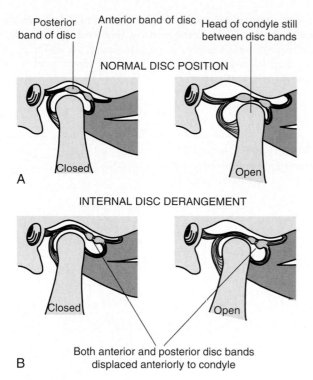

NORMAL DISC POSITION

Posterior band of disc   Anterior band of disc   Head of condyle still between disc bands

A
Closed   Open

INTERNAL DISC DERANGEMENT

B
Closed   Open

Both anterior and posterior disc bands displaced anteriorly to condyle

• **Figure 29.4 (A)** The condyle rides forward to the height of articular eminence. The anterior band of the disc stays forward of the condyle, and the posterior band stays behind the condyle. The jaw opens normally. **(B)** If the posterior band slips anterior to the condyle, then both the anterior and posterior bands of the disc are anterior to the condyle, and this becomes an internal disc derangement. If the posterior disc moves posterior to the condyle a popping noise might be heard as the disc jumps over the articular eminence as the jaw opens. If a second *reciprocal* click or pop is heard when the jaw closes, the posterior band is jumping anterior to the condyle and reproduces the internal derangement.

permanent damage to the components of the disc may occur. The posterior laminae may be torn and the disc permanently displaced anteriorly. The medial or lateral attachments of the disc to the poles of the condyle may be torn. If this happens, the tear is usually to the lateral pole attachment. Both circumstances will probably require surgery, which tends to be fairly successful (Fig. 29.4).

Subluxation

A condition in which a person opens his or her mouth too wide and is not able to close it again or closing it causes a popping back into position is called **subluxation**. This happens when the condyle glides too far forward and moves anterior to the articular eminence. If this happens the condyle cannot reposition itself in its proper place. The condyle remains forward, and when the patient tries to close his or her mouth, the condyle cannot move back because the muscles are trying to pull up and back, and the articular eminence does not allow the condyle to move back. If a patient cannot close the mouth, place your thumbs on the occlusal surface of mandibular posterior teeth with the index fingers beneath the inferior border of the mandible, and push down while guiding the jaw slowly back into its posterior position. It is advisable to wrap your thumbs in gauze so that they are protected in case the patient closes down on them. A posterior bite block is sometimes used to help relax the muscles and to allow a pivot

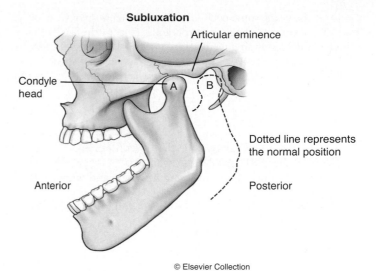

Subluxation

Articular eminence

Condyle head

A   B

Dotted line represents the normal position

Anterior   Posterior

© Elsevier Collection

• **Figure 29.5** A subluxation or partial dislocation of the joint occurs if the condyle comes so far anterior to the articular eminence that the condyle pops over the eminence and superior to it. At this point, the condyle cannot move back to its correct position, because it cannot jump back over the eminence. The condyle is trapped anterior to the eminence, and the jaw cannot be closed. The jaw remains in a locked open position until treated.

point to help manipulate the lower jaw. In general, there are several reasons for subluxation. One is the depth of the condylar fossa and the height of the articular eminence. Another is the position of the capsule around the joint, a factor that controls the amount of contraction of the lateral pterygoid muscle. This problem can be treated by surgically decreasing the height of the articular eminence (Fig. 29.5).

Bruxism

Many people grind their teeth; this is called **bruxism**. Most of the time this is done during sleep, although it does occur sometimes during waking hours. Over a long period, it may wear down teeth, but a more immediate result is a very tired and sore TMJ. Much of this tenderness has to do with the muscles of mastication tiring, yet it is the joint that seems to ache. One method of treatment is to make a plastic night guard to cover maxillary teeth. To a great extent, this eliminates excessive wear on teeth and tenderness of teeth caused by stress on the periodontal ligament. In other patients, tranquilizers may be used to relieve the tension that may contribute to the bruxism.

Arthritis and Other Pain in the TMJ

The TMJ is also subject to such conditions as **arthritis** and the pain that results from it. **Cortisone** may relieve arthritis, but the pain can still be a major problem. Other patients have a grinding sensation in the joint. Some contend that this is caused by excessive wear of the disc in the joint so that there is no longer a smooth gliding movement within the synovial cavities. This explanation seems very reasonable because the TMJ is a stress-bearing joint, and too much stress may cause it to wear out early in life and cause problems. However, there are reports of cases in which both condyles were fractured so severely that they had to be removed surgically, and the patients continued to function well without a real joint, which tells us that not enough is known about the TMJ and that it is more complex than was formerly believed.

Over the years, some occlusal surfaces of teeth may wear away, and the person may begin to experience pain in the TMJ. Many times, simply rebuilding teeth to their original height with crowns and onlays eases the pain. It is generally agreed that most of the problems in these cases do not arise in the joint itself but in the muscles of mastication, other head and neck muscles, and the occlusion of teeth. With changes in the relationship of the jaws caused by tooth wear, the muscles of mastication are no longer in their normal relaxed position. Therefore they might tend to go into **spasms** and cause pain.

Review Questions

1. What is a synovial cavity, and what is its function?
2. Describe the TMJ capsule and ligament.
3. What are the two TMJ movements? Where and when do they occur?
4. Describe the roles of the posterior laminae and the lateral pterygoid muscle in mastication.
5. What are some causes of TMJ pain?
6. What might cause TMJ sounds?
7. What is a disc derangement?

30
Muscles of Facial Expression

OBJECTIVES

- To name the various groupings or locations of the muscles of facial expression and their nerve innervations
- To describe the muscles of facial expression and their origins, insertions, and actions (not including the mouth)
- To name all the muscles surrounding the mouth and their origins, insertions, and actions
- To discuss the role of the buccinator muscle in mastication

The term *facial expression* in the chapter title may be a bit misleading because the muscles included in this chapter are located around the ears, scalp, neck, eyes, nose, and mouth. However, although some of them are not located in an area normally considered the face, they are located in areas that can physically display some kind of emotion or attentiveness. All these muscles are innervated by cranial nerve VII (facial nerve). Although most of the muscles are mentioned here, only the muscles around the oral cavity are discussed in great detail. These are the muscles you will be most concerned with in the dental office, and they are responsible for some functions related to speech and mastication.

Ears

The muscles around the ears are not well developed in humans. However, in lower forms of animals, they are better developed, and the ears can be easily moved and repositioned to better perceive sounds. There are three pairs of ear muscles (Fig. 30.1 and Table 30.1).

Anterior Auricular Muscle

The **anterior auricular muscle** arises from connective tissue of the scalp in front of the ear and runs posteriorly into the anterior part of the ear. The action of this muscle pulls the ear slightly forward.

Superior Auricular Muscle

The **superior auricular muscle** arises from connective tissue of the scalp above the ear, and the fibers run down and insert into the upper part of the ear. The action of this muscle raises the ear.

Posterior Auricular Muscle

The **posterior auricular muscle** arises from the **superior nuchal line** of the occipital bone and the mastoid area. The fibers run forward to insert into the posterior part of the ear. The action of this muscle pulls the ear back. This is probably the best developed of the ear muscles.

Scalp

The muscles of the scalp allow for its mobility both forward and backward (Table 30.2).

Occipitofrontalis (Epicranius)

The **occipitofrontalis (epicranius)** is a paired muscle with groups of fibers in front and back connected by a broad flat band of **fascia**. The anterior and posterior groups of muscle fibers take their origin from connective tissue of the scalp. This kind of attachment allows for either forward or backward movement of the scalp. The forward movement results in a frown or a squint, and the backward movement raises the forehead skin, as in surprise (see Fig. 30.1).

Neck

You may wonder how a muscle in the neck can show facial expression. However, pulling down the corners of the mouth, as in a grimace, is partly accomplished by the platysma muscle in the neck (Table 30.3).

Platysma

There is some disagreement as to which end of the **platysma** is the origin and which one the insertion. The upper end of the fibers attaches to the inferior border of the mandible, near the angles of the mouth and the skin of the face in that area. They pass down in a broad flat sheet to end in the skin of the chest area just below the clavicle. The muscle lies just below the skin of the neck; thus it moves the skin over the neck quite noticeably when it contracts, pulling the corners of the mouth down (see Fig. 30.1).

Eyes

Several muscles located around the eyes close the eyes and move the eyebrows (Table 30.4; see Fig. 30.1).

Orbicularis Oculi

Although the Latin term **orbicularis oculi** may be difficult to understand, by studying it carefully you can infer its meaning. The term *orbicularis* relates to the word *circular*, and it is easy to understand how the orbicularis oculi muscle encircles the eye.

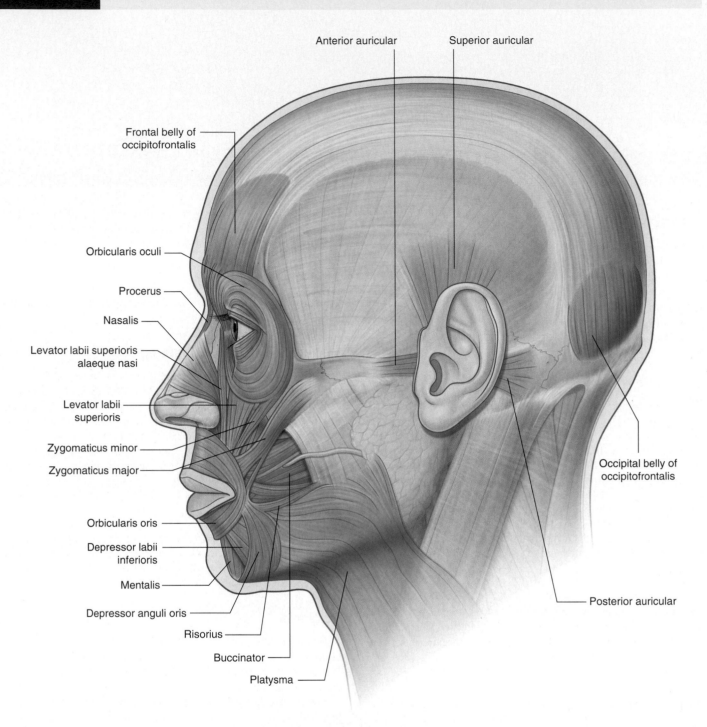

• **Figure 30.1** Muscles of facial expression lateral view. (From Drake R., Vogl, W. (2014). Gray's Anatomy for students, (3rd ed.). Churchill Livingston).

TABLE 30.1	**Muscles of the Ear**			
Muscle	**Origin**	**Insertion**	**Function**	**Nerve Innervation**
Anterior auricular muscle	Scalp in front of ear	Anterior ear	Pulls the ear forward	Cranial nerve VII
Superior auricular muscle	Scalp above ear	Upper ear	Raises ear	Cranial nerve VII
Posterior auricular muscle	Superior nuchal line	Posterior ear	Pulls ear back	Cranial nerve VII

TABLE 30.2 Muscle of the Scalp

Muscle	Origin	Insertion	Function	Nerve Innervation
Occipitofrontalis	Connective tissue of scalp		Moves scalp forward or backward	Cranial nerve VII

TABLE 30.3 Muscle of the Neck

Muscle	Origin	Insertion	Function	Nerve Innervation
Platysma	Skin below clavicle	Inferior border of mandible	Pulls corners of mouth down	Cranial nerve VII

TABLE 30.4 Muscles of the Eye

Muscle	Origin	Insertion	Function	Nerve Innervation
Orbicularis oculi	Medial and lateral edges of eye	Medial and lateral corners of eye	Closes eyelids	Cranial nerve VII
Corrugator	Bridge of nose	Lateral eyebrow	Pulls eyebrow medially and down	Cranial nerve VII
Procerus	Bridge of nose	Medial eyebrow	Pulls eyebrow down medially	Cranial nerve VII

There are two parts to the orbicularis oculi. The part that encircles the eye is the orbital part. It attaches to the skull at the medial and lateral edges of the orbit. The muscle fibers in the eyelid comprise the palpebral part. Their fibers also attach at the medial and lateral corners of the orbit. The action of the orbicularis oculi closes the eyelids and contracts the skin around the eye (see Fig. 30.2).

Corrugator

The **corrugator** runs from the bridge of the nose up and laterally to the lateral part of the eyebrow. It pulls the eyebrow medially and down, as in a frown (see Fig. 30.3).

Procerus

From the bridge of the nose, the fibers of the **procerus** extend up into the medial end of the eyebrow. They pull the eyebrow at the medial end down, as in a frown or a squint (see Figs. 30.1 and 30.2).

Nose

The muscles of the nose primarily encircle the opening of the nostrils (see Fig. 30.1). The nasalis is the muscle that opens and closes the nostrils. It is composed of two parts (Table 30.5).

Dilator Naris of the Nasalis

The **dilator naris** pulls down on the nostrils, causing them to flare or dilate.

Compressor Naris of the Nasalis

The **compressor naris** causes the nostrils to close or compress.

Mouth

The muscles grouped around the mouth influence expression and speech and aid in mastication. The pressure of these muscles on teeth helps hold teeth in alignment if the pressures are normal. Abnormal pressures caused by cheek biting, lip biting, and lip compression may cause them to move out of alignment (Table 30.6; see Figs. 30.2 and 30.3).

Orbicularis Oris

The **orbicularis oris** encircles the oral cavity in the tissue of the lip. It has some bony attachment at the anterior nasal spine and at the midline above the chin. The fibers encircle the lip like a purse string, and all the muscles surrounding the lips interlace with them. The action of the muscle is to close and compress the lips (see Figs. 30.1 and 30.3).

Levator Labii Superioris

The **levator labii superioris** elevates the upper lip. Its origin is just beneath the lower rim of the orbit. The fibers run down to be inserted into the fibers of the orbicularis oris of the upper lip, midway between the center of the lip and the corner of the mouth (see Figs. 30.1 and 30.3).

Zygomaticus Minor

The **zygomaticus minor** is a small muscle from the area of the zygomatic bone. The fibers run down and forward and insert into the orbicularis oris just lateral to the levator labii superioris. It also raises the upper lip, although it is usually a very poorly developed muscle and therefore does not exert great influence in this function (see Figs. 30.1 and 30.3).

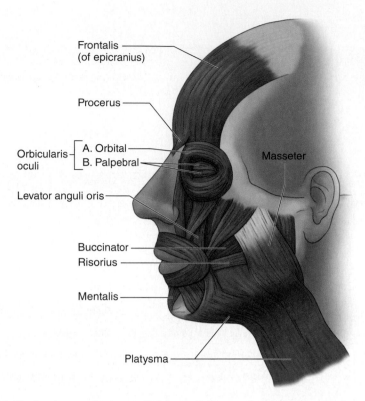

• **Figure 30.2** The levator anguli oris muscle is beneath the zygomaticus major muscle, which has been pushed aside to view the levator anguli oris muscle.

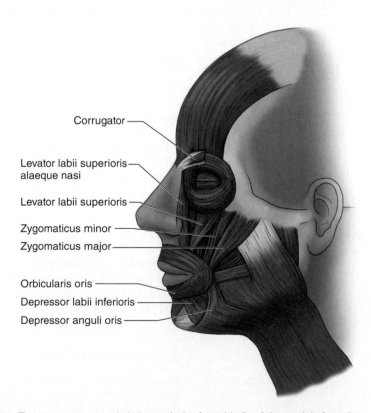

• **Figure 30.3** The corrugator muscle is beneath the frontal belly of the occipitofrontalis muscle and the orbicularis oculi muscle. A little of each of the latter two muscles is cut away to expose the corrugator muscle.

TABLE 30.5 Muscles of the Nose

Nasalis Muscle	Origin	Insertion	Function	Nerve Innervation
Dilator naris	Base of nose	Lateral of nose	Pulls nostrils down to flare	Cranial nerve VII
Compressor naris	Nasal septum	Lateral of nose	Compresses nostrils	Cranial nerve VII

TABLE 30.6 Muscles of the Mouth

Muscle	Origin	Insertion	Function	Nerve Innervation
Orbicularis oris	Anterior nasal spine	Skin of lip	Closes and compresses lips	Cranial nerve VII
Levator labii superioris	Lower orbit	Orbicularis oris	Elevates upper lip	Cranial nerve VII
Zygomaticus minor	Zygomatic bone	Orbicularis oris	Raises upper lip	Cranial nerve VII
Zygomaticus major	Zygomatic bone	Orbicular oris/angle of mouth	Elevates corners of mouth	Cranial nerve VII
Levator anguli oris	Maxilla	Orbicular oris/ corners of mouth	Pulls angle of mouth up toward the midline	Cranial nerve VII
Depressor labii inferioris	Inferior border of mandible	Orbicular oris/middle of lower lip	Pulls lower lip down	Cranial nerve VII
Depressor anguli oris	Inferior border of mandible	Orbicularis oris/corners of mouth	Pulls corners of mouth down	Cranial nerve VII
Mentalis	Anterior surface of mandible	Skin of chin	Pulls skin of chin up	Cranial nerve VII
Buccinator	Pterygomandibular raphe	Orbicular oris/corners of mouth	Pulls corners of mouth back and compresses cheeks	Cranial nerve VII
Risorius	Angle of mandible	Skin at the corner of mouth	Aids in smiling	Cranial nerve VII

Zygomaticus Major

The **zygomaticus major** is the larger muscle originating from the zygomatic bone. Its origin is lateral to the zygomaticus minor on the most prominent portion of the cheek and runs down and forward to insert into the orbicularis oris at the angle of the mouth. Its action is to elevate the corners of the mouth, as in a smile (see Figs. 30.1 and 30.3).

Levator Anguli Oris

The **levator anguli oris** lies deep to the levator labii superioris, the zygomaticus major, and the zygomaticus minor. It originates from the maxilla, just below the infraorbital foramen. The fibers run down and laterally to blend into the orbicularis oris at the corners of the mouth. This muscle pulls the angles of the mouth up and toward the midline (see Figs. 30.1 and 30.2).

Depressor Labii Inferioris

The origin of the **depressor labii inferioris** is the area beneath the angles of the mouth and just above the inferior border of the mandible. The fibers run up and medially to insert into the fibers of the orbicularis oris toward the middle of the lower lip. This muscle pulls the lower lip down, as in a pout (see Figs. 30.1 and 30.3).

Depressor Anguli Oris

The origin of the **depressor anguli oris** is from the same general area as that of the depressor labii inferioris, and the fibers of the former partly overlap the latter. From the origin, the fibers run up and converge in a triangular shape to blend into the orbicularis oris at the angle of the mouth. This muscle pulls the corners of the mouth down. Many of these fibers appear to be a continuation of the fibers of the platysma (see Figs. 30.1 and 30.3).

Mentalis

The **mentalis** originates on the anterior surface of the mandible, just beneath the lateral incisors. The fibers run down and toward the midline, where some even cross to meet the muscle on the opposite side, terminating with insertion into the skin of the chin. When the muscle contracts, it pulls this skin up (see Figs. 30.1, 30.2, and 30.4).

Buccinator

The **buccinator** is probably the most important muscle of the mouth (see Figs. 30.1, 30.2, and 30.4). Although it is a muscle of facial expression, it also plays a role in mastication. The muscle originates from a fibrous band (the **pterygomandibular raphe**), which runs from the pterygoid hamulus on the inferior portion of the medial pterygoid plate down to the medial surface of the

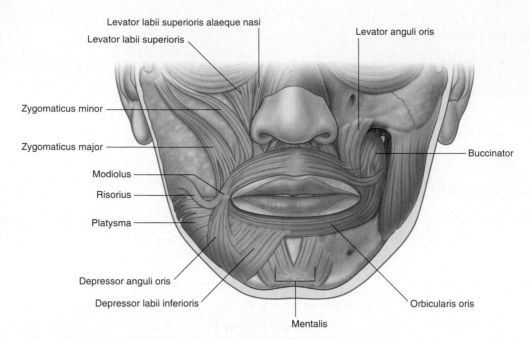

Levator labii superioris alaeque nasi
Levator labii superioris
Levator anguli oris
Zygomaticus minor
Zygomaticus major
Buccinator
Modiolus
Risorius
Platysma
Depressor anguli oris
Depressor labii inferioris
Orbicularis oris
Mentalis

• **Figure 30.4** The levator anguli oris and buccinator muscles are beneath the zygomatic and superioris muscles, which have been cut away on the right side of this picture. (From Drake R., Vogl, W. (2014). Gray's Anatomy for students, (3rd ed.). Churchill Livingston).

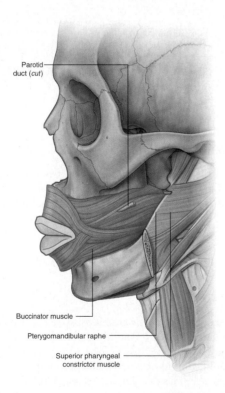

Parotid duct (cut)

Buccinator muscle
Pterygomandibular raphe
Superior pharyngeal constrictor muscle

• **Figure 30.5** Buccinator muscle. (From Drake R., Vogl, W. (2014). Gray's Anatomy for students, (3rd ed.). Churchill Livingston).

mandible near the posterior part of the mylohyoid line. The pterygomandibular raphe connects the anterior part of the **superior constrictor muscle** of the pharynx with the posterior part of the buccinator (see Fig. 30.5).

The buccinator also originates from the buccal alveolar bone of maxillary molars and from the corresponding area of mandibular molars. From these two bony origins and from the pterygomandibular raphe, the fibers of the buccinator run anteriorly, making up the musculature of the cheek. The fibers insert into the orbicularis oris at the corners of the mouth. When the muscle contracts, it pulls the corners of the mouth back and compresses the cheek. During chewing, the food is crushed and ground between the molars. As the food is squeezed out from the occlusal surfaces, some of the food is pushed onto the tongue, and the remainder is deposited into the buccal vestibule. The food on the tongue can be pushed back up onto the occlusal surface by the action of the tongue. The food that is forced out into the vestibule is pushed back up onto the occlusal surfaces, in part by the contraction of the buccinator muscle.

The buccinator muscle is frequently referred to as an *accessory muscle of mastication* because of the help it provides in chewing food. A person with paralysis of the facial muscles (Bell's palsy, or a stroke) would have difficulty chewing food. The food would pile up in the buccal vestibule and could not be forced back onto the chewing surfaces of the teeth. Because the buccinator cannot constrict, food is not forced out of the vestibule and up onto the occluding surfaces of the teeth.

The tongue acts as an oppositional muscle to the buccinator muscle in that the tongue forces food from the lingual toward the buccal and between the two muscles; food is kept balanced between the occluding surfaces of the teeth (see Chapter 24).

Risorius

The **risorius** is a small muscle that arises from the soft tissue near the angle of the mandible. It runs forward on the surface of the buccinator and inserts into the corner of the mouth. It aids in smiling but is usually very poorly developed. It also is an apparent continuation of the posterior fibers of the platysma muscle (see Fig. 30.2; Fig. 30.4).

All of the muscles of facial expression are innervated by cranial nerve VII (facial nerve).

Review Questions

1. Describe or name the head and neck locations of the muscles of facial expression.
2. Which nerve innervates the muscles of facial expression?
3. Of all the muscles of facial expression, which one is the most important for mastication? Why?

4. Describe where the following muscles enter the orbicularis oris muscle, the direction from which they enter, and their function:
   a. levator labii superioris
   b. zygomaticus minor
   c. zygomaticus major

31

Soft Palate and Pharynx

- To describe the origins, insertions, actions, and nerve supplies of the muscles of the soft palate and pharynx
- To describe the interrelationship of all of these muscles in chewing, swallowing, and speech

The muscles of the **soft palate** and **pharynx** are intricate in their arrangement and interrelationship. They share some common boundaries with the upper end of the digestive and respiratory systems and are important in the production of speech sounds. The soft palate forms the posterior end of the roof of the mouth. The pharynx has three components—the upper part, the nasal pharynx, is located at the posterior end of the nasal cavity; the middle part, the oral pharynx, is the back wall of the throat; and the lower part, the laryngeal pharynx, is below the tongue where the digestive and respiratory systems branch into their respective parts, the esophagus and the larynx.

Soft Palate

There are five pairs of muscles in the soft palate. These muscles help move the soft palate up and back to contact the posterior throat wall and seal off the nasal cavity from the oral cavity and also to narrow the space between the two palatine tonsils. This space is called the **fauces** and is used in swallowing. See Table 31.1 for muscles of the soft palate.

Palatoglossus Muscle

If you open the mouth and look at the area of the tonsils on the side of the throat wall, you will see that there is a vertical fold of tissue in front of and behind each tonsil. These are called the *anterior* and *posterior faucial pillars,* or the *palatoglossal* and *palatopharyngeal folds,* respectively. Beneath the palatoglossal fold is the **palatoglossus muscle**. It originates from the posterior end of the hard palate and the anterior end of the soft palate. The fibers run downward, laterally, and forward to insert into the posterolateral part of the tongue. When the palatoglossus muscle contracts, it pulls the sides of the tongue up and back, pulls the soft palate down on the lateral edges, and narrows the space between the left and right anterior faucial pillars. The nerve that supplies this muscle is a part of the eleventh cranial nerve (CN XI) running with branches of CN X (Figs. 31.1, 31.2).

Palatopharyngeus Muscle

The posterior faucial pillar is formed by the **palatopharyngeus muscle**. It originates from the posterolateral part of the soft palate and runs downward and laterally to insert into the pharyngeal constrictor muscle and the thyroid cartilage of the larynx. When it contracts, it narrows the posterior faucial pillar and elevates the pharynx and larynx. The nerve supply is also CNs X and XI (see Figs. 31.1 to 31.5).

TABLE 31.1 Muscles of the Soft Palate

Muscle	Origin	Insertion	Function	Nerve Innervation
Palatoglossus muscle	Posterior end of hard palate and anterior end of soft palate	Posterolateral part of tongue	Pulls sides of tongue back and down and pulls soft palate down, narrows space between fauces	Cranial nerve (CN) XI
Palatopharyngeus muscle	Posterolateral soft palate	Pharyngeal constrictor muscle and thyroid cartilage of larynx	Narrows posterior fauces pillar and elevates pharynx and larynx	CNs X and XI
Muscles of the uvula	Posterior end of hard palate	Soft palate	Shortens and broadens, changes contour of soft palate	CNs X and XI
Levator veli palatini	Temporal bone and medial wall of auditory canal	Posterior soft palate	Elevates posterior soft palate	CNs X and XI
Tensor veli palatini	Medial pterygoid plate and lateral wall of auditory canal	Posterior hard palate and anterior soft palate	Tenses anterior soft palate	CN V, division 3

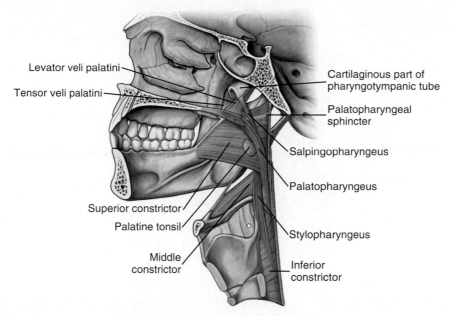

• **Figure 31.1** View of the lateral throat wall looking from the midline. The mucosa has been removed, and various muscles can be seen. Palatoglossal and palatopharyngeal muscles form anterior and posterior pillars, respectively; the palatine tonsil would lie between them. (From Drake RL, Vogl AW, Mitchell AWM, et al. *Gray's Atlas of Anatomy*. London, UK: Churchill Livingstone; 2008.)

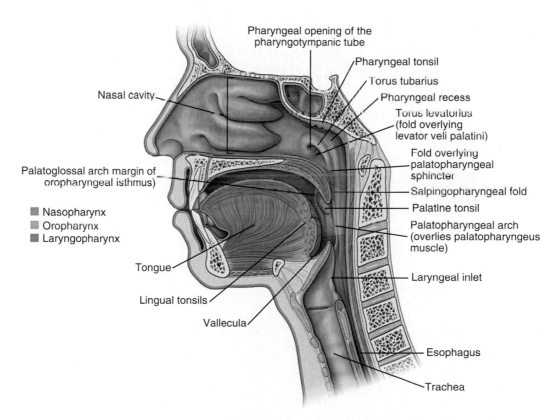

• **Figure 31.2** View of the lateral throat wall, similar to Fig. 31.1 but with the mucosa in place. Anterior and posterior pillars can be seen, as can the opening of the auditory tube in the nasal pharynx; the fold caused by the salpingopharyngeal muscle runs down from it. (From Drake RL, Vogl AW, Mitchell AWM, et al. *Gray's Atlas of Anatomy*. London, UK: Churchill Livingstone; 2008.)

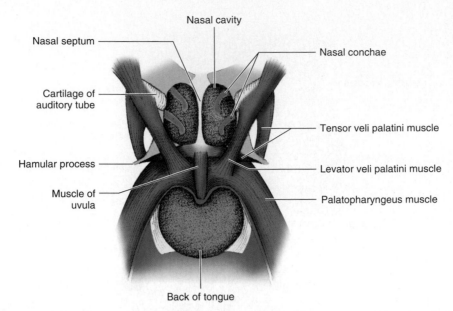

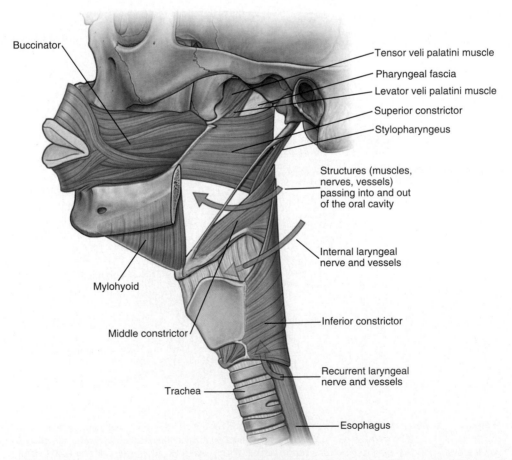

• **Figure 31.3** Posterior view of the muscles of the soft palate. The pharyngeal constrictor muscles have been removed, and the view is from behind the throat. Note especially how the levator veli palatine runs directly downward into the soft palate, whereas the tensor veli palatini runs downward and forward around the lateral side of the hamular process and then turns medially into the soft and hard palates. You can see how shortening of this muscle would help tense and raise the soft palate.

• **Figure 31.4** Lateral view of the pharyngeal constrictor muscles. Above them, you can see the tensor and levator veli palatini running downward into the soft palate. (From Drake RL, Vogl AW, Mitchell AWM, et al. *Gray's Atlas of Anatomy*. London, UK: Churchill Livingstone; 2008.)

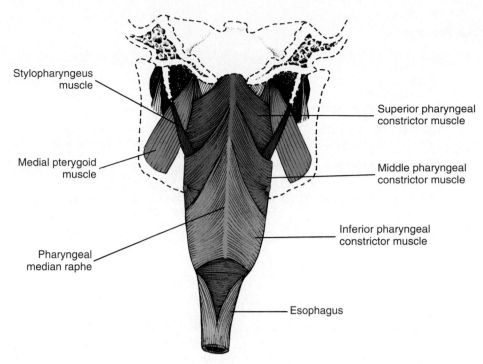

• **Figure 31.5** Posterior view of the pharyngeal wall. You can see overlapping of the pharyngeal constrictor muscles and the position of the stylopharyngeal muscle running down into them.

Muscle of the Uvula

The **uvula** is the small fold of tissue that hangs down in the throat from the posterior part of the soft palate. It is formed by two small bands of muscle, the left and right uvular muscles that originate from the posterior end of the hard palate and run back and down in the soft palate to form that structure. When the **muscle of the uvula** contracts, it shortens and broadens the uvula and changes the contour of the posterior end of the soft palate so that it adapts to the posterior throat wall when it is moved up against it. This muscle is also innervated by CNs X and XI (Fig. 31.3).

Levator Veli Palatini

The **levator veli palatini** elevates the posterior end of the soft palate. It originates from the petrous part of the temporal bone just anterior to the carotid canal and from the medial wall of the cartilagenous part of the auditory canal, or tube, which lies in the lateral wall of the nasal pharynx. The fibers run downward and slightly medially into the posterior part of the soft palate. When the muscle contracts, it pulls the posterior end of the soft palate up and back to contact the posterior pharyngeal (throat) wall. It also functions to help open the auditory tube if it is edematous and closed. The nerve supply to this muscle is also CNs X and XI (see Figs. 31.1, 31.2, and 31.4).

Tensor Veli Palatini

The last of the muscles of the soft palate is the **tensor veli palatini**. This muscle takes its origin from an area near the base of the medial pterygoid plate, where it meets the body of the sphenoid bone, as well as from the lateral wall of the cartilage of the auditory tube. The fibers run downward and forward to pass around

the lateral side of the hamular process on the medial pterygoid plate; as they pass around the hamular process, they turn medially and insert into the posterior edge of the hard palate and the anterior portion of the soft palate. As the name indicates, contraction of the muscle slightly tenses the anterior portion of the soft palate. Because very little tensing is achieved, it functions more to open the auditory tube when it is closed as a result of sinus infections. The nerve supply to this muscle is the third part of CN V and is usually denoted as V_3 (see Figs. 31.1, 31.3, and 31.4).

Pharynx

Pharyngeal Constrictors

The pharynx has two groups of muscles associated with it—one group that constricts the pharynx and another group that elevates and dilates the pharynx (Table 31.2). There are three pairs of pharyngeal constrictors, all of which insert into a midline tendon in the posterior throat wall known as the **median raphe**. These three muscles overlap one another in their insertion into this raphe (see Fig. 31.5).

Superior Pharyngeal Constrictor Muscle

The **superior pharyngeal constrictor muscle** originates in the lower part of the medial pterygoid plate and its hamular process, from the mandibular and maxillary alveolar processes on the buccal side just above the mylohyoid line, and from a tendinous band called the **pterygomandibular raphe**, which runs between these two areas. These points of origin are the same as for the buccinator muscle (see Chapter 30). The buccinator muscle runs forward, whereas the superior pharyngeal constrictor runs backward to insert into the base of the skull just in front of the foramen magnum and into the median raphe. As the muscle passes posteriorly,

<table>
TABLE 31.2	Muscles of the Pharynx			
Muscle	Origin	Insertion	Function	Nerve Innervation
Superior pharyngeal constrictor muscle	Hamular process of medial pterygoid plate and pterygomandibular raphe	Median raphe	Constricts upper pharynx, forces bolus into esophagus	CNs X and XI
Middle pharyngeal constrictor muscle	Upper hyoid bone and styloid process of temporal bone	Median raphe	Constricts upper pharynx, forces bolus into esophagus	CNs X and XI
Inferior pharyngeal constrictor muscle	Thyroid cartilage of larynx	Median raphe	Constricts upper pharynx, forces bolus into esophagus	CNs X and XI
Stylopharyngeus muscle	Medial side of styloid process	Lateral pharyngeal wall and thyroid cartilage of larynx	Dilates pharynx, lifts pharynx in swallowing	CN IX
Salpingopharyngeus muscle	Auditory tube in nasal pharynx	Thyroid cartilage of larynx	Dilates pharynx, lifts pharynx in swallowing	CNs X and XI
</table>

its fibers fan out, upward, and downward. When the muscle contracts, it constricts the upper part of the pharynx and is able to force the contents of the pharynx downward. The muscle is supplied by CNs X and XI (see Figs. 31.4 and 31.5; Fig. 31.6), which make up the **pharyngeal plexus of nerves** for most of these muscles.

Middle Pharyngeal Constrictor Muscle

The **middle pharyngeal constrictor muscle** originates from the posterior, upper part of the hyoid bone and from the stylohyoid ligament, which runs from the styloid process of the temporal bone to the tip of the hyoid bone in the neck below the larynx. The fibers run backward, fanning out and overlapping the superior constrictor muscle above and underlying the inferior constrictor muscle below as it inserts into the median raphe. When the muscle contracts, it also constricts the pharyngeal opening and forces the food down toward the esophagus. This muscle is also supplied by CNs X and XI (see Figs. 31.4 and 31.5).

Inferior Pharyngeal Constrictor Muscle

The **inferior pharyngeal constrictor muscle** takes its origin from the posterior part of the thyroid cartilage of the larynx. The fibers run backward, overlying the middle pharyngeal constrictor, and insert into the median raphe. The lowest of these fibers blend in with the upper part of the wall of the esophagus so that contraction of this muscle also constricts the lower end of the pharynx and forces the food into the esophagus, which then continues the movement of the food toward the stomach. The nerve supply to this muscle is CNs X and XI (see Figs. 31.4 and 31.5).

Pharyngeal Elevators and Dilators

The second group of muscles in the pharynx aids in elevating and dilating the pharynx.

Palatopharyngeus Muscle

Although the palatopharyngeus muscle has already been listed as a muscle of the soft palate, you can see from its action that it also has the ability to elevate the pharynx. This action is necessary to receive the food that is to be swallowed.

Stylopharyngeus Muscle

The **stylopharyngeus muscle** takes its origin from the base of the styloid process on the medial side. It then runs downward and medially to enter the pharyngeal constrictors between the superior and middle constrictor to blend in with fibers of the palatopharyngeal muscle, which then insert into the lateral pharyngeal wall and the thyroid cartilage of the larynx. Contraction of the muscle causes dilation and elevation of the pharynx. *This is the primary dilator of the pharynx.* The nerve supply to this muscle is CN IX (see Figs. 31.4 and 31.5).

Salpingopharyngeus Muscle

The **salpingopharyngeus muscle** takes its origin from the end of the auditory tube in the lateral wall of the nasal pharynx. The fibers run downward to blend in with the **palatopharyngeus muscle** and the lateral pharyngeal wall. Contraction of the muscle primarily lifts the pharyngeal wall in the act of swallowing, as does contraction of the other muscles listed previously. The nerve supply to this muscle is CNs X and XI (see Figs. 31.1 and 31.2).

Actions

Speech

When we speak, the soft palate is pulled up and back to contact the posterior pharyngeal wall. This is accomplished primarily by the levator veli palatini and the muscles of the uvula. If the soft palate is unable to adapt well to the posterior pharyngeal wall, the speech will have a nasal sound. A common example of this occurs when a person has enlarged adenoids (pharyngeal tonsils), which are in the posterior pharyngeal wall just where the soft palate contacts it. These enlarged adenoids give the voice a definite nasal tone because of the rough surface of the adenoids letting air escape between the soft palate and the adenoids. For another example, if there is a large open contact region, as occurs in a cleft palate, the voice may be unintelligible.

Swallowing

While we are considering the act of swallowing, let us look at what precedes it and follow it through to completion, using the

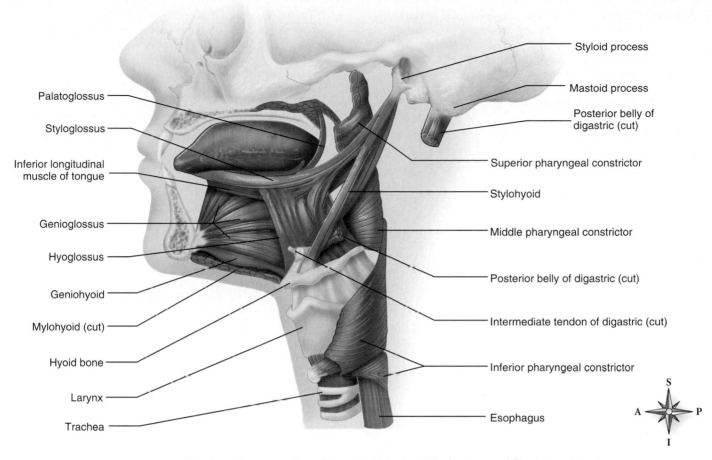

Palatoglossus

Styloglossus

Inferior longitudinal muscle of tongue

Genioglossus

Hyoglossus

Geniohyoid

Mylohyoid (cut)

Hyoid bone

Larynx

Trachea

Styloid process

Mastoid process

Posterior belly of digastric (cut)

Superior pharyngeal constrictor

Stylohyoid

Middle pharyngeal constrictor

Posterior belly of digastric (cut)

Intermediate tendon of digastric (cut)

Inferior pharyngeal constrictor

Esophagus

• **Figure 31.6** Muscles of the mouth. (From Patton KT, Thibodeau GA. *Anatomy and Physiology*, 8th ed. St. Louis, MO: Mosby; 2013.)

example of meat. Meat is incised by anterior teeth and ground up by posterior teeth. While this happens, the meat is also being mixed with saliva. When it reaches the proper consistency, it is shaped into a ball of food by the teeth, cheeks, and tongue; this ball is referred to as a **bolus of food**.

The bolus is placed on the tongue, the tongue moves up and back, and the bolus is shifted onto the posterior part of the tongue and moved back into the oral pharyngeal area. As the tongue moves up and back, the muscles of the soft palate raise the posterior end of the soft palate to contact the posterior pharyngeal wall and narrow the fauces so that they press tightly against the sides of the tongue, sealing off the back part of the tongue and the oral pharynx from the front part of the tongue and the oral cavity.

If we look at the action of the pharyngeal muscles in this swallowing process, we see that the elevators and dilators of the pharynx lift and widen the pharynx to receive the bolus of food that has just been moved back into the oral pharynx. Next, the constrictors compress the upper part of the oral pharynx and push the food down into the laryngeal pharynx. As this happens, some of the pharyngeal muscles elevate the thyroid cartilage of the larynx with assistance from the thyrohyoid muscle and a number of other muscles. This allows the epiglottis to shelter the laryngeal opening from food moving into it, and the food moves down into the upper end of the esophagus. The upper half of the esophagus is also a voluntary skeletal muscle, and a person can willfully move food about halfway down the esophagus before the further movement is taken over by involuntary smooth muscle, which creates wavelike constrictions of the digestive tube, known as **peristaltic contractions**. At one time or another, we have all moved too much food into the esophagus too quickly and have felt as if it was stuck halfway down. In essence, this is true because we can move the food only that far voluntarily; then it has to stop and wait for the involuntary peristaltic waves to take it the rest of the way; these waves proceed at a much slower rate than the voluntary waves of contraction that we can create.

Review Questions

1. What are the muscles of the soft palate that narrow the fauces, and what other actions can they accomplish? Describe their origins and insertions.

2. Which muscles of the pharynx aid in elevation and dilatation of the pharynx? Which nerves supply them?

3. Name the origins and insertions of the pharyngeal constrictors as well as their nerve supplies.

4. What creates nasal sounds in a person's speech?

5. What muscle closes off the oral pharynx from the nasal pharynx in speech, and what is its nerve supply?

6. List the sequence of events that take place when food is masticated and swallowed.

7. Why do we sometimes feel as though food is caught halfway down our throats?

32

Arterial Supply and Venous Drainage

OBJECTIVES

- To trace blood from the time it returns from the vena cava to the heart, out, and back until it returns again from the entire body
- To trace blood supply from the heart to all areas of the oral cavity, including teeth
- To trace venous drainage from teeth and oral cavity back to the heart
- To define *hematoma*
- To discuss the possible problems associated with a posterior superior alveolar injection

A student of anatomy should have a clear picture of blood flow through the entire body. Blood enters into the right atrium of the heart from the body. From the right atrium, it travels through the right atrioventricular valve (tricuspid valve) to the right ventricle. The right ventricle pumps it out through the pulmonary valve into the **pulmonary artery** and then to the lungs. There it picks up oxygen and returns to the left atrium of the heart through paired **pulmonary veins** on each side. From the left atrium, blood passes through the left atrioventricular valve (bicuspid or mitral valve) to the left ventricle, and the left ventricle pumps it out through the aortic valve into the **aorta**. From the aorta, blood flows through the thorax and the abdomen. In the pelvis, the aorta ends as paired common iliac arteries. The common iliac arteries split into internal and external iliac arteries. The internal iliac arteries mainly supply the pelvis and nearby areas, whereas the external iliac arteries continue as femoral arteries down into the leg. Internal, external, and common iliac veins bring blood back from those regions until it reaches the abdomen, where the veins become the inferior vena cava, which returns blood to the right atrium.

Within the head and neck region are many blood vessels, each with numerous branches. In this chapter, we will concentrate on those vessels that supply and drain teeth and the oral cavity, starting with the heart and tracing blood into the head and neck region and then back to the heart again.

Arterial Supply

The pathways to the right and left sides of the head and neck region are slightly different. On the right side, the **brachiocephalic artery** (*brachio* meaning "arm"; *cephalic* meaning "head") branches off the arch of the aorta. Coming off the brachiocephalic artery are the right subclavian artery to the right arm, and the right common carotid artery to the right side of the head. The left common carotid artery comes directly off the arch of the aorta on the left side, and the left subclavian artery comes off the arch of the aorta lateral to the left common carotid artery.

Common Carotid Artery

In the neck, on both sides, the **common carotid artery** runs within the carotid sheath, along with the internal jugular vein and the vagus nerve, and lies beneath the sternocleidomastoid muscle, which runs along the side of the neck. At about the level of the larynx, the common carotid divides into the **external carotid artery** and the **internal carotid artery**.

The internal carotid artery has no branches in the neck but goes up to enter the skull. Once inside the skull, it branches to supply the eyes, the brain, and some limited regions of the coverings of the brain (Fig. 32.1).

Unlike the internal carotid artery, the external carotid artery has several branches in the neck, as shown in Figs. 32.1 and 32.2. The best way to study these arteries is by understanding the directions and the order in which they come off of the external carotid artery.

Anterior branches: There are three anterior branches. In order of lowest to highest, they are (1) the **superior thyroid artery** to the thyroid gland and larynx; (2) the **lingual artery** to the tongue and floor of mouth; and (3) the **facial artery** that supplies the submandibular salivary gland, the area beneath the chin, and the face.

Medial branches: There is only one medial branch, the **ascending pharyngeal** artery to the pharyngeal wall and tonsil area.

Posterior branches: There are two posterior branches, (1) the **occipital artery** to the occipital region, and (2) the **posterior auricular artery** to the area behind the ear.

The external carotid artery ends by dividing into the **maxillary artery** and the **superficial temporal arteries**. However, we will consider in detail only the **lingual, facial**, and **maxillary arteries** (Table 32.1).

Lingual Artery

The lingual artery branches off the external carotid artery below the facial artery. The lingual artery then travels forward and deep, going beneath the hyoglossus muscle of the tongue and ending in three branches: the **dorsal lingual artery** to the deep posterior part of the tongue, the **deep lingual artery** to the deep anterior part of the tongue, and the sublingual artery to the ventral surface of tongue and floor of the mouth. **The lingual artery** supplies the tongue and the tissue in the floor of the oral cavity (Table 32.2). If you have ever cut your tongue, you know that there is well-developed blood supply within this tissue, which is completely supplied by the lingual artery (Fig. 32.3). Quite frequently the

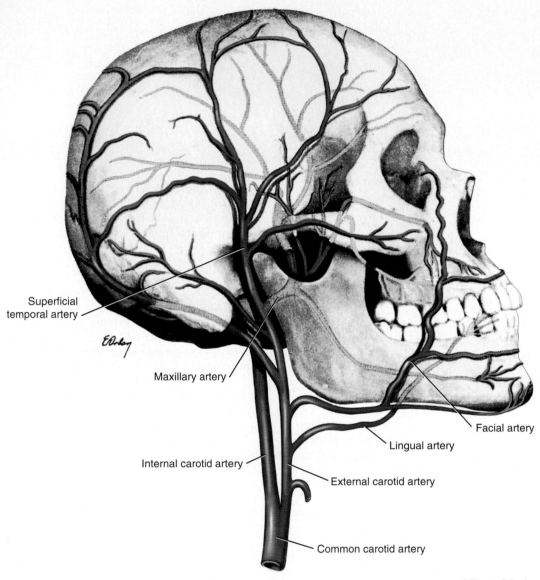

• **Figure 32.1** General distribution of arteries from the lower part of the neck up through the skull area. (From DuBrul EL. *Sicher's Oral Anatomy.* 7th ed. St. Louis, MO: Mosby; 1980.)

lingual and facial arteries come off the external carotid as one branch and then split. This branch is referred to as the *linguofacial trunk*.

Facial Artery

The facial artery ascends the side of the neck, runs deep to the submandibular gland, supplying the gland, and crosses the lower border of the mandible just in front of the angle of the mandible. (You can feel a small depression on the lower border of the mandible. At this point, the artery gives off a submental branch, which runs along the inferior border of the mandible to the chin. After giving off this branch, the facial artery and vein cross the mandible. It is at this point that you can compress the vessels to act as a pressure point for facial bleeding.) After crossing the mandible, the artery travels across the face, ending near the inner corner of the eye as the angular artery. On its way, it supplies blood to skin and the muscles of facial expression. It also sends

branches to the maxillary and mandibular lips and to the sides of the nose (Table 32.3).

Maxillary Artery

The maxillary artery, along with the superficial temporal artery, is a terminal branch of the external carotid artery. It diverges from the external carotid at the level of the neck of the condyle on its deep surface. There are about 15 branches of this artery, but in our discussion, we will only be concerned with a little more than half of them. In general, this artery supplies the muscles of mastication, teeth, the oral and nasal cavities, the coverings of the brain, and several smaller areas (see Table 32.4). From its beginning, where it branches off the external carotid artery, the maxillary artery runs forward in an area known as the **infratemporal fossa**, where it crosses the surface of the lateral pterygoid muscle to enter the **pterygopalatine fossa** behind and below the eye (Fig. 32.4).

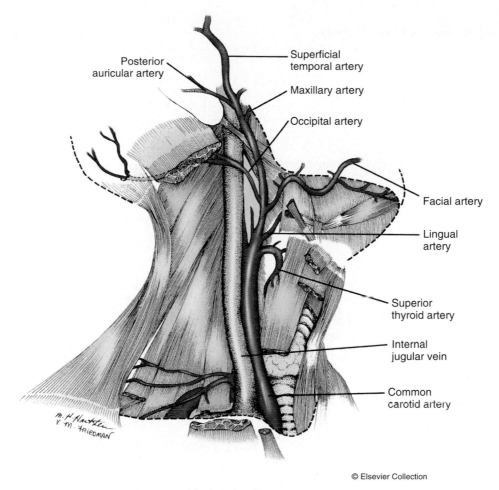

Posterior auricular artery

Superficial temporal artery

Maxillary artery

Occipital artery

Facial artery

Lingual artery

Superior thyroid artery

Internal jugular vein

Common carotid artery

• **Figure 32.2** Branches of the external carotid artery.

Infratemporal Fossa Branches

The more important branches of the maxillary artery in the infratemporal fossa are the **inferior alveolar, temporal, masseteric, pterygoid, middle meningeal**, and **buccal branches** (see Fig. 32.4).

Inferior Alveolar Artery with Mental Branch. The inferior alveolar branch runs down to enter the mandibular foramen and runs in the mandibular canal. It sends off branches to each of the mandibular teeth, their periodontal ligaments, and to the bone. In the premolar region, the inferior alveolar artery sends off a small branch called the **mental artery**, which exits from the mandible through the mental foramen. It supplies the mandibular buccal gingiva and mucosa from the premolars to the incisors and also supplies the mucosa of the mandibular lip and chin.

The inferior alveolar continues *inside* the mandibular canal as the **incisive artery**. The incisive artery supplies the mandibular anterior teeth and their labial gingiva and periodontium. The incisive artery of one side crosses the midline to anastomose with the incise artery of the opposite side (Table 32.5).

Deep Temporal Branches. Two temporal branches arise from the maxillary artery to supply the temporal muscle: the anterior and posterior deep temporal arteries.

Masseteric Branch. The masseteric branch comes off the maxillary artery and runs laterally through the coronoid notch of the ramus, entering the deep surface of the masseter muscle to supply it with blood.

Pterygoid Branches. There may be one or more pterygoid branches that extend to the medial and lateral pterygoid muscles. Their courses and directions vary among individuals.

Middle Meningeal Artery. The middle meningeal artery comes off the maxillary, generally opposite the inferior alveolar artery, and runs up through the foramen spinosum to be the major blood supply to the meninges of the brain.

Buccal Branch. The buccal branch runs down and forward to supply the mucosa of the cheek and the buccal mucosa and gingiva of maxillary and mandibular posterior teeth (see Fig. 32.4).

Pterygopalatine Fossa Branches

At the anterior part of the infratemporal fossa, the maxillary artery reaches the pterygopalatine fossa, entering it through the pterygomaxillary fissure, the opening between the maxillary tuberosity and the pterygoid process of the sphenoid bone. The pterygopalatine fossa lies behind and slightly below the orbital cavity. From there, branches divide into five general directions: backward to the nasal pharynx, down to the palate, medially into the nasal cavity and eventually to the anterior palatal area, laterally to the maxillary tuberosity, and forward into the infraorbital area of the face (see Fig. 32.4; Fig. 32.5).

Descending Palatine Artery. The **descending palatine artery** extends down from the maxillary artery to the posterior hard palate through the pterygopalatine canal. There it splits into two branches: the **lesser palatine artery**, which supplies the soft palate, and the **greater palatine artery**, which travels forward along the lateral part of the hard palate to supply the palatal mucosa and maxillary lingual gingiva. These vessels emerge into the palatal area through the lesser and greater palatine foramina, respectively (see Fig. 32.5).

TABLE 32.1   Branches of the External Carotid Artery

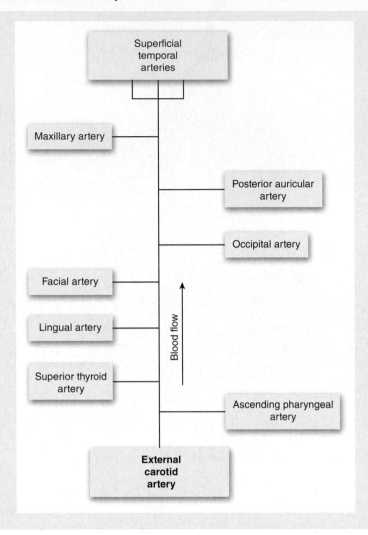

TABLE 32.2   Branches of the Lingual Artery

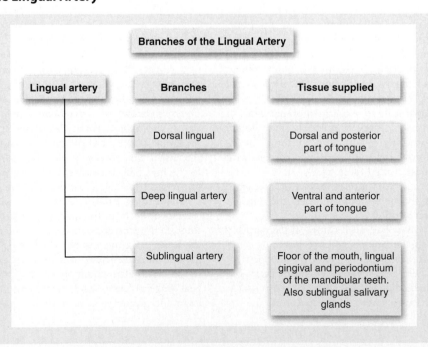

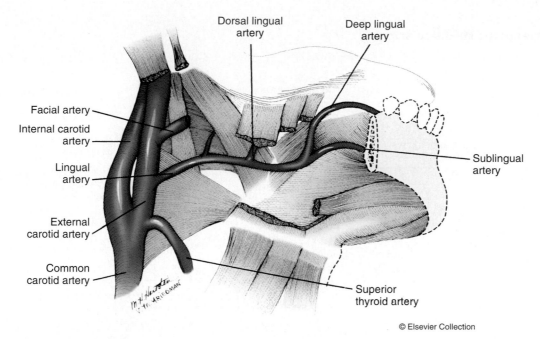

• **Figure 32.3** Lingual artery branches that supply blood to the tongue.

© Elsevier Collection

TABLE 32.3   **Branches of the Facial Artery**

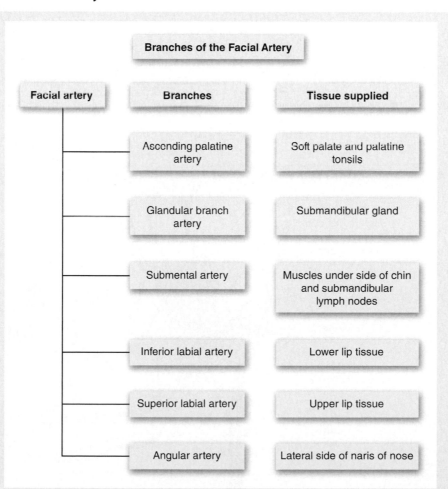

Branches of the Facial Artery

Facial artery	Branches	Tissue supplied
	Ascending palatine artery	Soft palate and palatine tonsils
	Glandular branch artery	Submandibular gland
	Submental artery	Muscles under side of chin and submandibular lymph nodes
	Inferior labial artery	Lower lip tissue
	Superior labial artery	Upper lip tissue
	Angular artery	Lateral side of naris of nose

TABLE 32.4 Branches of the Maxillary Artery

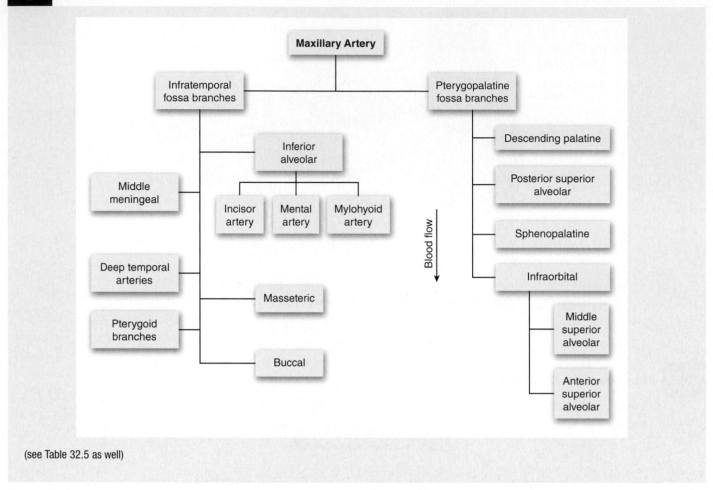

(see Table 32.5 as well)

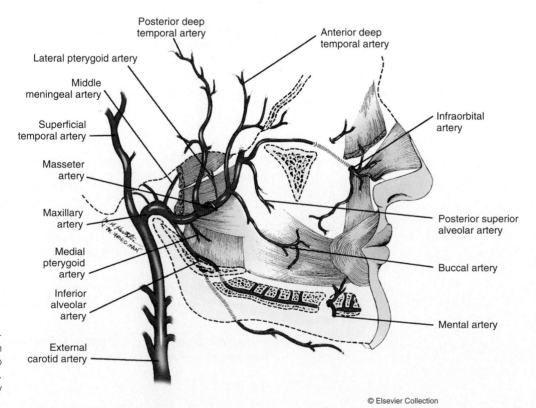

• **Figure 32.4** Cut-away section showing the origin of the maxillary artery from the external carotid artery just medial to what would be the neck of the condyle. Most branches of the maxillary artery can be seen.

TABLE 32.5   **Branches of the Maxillary Artery and the Areas They Supply**

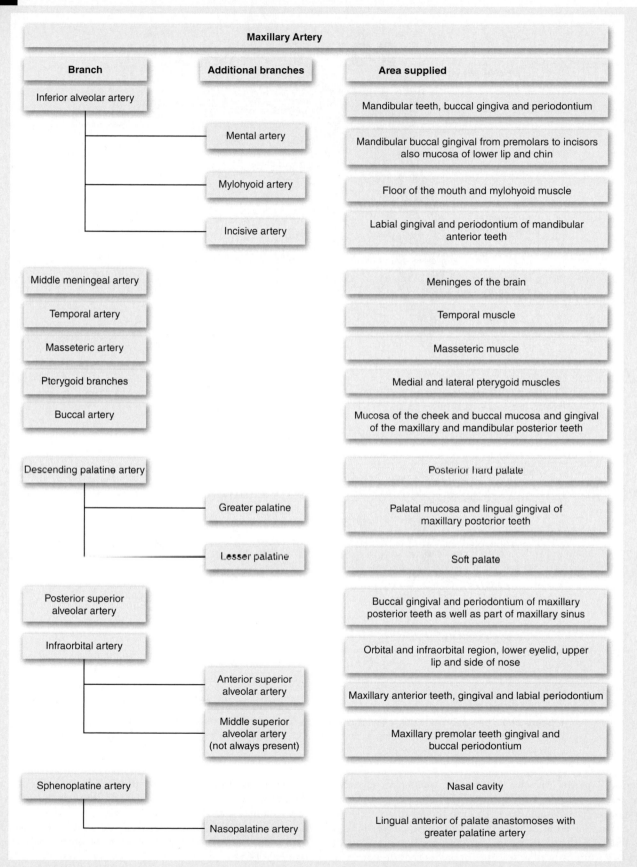

Maxillary Artery		
Branch	**Additional branches**	**Area supplied**
Inferior alveolar artery		Mandibular teeth, buccal gingiva and periodontium
	Mental artery	Mandibular buccal gingival from premolars to incisors also mucosa of lower lip and chin
	Mylohyoid artery	Floor of the mouth and mylohyoid muscle
	Incisive artery	Labial gingival and periodontium of mandibular anterior teeth
Middle meningeal artery		Meninges of the brain
Temporal artery		Temporal muscle
Masseteric artery		Masseteric muscle
Pterygoid branches		Medial and lateral pterygoid muscles
Buccal artery		Mucosa of the cheek and buccal mucosa and gingival of the maxillary and mandibular posterior teeth
Descending palatine artery		Posterior hard palate
	Greater palatine	Palatal mucosa and lingual gingival of maxillary posterior teeth
	Lesser palatine	Soft palate
Posterior superior alveolar artery		Buccal gingival and periodontium of maxillary posterior teeth as well as part of maxillary sinus
Infraorbital artery		Orbital and infraorbital region, lower eyelid, upper lip and side of nose
	Anterior superior alveolar artery	Maxillary anterior teeth, gingival and labial periodontium
	Middle superior alveolar artery (not always present)	Maxillary premolar teeth gingival and buccal periodontium
Sphenoplatine artery		Nasal cavity
	Nasopalatine artery	Lingual anterior of palate anastomoses with greater palatine artery

(see Table 32.4 as well)

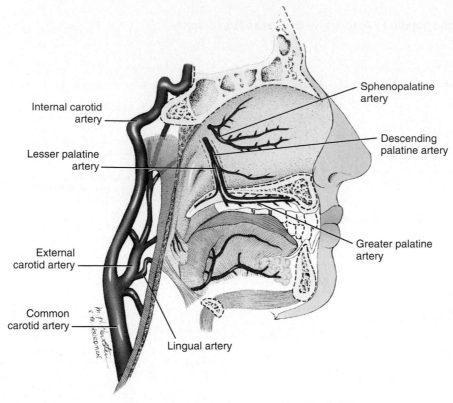

© Elsevier Collection

• **Figure 32.5** Section of the lateral part of the hard palate, showing blood supply to the hard and soft palates and to the nasal cavity area.

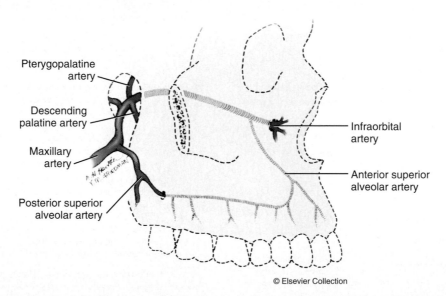

© Elsevier Collection

• **Figure 32.6** The infraorbital artery extending across the floor of the orbit, with the anterior superior alveolar artery branching off and supplying anterior teeth and possibly premolars. The anterior and posterior superior alveolar arteries anastomose with one another.

Posterior Superior Alveolar Artery. The **posterior superior alveolar artery** comes out of the pterygopalatine fossa through the pterygomaxillary fissure, descends onto the maxillary tuberosity, and enters the bone behind the third molar. From there it supplies blood to all the maxillary posterior teeth and to part of the maxillary sinus, as well as to some branches that do not enter bone but rather supply the posterior buccal mucosa of the upper posterior teeth (Fig. 32.6, and see Fig. 32.4).

Sphenopalatine Artery. The **sphenopalatine artery** comes off the maxillary artery and runs medially through the sphenopalatine foramen into the nasal cavity, supplying most parts of the nasal cavity. It finally emerges from the incisive foramen as the nasopalatine artery to anastomose with the greater palatine artery (see Fig. 32.5).

Infraorbital Artery. The **infraorbital artery** is the end part of the maxillary artery. From its location in the floor of the orbital cavity, it sends a branch, the **anterior superior alveolar artery**, down into the bone in front of the maxillary sinus, supplying maxillary anterior teeth. It also anastomoses with the posterior superior alveolar artery in the wall of the sinus. The remainder of the infraorbital artery emerges through the infraorbital foramen onto the face and supplies the maxillary lip and its mucosa, maxillary labial gingiva, lower eyelid, and sides of the nose (see Figs. 32.4 and 32.6).

Sometimes there is a second branch, the **middle superior alveolar artery**. It is not always present, but when present it branches from the infraorbital artery and runs inferiorly along the lateral wall of the maxillary sinus. It supplies the premolar teeth and their buccal gingiva and periodontium. It anastomoses with the posterior and anterior superior alveolar arteries. When it is not present, this area is covered by the anterior superior alveolar as it anastomoses with the posterior superior alveolar artery.

Venous Drainage

Now that we have studied how blood reaches the head and neck region, in particular the oral cavity, we will examine the return of blood to the heart. In general, veins follow the same pathways as those of arteries and, in most instances, have the same names. For this reason, the majority of discussion in most anatomic texts is devoted to blood supply, or arteries, and focuses less on the veins.

Jugular Veins

In the head and neck region, the names of the veins vary slightly from those of the arteries. Instead of internal and external carotid veins, they are designated as **internal** and **external jugular veins**. The internal jugular vein drains the entire brain area and passes out of the skull through the jugular foramen. The internal jugular vein, in general, drains much of the area from the front of the ear to the front of the face through veins that correspond to arteries—for example, the facial, lingual, and part of the superficial temporal veins.

The maxillary vein is formed by an intertwining network of veins known as the **pterygoid plexus of veins**. These veins are so close to the maxillary tuberosity that there is a risk of piercing them if the angulation of the needle is incorrect during posterior superior alveolar nerve blocking. When this happens, blood escapes into the tissue spaces, and a **hematoma** occurs—a swelling and discoloration of the area that can cause great concern to the patient. In general, after initial use of cold packs, the application of moist heat will help dissipate the swelling and discoloration.

The superficial temporal vein and the maxillary vein form the **retromandibular vein** (*retro* meaning "behind"). The retromandibular vein divides into a posterior retromandibular vein and an anterior retromandibular vein. The posterior retromandibular vein joins with the posterior auricular vein to form the external jugular vein. The external jugular vein descends, crossing the lateral surface of the sternocleidomastoid muscle, and ends by emptying into the subclavian vein, which drains part of the temporal, maxillary, and posterior auricular areas. The anterior retromandibular vein joins with the facial vein and forms the common facial vein, which enters the internal jugular vein. The common facial vein then drains part of the superficial temporal and maxillary area as well as the facial region (Figs. 32.7 and 32.8).

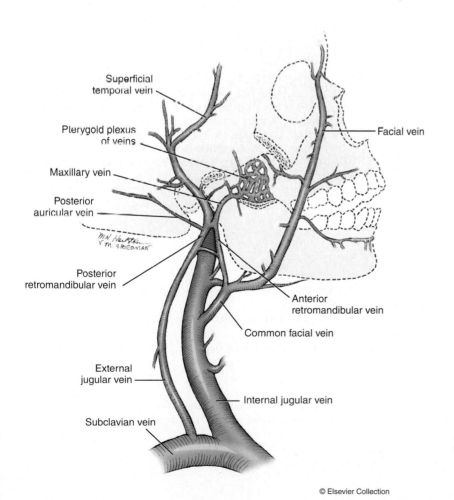

• **Figure 32.7** General drainage areas of the internal and external jugular veins. The retromandibular vein connects the internal and external jugular veins and distributes blood between them.

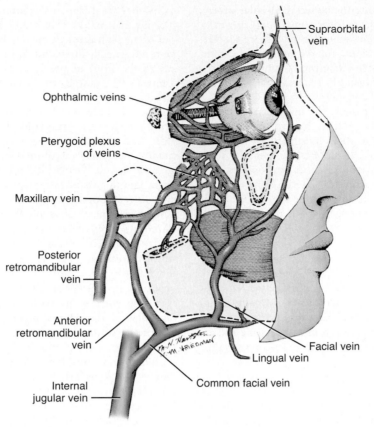

Supraorbital
vein

Ophthalmic veins

Pterygoid plexus
of veins

Maxillary vein

Posterior
retromandibular
vein

Anterior
retromandibular
vein

Internal
jugular vein

Facial vein

Lingual vein

Common facial vein

© Elsevier Collection

• **Figure 32.8** The pterygoid plexus of veins just behind the maxillary tuberosity. It may be injured during injection of that area of maxillary molars.

Either the posterior or the anterior branch of the retromandibular vein is often missing. This causes more blood to shunt to either the external or internal jugular vein, causing differences in the sizes of these two veins.

The external jugular veins empty into the **subclavian veins** from the arm. These veins join the internal jugular veins, forming the brachiocephalic veins, and flow into the **superior vena cava** and on into the right atrium of the heart. The supply to and from the head and neck region is then complete, and the blood can flow out to the lungs again.

Review Questions

1. Trace the path of blood (through chambers, valves, and vessels) from the time it first enters the heart until it returns to the heart.
2. What route does blood take from the heart into the head and neck region?
3. What are the two divisions of the common carotid artery?
4. Which branches of the external carotid artery supply all teeth and the oral cavity?
5. Where does the blood supply to the muscles of mastication originate?
6. Name the individual vessels that supply all areas of the oral cavity.
7. What is the major vein that drains most of the head and neck region?
8. What is the pterygoid plexus of veins, what does it form, and what is its significance?
9. Trace the pathway of venous blood from the neck back to the heart.
10. What happens to the jugular veins if either the anterior or the posterior retromandibular vein is missing?

33

Salivary Glands

As you may recall from Chapter 17, the glands of the body are classified in a number of ways. Salivary glands are classified as exocrine, merocrine, compound tubuloalveolar, serous, mixed, or mucous. They are also divided into major salivary glands, which are the three pairs of large glands, and minor salivary glands, which are found throughout the oral cavity (Table 33.1).

Major Salivary Glands

The major salivary glands are three pairs of glands that produce the bulk of the fluid in the mouth. This fluid is saliva, which mixes with food to make it easy to swallow and begins to break down starches into smaller carbohydrate units; further food breakdown takes place in the stomach. Saliva also keeps the mucosa in the oral cavity from drying out and aids in swallowing and speech (review Chapter 25 for the other functions of saliva). The three gland pairs are the parotid, the submandibular, and the sublingual salivary glands.

Parotid Gland

The **parotid gland** is located on the surface of the masseter muscle, behind the ramus of the mandible on the medial side of the ramus (see Chapter 26). It is composed of many grapelike clusters of cells that secrete into a system of tubes leading to the oral cavity. If you look at the cells of the secretory part of the gland through a microscope, you will see that the cells are all the same type—they produce a thin, watery secretion referred to as **serous secretion**. Although these glands are the largest of the salivary glands, the pair produces only about 25% of the total resting salivary volume. Fig. 33.1 shows the location of the gland. You can see that the duct leading from the gland travels anteriorly across the master muscle (see Chapter 28) and pierces the buccinator muscle (see Chapter 30) to open into the oral cavity opposite the maxillary second molar via Stenson's duct.

If Stenson's duct, or Stenson's papilla, becomes blocked for any reason, such as salivary duct stone or injury, the flow of saliva is stopped and saliva backs up to the salivary gland. This causes pain upon eating and swelling of the parotid gland. Treatment includes milking the salivary papilla until the stone is expelled. If this treatment fails, surgery is required.

Submandibular (Submaxillary) Gland

The **submandibular (submaxillary) gland** provides about 60% to 65% of the total resting salivary volume. It is called a *mixed gland* because it includes both serous and mucus cells. Mucus is thicker and stickier than serum, and although almost two-thirds of the cells in the submandibular gland are serous, the mucus component results in a slightly viscous secretion. The gland is located below and toward the posterior part of the body of the mandible (see Chapter 26). Place your finger on the inferior border of the mandible and run it back toward the angle of the mandible. As you near the angle, you will feel a slight depression in the inferior border where the facial artery and vein cross the mandible. If you move your finger medially from that point, you may feel a lump in the neck: the submandibular gland. The gland is wrapped around the mylohyoid muscle in the neck (see Chapter 28). Most of the gland lies on the superficial side, and part of it lies on the deep side of the muscle in the posterior and lateral floor of the mouth. The duct extends from the deep part of the gland and runs forward in the floor of the mouth to open onto a small elevation called the *sublingual caruncle*. This is located at the base of the lingual frenum, the fold of tissue that attaches the tongue to the floor of the mouth (Figs. 33.2 and 33.3).

Sublingual Gland

The **sublingual gland** is the smallest of the three pairs of glands and contributes only 10% of the total salivary volume. It is composed of mostly mucus cells with some serous cells; therefore, the secretion of this gland is even more viscous than that of the submandibular gland. It is also easier to see serous demilunes capping the mucus acini in this gland, as described in Chapter 25. It is located in the anterior floor of the mouth next to mandibular canines. It has one major duct, which opens with the submandibular duct, and several smaller ducts, which open in a line along the fold of tissue beneath the tongue, known as the *sublingual fold*

TABLE 33.1	Salivary Glands	
Name	**Location**	**Type of Secretion**
Major Salivary Glands		
Parotid	Anterior ear	Serous
Submandibular	Angle of mandible	Mixed serous
Sublingual	Anterior floor of mouth	Mucous
Minor Salivary Glands		
Labial	Lips	Mixed
Buccal	Cheeks	Mixed
Palatine	Hard and soft palates	Mucous
Lingual	Anterior tongue	Mixed
	Middle tongue	Serous
	Posterior	Mucous

(see Figs. 33.2 and 33.3). This gland is surrounded by minor sublingual glands, which are discussed later in this chapter.

All these glands should be palpated in intraoral and extraoral examinations, and any enlargement of these glands should be further investigated. If a patient has lost all of their teeth, as well as most of the mandibular ridge of bone, the sublingual gland will appear to bulge up into the floor of the mouth when the mouth is opened wide. This is not unusual and is no cause for alarm as long as the new denture replacing the lost teeth does not press on the gland.

Minor Salivary Glands

The structure of the minor salivary glands is similar to that of the major glands, but the minor salivary glands are much smaller and have less branching. The primary differences between the two classifications are size, the number of secretory units or acini, and the number of ducts. The function of the minor glands is not to produce saliva for mixing with food but, rather, to secrete minor amounts of saliva onto the surface to keep the mucosa moist. Some of these glands are pure serous cells, most are pure mucous cells, and the rest of them are mixed but mostly mucous. They do not have a long ductal system; thus there are many clusters of these glands throughout the mouth, each with its own ductal opening. They are located labially, buccally, palatally, glossopalatally, and lingually.

Labial Glands

In maxillary and mandibular lips are the **labial glands**, opening onto the inner surface. These are mixed glands but mostly mucus. You can see them in a mirror by pulling the lip out and looking at its inner surface, where they are present beneath the epithelium. This is also a good place to see the distribution of ductal openings. Gently pull your mandibular lip out while standing in front of a mirror and dry off the inner surface with a tissue. Then pull the lip tight, and watch for tiny drops of moisture to appear

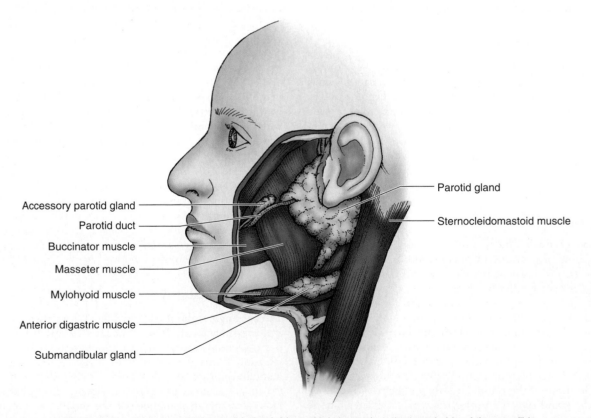

• **Figure 33.1** Lateral view of the parotid gland. Most of it is located on the lateral side of the mandible and masseter muscle, wrapping around the back of the mandible. The duct pierces the buccinator muscle as it opens into the oral cavity.

Accessory parotid gland
Parotid duct
Buccinator muscle
Masseter muscle
Mylohyoid muscle
Anterior digastric muscle
Submandibular gland
Parotid gland
Sternocleidomastoid muscle

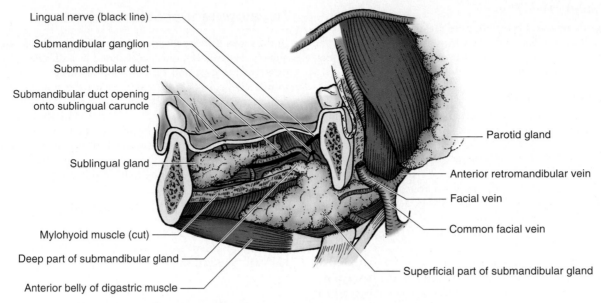

• **Figure 33.2** The submandibular gland has a superficial part that can be palpated and a deep part from which the duct runs forward to the sublingual caruncle. *Dotted line,* path of duct.

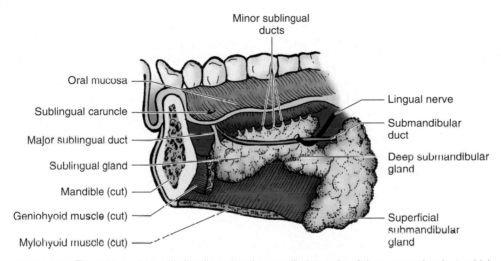

• **Figure 33.3** The sublingual gland is just lingual to the mandibular canine. It has one major duct, which joins with the submandibular gland, and many minor ducts, which open into the sublingual fold.

on the lip surface. These drops indicate the location of the labial gland ducts.

Buccal Glands

On the inner cheek region are the **buccal glands**. They are similar to the labial glands, differing only in location.

Palatine Glands

Located in the soft palate and in the posterior and lateral parts of the hard palate are the **palatine glands**. They are purely mucous in nature. Because there are no minor salivary glands in the anterior part of the hard palate to keep it moist, the drying effect tends to cause the epithelium there to be more keratinized than in the posterior and lateral parts of the hard palate.

Glossopalatine Glands

Continuing from the posterior lateral parts of the palate down into the anterior fold of tissue in front of the palatine tonsil, you will find the **glossopalatine glands**. These are also purely mucous in nature.

Lingual Glands

The **lingual glands** are divided into several groups: anterior lingual glands, lingual glands of von Ebner, and posterior lingual glands.

Anterior Lingual Glands

These glands are found near the tip of the tongue and open onto the under or ventral surface. They are mostly mucous in nature.

Lingual Glands of von Ebner

Lingual **glands of von Ebner** are pure serous glands located beneath the vallate papillae and open into the trough around the gland. These glands function to wash off the taste buds so that they can perceive new tastes.

Posterior Lingual Glands

The posterior lingual glands are located around the lingual tonsils on the posterior third of the tongue. They are purely mucous in nature.

Sublingual Glands

Although these are not usually listed separately, the sublingual glands are small individual glands that surround the major sublingual gland. They open into a row of ducts running back along the sublingual fold in the floor of the mouth. They are mainly mucous in nature.

   All of these glands, whether major or minor, are controlled by the **autonomic nervous system**. To be specific, the **parasympathetic nervous system** within the autonomic nervous system is the main stimulus for salivation. Although the sympathetic nervous system does not itself play a major role in salivation, it does control blood flow, which is important in saliva production. Stimulation of the sympathetic nervous system decreases the flow of blood to the glands and slows the production of saliva. The smell of food or the presence of something in the mouth, even something without a pleasant taste, will stimulate the glands. Even chewing on plain paraffin can cause secretion. A number of medications can cause overstimulation or understimulation of these glands, and a history of the patient's medications will help you understand why there may be more or less saliva in the mouth than you would expect and how the consistency might be different. You should also realize that "normal" amounts of saliva vary considerably from one person to another. Saliva also is affected by dehydration. If the body does not contain enough water, salivary glands will shut down production in an effort to conserve water, causing the patient to have a dry mouth.

Development of Salivary Ducts

In the major salivary glands, we are looking at the development of a ductal system. The duct starts out at as a dimple at the point of origin of the duct and then develops a cluster of small balls that form a solid cord of cells until it reaches the point where glandular cells begin to develop. This solid cord begins to break down in the middle cells, and a duct is formed. Fig. 33.1 shows that part way along the duct, there are small units that increase the secretory capacity of the gland as well as the distribution of saliva. Figs. 33.1, 33.2, and 33.3 show that there may be a significant distribution of saliva as the duct goes along to its termination.

Innervation of Salivary Glands

Salivary glands are innervated by the autonomic nervous system, primarily by the cranial nerve VII (CN VII). The mere sight of food will cause saliva to begin to flow.

Clinical Considerations

Xerostomia (dry mouth) is caused by reduction in saliva production. It is commonly seen in older individuals and patients "taking certain medications and undergoing cancer treatments (radiation or chemotherapy)." It results in the mouth being dried out and makes eating and swallowing difficult. Teeth become prone to decay because they have lost the protection afforded by saliva, which cleans their surfaces and dilutes the acids produced by bacteria.

   Salivary stones are calcium products formed within salivary glands. Most of these are flushed out by saliva, but if a stone gets too large, it can block the salivary gland. This results in a painful condition wherein when the patient tries to eat, saliva is produced but cannot come out of the blocked salivary duct, so it backs up into the salivary gland. This causes pain when eating or even looking at food. The salivary gland is swollen and painful upon palpation. Surgery may be required if the stone cannot be extracted by *milking* the duct.

Review Questions

1. What are the major salivary glands, and where do their ducts open?
2. What are the minor salivary glands, and where do their ducts open? What type of mucus do they secrete?
3. What is the function of saliva, as discussed in this chapter?
4. List the three groups of lingual salivary glands.
5. Why is the soft tissue on the anterior hard palate more keratinized than that on the soft palate?

6. If a patient presents with a swollen parotid gland, pain upon eating, tenderness upon palpation, and a diminished salivary flow, what are some of the possible causes?
   a. blocked salivary gland
   b. mumps
   c. radiation treatment
   d. dehydration
   e. all of the above

34

Nervous System

OBJECTIVES

- To name the basic components of the nervous system
- To describe the general makeup of a spinal nerve
- To describe how a sensory impulse causes a motor response
- To name the 12 cranial nerves and their general function
- To describe the components and general function of the autonomic nervous system
- To name the specific branches of the trigeminal nerve and which areas of the face, teeth, and oral cavity each branch supplies
- To describe the nerves and areas involved in general and special sensation of the tongue
- To discuss the nerves and pathways involved in parasympathetic innervation to major salivary glands

The nervous system has many routine functions. It relays messages from distant parts of the body to let the brain know exactly what is happening in each part. The brain may file the information in its memory for future reference, or it may react immediately to that message. The brain coordinates and sends out messages that cause muscles to contract, stimulates glands to secrete, regulates numerous functions, and performs many of these tasks without true consciousness on our part. To accomplish all of this, the nervous system has tremendous organization and potential. Some authorities have theorized that we normally use only 10% of our mental capacity. There are clearly more cells in the brain than we could ever use, and sometimes when there is brain damage, these unused cells can be called upon to reestablish damaged pathways.

The nervous system is divided into two major categories: the **central nervous system**, consisting of the brain and spinal cord, and the **peripheral nervous system**, which comprises all nerves that extend outward from the brain and spinal cord (Fig. 34.1).

Remember from Chapter 17 that a neuron or a group of neurons transmits a message or impulse in only one direction. Therefore it is necessary to have both sensory and motor neurons. A nerve is actually a bundle of neurons, some of which are sensory neurons and some of which are motor neurons. These neurons are what enable messages to travel to and from the brain. Most nerves have both motor and sensory neurons, although some nerves may be either purely motor or purely sensory.

Central Nervous System

The brain and the spinal cord are made up of motor or sensory neurons, but they are only part of the chain. Imagine that you

have caught your finger in a desk drawer. You feel pain and quickly pull your finger out of the drawer. Neurologically, a pain receptor or free nerve ending in the finger has picked up the message and carried it to the spinal cord. A second neuron has carried the message up the spinal cord to the lower parts of the brain, and a third neuron has taken it to the surface of the brain, where it was recognized as pain. The pain was interpreted by the brain, and past experience stored in the brain triggered the information that the finger should be removed from the drawer so that it would no longer be crushed. A motor message then left the brain and traveled down the spinal cord, and a second motor neuron carried the message out of the spinal cord and along a peripheral nerve to muscles that pulled the finger out of the drawer (Fig. 34.2).

The nervous system also builds in a shortcut to this system known as a **reflex arc**. This shortcut takes place in the spinal cord between the sensory neuron, as it enters the spinal cord, and the motor neuron, as it leaves the spinal cord. A shorter neuron, called the *intercalated neuron,* runs between the two neurons and carries the message from the sensory side to the motor side without the message having to go to the brain. The action is actually accomplished before the person thinks about it. When you touch a hot stove, what happens? You usually pull your hand away before you actually realize the stove is hot or before you consciously tell yourself to remove your hand from the stove (Fig. 34.3).

The brain and the spinal cord are only a part of the sensory chain. The spinal cord and the brain are the center of nervous activity, but they cannot act alone. They need the contributions of the peripheral nervous system.

Peripheral Nervous System

The peripheral nervous system is traditionally grouped into three components: **spinal nerves**, **cranial nerves**, and the **autonomic nervous system**.

Spinal Nerves

The spinal nerves extend from the spinal cord to distant parts of the body. These nerves generally have both motor and sensory neurons in them. There are 31 pairs of spinal nerves: 8 in the **cervical**, or neck, region; 12 in the **thoracic**, or chest, region; 5 in the **lumbar**, or lower back, region; 5 in the **sacral**, or hip, region; and 1 in the **coccygeal**, or tailbone, region (Fig. 34.4). These nerves are distributed by region from the neck to the toes. Several of the cervical nerves innervate some of the hyoid muscles that depress the mandible and raise the larynx.

The central speckled area of the spinal cord is known as **gray matter** (see Fig. 34.3). This gray matter is made up of the cell bodies of both motor and sensory neurons, which are arranged in the shape of a butterfly in the central area of the spinal cord. The

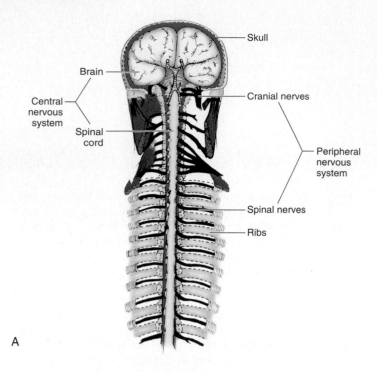

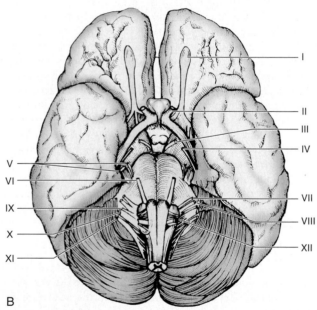

• **Figure 34.1** **(A)** The central nervous system (brain and spinal cord) and spinal segments and a few cranial nerves of the peripheral nervous system. **(B)** Inferior view of the brain, showing the origin of 12 pairs of cranial nerves. (Modified from Goss CM. *Gray's Anatomy of the Human Body*, 29th ed. Philadelphia: Lea & Febiger; 1973.)

area around the gray matter is referred to as **white matter** and is made up of myelinated axons of both motor and sensory neurons. The spinal nerve has a **dorsal root**, which is the sensory root. The dorsal root has a **dorsal root ganglion**, which is a collection of cell bodies of the sensory neurons entering the spinal cord at that level. There is also a **ventral root**, which is the motor root. The point where the dorsal and ventral roots meet is the beginning of the **spinal nerve**, and at that point the spinal nerve contains both motor and sensory neurons. The spinal nerve then divides into a

small **dorsal primary ramus** and a larger **ventral primary ramus**. Both of these primary rami are mixed motor and sensory nerves. The dorsal primary ramus carries sensation from the skin in a narrow band at the midline of the back, which is only a few inches wide, and also supplies the back muscles that lie immediately next to the vertebrae in the back. There are only a few dorsal primary rami that we can easily identify as nerves, and those are purely the sensory parts of the dorsal rami. The ventral primary rami are what we normally see as nerves in the body.

These nerves may be subject to damage in many ways. They exit from the spinal canal in the spinal vertebrae through intervertebral foramina. These foramina are formed as two semicircular openings, one from the vertebra above and one from the vertebra below. Damage to the vertebral discs between the vertebrae, or their slow compression with age, may cause pinching of the spinal nerve at that level. Sometimes this causes some pain and/or numbness and possibly some muscle weakness. If this condition is not corrected, the nerve will deteriorate from the damaged area out to its peripheral ending. If the pinched nerve is relieved by surgery, regrowth might occur out from the area of damage and thus reestablishment of function is achieved. The nerves within the spinal cord do not regenerate well, and damage to the spinal cord is usually permanent. Much research is being done to find a way to stimulate regrowth of nerves in the spinal cord and brain.

Cranial Nerves

The cranial nerves (CNs) attach directly to the brain. There are 12 pairs of these nerves, each with a separate function. When referring to these nerves, it is proper to use Roman numerals.

I, olfactory nerve—sensory; provides special sense of smell from the nose to the brain.

II, optic nerve—sensory; provides special sense of sight from the eye to the brain.

III, oculomotor nerve—motor; supplies most of the muscles that move the eye in different directions and one that raises the upper eyelid; parasympathetic innervation to the eye causes the pupil to contract and the lens to change shape and become more rounded for close vision.

IV, trochlear nerve—motor; supplies the **superior oblique muscle**, the muscle that moves the eyes downward and laterally.

V, trigeminal nerve—motor and sensory; sensory innervation for all teeth, the oral cavity, the anterior two-thirds of the tongue, the maxillary sinuses, the nasal cavity, and most of the skin of the front anterior face and head; motor innervation to the muscles of mastication, a soft palate muscle (**tensor veli palatini**) as well as the **tensor tympani muscle** of the middle ear. The **trigeminal** nerve is the most important nerve for our consideration and will be covered in greater detail later.

VI, abducens nerve—motor; supplies the **lateral rectus muscle**, the muscle that moves the eye laterally.

VII, facial nerve—motor and sensory; motor innervation to the muscles of facial expression, the stylohyoid and posterior belly of the digastric muscles, as well as the stapedius muscle of the middle ear; parasympathetic innervation to the submandibular and sublingual salivary glands, and the lacrimal gland of the eye (autonomic); sensory innervation from some areas behind the ear, and taste from the anterior two-thirds of the tongue.

VIII, statoacoustic nerve—sensory; for hearing and balance (equilibrium).

IX, glossopharyngeal nerve—motor and sensory; motor innervation to one of the muscles of the pharynx, the **stylopharyngeus**;

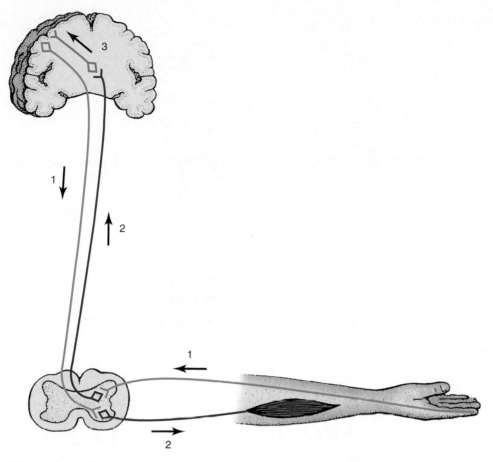

• **Figure 34.2** Multiple neurons at various levels necessary to complete a conscious sensorimotor reaction.

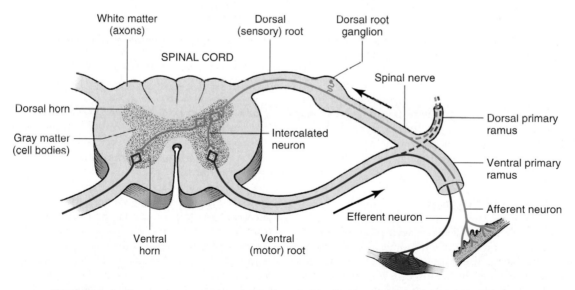

• **Figure 34.3** A reflex arc. A message travels into the spinal cord and out again without reaching the brain.

parasympathetic innervation to the parotid salivary gland; sensory innervation to the posterior one-third of the tongue for taste, as well as general sensations, such as pain, pressure, heat, and cold; also provides sensation to most of the mucosa of the pharynx and to a small area of the skin of the ear.

X, vagus nerve—motor and sensory; motor innervation to the muscles of the pharynx and larynx and most of the muscles of the soft palate; parasympathetic innervation controls most of the smooth muscles of the body, the cardiac muscle, and many of the glands of the body; sensory innervation from the skin around the ear and taste and general sensation from the root of the tongue and epiglottis.

XI, accessory (spinal accessory) nerve—motor; supplies the **trapezius muscle** and the **sternocleidomastoid muscle** in the

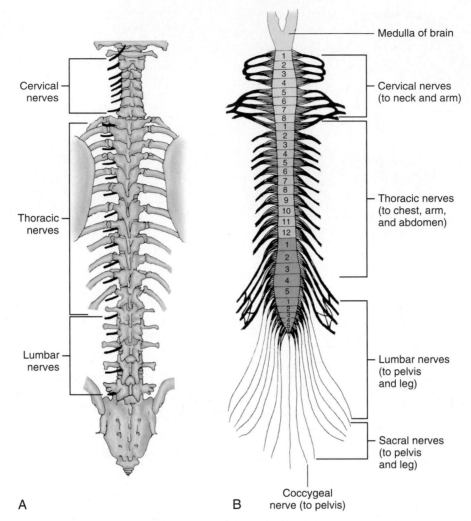

Medulla of brain

Cervical nerves

Cervical nerves (to neck and arm)

Thoracic nerves

Thoracic nerves (to chest, arm, and abdomen)

Lumbar nerves

Lumbar nerves (to pelvis and leg)

Sacral nerves (to pelvis and leg)

A

B

Coccygeal nerve (to pelvis)

• **Figure 34.4** **(A)** Some spinal nerves as they emerge from the vertebral column. **(B)** General arrangement of spinal nerves as they are grouped by regions. (Modified from Chusid JG, McDonald JJ. *Correlative Neuroanatomy and Functional Neurology*, 17th ed. Los Angeles: Lange Medical Publications; 1979.)

neck. Some parts of this nerve run with the vagus nerve and supply most of the soft palate, larynx, and pharynx muscles.

XII, hypoglossal nerve—motor; supplies most of the intrinsic and extrinsic muscles of the tongue except the **palatoglossus**, which is supplied by CNs X and XI.

Autonomic Nervous System

Before we continue with a more detailed description of some of these CNs, a brief discussion of the autonomic nervous system and its function is necessary. The autonomic system is sometimes called the *automatic nervous system* because it is not controlled by will. The system has motor and sensory fibers; the motor fibers supply smooth and cardiac muscle and glands, and the sensory fibers carry what is called **visceral sensation**. This is sensation from the various viscera or organs of the body, as well as from the mucous membrane from the tonsils on down through the digestive and respiratory tracts. Much of this visceral sensory pain is not well-isolated pain but pain of a more diffuse nature.

The autonomic nervous system has two parts: the **sympathetic system**, also known as the **thoracolumbar outflow** or the "**fight-or-flight mechanism**," and the **parasympathetic system**, also

known as the **craniosacral outflow**. Each of these components innervates all parts of the body, and therefore each organ generally has a sympathetic nerve supply and a parasympathetic nerve supply. These systems are **antagonists**, which means they have opposite actions.

Consider the action of the sympathetic nervous system. If someone frightens you, the sympathetic nervous system is stimulated, and you might find that the following things happen: your heart beats very fast and strong because of the release of **adrenalin** (or **epinephrine**); you become pale, and your skin feels cold and clammy as a result of shutdown of the surface capillaries; and you feel a knot in your stomach because of shutdown of blood supply to the digestive tract. All of this blood is being shunted to the skeletal muscles of the body; your heart beats faster; and you are breathing faster so that you are getting more oxygen into the body, which then goes to the muscles. The adrenalin aids the actions of the heart and lungs and enables the body to meet stressful situations. You may also find that your mouth becomes dry from shutdown of salivary glands, and the pupil of your eye dilates to let in more light so that you can better see the situation that has caused the stress. This reaction is referred to as the *fight-or-flight mechanism*.

Stimulation of the parasympathetic nervous system and the resultant actions tend to be the opposite of those of the sympathetic nervous system. The parasympathetic nervous system is referred to as the **vegetative system** because it relates to the process of digestion. Stimulation of this system slows down the heart and respiration; increases blood flow to the digestive system; increases **peristaltic contractions**; and stimulates secretion of the glands of the body, including that of the salivary glands.

Where do the terms *craniosacral* and *thoracolumbar* come from? Parasympathetic fibers come off the brain with CNs III, VII, IX, and X and off the spinal cord at the sacral levels (S2 to S4), hence the name **craniosacral outflow** (Fig. 34.5). As you look at the functions of the CNs, note the parasympathetic functions of CN III, VII, IX, and X. CN X has virtually no parasympathetic function that affects the head and neck region, but it affects structures within the thorax and the abdomen. The

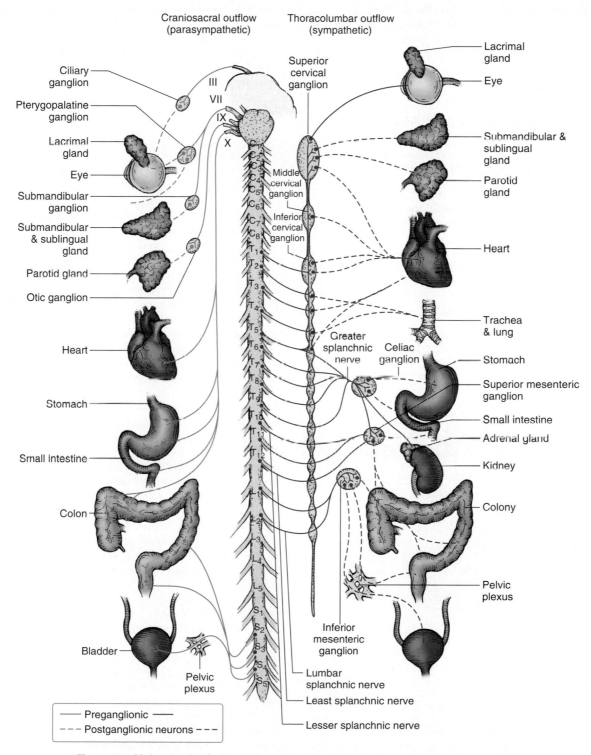

• **Figure 34.5** Various levels of origin of the autonomic nervous system and some areas supplied.

sympathetic system comes off the spinal cord at the 12 thoracic levels (T1 to T12) and the first two lumbar levels (L1 and L2), hence the name *thoracolumbar outflow*. The sympathetic nerves get to the head by running upward in a chain from the upper thoracic levels and then breaking off to run along the surfaces of the carotid arteries to virtually every part of the head. Sympathetic fibers also go back into the spinal nerves at all levels and run to the blood vessels, sweat glands, and smooth muscles, all of which are innervated by sympathetic fibers only.

The autonomic nervous system is a two-neuron system—a **preganglionic neuron** and a **postganglionic neuron**. As the names indicate, these neurons synapse in a **ganglion**, which is an accumulation of cell bodies of the postganglionic neurons outside the central nervous system. A number of parasympathetic ganglia are associated with the trigeminal nerve, the glossopharyngeal nerve, and the oculomotor nerve.

Nerves to the Oral Cavity and Associated Structures

Trigeminal Nerve (Cranial Nerve V)

The trigeminal nerve has three main branches, usually denoted as the **ophthalmic division (V$_1$)**, the **maxillary division (V$_2$)**, and the **mandibular division (V$_3$)**. The first two divisions of the trigeminal nerve are purely sensory. One of the overall functions of these three divisions is the innervation of the skin of the anterior face and head region. Fig. 34.6 shows where each of these three divisions supplies the face. Note that it does not supply the skin over the angle of the mandible. That area (L) is supplied by the **greater auricular nerve** of the cervical plexus of the neck (see Table 34.1).

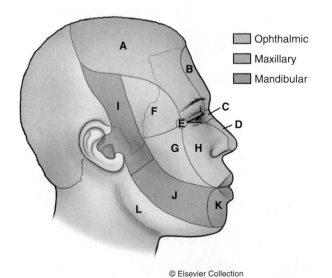

© Elsevier Collection

• **Figure 34.6** Areas of distribution on facial skin of the three divisions of the trigeminal nerve: ophthalmic, maxillary, and mandibular. Cutaneous innervation of the face; the letters indicate branches of the main divisions of the fifth cranial nerve: **(A)** supra-orbital nerve; **(B)** supratrochlear nerve; **(C)** infratrochlear nerve; **(D)** external nasal nerve; **(E)** lacrimal nerve; **(F)** zygomaticotemporal nerve; **(G)** zygomaticofacial nerve; **(H)** infraorbital nerve; **(I)** auriculotemporal nerve; **(J)** buccal nerve; **(K)** mental nerve; **(L)** greater auricular nerve (not a part of the trigeminal nerve).

Ophthalmic Division (V$_1$)

The ophthalmic division of the trigeminal nerve leaves the skull through the superior orbital fissure and enters the orbital cavity. It has three major branches, one of which is the **frontal nerve**. The frontal nerve travels forward in the roof of the orbit and breaks into two branches: the supraorbital nerve and the supratrochlear nerve. The **supraorbital nerve** emerges through the supraorbital notch and supplies the skin above the eye and up into the forehead. The **supratrochlear nerve** supplies the skin of the upper medial corner of the eye (Fig. 34.7). Another major branch of the ophthalmic division is the **lacrimal nerve**, which carries sensory responses from the skin above the lateral eye area and the lacrimal gland. The third major branch of the ophthalmic division is the **nasociliary nerve**, which sends **anterior** and **posterior ethmoidal nerve** branches into the nasal cavity and sends an **infratrochlear nerve** to the inferior, medial corner of the eye. One of the ethmoid branches, the anterior ethmoid, also has a branch that comes out onto the skin of the nose as an **external nasal nerve**.

Maxillary Division (V$_2$)

The maxillary division of the trigeminal nerve exits from the skull through the foramen rotundum and lies in the pterygopalatine fossa behind and below the eye. The branches follow the same kind of distribution pattern as the maxillary artery does—that is, to maxillary teeth and the oral cavity, the nasal cavity, the skin of the cheek, the midface, and the temporal region. These branches have basically the same names and pathways as those of the arterial supply to that area, thereby giving you some idea of their distribution. In the pterygopalatine fossa, the maxillary division splits into the following branches.

Posterior Superior Alveolar Nerve

The **posterior superior alveolar nerve** emerges laterally from the pterygopalatine fossa through the pterygomaxillary fissure and travels along the posterior portion of the maxillary tuberosity. It supplies the maxillary buccal gingiva of premolars and molars. It then enters the bone to supply second and third maxillary molars and usually the distobuccal and lingual roots of the first maxillary molar. It also supplies part of the maxillary sinus (Fig. 34.8).

Sphenopalatine Nerve

The **sphenopalatine nerve** branch comes off the maxillary division, goes through the sphenopalatine foramen, and supplies the lateral walls of the nasal cavity via **superior lateral nasal nerves**. It then goes up and comes down and forward across the nasal septum and leaves the nasal cavity through the incisive foramen as the **nasopalatine nerve** in the anterior palate, where it supplies the lingual gingiva adjacent to maxillary central and lateral incisors (Fig. 34.9).

Pterygopalatine Nerves

There are two small nerves that descend from the maxillary division and are known as the **pterygopalatine nerves**. These nerves connect the **pterygopalatine ganglion** with the maxillary nerve. This ganglion is a parasympathetic ganglion that is supplied via the **greater petrosal nerve**, a preganglionic nerve from CN VII. The postganglionic nerve coming out of the ganglion travels in the zygomatic nerve to provide parasympathetic innervation to the lacrimal gland. A sympathetic nerve, the **deep petrosal nerve**, passes through the ganglion and is destined mainly to blood vessels (Figs. 34.10 and 34.11).

TABLE 34.1   Branches of the Trigeminal Nerve: A Flow Chart

V₁. Ophthalmic division—enters orbit via superior orbital fissure. All branches are sensory.
1. Lacrimal nerve—sensory from lacrimal gland and skin above upper lateral corner of eye.
2. Frontal nerve—runs in roof of orbit and near front breaks into two branches.
   A. Supraorbital nerve—out through supraorbital notch or foramen to skin of forehead.
      1. Medial branch
      2. Lateral branch
   B. Supratrochlear nerve—comes medially off frontal and runs to inner corner of the eye above the trochlea for the superior oblique muscle. Supplies the skin over upper medial corner of eye.
3. Nasociliary nerve—travels lower in the orbit close to the optic nerve.
   A. Ciliary ganglion attaches to this part, and long and short ciliary nerves run to supply sensation to the cornea of the eye.
   B. Posterior ethmoid nerve goes through foramen of same name into posterior ethmoid region.
   C. Anterior ethmoid nerve enters the anterior ethmoid foramen and anterior ethmoid area. Supplies the anterior ethmoid air cells.
      1. Infratrochlear nerve—comes off anterior ethmoid nerve before it enters foramen. Travels below trochlea in medial corner of eye. Supplies skin in lower medial corner of eye.
      2. External nasal nerve—comes off anterior ethmoid nerve and travels to skin of nose just below nasal bones

V2. Maxillary division—exits skull through foramen rotundum and enters the pterygopalatine fossa behind and below the orbit, where it is attached to the pterygopalatine ganglion. It is also all sensory.
1. Posterior superior alveolar nerve—comes out of the pterygopalatine fossa through the pterygomaxillary fissure and onto tuberosity of maxilla. It supplies posterior upper molars and adjacent mucosa and maxillary sinus.
2. Zygomatic nerve—travels up into orbit and exits through zygomatico-facial and zygomatico-temporal foramen to supply skin over zygoma.
3. Pharyngeal nerve—back into upper wall of pharynx to mucosa.
4. Descending palatine nerve—descends down toward hard and soft palate and becomes:
   A. Greater palatine nerve—comes through greater palatine foramen to supply hard palate up to incisive foramen.
   B. Lesser palatine nerve—comes through lesser palatine foramen to supply the soft palate.
5. Sphenopalatine nerve—goes through the sphenopalatine (pterygopalatine) foramen into nasal cavity and has two branches:
   A. Posterior superior lateral nasal nerve—to that part of the nasal cavity.
   B. Nasopalatine nerve—travels down and forward on nasal septum, supplying that structure, then exits through incisive foramen and supplies gingiva lingual to anterior maxillary teeth.
6. Infraorbital nerve—the continuation of V₂ that runs along floor of orbit. There are three branches:
   A. Middle superior alveolar nerve—comes off infraorbital, running in wall of maxillary sinus to supply the sinus and upper premolars.
   B. Anterior superior alveolar nerve—comes off infraorbital nerve and runs down in maxillary bone to supply upper anterior teeth
   C. Infraorbital nerve—continues forward in floor of orbit and exits skull through infraorbital foramen. It has three branches:
      1. Lateral nasal—to side of nose
      2. Inferior palpebral—to skin of lower eyelid
      3. Superior labial—to skin and mucosa of upper lip

V₃. Mandibular division—this part of the trigeminal is *both* sensory and motor; compare these branches to the anterior and posterior division of the nerve.
A. Motor
   1. Nerve to tensor tympani—keeps eardrum taut
   2. Nerve to tensor veli palatini—helps tense soft palate
   3. Anterior and posterior deep temporal nerves—to temporalis muscle
   4. Nerve to masseter muscle
   5. Nerves to medial and lateral pterygoid muscles
   6. Mylohyoid nerve—off inferior alveolar nerve—supplies mylohyoid muscle and anterior digastric muscle
B. Sensory
   1. Buccal nerve to skin and mucosa of cheek
   2. Inferior alveolar nerve—to lower teeth
   3. Mental nerve—comes out through mental foramen to supply lower lip and skin of chin
   4. Lingual nerve—general sensation to anterior two-thirds of tongue
   5. Auriculotemporal nerve—to skin anterior and superior to the ear

The **descending palatine nerve** runs off the pterygopalatine ganglion straight down to the posterior part of the hard palate. There it separates into two branches: the **lesser palatine nerve**, which supplies the soft palate, and the **greater palatine nerve**, which supplies all the mucosa of the hard palate except the small area supplied by the nasopalatine branch of the sphenopalatine nerve. The greater palatine nerve extends along the lateral portion of the hard palate; the greater and lesser palatine nerves enter the palatal areas through the greater and lesser palatine foramina (see Figs. 34.8 and 34.10). They also supply the glands of the palate.

Zygomatic Nerve

The **zygomatic nerve** comes off the maxillary division, goes up into the orbit, and exits to supply the skin over the cheek and temple. It also carries postganglionic fibers from the pterygopalatine ganglion to provide parasympathetic innervation to the lacrimal gland (see Figs. 34.8 and 34.10).

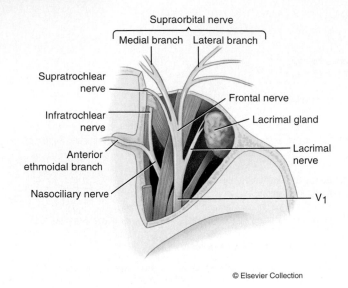

• **Figure 34.7** Supraorbital nerve of the first division of the trigeminal nerve as it comes out through the supraorbital notch to supply the skin of the forehead.

Infraorbital Nerve

The **infraorbital nerve** runs forward in the floor of the orbit to exit onto the face through the infraorbital canal and foramen. It supplies the skin of the nose, the lower eyelid, the skin and mucosa of the maxillary lip, and the maxillary labial gingiva. Although in the floor of the orbit, it sends two branches down to supply the rest of the maxillary teeth. The first branch to come off as the nerve travels forward is the **middle superior alveolar nerve**, which lies in the wall of the sinus to supply the premolars and usually the mesiobuccal root of the maxillary first molar. This nerve also supplies part of the maxillary sinus. The **anterior superior alveolar nerve** extends down, anterior to the wall of the sinus, to supply the maxillary anterior teeth (see Fig. 34.8). Other branches of the maxillary division go back to supply the area of the nasal pharynx.

Mandibular Division (V₃)

The mandibular division of the trigeminal nerve leaves the skull through the foramen ovale, traveling downward. As it leaves the skull, it enters an area known as the *infratemporal fossa,* adjacent to the pterygoid muscles of mastication. It then breaks off into anterior and posterior divisions.

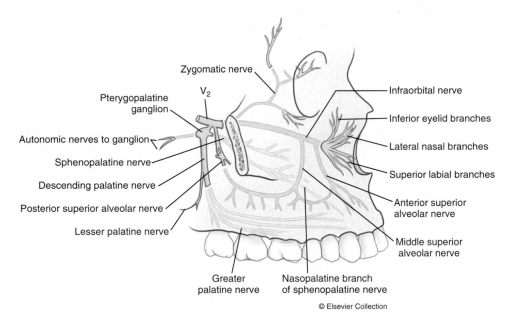

• **Figure 34.8** General distribution of the maxillary division of the trigeminal nerve. The posterior superior alveolar nerve can be seen coming off the main trunk of V₂, and the middle and anterior superior alveolar nerves can be seen coming off the infraorbital nerve.

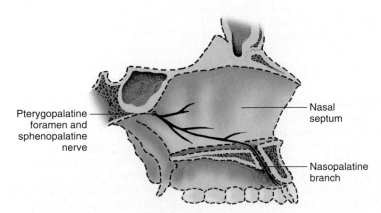

• **Figure 34.9** The sphenopalatine nerve enters the nasal cavity and one branch, the nasopalatine branch, travels down the nasal septum and exits through the incisive foramen to the anterior palatal mucosa.

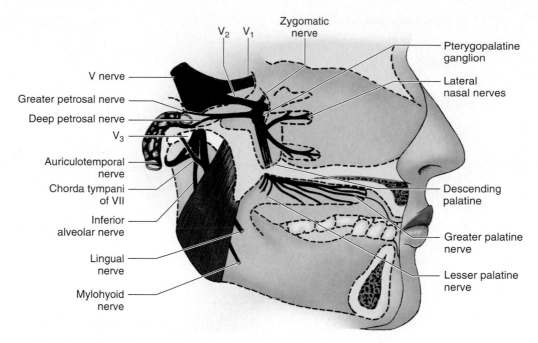

• **Figure 34.10** Partial diagram of V₂ and V₃. Note the descending palatine nerve and its greater and lesser palatine branches going to the hard and soft palates, respectively.

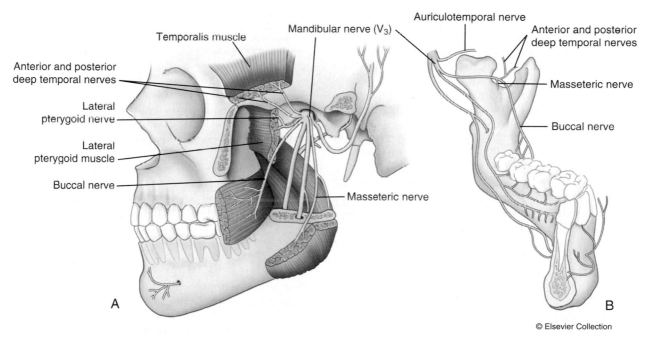

© Elsevier Collection

• **Figure 34.11** The anterior trunk of the mandibular nerve (the third division of the trigeminal nerve). **(A)** Lateral view. **(B)** Medial view.

Anterior Division

The anterior division breaks off into a number of branches. There are five motor nerves for the muscles of mastication: two to the temporal muscle and one each to the masseter muscle and the medial and lateral pterygoids. The last branch of the anterior division is the buccal nerve.

Buccal Nerve. The **buccal nerve** spreads out on the surface of the buccinator muscle and then penetrates the muscle. The lowest of its branches is frequently referred to as the **long buccal nerve**

and lies in the posterior portion of the mandibular mucobuccal fold. There it supplies the buccal mandibular gingiva up to the mental foramen. The remainder of the buccal nerve supplies the skin and mucosa of the cheek and most of the maxillary buccal gingiva (see Fig. 34.11).

Posterior Division. The posterior division of the mandibular division of the trigeminal nerve has three major sensory branches and one motor branch (Fig. 34.12).

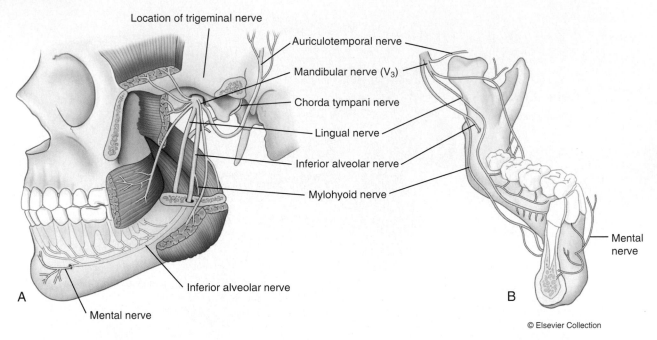

Location of trigeminal nerve

Auriculotemporal nerve

Mandibular nerve (V₃)

Chorda tympani nerve

Lingual nerve

Inferior alveolar nerve

Mylohyoid nerve

Mental nerve

Inferior alveolar nerve

Mental nerve

A

B

© Elsevier Collection

• **Figure 34.12** The posterior trunk of the third division of the trigeminal nerve (mandibular nerve). **(A)** Lateral view. **(B)** Medial view.

Lingual Nerve. The **lingual nerve** is one of the largest branches of the mandibular division. It supplies sensation to the floor of the mouth, the lingual mandibular gingiva, and the anterior two-thirds of the tongue. Not too far below the foramen ovale, the lingual nerve is joined by a branch from the seventh cranial nerve (facial), known as the **chorda tympani**. This small branch of nerve VII has parasympathetic (secretomotor) fibers to supply the submandibular and sublingual salivary glands and also carries special sensory fibers of taste perception from the anterior two-thirds of the tongue. Thus, in the floor of the mouth, where the lingual nerve is located, there are actually fibers from CN V and from CN VII all wrapped together, looking like one nerve. This juxtaposition also means that when the lingual nerve is inadvertently anesthetized during injection to mandibular teeth, the patient not only loses general sensation but also loses taste sensation in the anterior two-thirds of the tongue. Just above the submandibular gland, the **submandibular ganglion** is suspended from the lingual nerve. This parasympathetic ganglion is part of CN VII to supply the submandibular and sublingual salivary glands (see Fig. 34.12). These parasympathetic fibers come from the chorda tympani.

Inferior Alveolar Nerve. The **inferior alveolar nerve** primarily serves mandibular teeth, although it has a small motor branch called the **mylohyoid nerve**, which supplies the mylohyoid muscle and the anterior belly of the digastric muscle. Just beyond the point where the mylohyoid nerve branches off, the inferior alveolar nerve enters the mandible through the mandibular foramen and supplies all mandibular teeth and the periodontal ligaments of those teeth (see Figs. 34.12 and 34.13). Between mandibular premolars, a small branch known as the **mental nerve** comes out laterally through the mental foramen to supply the mucosa of the lip and labial gingiva in the anterior mandible area. It also supplies the skin of the mandibular lip and chin. This

accounts for numbing of the mandibular lip and chin during anesthetization of mandibular teeth because they are all innervated by the same nerve.

Auriculotemporal Nerve. The **auriculotemporal nerve** runs backward to supply the area above and in front of the ear. Lying on the medial surface of the mandibular division, just below the foramen ovale, is the **otic ganglion**, and coming off the ganglion are regular motor fibers to the tensor veli palatini and the tensor tympani muscles. There is also a preganglionic nerve, the **lesser petrosal nerve** from CN IX, which comes down from the brain through the foramen ovale and synapses in the otic ganglion. Postganglionic fibers travel with the auriculotemporal nerve and provide parasympathetic innervation to the parotid gland (see Figs. 34.10, 34.12, and 34.13).

Facial Nerve (CN VII)

Most of the facial nerve exits the brain through the stylomastoid foramen behind the ear. It comes forward and is found within the substance of the parotid gland. Inside the gland, it separates into a number of branches to provide motor innervation to the muscles of facial expression. The distribution of these branches varies from person to person, but there generally is a temporal branch, a zygomatic branch, one buccal branch or more, a mandibular branch, and a cervical branch (Fig. 34.14). The cervical branch supplies the platysma muscle in the neck. Before the nerve enters the parotid gland, a small nerve branches to the skin behind the ear, the auricular muscles, and the stylohyoid and posterior digastric muscles. Although the facial nerve is still inside the skull, a branch extends through the middle ear and out of the skull as the chorda tympani. As mentioned previously, this nerve carries parasympathetic (secretomotor) fibers to the submandibular and sublingual glands and special taste fibers from the anterior

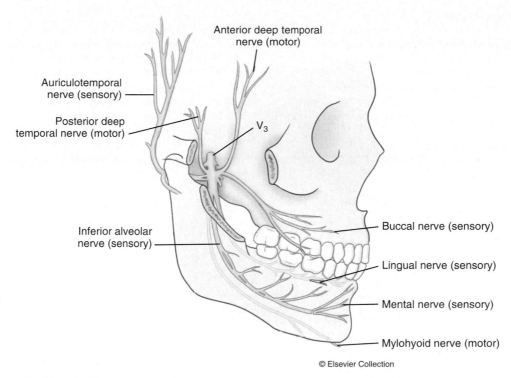

Anterior deep temporal nerve (motor)

Auriculotemporal nerve (sensory)

Posterior deep temporal nerve (motor)

V_3

Buccal nerve (sensory)

Inferior alveolar nerve (sensory)

Lingual nerve (sensory)

Mental nerve (sensory)

Mylohyoid nerve (motor)

© Elsevier Collection

• **Figure 34.13** The inferior alveolar nerve (V_3) enters the mandible through the mandibular foramen, and the mental nerve branches off it in the premolar region. The auriculotemporal nerve extends back over the ear.

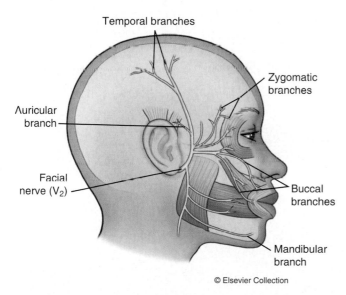

Temporal branches

Zygomatic branches

Auricular branch

Facial nerve (V_2)

Buccal branches

Mandibular branch

© Elsevier Collection

• **Figure 34.14** Branches of the facial nerve that supply the muscles of facial expression.

two-thirds of the tongue. Again, these fibers run in the same bundle with the lingual nerve (see Figs. 34.12 and 34.13). Remember that the facial nerve also sends off a branch, the greater petrosal nerve, which goes to V_2 to carry parasympathetic innervation to the lacrimal gland.

Glossopharyngeal Nerve (CN IX)

The glossopharyngeal nerve exits the skull along with the vagus and accessory nerves through the jugular foramen. It then sends one branch to a pharyngeal muscle, the stylopharyngeus, and branches to the mucosa of the constrictor muscles of the pharynx, which help accomplish swallowing. Another branch goes to the posterior one third of the tongue to supply both general sensation and taste to that region. As indicated previously, the lesser petrosal branch of CN IX provides parasympathetic innervation to the parotid gland (see Fig. 34.10).

Vagus Nerve (CN X)

The vagus nerve affects more areas of the body than any other CN. It sends fibers down to the heart, lungs, kidneys, and most of the digestive tract. Its branches to the pharynx, larynx, and tongue are of the greatest importance to our discussion. The vagus nerve sends a small branch to the base of the tongue, where it innervates the base of the tongue and the epiglottis. This branch carries general sensation and has a few taste fibers. There are two branches that go to the larynx—the superior and the inferior laryngeal (or recurrent laryngeal) nerves. These provide general sensation and motor activity to the muscles of the larynx. There is also a motor branch to the muscles of the soft palate and pharynx. All of these are accompanied by the cranial portion of CN XI, which is believed to supply most of the previously mentioned structures. Refer to the table Nerve Supply to the Oral Cavity, located at the end of Chapter 36.

Review Questions

1. What are the two subdivisions of the nervous system?
2. What are the parts of a spinal nerve? What are the two parts seen in a cross-section of the spinal cord?
3. What happens when the sympathetic nervous system is stimulated?
4. What happens when the parasympathetic nervous system is stimulated?
5. Name the 12 cranial nerves and their general functions.
6. Which nerves carry parasympathetic fibers?
7. Which nerves supply each tooth?
8. Name the nerves supplying each area of oral mucosa.
9. Name the nerve supply to the major salivary glands, and describe their pathway to the glands.
10. Which nerve is responsible for the sensation of taste to the anterior two-thirds of the tongue?
11. If CN VII was damaged emerging from the brain, which glands would be affected?
12. If the parotid gland had a tumor and had to be removed, what nerve might be affected, and what would be the result?

35

Lymphatics and the Spread of Dental Infection

OBJECTIVES

- To briefly discuss the function of the lymphatic system
- To diagram and label the major groups of lymph nodes that drain teeth and the oral cavity
- To define the terms *primary*, *secondary*, and *tertiary nodes of involvement* as they relate to lymph drainage
- To name the primary lymph drainage of all teeth
- To briefly discuss the concept of fascial space infection
- To explain how a fascial space infection may spread from the oral cavity to the thorax
- To define Ludwig's angina

Lymphatic System

The lymphatic system is a part of the overall lymphoid system of the body and a component of the immune system of the body. It is an accumulation of tiny channels or tubules with small nodular structures called **lymph nodes** interconnecting them. The system functions by returning fluids to the bloodstream from the various tissues of the body. A filtrate of blood plasma flows out of the capillaries into the surrounding tissues, where it becomes extracellular fluid. It is eventually picked up by lymphatic vessels or tubules. The extracellular fluid, now referred to as **lymphatic fluid**, flows through tubules, then through nodes, back through tubules, and generally through some more nodes. It finally empties into the venous system at the junction of the internal jugular and subclavian veins on the right side of the neck and on the left side into the thoracic duct, and travels eventually back to the heart. This kind of fluid circulation repeats itself continually. The lymph nodes act as filters for the fluids, and the lymphocytes produced within the lymph nodes combat infections that might spread through the lymphatic channels. Most tissues, including the tooth pulp, have lymph vessels in them. The distribution of these vessels has been well determined, and this information can be used as a diagnostic tool in the study of oral infections and as a means of slowing the spread of cancers.

Distribution Pattern

Five **superficial groups** of lymph nodes in the head and neck could eventually allow lymph infection to reach the heart (see Fig. 35.1).

1. The **occipital node**—located behind the ear and drains the crown of the head, and if not stopped there, the infection drains into deeper nodes.

2. **Posterior auricular (mastoid nodes)**—also behind the ear. From there it can go to into a larger node below, and a bit behind the **parotid gland**, following the facial artery where they drain the posterior side of the scalp.

3. **Preauricular/parotid node**—drains from the anterior head above the eyes into nodes on the lateral side of the parotid gland.

4. **Submandibular nodes**—these are below and behind the chin, and they drain and follow the course of the **facial artery from the forehead**, draining the gingiva, teeth, and tongue.

5. **Submental nodes**—drain inferior chin, floor of mouth, tongue tip, and lower incisors.

The **jugulodigastric node**, a large node found at the angle of the mandible, borders on the posterior of the parotid gland. It receives drainage from a potential number of nodes that drain the anterior ear, anterolateral scalp, upper face, gingiva, eyelids, and cheek region.

The pre-auricular/parotid node drains a very small accumulation of nodes, the submental nodes, which are found beneath the chin. Several areas around the chin drain into these nodes. Any infection in these areas would generally cause some tenderness and enlargement of the nodes. These nodes tend to drain into the submandibular nodes or directly down and across the neck to the deep cervical nodes.

Submandibular Nodes

The **submandibular nodes** are found grouped around the submandibular gland near the angle of the mandible. The easiest way to locate the gland and the nodes is to place a finger on the inferior border of the mandible near the angle. Run the finger back and forth until you feel the depression in the inferior border of the mandible. This is the point at which the facial artery and vein cross the inferior border. Just medial to this depression is the submandibular gland, and the **submandibular lymph nodes** are grouped around it.

The areas that drain into these nodes are all of the maxillary teeth and the maxillary sinus, with the exception of the maxillary third molars; the mandibular canines and all mandibular posterior teeth, with the possibility that the mandibular third molars may not drain here; the floor of the mouth and most of the tongue; the cheek area; the hard palate; and the anterior nasal cavity. As mentioned before, the submental nodes also drain into these nodes. Any infections in these areas tend to cause enlargement and tenderness of the submandibular nodes. This condition of tenderness and enlargement is referred to as **lymphadenopathy**. There is significant variation in the path of these nodes. The above nodes may be palpable because they are more superficial, but the deep

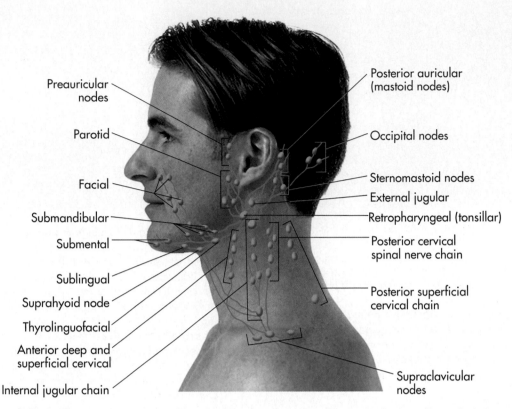

Preauricular nodes

Parotid

Facial

Submandibular

Submental

Sublingual

Suprahyoid node

Thyrolinguofacial

Anterior deep and superficial cervical

Internal jugular chain

Posterior auricular (mastoid nodes)

Occipital nodes

Sternomastoid nodes

External jugular

Retropharyngeal (tonsillar)

Posterior cervical spinal nerve chain

Posterior superficial cervical chain

Supraclavicular nodes

• **Figure 35.1** Location of palpable superficial lymph nodes. Elsevier collection. (From Darby's *Comprehensive Review of Dental Hygiene* 9th Edition Fig 4.10.)

cervical nodes to follow are much deeper inside the neck and unable to palpate.

Superior Deep Cervical Nodes

The **superior deep cervical nodes** are located on the lateral surface of the internal jugular vein and lie just beneath the anterior border of the sternomastoid muscle, about 2 inches below the ear. A number of other nodes drain into this group—the submandibular nodes; the nodes behind the back throat wall, known as the **retropharyngeal nodes**; the parotid nodes in front of the ear and the parotid gland; and others. This is the group affected when a person has a particularly sore throat. When a throat infection begins, the first group of nodes involved is the retropharyngeal nodes because they are behind the throat wall. Because palpating these nodes is impractical, the next group of nodes generally involved in a throat infection, the upper deep cervical nodes, is the first to be noticed. Many patients with sore throats first notice tenderness in the upper deep cervical nodes. The superior deep cervical group also drains both maxillary and mandibular third molar regions, the base of the tongue, the tonsillar area, the soft palate, and the posterior nasal cavity region. Therefore tenderness in the upper deep cervical nodes without a sore throat should cause you to look in a number of areas to discover the source of the infection.

Inferior Deep Cervical Nodes

The **inferior deep cervical nodes** are also found on the lateral surface of the internal jugular vein and beneath the anterior border of the sternomastoid muscle. These nodes are also around the internal jugular vein, although much lower down the vein than the superior deep cervical. For that reason, in some texts they are referred to as upper and lower deep cervical nodes (see Fig. 35.2). The inferior deep cervical nodes are located about 2 inches above the clavicle. They drain the superior (upper) deep cervical nodes and many of the nodes at the back of the neck, frequently referred to as *occipital nodes*, as well as some glands in the anterior neck. From the inferior (lower) deep cervical nodes, the lymphatic fluid drains into the junction of the subclavian and internal jugular veins.

Node Groups Affected by Disease

The terms **primary nodes**, **secondary nodes**, and **tertiary nodes** are often used in discussions about infections and cancer, both of which spread through lymphatic channels. These terms refer to the groups of nodes that are affected in a disease process. If an infection is not stopped by the first (primary) group of nodes, it will spread to the second (secondary) group. If it is not stopped there, it may spread to the third (tertiary) group. One node or group of nodes can be primarily involved in one source of infection, and the same group of nodes can be involved at the secondary or tertiary level in another source of infection. Look at the deep cervical nodes (see Fig. 35.2). They are divided into a superior (upper) and an inferior (lower) deep cervical group; the upper (superior) group eventually may drain into the lower (inferior) group.

An infection of the third molars may involve these nodes first—the primary group involved. If the infection were in a second mandibular molar, the initial sign of infection would be in the submandibular nodes. If it were not successfully combated there, it would spread secondarily to the superior deep cervical nodes.

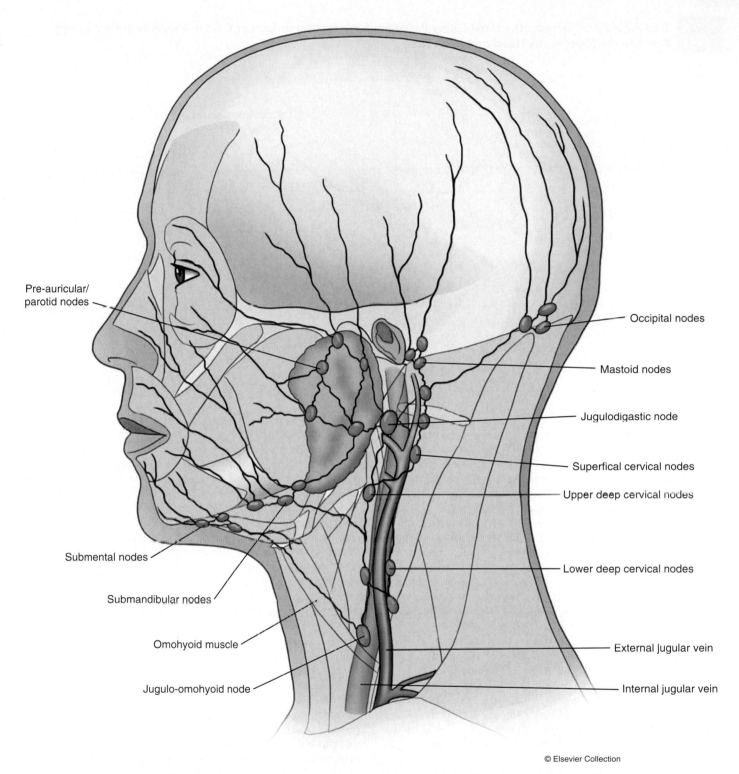

Pre-auricular/
parotid nodes

Occipital nodes

Mastoid nodes

Jugulodigastic node

Superfical cervical nodes

Upper deep cervical nodes

Lower deep cervical nodes

Submental nodes

Submandibular nodes

Omohyoid muscle

Jugulo-omohyoid node

External Jugular vein

Internal jugular vein

© Elsevier Collection

• **Figure 35.2** Locations of some of the major groups of lymph nodes that drain the head and neck. The retropharyngeal group is not visible because of its location behind the throat. The deep cervical chain lies on the internal jugular vein beneath the sternomastoid muscle (not depicted), which has been removed in this view.

Infections originating in the middle of the lower lip would spread first to the submental nodes, secondarily to the submandibular nodes, and then to the superior deep cervical nodes, which, in this instance, would be tertiary nodes of involvement. Keep in mind that in infections, any group of nodes may overcome the infection if it is not too severe, and the infection may go no further. Table 35.1 shows the most likely pathways of infections as they drain from one set of nodes to another. In the case of cancers, spreading to each deeper and more inferior node implies that the chances of the cancer metastasizing (spreading) are more likely.

| TABLE 35.1 | This Flow Chart Depicts the Most Likely Pathways for Infection or Cancer Cells to Move from One Lymph Node to the Next in the Head and Neck Area |

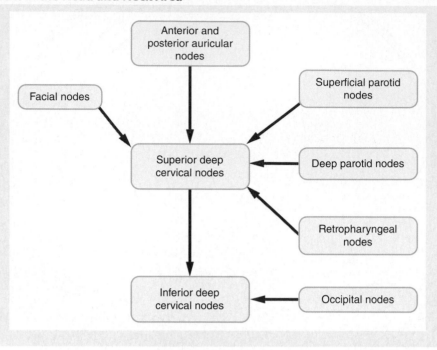

An understanding of this concept is necessary to comprehend the spread of oral cancer. Each group of nodes acts as a resistance barrier against the spread of cancer. The nodes slow the spread, and if the cancer is detected early enough, it can be treated with greater success. Once the infection or the cancer reaches the lower deep cervical nodes and passes through them, it enters the bloodstream, moving directly into the heart and then throughout the body. With this in mind, it is easy to understand why cancer on the tip of the tongue has a lower **mortality rate** compared with cancer that begins farther back on the tongue or in the throat. The tip of the tongue generally drains through three or four groups of nodes before the cancer enters the bloodstream and spreads throughout the body, whereas cancer in the posterior portion of the tongue or in the throat travels to the upper deep cervical nodes, onto the lower deep cervical nodes, and into the bloodstream. In that area, there are generally only two groups to stop the spread of the disease. When cancer is detected, knowing the location of the cancer and having knowledge of the nodes involved allows the surgeon to do a biopsy of the next group of nodes in the chain to see if there is cancer in them. If these nodes are free of cancer, it can be a good sign that the cancer has not spread any further and generally means a more favorable prognosis for the patient.

Spread of Infection in Fascial Spaces

Another way through which infections may spread is through **fascial spaces**. Although infection spread through fascial spaces is much less common, it displays much more dramatic clinical symptoms. The spaces between muscle and tissue layers are referred to as **fascial layers**, or fascial planes, and infections may spread to this area. You may have seen a patient with a large swollen jaw or with a swollen area beneath the eye. In this situation, the infection of dental origin is not spreading through the small lymphatic channels but has broken out of the bone around the tooth and is spreading between tissue or muscle layers.

This kind of infection spread will follow certain predictable pathways, depending on its location. In general, dental infections start in the maxillae or the mandible at the apex of a tooth or in the periodontal space around a tooth. Most periodontal space infections cause a swelling of gingival or mucosal tissue within the oral cavity. Infections at the apices of the teeth cause swelling in one of two directions: buccal or lingual. Most buccal swellings also lead to a swelling in the vestibule of the oral cavity. This swelling is sometimes referred to as a **gumboil**. The infection comes to a pointed head, breaks through the mucosa, and drains into the oral cavity. If a mandibular infection spreads not in the buccal but in the lingual direction, it will travel to the tissue spaces in two specific areas—above the mylohyoid muscle in the floor of the mouth or beneath the mylohyoid muscle in the tissue beneath the chin—depending on its point of origin.

How can one predict where the infection will go? Refer to Fig. 35.3, a lateral view of the body of the mandible, which displays the lengths of the roots of individual teeth. The mylohyoid muscle attaches at the mylohyoid ridge on the mandible (refer back to Fig. 26.17). Look at the mylohyoid ridge on the mandible and note its location relative to the apices of the roots. You can see in Fig. 35.2 that the apices of the mandibular second and third molar teeth are inferior to the mylohyoid muscle, whereas the apices of the roots of premolars, anterior teeth, and usually the first molar are above the mylohyoid muscle. Therefore a mandibular second or third molar infection will tend to break out of the bone below the mylohyoid muscle and spread to the floor of the mouth beneath the mandible, referred to as the **submandibular space**.

Infections of the first molar and premolar teeth will tend to break out of bone above the mylohyoid muscle. They spread to the spaces beneath the tongue but above the mylohyoid muscle, referred to as the **sublingual space**.

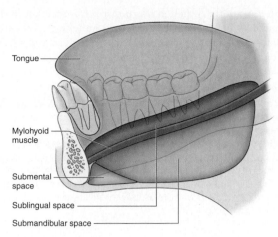

• **Figure 35.3** Medial lateral view of mandible displaying location of the mandibular teeth root tips in relationship to the mylohyoid muscle and submandibular spaces.

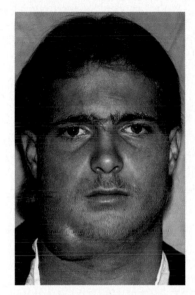

• **Figure 35.4** Ludwig's angina: the swelling under and to the right side of the patient's mandible is not only uncomfortable but dangerous. The same pressure that distends the tissue outside of the face also pushes the tongue backward in the mouth. This starts to suffocate the patient by blocking the airway in his throat. (From Misch's avoiding complications in Oral implantology.)

Infection from the anterior teeth will tend to spread into the submental space below the chin. This will cause a swelling beneath the chin.

All the spaces communicate with each other. If one space swells up too much some of its infected material will find a way into an adjacent space. If a third molar infection causes a cellulitis that produces too much pressure to confine it to just the submandibular space, then the cellulitis will also move into the adjacent sublingual space or even the parapharyngeal space.

Infections from the submandibular and sublingual spaces sometimes form a serious life-threatening cellulitis referred to as **Ludwig's angina** (Fig. 35.4). These infections continue to spread by gravity, if not treated. Whether these infections occur above or below the mylohyoid muscle, as they spread down and back, they reach the posterior end of the mylohyoid muscle. Both kinds of

infection eventually reach the side of the neck next to the pharynx, which is referred to as the **lateral pharyngeal** or **parapharyngeal space**. This causes swelling on the side of the neck, if left untreated. From here the infection may spread around the pharynx to its posterior border, which is referred to as the **retropharyngeal space**, and from there to the **posterior mediastinum**, which is in the back of the chest, or thoracic cavity. If the infection reaches this point, the person may die within a short period. With the advent of antibiotics, these infections are not seen as frequently as they were in the past but are still often encountered.

The term *angina* means tortured, twisted, or painful. In the case of Ludwig's angina, it refers to the fact that patients can die from asphyxiation. The tongue is pushed posteriorly toward the back of the mouth. This starts to close off the pharynx, preventing the patient from breathing and causing the patient to suffocate. This can happen in a matter of hours, so patients with Ludwig's angina must undergo immediate treatment and probable hospitalization. Before the advent of antibiotics Ludwig's angina was 50% fatal. Even now with antibiotics and surgical intervention the mortality rate is 8%. Ninety percent of the time Ludwig's angina is caused by infections from just two teeth, the mandibular second and third molars. The other ten percent are from things like infected oral piercings, broken jaws, mouth lacerations, and oral tissue infections, even other teeth.

When mandibular anterior and premolar and first molars abscess, they usually abscess buccally. If they abscess lingually the infected tissue goes into the sublingual space above the mylohyoid muscle. If this sublingual infection is severe enough the infected tissue could find its way into the submandibular space. This, however, is rare compared to the number of infections in this area occurring from mandibular second and third molars. The importance of this section is not to completely describe or define the boundaries of these spaces or **potential spaces** but to understand how the origin or location of the original infection determines the pathway it will follow and the potential outcome if left untreated.

One more space that should be mentioned is the pterygomandibular space. This space is located medial to the ramus of the mandible starting from the retromandibular pad posteriorly and superiorly (see Fig. 35.5). It is most often associated with

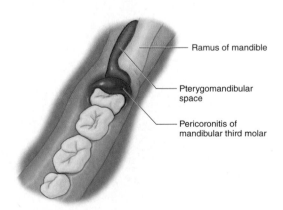

• **Figure 35.5** Pericoronitis is the infection of the periodontal tissues surrounding a mandibular third and sometimes second molar. The gingival tissue swells up with so much suppuration (pus) that it literally covers over a large portion of the crown. In this depiction, the posterior half of the crown of the third molar is covered with swollen gingiva. If left to fester, this infection could easily spread to the pterygomandibular space behind the retromolar pad. The tissue is cut away to show the location of the pterygomandibular space in relation to the third molar and the ramus of the mandible.

pericoronitis from periodontal infections of third and sometimes second molars. The pterygomandibular space communicates with the parapharyngeal and submandibular spaces, which makes it a location for potentially serious even life-threatening outcomes.

Other Maxillary Infections

Maxillary infections react slightly differently because of the anatomic features of the area. If the infection does not open into the maxillary buccal vestibule or onto the palate, it may spread toward three areas—the nasal cavity, the maxillary sinus, or the soft tissue spaces of the cheek or the area below the eye. The area involved is related to the tooth involved. Swelling below the eye is usually related to infection from an anterior tooth, usually the maxillary canine, whereas swelling in the cheek is usually related to infection

in a posterior tooth. Although it is possible for infection to spread to the nasal cavity or maxillary sinus, it is rather rare. These maxillary infections around the eye or cheek can also spread to the lateral pharyngeal space and from there to other areas.

Brain Buster

- Perform a head and neck exam on fellow classmates. Compare and contrast findings.
- Ludwig's angina has been linked to oral piercing. Educate individuals who may be considering getting an oral piercing. Have the individual ask questions about the sterilization method being used in their establishment.
- When scaling mandibular third and second molars, pay particular attention to teeth whose crowns are partially covered by gum tissue. This could indicate pericoronitis.

Review Questions

1. What is the function of lymph nodes?
2. What are the major groups of lymph nodes in the head and neck?
3. Name the structures that drain primarily into each group of lymph nodes.
4. What are fascial spaces?
5. Where can fascial space infections eventually end up if left untreated, and how serious can this be?
6. Submental space infections come from which group of teeth?
7. Swelling below the eye would come from infection in which teeth?
8. What group of nodes could be palpated as being painful in a throat infection?

36

Anatomic Considerations of Local Anesthesia

OBJECTIVES

- To understand the anatomy of the maxillary nerve as it relates to administration of local anesthesia
- To understand the anatomy associated with mandibular blocks
- To understand the different areas anesthetized by the maxillary and mandibular nerve blocks
- To understand the major concerns associated with different local anesthetic nerve blocks
- To understand the anatomic considerations during administration of local anesthesia
- To understand the anatomy involved in local infiltration and nerve block injections

Dental Local Anesthetics

Dental local anesthetics are used to anesthetize teeth and gingivae. They are divided into local **infiltration injections (supraperiosteal injections)** and **regional nerve blocks.** Local *infiltration anesthesia* affects the tissue in a very small area, the area where the anesthetic is delivered. The anesthetic must penetrate the periosteum in order to anesthetize the periodontium, teeth, and gingiva. Otherwise only the gingiva may be anesthetized and not necessarily the teeth in the immediate area. The *supraperiosteal injection* affects teeth, the periodontium, and gingivae.

The anesthetic is delivered close to a main nerve trunk in a *regional block.* The regional nerve block affects a much larger area and more teeth because it affects a number of nerves rather than just a single nerve. Regional blocks may affect an area far removed from the original injection site. A regional block may or may not affect teeth but definitely affects the periodontium and gingiva of a large or small area because the area anesthetized is close to a nerve trunk.

Local Infiltration or Supraperiosteal Injection

Local Infiltration

Local infiltration is the term used for anesthesia of a small soft tissue area and not necessarily teeth or bone. The anesthetic is deposited into the soft tissue, and only the soft tissue in the area where anesthetic is deposited will be anesthetized. The term is often confused with *supraperiosteal injection,* where the roots of

teeth are anesthetized as well as soft tissue. The needle in the local infiltration injection pierces the gingiva and stops before it hits the bone. Anatomic concerns are limited to how much anesthetic can be deposited into the tissue without tearing or stretching the tissue. Attached gingiva can be stretched too far, whereas free gingiva or buccal mucosa can absorb more anesthetic. Hitting a nerve or blood vessel or tearing the periosteum is unlikely because the needle stops as soon as it pierces the gingiva. Local infiltration can be used in the interdental papilla, free gingiva, or attached gingiva to control bleeding if a vasoconstrictor is added to the anesthetic agent (Fig. 36.1).

In reality, in the **maxilla** it is hard to anesthetize soft tissue only because the anesthetic infiltrates into the bone and anesthetizes the bone. If the anesthetic is delivered above the roots of the maxillary teeth, as a local injection, it becomes a supraperiosteal injection and anesthetizes the teeth as well. This is different in the **mandible,** and an infiltration injection of **most** local anesthetics does not penetrate the mandibular bone and therefore does not become a supraperiosteal injection because it does not anesthetize the teeth.

For our purposes, the terms local infiltration and supraperiosteal injection are interchangeable in the maxilla but not in the mandible.

Supraperiosteal Injection

The **buccal** bone of the maxilla is much more porous than that of the mandible. This makes it easier for the anesthetic solution to penetrate the buccal bone of the maxilla and reach the apices of maxillary teeth. To do this the anesthetic solution must be delivered above the apexes of the roots of the teeth. It then moves through the bone and drops the solution into the root apexes via the blood vessels. It is here at the root apex that the nerve exits the tooth. If the anesthetic solution reaches this area, it will anesthetize the tooth. The bone and its surrounding gingiva on the facial side of the tooth are anesthetized as the solution penetrates bone and reaches the terminal branches of nerve in the gingiva and alveolar bone.

The **lingual** gingiva of maxillary teeth will require separate lingual local infiltration. This attached tissue is much denser and does not allow room for much anesthetic solution. Consequently the gingiva can be anesthetized, but there is usually not enough solution to penetrate bone at the root apex. Most dental procedures only require the facial supraperiosteal injection unless the lingual gingiva is involved as in periodontal debridement, an extraction, or periodontal surgery.

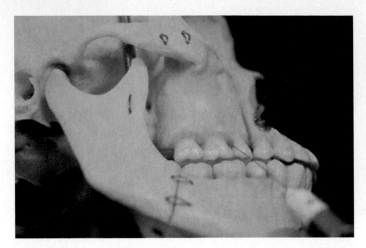

• **Figure 36.1** The needle in the interdental papillary is inserted into the dental papilla and stops before it touches the interdental bone.

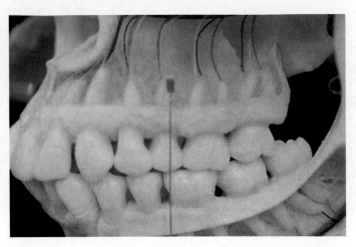

• **Figure 36.2** The needle tip of the maxillary supraperiosteal injection stops just short of alveolar bone at a height just above the target root apex. The red square at the end of the needle helps to identify its tip location.

Maxillary Supraperiosteal Injection

The anatomic considerations for **maxillary supraperiosteal injection** are mainly puncturing of an artery or vein in the mucosa. The injection is made in the unattached vestibular tissue at the height of the mucobuccal fold, and the needle continues to penetrate to just above the height of the targeted maxillary root apex. The anesthetic solution penetrates the gingiva and bone and drops down via gravity into the area of the root apex (Fig. 36.2). The local anesthetic is quite predictable but only anesthetizes the tooth below the injection and its buccal tissue. It is necessary to have a good understanding of the root's length to properly perform supraperiosteal injections.

In Fig. 36.3 the needle is far above and posterior to the roots of the molars. This injection site is for a regional block and not a supraperiosteal injection (see Fig. 36.3).

Mandibular Supraperiosteal Injection

The mandibular bone is much denser and less porous than the maxillary bone. Therefore, only certain local anesthetics can penetrate it. It requires more time to take effect and a different target location, compared with maxillary supraperiosteal injection.

The **mandibular supraperiosteal injection** is similar to the maxillary supraperiosteal injection with three exceptions. First, only a few anesthetics can penetrate the denser mandibular bone. Lidocaine, mepivacaine, or prilocaine, which are the most common local anesthetic agents, cannot be used. Only articaine effectively penetrates mandibular bone.

Second, the injection site is not directly above the target area but one-half tooth distal to the target. If the mandibular first molar needs to be anesthetized, the injection site would be between the mandibular first and second molar (one-half tooth farther distal to the target site). This is because the anesthetic solution needs to penetrate bone and arrive at the inferior alveolar nerve in a location posterior to the target area. All mandibular teeth are innervated by the inferior alveolar nerve. The anesthetic solution needs to be delivered posterior to the target area so that the agent can intercept the transmission of the nerve impulses that are sent posteriorly, back toward the trigeminal nerve ganglion.

Third, the needle must go to the height of the root apex or just above the root apex in mandibular teeth, and gravity will carry the anesthetic *down* to the area of the root as the anesthetic agent penetrates this denser bone (Fig. 36.4).

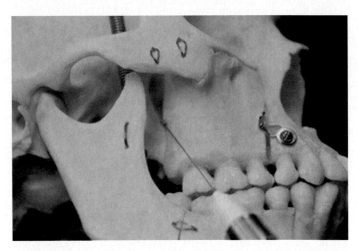

• **Figure 36.3** The target area for the posterior superior alveolar injection is the posterior alveolar nerve. This nerve emerges from the posterior superior alveolar foramen, which is found on the posterior superior area of the maxillary tuberosity above the maxillary second molar.

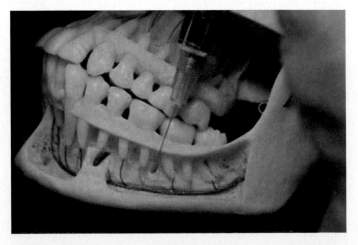

• **Figure 36.4** Mandibular supraperiosteal injection site is distal to and about the height of the apex of the target tooth.

Regional Nerve Blocks

Maxillary Nerve Blocks

Maxillary nerve blocks anesthetize a broader area of tissue compared with supraperiosteal injections. A local anesthetic is deposited in the vicinity of a major nerve trunk, and it anesthetizes the area the nerve innervates from that point on. The maxillary branch of the fifth cranial nerve (CN V) gives off the posterior superior alveolar branch in the area posterior and superior to the maxillary tuberosity (Fig. 36.5). The remaining branch continues on to become the middle superior alveolar nerve branch (See Table 36.1). The middle superior alveolar nerve continues on to join with the anterior superior alveolar nerve. Both of these latter nerves also have branches that ascend upward to meet the infraorbital nerve, which emerges from the infraorbital foramen.

Four maxillary nerve blocks are delivered from the facial side, as discussed here.

1. The **posterior alveolar nerve block** anesthetizes maxillary molars and their associated bone, gingiva, and buccal periodontium. The one exception is the mesiobuccal root of the maxillary first molar. At this point refer to Fig. 36.6 and note the areas covered by regional blocks.
2. The **middle superior alveolar nerve block** anesthetizes maxillary premolars, their associated bone, gingiva, buccal periodontium, and the mesiobuccal root of the maxillary first molar.
3. The **anterior superior alveolar nerve block** anesthetizes maxillary anterior teeth (canine, lateral, and central) along with their associated bone, gingiva, buccal periodontium, and the maxillary lip to the midline.
4. The **infraorbital nerve block** anesthetizes both areas covered by the middle and anterior superior alveolar nerve blocks. It covers maxillary anterior teeth, premolars, and the mesiobuccal root of the maxillary first molar. It also covers their associated bone, gingiva, facial periodontium of these maxillary teeth to the midline, and part of the cheek.

In performing any of these nerve blocks, a long needle is first inserted into the maxillary buccal fold and continued up much farther than one would go with the supraperiosteal injection. If the needle hits bone, back off slightly so that the periosteum is not torn. Tearing the periosteum could be instantly painful as well as uncomfortable postoperatively. It is easy to inadvertently perform a superior alveolar nerve block when trying to perform a supraperiosteal injection if the needle point is carried too far above the desired target area (Fig. 36.7).

The major concerns with all nerve blocks are injecting into a blood vessel, tearing a blood vessel, or puncturing a nerve. Anesthetic solution injected into a blood vessel continues on the path of that blood vessel. Anesthetic delivered into the posterior alveolar vein travels into the facial vein and the maxillary vein, both leading into the internal jugular vein and then into the brachiocephalic vein and eventually to the lungs and the heart, from where the anesthetic is pumped all over the body. A patient could therefore feel numbness in the toes, ears, or even fingers. If this

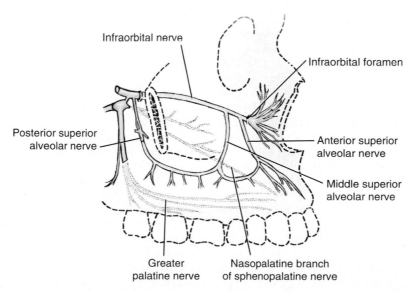

Infraorbital nerve

Infraorbital foramen

Posterior superior alveolar nerve

Anterior superior alveolar nerve

Middle superior alveolar nerve

Greater palatine nerve

Nasopalatine branch of sphenopalatine nerve

• **Figure 36.5** Right maxilla showing the superior alveolar nerve as its branches continue from anterior to posterior while joining up with the infraorbital nerve and ultimately the maxillary branch of the fifth cranial nerve (V_2).

TABLE 36.1	Nerve Supply of Oral Cavity		
	Mucosa	**Teeth**	**Sinus**
Maxillary Division (V₂)			
Posterior superior alveolar	Buccal; maxillary gingiva	Maxillary molars	Maxillary sinus
Middle superior alveolar	—	Maxillary premolars and mesiobuccal root of first molar	Maxillary sinus
Anterior superior alveolar	Labial gingiva of maxilla	Maxillary anteriors	—
Infraorbital (superior labial)	Labial gingiva of maxilla	—	—
Nasopalatine	Lingual gingiva of maxillary incisors	—	—
Descending Palatine			
Greater palatine	All hard palate except lingual gingiva of maxillary incisors	—	—
Lesser palatine	Soft palate	—	—
Mandibular Division (V₃)			
Inferior alveolar	—	All mandibular teeth	—
Mental	Facial gingivae from mandibular premolar to central incisor, mucosa, and skin of lower lip	—	—
Lingual	All mandibular lingual gingivae, floor of mouth, and anterior two-thirds of tongue	—	—
Buccal	Cheek and mandibular buccal gingivae from first premolar on back	—	—
Facial Nerve (VII)			
Chorda tympani	Taste in anterior two-thirds of tongue	—	—
Glossopharyngeal nerve (IX)	Taste and sensation to posterior third of tongue	—	—

anesthetic contained a vasoconstrictor, unwanted serious cardiovascular events—from fainting to a stroke or even a heart attack—could occur, although these consequences are rare.

The ***posterior superior alveolar nerve block*** anesthetizes maxillary molars and their associated bone, gingiva, and buccal periodontium. The one exception is the mesiobuccal root of the maxillary first molar, which is usually innervated by the middle alveolar nerve. The posterior superior alveolar nerve, artery, and vein are all located together within the pterygopalatine fossa just distal and superior to the tuberosity of the maxilla (Fig. 36.8). They are not covered by bone at this point. You can see that a needle could easily puncture or barely scrape a nerve, artery, or vein. If this occurs, it would cause not only pain but also bleeding from a blood vessel; if the nerve is punctured or even touched, an extremely painful reaction (**"nerve shock"**) results. If bleeding occurs, swelling followed by a hematoma will result. If the needle is taken farther distally, even more serious bleeding and other traumatic events could occur.

The consequences magnify as the size of the blood vessels increase and more anesthetic solution is deposited within these blood vessels. The presence of a vasoconstrictor also increases the seriousness of the consequences because the vasoconstrictor is then spread around the body.

The ***middle superior alveolar nerve block*** anesthetizes maxillary premolars and their associated bone, gingiva, buccal periodontium, and the mesiobuccal root of the maxillary first molar. The injection for this block is given more superiorly than a premolar supraperiosteal injection. The area affected is greater because the anesthetic is deposited closer to the nerve trunk.

Injection for the middle superior nerve block is given immediately above the second premolar, and the needle is taken higher than a maxillary premolar supraperiosteal injection. The superior dental plexus is the target area and is located above the maxillary second premolar (Fig. 36.9).

The ***anterior superior alveolar nerve block*** anesthetizes maxillary anterior teeth (canine, lateral and central) along with their associated bone, gingiva, buccal periodontium to the midline, and half the maxillary lip. The injection for this block is given in the mucogingival fold immediately above the maxillary canine, just mesial to the canine eminence (Fig. 36.10). The needle is taken higher than with a supraperiosteal injection, and thus the anesthetic is delivered closer to the nerve trunk and thus affects a greater area than the supraperiosteal injection. Both the anterior and the middle superior alveolar nerve blocks are relatively free from complications because they are not administered in highly vascular areas. However, great care must be taken to keep the tip of the needle above the canine. If the tip of the needle goes too far mesially above the maxillary lateral incisor, a highly vascular area that is rich in nerves and blood vessels could be encountered. This is the area below the infraorbital foramen. It is here that the infraorbital nerve, artery, and vein emerge from the infraorbital foramen.

The ***infraorbital nerve block*** anesthetizes both areas covered by the middle and anterior superior alveolar nerve blocks. It covers maxillary anterior teeth, premolars, and mesiobuccal root of the maxillary first molar, as well as their associated bone, gingiva, buccal periodontium, the maxillary lip to the midline, and part of the cheek. It also covers the lateral of the nose and the lower eyelid (see Fig. 36.5).

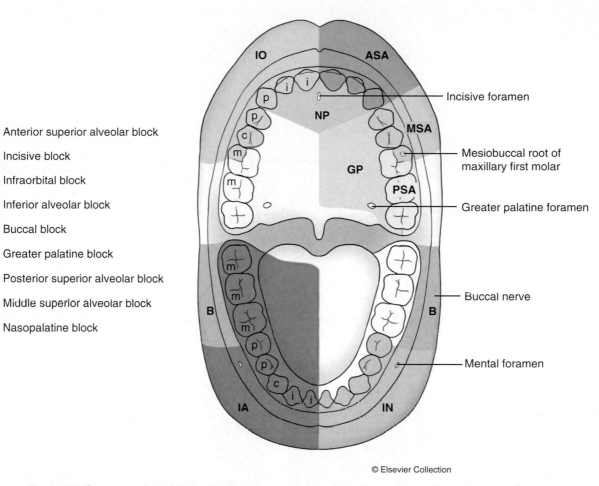

ASA | Anterior superior alveolar block
IN | Incisive block
IO | Infraorbital block
IA | Inferior alveolar block
B | Buccal block
GP | Greater palatine block
PSA | Posterior superior alveolar block
MSA | Middle superior alveolar block
NP | Nasopalatine block

© Elsevier Collection

• **Figure 36.6** Structures affected by local anesthetic nerve blocks. Note the mesiobuccal root of the maxillary first molar has innervation different from the rest of this molar.

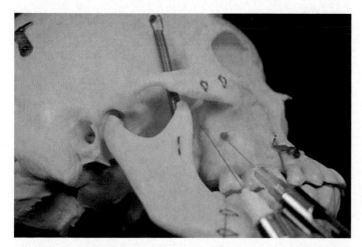

• **Figure 36.7** Maxillary tuberosity showing the location of the supraperiosteal injection versus the location of the posterior superior alveolar block injection (PSA). The supraperiosteal injection is mesial to the PSA block. One can see that taking the needle tip slightly more superior and distally with the supraperiosteal injection could become a superior alveolar block. The main concern is not the nerve anesthesia but the much greater vascular area to be encountered. Both injections could have the same insertion point above the second molar.

The infraorbital nerve branches out from the infraorbital foramen, and so do the branches of the infraorbital artery and vein (see Fig. 36.6). Blood vessels and branches of the nerve are larger closer to the foramen. There are many potential complications because of this area being rich in blood vessels and nerves. If the foramen is entered, it is easy to puncture any of these. It is possible even to enter the orbit of the eye. The target area for depositing the anesthetic solution is as close to the foramen as possible without entering it or damaging any of its structures (Fig. 36.11). The anesthetic is then massaged into the foramen by manipulating the tissues with a finger and using gentle pressure. This block can be painful and can cause a hematoma in the injection area and even in the lower eyelid, so the clinical conditions must warrant the risk associated with this block. The same area could be anesthetized with two blocks, the anterior and the middle superior alveolar nerve blocks (see Table 36.1).

Clinical Considerations

Zygomatic bone is denser than alveolar bone, and the anesthetic solution does not penetrate zygomatic bone as easily as it can penetrate alveolar bone. In addition, zygomatic bone may be lower than the root apices of molars and premolars. This situation makes it difficult to perform a superior alveolar nerve block or even a supraperiosteal injection. In these cases, it is necessary to make several injections anterior and distal to the desired target area.

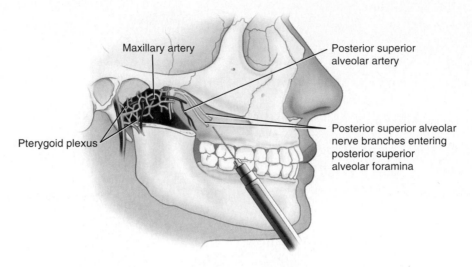

• **Figure 36.8** The pterygoid plexus is an area rich in vascular and nerve tissues. It is essential to proceed slowly with the needle so as to not tear or disrupt this tissue. Ideally the needle tip will not be in this area but anterior and slightly inferior to it. However, you must be prepared to be in this area by accident and know how to avoid complications.

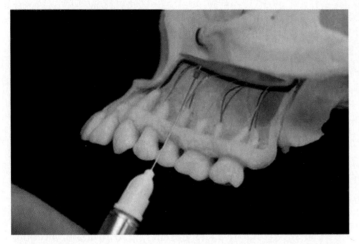

• **Figure 36.9** The middle superior alveolar injection is above the maxillary second premolar. The needle tip should end slightly above the apex of the premolar just short of the zygomatic process. When this process extends more inferiorly, this block, in essence, can be accomplished with two supraperiosteal injections, one anterior and one posterior to the second premolar.

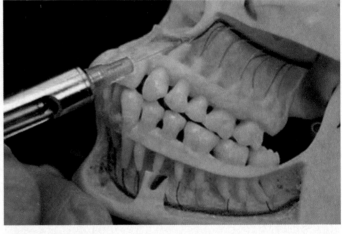

• **Figure 36.10** The anterior superior alveolar nerve block is given immediately above the canine. The anesthetic solution is delivered well above the apex of the canine root. In this way, more branches of the infraorbital nerve can be intercepted so that a larger soft tissue area is affected.

If nerves and blood vessels do not stop at the midline, a **crossover effect** occurs. A *crossover* occurs when some nerve branches cross over into an area innervated by another adjacent nerve. For instance, at the midline, if the nerve crosses over from the right side, it innervates something on the left side. Giving an anesthetic on the left side, in this case, does not work because the nerve that crossed over from the right innervates this area. So when dealing with anesthetics in the areas of the central incisors, it is sometimes necessary to anesthetize both sides because of this crossover effect. Crossover of nerves occurs not only at the midline but between areas affected by different nerve branches. A crossover effect can also occur at the junction between areas that are adjacent to each other but are typically innervated by two different nerve branches. If one nerve block does not affect the desired target area, a second

nerve block (that normally serves the adjacent area) may be required.

Palatal Nerve Blocks

There are two palatal nerve blocks that provide anesthesia to the palatal periodontium and gingiva. Neither of these two blocks anesthetizes the tooth pulp or the associated buccal periosteum and gingiva. They affect only the lingual tissues. The **nasopalatine nerve block** affects the hard and soft tissues of the palatal periodontium and gingiva of the six anterior teeth (canine to canine). All six anterior teeth are affected by one anesthetic nerve block (Fig. 36.12).

The **greater palatine nerve block** (Fig. 36.13) affects the hard tissue of the posterior palate, palatal periodontium, and palatal

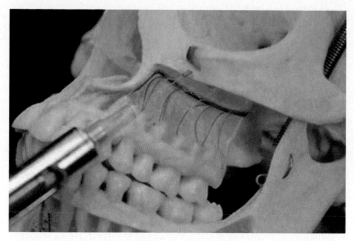

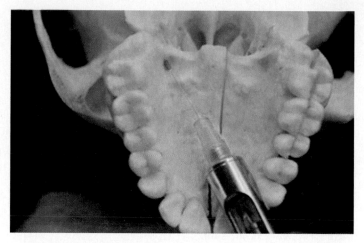

• **Figure 36.11** The infraorbital injection is given at the infraorbital foramen above the maxillary first premolar. Care must be used not to enter the foramen with the needle. Note in the illustration the infraorbital foramen just above the green tip placed at the end of the needle. The blue, red, and yellow indicate the blood vessels and nerves exiting the foramen.

• **Figure 36.13** The greater palatine block is given as close to the greater palatine foramen as possible without entering it. This block may require two injections, and the first one should be slightly mesial and anterior to the foramen, and the second as close to the foramen as possible.

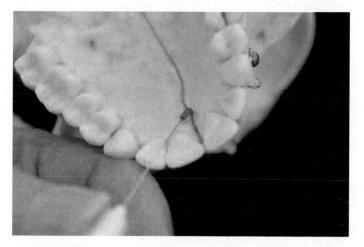

• **Figure 36.12** The nasopalatine block affects the lingual tissue of all six anterior teeth. This can be a painful injection, so anesthetic is slowly deposited into the incisive papilla just lingual to the centrals. The tissue is firm here, so only drops of anesthetic are deposited at a time. Once some anesthetic has taken effect, then more is deposited right at the incisive foramen. This may require two separate injections. Do not enter the foramen.

injection should be given slowly, allowing time for the anesthetic to be dispersed into the surrounding tissue.

The *nasopalatine nerve block* anesthetizes the nasopalatine nerves as they enter the incisive foramen as they return from the mucosa of the anterior palate. The incisive foramen is located immediately lingual and between the two maxillary central incisors. One injection can anesthetize the anterior hard palate, all of the lingual gingival tissues, and the periodontium of the six maxillary anterior teeth (canine to canine).

The *greater palatine nerve block* anesthetizes the posterior lateral hard palate, palatal gingiva, and periodontium of maxillary posterior teeth. There is a crossover area between canines and maxillary first premolars. This is where a plexus forms between the greater palatine nerves and the nasopalatine nerves. Tissues in this area may require both blocks. The greater palatine foramen are depressions located on the posterior of the hard palate at the junction of the hard palate and alveolar process of the maxilla, one on each side. They are usually superior to the root apices of third molars in adults (deciduous second molars in children).

The goal of local anesthesia is to block the innervation from the nerve branches as they try to send their messages back to the brain through the nerves.

To do this, the anesthetic solution must reach the nerve branch somewhere between the targeted area to be anesthetized and the nerve trunk.

The closer the anesthetic is to the nerve trunk, the more area is affected by the anesthetic. If the anesthetic agent is deposited at the incisive foramen, the lingual of six anterior teeth will be affected. However, if the anesthetic agent is deposited distal or medial to the greater palatine foramen, the desired target area might not be affected. That is because the lingual area of the desired tooth may not be served by these branches of nerve.

To give a palatal nerve block or even a palatal periosteal injection, the needle needs to be inserted about 5 mm anteriorly and laterally to the greater palatine foramen but in a direct line toward the desired target area. The solution should be deposited between the target area and the greater palatine foramen. The anesthetic may not last as long, but there is more assurance of getting the target anesthetized. A second injection can always be given closer to the foramen after the first injection has taken effect. This makes

gingiva of the maxillary molar and premolar areas. There is often a crossover effect in the area of the first premolar, where branches of the nasopalatine nerve block innervate the gingiva of maxillary first premolars.

Both these injection areas are covered with hard dense gingival tissues. This gingiva is firmly attached to palatal bone and allows very little room for deposit of the anesthetic solution. These injections can be painful, and to avoid this, they are administered slowly under light pressure. Care must be taken not to over-distend the tissue, or it will cause postoperative pain. There is no need to enter the incisive foramen or greater palatine foramen; doing so is painful and can damage nerves and blood vessels. The palatal tissue overlying the incisive foramen is denser and more firmly attached compared with the tissues overlying the greater palatine foramen. Depositing enough anesthetic solution in this area is more difficult and causes more pain to the patient. This

this process more comfortable for the patient and allows more anesthetic solution to be deposited at the injection site. Giving enough solution in this dense mucosa with just one injection usually causes pain to the patient.

There are two popular ways to lessen the pain from injecting into tissue without using a topical anesthetic. The first is to inject very slowly. This allows the anesthesia solution to be absorbed into the tissue and eliminates a burning sensation. The second is the use of pressure anesthesia. The latter requires putting pressure on the injection site before injecting the solution. A cotton-tipped applicator is applied to the injection site for 30 to 60 seconds before the injection, during the injection, and a few seconds after the injection. This causes nerve innervations to respond to the pressure long enough to cause slight numbness. If the pressure is relieved in any way, there is immediate recovery of sensation, and the patient will feel the pain.

Both the nasopalatine and greater palatine nerve blocks require slow injection flow and pressure anesthesia. These blocks can still be somewhat uncomfortable for the patient. In each situation topical anesthetic is also highly recommended.

A better way to lessen the pain of the injection is topical anesthetic. Topical anesthetic such as pressure anesthesia takes time to work. First the tissue is wiped dry and then the topical is applied, usually as a spray, gel, or liquid. Wait the amount of time recommended by the manufacturer before inserting the needle for the injection. During this waiting time a Q-tip could be used to apply pressure anesthetic at the target injection site.

Mandibular Nerve Blocks

The mandibular branch of CN V (V$_3$), which is called the *trigeminal nerve,* serves mandibular teeth, the facial and lingual

periodontium, and related gingiva. There are several areas where anesthetic solution can be deposited to reach these nerve branches, each anesthetizing specific areas.

The mandible is denser, and it is harder for the anesthetic solution to penetrate it compared with the maxilla. Articaine is the main anesthetic solution that seems to function as a mandibular supraperiosteal injection. It is more effective in the anterior region of the mandible than in the posterior region. The entire half of the mandible can be anesthetized by an inferior alveolar nerve block, and many different anesthetic solutions can be used to do this.

The most common mandibular block is the **inferior alveolar nerve block** (Fig. 36.14). This injection anesthetizes both the inferior alveolar nerve and the lingual nerve. It anesthetizes all mandibular teeth on one side to the midline, along with the associated lingual periodontium and gingiva. This block also affects the facial periodontium and gingiva of premolars and anterior teeth to the midline, floor of the mouth to the midline, and the anterior two-thirds of the tongue to the midline. There sometimes is a slight crossover effect at the midline. The lingual nerve is anesthetized because of its close anatomic relationship to the inferior alveolar nerve. To achieve anesthesia on the buccal gingiva and periodontium, most clinicians will follow this nerve block injection with a local infiltration of the long buccal nerve.

The **lingual block** anesthetizes lingual tissues and not teeth or buccal tissues. It affects only the lingual nerve, and the anesthetic is deposited anterior to and lingual to the inferior alveolar block. The lingual block anesthetizes the lingual gingiva, the lingual periodontium of mandibular teeth to the midline, the anterior two-thirds of the tongue to the midline, and the floor of the mouth to the midline (Fig. 36.15). The lingual block can be given while doing a mandibular block. The operator deposits some

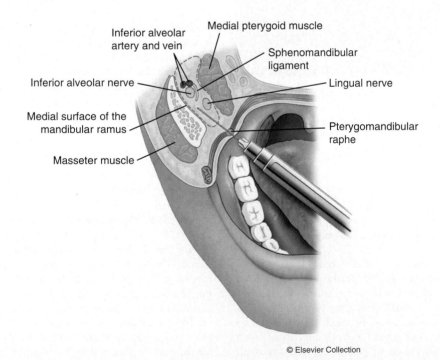

Inferior alveolar artery and vein

Medial pterygoid muscle

Inferior alveolar nerve

Sphenomandibular ligament

Lingual nerve

Medial surface of the mandibular ramus

Pterygomandibular raphe

Masseter muscle

© Elsevier Collection

• **Figure 36.14** The target area of the inferior alveolar nerve block is the inferior alveolar nerve just before it enters the mandibular foramen in the center of the ramus of the mandible. Anesthetic solution is deposited into the pterygomandibular space just superior to the lingua anterior to the foramen. The solution drifts down and intercepts the inferior alveolar nerve. Even before this, the anesthetic solution is deposited as the needle is advanced and the lingual nerve is anesthetized.

The **Gow-Gates mandibular nerve block** affects more tissue area than the inferior alveolar nerve block but requires more time to initiate and become effective. The **Vazirani-Akinosi mandibular nerve block** also affects a large area of tissue; it is usually used when patients have trismus or difficulty opening the mouth. This injection also takes additional time to take effect because the local anesthetic solution needs to travel farther down to the nerve.

Inferior Alveolar Nerve Block

The inferior alveolar nerve block, also called the **mandibular nerve block**, affects mandibular teeth, lingual periodontium and gingiva, and the facial periodontium and gingiva of anterior teeth. The anesthetic solution is deposited anterosuperior to the mandibular canal, which is located on the mesial surface of the ramus. The anterosuperior edge of the mandibular canal has a slight projection of bone, called the *lingula*. The anesthetic solution is deposited above this area, and the solution drops posteriorly and inferiorly down into the area above the mandibular foramen. Here the anesthetic intercepts the inferior alveolar nerve just as it enters the mandibular canal and before it enters bone.

The lingual nerve is located anterior and lingual to the mandibular canal and can be anesthetized by the mandibular nerve block because of its closer relationship to the inferior alveolar nerve. As the solution is injected and absorbed by tissues, some solution will diffuse to the lingual nerve (see Figs. 36.14 and 36.15). The lingual nerve block helps anesthetize the lingual gingival tissues for periodontal debridement, gingival curettage, extractions, and periodontal surgery. The lingual nerve block uses the same injection site as the mandibular inferior alveolar nerve block and can be given at the beginning of performing this block. The clinician proceeds as if performing the mandibular inferior alveolar nerve block and deposits anesthetic solution when the needle is halfway between the ramus and the injection site.

When performing the *inferior alveolar block*, the syringe barrel is over the second premolar at the corner of the mouth opposite the side being injected. The needle is inserted on a horizontal line, one-half to two-thirds of the way from the coronoid notch on the anterior of the ramus, to the pterygomandibular raphe (Fig. 36.16). The needle continues posteriorly on a plane parallel to the occlusal plane, about 10 mm above the occlusal plane. The

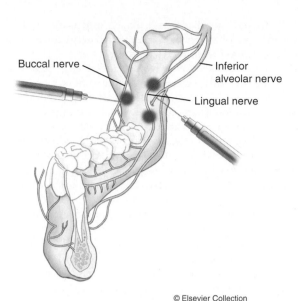

Buccal nerve

Inferior alveolar nerve

Lingual nerve

© Elsevier Collection

• **Figure 36.15** The lingual block can be given as a separate block; the needle does not have to go anywhere near the ramus of the mandible because the lingual nerve is closer to the injection site. The red areas indicate where anesthetic is to be deposited to affect the following nerves: inferior alveolar (top right), long buccal (middle left), and the lingual nerve (lower right).

anesthetic solution prior to delivering the rest of the solution at the mandibular foramen (see Fig. 36.17).

The **mental block** affects the facial periodontium and gingiva of the mandibular premolars and anterior teeth to the midline. It does not affect teeth.

To anesthetize teeth, a variation of the *mental block*, the **incisive block**, is used. It differs from the mental block in that manual pressure is applied at the injection site to force or massage the anesthetic solution into the mental canal. This allows premolars and anterior teeth to the midline to be anesthetized. If enough anesthetic can enter the canal, the following tissues will become numb: premolars and anterior three teeth and their associated facial periodontium and gingiva, but not their lingual tissues.

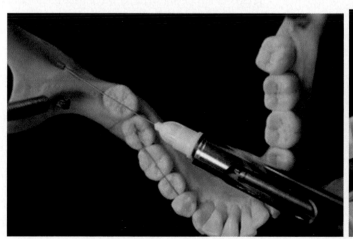
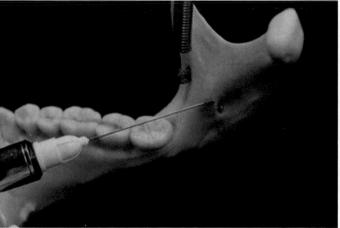

• **Figure 36.16** Two views of the same injection. The position of the syringe when performing an inferior alveolar block. The path of the needle is 6 to 10 mm above the occlusal plane and about the same height above the coronoid notch. Note the end of the needle is mesial to and slightly above the mandibular foramen. The anesthetic is deposited just anterior and superior to the lingula of the ramus.

coronoid notch can be used as a landmark; the injection path is about 6 to 10 mm higher than the coronoid notch.

The target area for the inferior alveolar injection is the *lingula* just anterior to and above the mandibular canal (Figs. 36.15 and 36.16). The needle is placed on a trajectory from the second premolar to the mandibular canal until it touches the ramus of the mandible. It is then pulled back and the syringe aspirated to make sure the needle is not in a blood vessel and then the anesthetic is deposited.

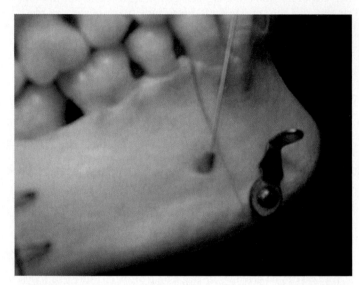

• **Figure 36.17** For the mental block and incisive block, the anesthetic is deposited just above and anterior to the mental foramen. Do not enter the foramen with the needle. If you want an incisive block, gently massage the anesthetic solution into the foramen using slight constant pressure. A second anesthetic is often required and can be delivered without causing pain after the first has taken effect. These techniques are learned with practice and patience over time.

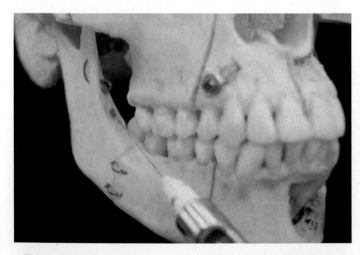

• **Figure 36.18** The buccal or long buccal block is administered in the buccal mucosa distal and buccal to the posterior-most molar. The injection is made just deep enough to catch the buccal nerve as it crosses over the anterior border of the mandibular ramus. This is slightly lateral to the retromandibular pad. The red indicator at the end of the needle might be a little too high or too posterior. A second injection if needed could be lower and more mesial.

If a second anesthetic injection is necessary, it is usually delivered superior to the first, because the most likely error is to administer it too low to the target area.

Bilateral blocks are to be avoided unless absolutely necessary because the body of the tongue, floor of the mouth, and the entire mandibular lip are anesthetized. This makes it hard for the patient to swallow, scares the patient, and makes it too easy for the patient to bite the tongue or lip after the clinical procedure is finished. This is especially true in the case of children or adults with special needs. They cannot feel the lip or tongue and can bite through these tissues.

The major anatomic concerns are hematomas (puncturing of blood vessels) and directly touching the nerve (nerve shock of the lingual nerve). It is very important to aspirate the syringe in all the mandibular blocks. If the needle is advanced too far into soft tissue and is not positioned near the mandibular foramen of the ramus, anesthesia could be injected into the parotid gland, which will anesthetize the patient's facial nerve. It is also possible to inject into a muscle or tendon, causing pain in both.

Mental Block

The **mental nerve block** anesthetizes the mental nerve branches as it exits the mental foramen. This block provides anesthesia to the associated facial periodontium and gingiva of the mandibular premolars and anterior teeth. The anesthetic is delivered as close to the mental foramen as possible without entering the canal. In essence, this is a form of local infiltration but in an area of major nerve branches, and thus a large area of tissue is affected (Fig. 36.17).

Incisive Nerve Block

The **incisive nerve block** is the same as the mental nerve block except that the goal is to get the anesthetic into the mental canal. Pressure is applied directly to the injection area, which forces anesthetic into the canal. Mandibular premolars and anterior teeth, as well as their associated facial tissues, are then anesthetized. This nerve block is easier to perform if articaine is employed because it penetrates mandibular bone better compared with other local anesthetic agents. In no case should the needle be placed directly into the mental canal because blood vessels and nerves can be damaged by forcing a needle into this very restricted space. Instead, the anesthetic solution should be deposited slightly superior to the mental foramen and be allowed to diffuse into the foramen by applying pressure and a massaging action.

The anatomic major concern with either the mental block or the incisive block is a hematoma, nerve shock, or puncturing of a blood vessel.

Buccal Nerve Block

If anesthesia of the buccal gingiva and periodontium of molar teeth is required, a buccal nerve block is used. The *buccal nerve* can be reached in the retromolar area just posterolateral to the most posterior molar. This **buccal block**, also called *long buccal block,* is a shallow injection as the buccal nerve is not covered by bone in this area (Fig. 36.18). The buccal (long buccal) block affects the buccal periodontium and gingiva of the molar teeth area but does not anesthetize the molars.

Gow-Gates Nerve Block

The *Gow-Gates block* can anesthetize the following nerves: inferior alveolar, mental, buccal, lingual, incisive, mylohyoid, and auriculotemporal nerves. This nerve block anesthetizes all mandibular teeth on one side, their lingual periodontium and gingiva, the periodontium and gingiva of premolars and anterior teeth, the floor of the mouth and lip on one side, and the anterior two-thirds of the tongue. In addition, this block also anesthetizes the soft tissues covering zygomatic bone, some temporal areas, and the digastric and mylohyoid muscles.

This block is useful in patients with a history of failure with the inferior alveolar nerve block. It requires more skill to perform and takes more time to take effect. It is not as easy to learn or master as the inferior alveolar nerve block.

Clinical Considerations

It is important to consider the feelings of the patient in determining an anesthetic technique. Most patients do not want half of their mouth made numb when a smaller, more targeted area can be anesthetized. Patients prefer a quick procedure and pain-free injection. They feel very uncomfortable if swallowing becomes difficult during and after the procedure. It is important to remember that children can easily bite their lip, cheek, or gums when they are numb. Have them bite on a cotton roll until their tissue is no longer numb.

The *Vazirani-Akinosi nerve block* is used when patients cannot open the mouth very wide. This is usually caused by **trismus**, injury, or temporomandibular joint dysfunction. This inability to open the mouth usually contraindicates any treatment other than that directed toward correcting these symptoms. This nerve block requires more skill to perform and takes more time to take effect. It is not as easy to learn or master as the inferior alveolar nerve block or the Gow-Gates nerve block.

The *Vazirani-Akinosi nerve block* is a closed-mouth anesthetic technique that can be painful if the bone of the maxilla or coronoid process is scraped; the additional risk is piercing of muscles or the tendons of muscles. This block may cover the same areas as that covered by the Gow-Gates block but it does not affect the auriculotemporal nerve.

Clinical Considerations

Anesthetic nerve blocks fail for a wide variety of reasons besides poor technique. If the patient's tissue pH is too low, the anesthetic solution will not release its free base, and it will not be able to anesthetize the nerve. This can be a normal everyday occurrence for some individuals, but it also occurs at infection sites. Infection sites exhibit a lower pH; they are acidic.

The tissue also becomes more acidic with each injection because the anesthetic solution itself is acidic. It makes it more difficult for subsequent deposits of anesthetic to release their free base because the area is becoming more acidic. Therefore it makes no sense to keep administering anesthetic to the same target area. Change the target area for better results.

If the anesthetic solution is penetrating a nerve with numerous fibers, some of the nerve fibers in the middle or opposite side of the nerve may not be affected, whereas other fibers closer to the solution may be affected.

If anesthetic solution is deposited in the area of a vein, the solution could be withdrawn from the area by the vein before the anesthetic has a chance to exert its effect.

There is much anatomic variety among individuals. Nerves and blood vessels are not always where they are supposed to be. There is no one technique that works for all of the patients all of the time.

This chapter is not a "how-to" guide on giving injections but, rather, is about applied anatomy. Much more complete education on patient evaluation, drugs, techniques, complications, and drug interactions is necessary before one can begin to administer local anesthetics. Mastering the techniques of local anesthesia is an ongoing effort and requires constant updating of knowledge. Anatomy may not change, but techniques, drugs, and interactions frequently do.

Review Questions

1. A supraperiosteal injection, if successful, anesthetizes
   a. only teeth
   b. only soft tissue
   c. soft tissue and teeth
   d. none of the above
2. A supraperiosteal injection is usually more successful in the
   a. maxillary
   b. mandibular
   c. inferior alveolar nerve
   d. a and b
   e. b and c
3. If a patient is allergic to sulfites, which anesthetic solution should not be administered?
   a. local anesthetics with vasoconstrictors
   b. anesthetics that do not contain vasconstrictors.
   c. anesthetics that contain epinephrine
   d. a and c
   e. a, b, and c
4. Which of the following is *not* a maxillary nerve block?
   a. posterior superior alveolar block
   b. infraorbital block
   c. nasopalatine block
   d. mental nerve block

5. Which covers a broader area?
   a. an infiltration
   b. a supraperiosteal injection
   c. a nerve block
   d. a topical anesthetic
6. Which are methods to help lessen pain while administering a local anesthetic?
   a. pressure anesthesia
   b. topical anesthetic
   c. injecting the anesthetic solution slowly
   d. all of the above
7. A successful infraorbital block can anesthetize
   a. the lateral tissue of the nose
   b. the lower eye lid
   c. premolars
   d. mesiobuccal root of the first molar
   e. anterior teeth
   f. all of the above
8. If your needle touches a nerve while giving an injection, you could expect the patient to
   a. experience a burning sensation
   b. experience severe pain
   c. jump out of the chair
   d. experience nerve shock
   e. any or all of the above

9. What are some of the consequences of puncturing a blood vessel?
   a. pain
   b. hematoma
   c. swelling
   d. numbness of other body parts
   e. any or all of the above

10. What do you do if a hematoma occurs during treatment?
    a. apply heat
    b. apply pressure
    c. do nothing
    d. a and b

11. A mental nerve block differs from an incisive block in what way?
    a. The mental block numbs teeth only.
    b. The incisive block anesthetizes gingival tissue only.
    c. The mental block numbs teeth and soft tissue.
    d. The incisive block anesthetizes teeth and soft tissue.

12. Which block requires pressure and massage of the tissue to take affect?
    a. infraorbital block
    b. mental block
    c. incisive block
    d. a and c
    e. b and c

13. Which of the following blocks requires the needle to enter the foramen?
    a. mental block
    b. infraorbital block
    c. incisive block
    d. none of the above

14. What single injection can achieve two separate blocks?
    a. middle superior alveolar block injection
    b. injection for the posterior superior alveolar block
    c. injection for the inferior alveolar nerve block
    d. injection for the anterior superior alveolar nerve block

15. Which block affects only soft tissue?
    a. mental block
    b. buccal block
    c. greater palatine nerve block
    d. lingual nerve block
    e. all of the above

16. Which nerve block could be used in a situation where the patient cannot open the mouth?
    a. Gow-Gates mandibular block
    b. inferior alveolar nerve block
    c. Vazirani-Akinosi mandibular block
    d. all of the above

Unit IV Test

1. Excluding the ear ossicles, there are _____ bones in the skull.
   a. 8
   b. 14
   c. 12
   d. 22

2. The nasal septum is formed by the _____ bone.
   a. sphenoid
   b. ethmoid
   c. vomer
   d. both b and c

3. Which of the following bones is *not* a part of the neurocranium?
   a. sphenoid
   b. ethmoid
   c. temporal
   d. frontal
   e. occipital
   f. maxilla

4. The mental foramen is located in the
   a. body of the maxilla
   b. ramus of the mandible
   c. body of the mandible
   d. alveolar process of the maxilla

5. The posterior nasal spine is a part of the _____ bone.
   a. nasal
   b. maxillary
   c. mandibular
   d. palatine
   e. none of the above

6. Which of the following statements is *true* concerning the sphenoid?
   a. It can be seen from a lateral view of the skull.
   b. It can be seen from an internal view of the skull.
   c. It can be seen in the orbit.
   d. both a and b
   e. both a and c
   f. all of the above

7. What two sutures meet at the Bregma?
   a. frontotemporal suture
   b. coronal suture
   c. sagittal suture
   d. b and c
   e. a and c

8. In which of the following bones would you find the external auditory meatus?
   a. the mastoid bone
   b. the temporal bone
   c. the occipital bone
   d. both a and c
   e. none of the above

9. Sella turcica is found in the
   a. sphenoid bone
   b. mastoid process
   c. lacrimal bone
   d. inferior meatus
   e. none of the above

10. Which of the following opens into the maxillary sinus?
    a. frontal sinus
    b. inferior meatus
    c. anterior ethmoid sinus
    d. nasolacrimal duct
    e. hiatus semilunaris

11. Which of the following teeth would *not* be found in proximity to the floor of the maxillary sinus?
    a. maxillary first molar
    b. maxillary lateral incisor
    c. maxillary first premolar
    d. maxillary third molar
    e. none of the above
12. Where is the opening of the maxillary sinus into the nasal cavity found?
    a. in the floor of the sinus
    b. in the roof of the sinus
    c. two-thirds of the way up the lateral wall
    d. two-thirds of the way up the medial wall
    e. none of the above
13. The ethmoid bulla is found in the
    a. inferior meatus
    b. superior meatus
    c. sphenoethmoidal recess
    d. middle meatus
    e. none of the above
14. What space communicates with the anterior ethmoid?
    a. inferior nasal concha
    b. opening of nasolacrimal duct
    c. hiatus semilunaris
    d. none of the above
15. Posterior part of the nasal septum may be known as the
    a. choana
    b. sphenoethmoidal recess
    c. posterior nasal aperture
    d. both a and b
    e. both a and c
    f. all of the above
16. What is the function of the temporalis muscle?
    a. depress the mandible
    b. elevate the mandible
    c. protrude the mandible
    d. retrude the mandible
    e. depress and protrude the mandible
    f. elevate and retrude the mandible
17. Which of the following is *not* the origin of the medial pterygoid muscle?
    a. maxillary tuberosity
    b. pterygoid fossa
    c. pterygoid plate
    d. zygomatic arch
18. Which of the following muscles directly affects the movement of the temporomandibular joint (TMJ)?
    a. temporalis
    b. masseter
    c. pterygoid plate
    d. zygomatic arch
    e. both a and b
19. The muscles of mastication are innervated by the _____ cranial nerve.
    a. V
    b. VII
    c. IX
    d. X
20. What muscles function in the closing of the jaws?
    a. masseter muscle
    b. temporalis muscle
    c. medial pterygoid muscle
    d. a, b, and c
    e. both a and b

21. Which of the following muscles is capable of retruding the mandible?
    a. temporalis
    b. digastric
    c. mylohyoid
    d. lateral pterygoid
    e. a and b
22. Which of the following is *not* an infrahyoid muscle?
    a. sternohyoid
    b. omohyoid
    c. mylohyoid
    d. thyrohyoid
    e. none of the above
23. Which of the following statements is *not* true about the sternocleidomastoid and trapezius muscles?
    a. They can both assist in movements of the head.
    b. They can be involved in referred pain.
    c. Spasms in either muscle can refer pain to the TMJ.
    d. They both have similar insertions.
24. The disk of the TMJ is attached laterally and medially to the
    a. medial pterygoid muscle
    b. lateral pterygoid muscle
    c. poles of the condyle
    d. retrodiscal pad
    e. none of the above
25. The temporomandibular ligament functions to
    a. pull the disk posteriorly
    b. pull the disk anteriorly
    c. keep the condyle from being pulled too far posteriorly
    d. keep disk from being pulled too far anteriorly
26. The temporomandibular ligament is found in the
    a. posterior part of the capsule
    b. medial part of the capsule
    c. anterior part of the capsule
    d. lateral part of the capsule
27. Pain in the area of the TMJ coming from another area, not related directly to the TMJ, is known as _____ pain.
    a. myofascial
    b. referred
    c. false
    d. none of the above
28. Dislocation of the TMJ is referred to as
    a. protraction
    b. retrusion
    c. subluxation
    d. depression
29. When the disk of the TMJ is deranged, it is usually
    a. immobile
    b. displaced posteriorly
    c. displaced anteriorly
    d. none of the above
30. The muscles of facial expression are innervated by the _____ cranial nerve.
    a. V
    b. VII
    c. IX
    d. X
    e. XI
31. Which two muscles play a role in smiling?
    a. levator labii superioris
    b. depressor labii inferiors
    c. zygomatic major
    d. mentalis
    e. orbicularis oris

32. Which muscle plays a role in keeping the food on the occlusal surfaces during mastication?
    a. orbicularis oris
    b. buccinator
    c. zygomaticus major
    d. mentalis
    e. none of the above

33. Which group of muscles of facial expression is the *most* poorly developed?
    a. orbicularis oris
    b. mentalis
    c. risorius
    d. levator anguli oris
    e. buccinator

34. Which muscle plays a major role in frowning?
    a. nasalis
    b. orbicularis oculi
    c. corrugator
    d. orbicularis oris
    e. none of the above

35. Which muscle plays a major role in pulling the lip down?
    a. procerus
    b. zygomaticus minor
    c. depressor anguli oris
    d. depressor labii inferioris
    e. none of the above

36. Which palatal muscle is innervated by the fifth cranial nerve (CN V)?
    a. uvula
    b. palatopharyngeus
    c. palatoglossus
    d. levator veli palatini
    e. tensor veli palatini

37. What is the function of the stylopharyngeus muscle?
    a. elevates the pharynx
    b. dilates the pharynx
    c. depresses the pharynx
    d. pulls the pharynx anteriorly
    e. elevates and dilates the pharynx

38. Which muscle pulls the soft palate into contact with the posterior pharyngeal wall?
    a. uvula
    b. palatopharyngeus
    c. palatoglossus
    d. levator veli palatini

39. Which muscle helps move the bolus of food upward and backward to the oral pharynx?
    a. tongue
    b. palatopharyngeus
    c. levator veli palatini
    d. tensor veli palatini

40. What muscle would help open the auditory tube if it was closed because of edema?
    a. palatoglossus
    b. styloglossus
    c. uvula
    d. levator veli palatini
    e. all of the above
    f. none of the above

41. Which muscle causes dilation and elevation of the pharynx?
    a. stylopharyngeal muscle
    b. palatoglossus
    c. tensor veli palatini
    d. salpingopharyngeus
    e. all of the above

42. Which pharyngeal constrictor muscle has its origin on the thyroid cartilage?
    a. superior constrictor muscle
    b. middle constrictor muscle
    c. inferior constrictor muscle
    d. both a and b

43. Which artery does not supply blood to the oral cavity?
    a. lingual artery
    b. maxillary artery
    c. palatal artery
    d. mental artery
    e. They all supply blood to the oral cavity.

44. Which of the following are branches of the external carotid artery?
    a. lingual
    b. maxillary
    c. superficial temporal
    d. facial
    e. all of the above
    f. none of the above

45. The _____ artery supplies blood to the muscles of mastication.
    a. mental
    b. facial
    c. lingual
    d. maxillary
    e. superficial temporal

46. What vein may be injured during the administration of anesthesia to the posterosuperior alveolar nerve?
    a. retromandibular vein
    b. pterygoid plexus of veins
    c. facial vein
    d. temporal vein

47. If the posterior retromandibular vein is absent on one side, which of the following statement(s) is/are true?
    a. The external jugular vein will be smaller than normal.
    b. The internal jugular vein will be larger than normal.
    c. All blood from the maxillary vein will enter the common facial vein.
    d. both a and b
    e. both b and c
    f. all of the above

48. If the posterior superior alveolar artery were blocked, how would blood get to the maxillary molars?
    a. via the greater palatine artery
    b. via the anterior superior alveolar artery
    c. via the nasopalatine artery
    d. via the sphenopalatine artery
    e. none of the above

49. The _____ gland's duct opens into the vestibule opposite the maxillary second molar.
    a. parotid
    b. submandibular
    c. sublingual
    d. buccal

50. Which of the following major salivary glands is mostly serous with some mucous acini?
    a. buccal
    b. sublingual
    c. parotid
    d. submandibular
51. Where does the submandibular gland open into the oral cavity?
    a. opposite the maxillary second molar
    b. on the sublingual caruncle
    c. at the base of the labial frenum
    d. b and c
52. The serous glands of von Ebner are found
    a. in the cheek
    b. in the palate
    c. in the floor of the mouth
    d. in the tongue
53. The nerve supply to all salivary glands comes from the
    a. autonomic nervous system
    b. parasympathetic nervous system
    c. sympathetic nervous system
    d. voluntary nervous system
    e. a and b
    f. a and c
54. Which major salivary gland has more than two ducts?
    a. parotid
    b. submandibular
    c. sublingual
    d. both a and b
    e. both b and c
55. There are _____ pairs of cranial nerves.
    a. 5
    b. 7
    c. 9
    d. 12
56. Which cranial nerve is involved in taste?
    a. glossopharyngeal
    b. vagus
    c. facial
    d. all of the above
    e. none of the above
57. The second division of the trigeminal nerve is known as the
    _____.
    a. mandibular division
    b. ophthalmic division
    c. pharyngeal division
    d. maxillary division
58. What nerve innervates the lingual gingiva of the maxillary central incisors?
    a. greater palatine nerve
    b. inferior alveolar nerve
    c. posterior superior alveolar nerve
    d. nasopalatine nerve
59. What nerve innervates the mucosa of the mandibular lip?
    a. lingual nerve
    b. anterior superior alveolar nerve
    c. buccal nerve
    d. mental nerve
    e. both a and d

60. What nerve innervates the maxillary central incisor?
    a. anterior superior alveolar nerve
    b. middle superior alveolar nerve
    c. inferior alveolar nerve
    d. lingual nerve
    e. nasopalatine nerve
61. Which of the following cranial nerves does *not* have parasympathetic fibers in its origin?
    a. III
    b. V
    c. VII
    d. IX
    e. X
    f. none of the above
62. What clinical sign would you *not* find in stimulation of the sympathetic nervous system?
    a. increased heart rate
    b. increased respiration
    c. decreased blood supply to skin
    d. decreased blood supply to the gastrointestinal (GI) tract
    e. constriction of the pupil of the eye
    f. All of the above signs appear in stimulation of the sympathetic nervous system.
63. What is the function of lymph nodes?
    a. help return intercellular fluids to the bloodstream
    b. produce lymphocytes
    c. fight infection
    d. prevent spread of infection
    e. all of the above
64. A secondary node of involvement for an infection of a maxillary first molar would be
    a. submental
    b. upper deep cervical
    c. submandibular
    d. lower deep cervical
    e. none of the above
65. The primary nodes of drainage for a maxillary central incisor are the
    a. submental nodes
    b. submandibular nodes
    c. retropharyngeal nodes
    d. upper deep cervical nodes
    e. none of the above
66. A fascial space infection in the oral cavity region could ultimately spread to the
    a. floor of the mouth
    b. side of the throat
    c. region behind the throat
    d. posterior mediastinum
    e. none of the above
67. Cancer of the _____ area would likely have the best prognosis.
    a. posterolateral border of tongue
    b. maxillary sinus
    c. maxillary lip
    d. tip of tongue
    e. submandibular salivary gland
68. An infection into the submental space causing a swelling beneath the chin is called
    a. an abscess
    b. sinus infection
    c. Ludwig's angina
    d. parotid space infection

69. To achieve anesthesia of the maxillary first molar, which two maxillary nerve blocks might need to be administered?
    a. middle superior alveolar and posterior superior alveolar
    b. posterior superior alveolar and anterior superior alveolar
    c. middle superior alveolar and anterior superior alveolar
    d. infraorbital and posterior superior alveolar

70. What anatomic landmark is the visual target location for the nasopalatine nerve block?
    a. dimple of tissue covering the greater palatine foramen
    b. soft palate and the nasopalatine foramen under it
    c. incisive papilla and the nasopalatine foramen beneath it
    d. height of the mucobuccal fold

71. Which of the following is *true* of mandibular nerve blocks?
    a. Supraperiosteal injections are more difficult because mandibular bone is denser than maxillary bone.
    b. Mandibular injections affect portions of the trigeminal nerve.
    c. There may be crossover effect with nerves at the midline of the mandible.
    d. all of the above

72. What anatomic landmark is the target location for the inferior alveolar nerve block?
    a. mandibular foramen
    b. mental foramen
    c. coronoid notch
    d. zygomatic bone

73. What makes supraperiosteal injections more effective in the maxilla compared with the mandible?
    a. The bone is more dense in the maxilla.
    b. The bone is less dense in the maxilla.
    c. Anesthetic penetrates the mandible faster.
    d. Only anesthetics with vasoconstrictors can be used in the maxilla.

74. What is not anesthetized by an infraorbital nerve block?
    a. maxillary incisor teeth
    b. premolar teeth
    c. lingual periodontia of maxillary canine teeth
    d. labial gingiva of maxilla

75. Which of the following is not true of a mental nerve block?
    a. The lower inferior alveolar covers this same area and more.
    b. The mandibular premolar teeth are also anesthetized.
    c. The labial gingiva of the mandible is anesthetized.
    d. One-half of the lower lip is anesthetized.

Unit IV Suggested Readings

Christensen JB, Telford IR. *Synopsis of Gross Anatomy*. 5th ed. Hagerstown, MD: Lippincott; 1988.

DuBrul E. *Sicher's Oral Anatomy*. 8th ed. St Louis, MO: Ishiyaku Euro; 1988.

Fehrenbach MJ. *Illustrated Anatomy of the Head and Neck*. 5th ed. St. Louis, MO: Elsevier; 2017.

Fried LA. *Anatomy of the Head, Neck, Face and Jaws*. 2nd ed. Philadelphia, PA: Lea & Febiger; 1980.

Friedman SM. *Visual Anatomy*. Vol. 1: Head and Neck. Hagerstown, MD: Harper & Row; 1970.

Gardner M. *Basic Anatomy of the Head and Neck*. Baltimore, MD: Williams & Wilkins; 1992.

Gartner LP, Hiatt JL. *Textbook of Head and Neck Anatomy*. 3rd ed. Philadelphia, PA: Lippincott, Williams & Wilkins; 1987.

Logothetis DD. *Local Anesthesia for the Dental Hygienist*. St. Louis, MO: Elsevier; 2017.

McClintic JR. *Human Anatomy*. St. Louis, MO: Mosby; 1983.

McMinn RMH, Hutchings R, Logan B. *Colour Atlas of Head and Neck Anatomy*. 2nd ed. St. Louis, MO: Mosby; 1994.

Paff GH. *Anatomy of the Head and Neck*. Philadelphia, PA: WB Saunders; 1973.

Reed GM, Sheppard VF. *Basic Structures of the Head and Neck*. Philadelphia, PA: WB Saunders; 1976.

Seeley RR, Stephens TD, Tate PP. *Anatomy and Physiology*. 2nd ed. St. Louis, MO: Mosby; 1996.

Short MJ. *Head, Neck and Dental Anatomy*. 2nd ed. New York, NY: Delmar; 1994.

Thibideau G, Patton K. *Anatomy and Physiology*. 3rd ed. St. Louis, MO: Mosby; 1996.

Wilson-Pauwerls L, et al. *Cranial Nerves: Anatomy and Clinical Comments*. St. Louis, MO: Mosby; 1988.

Wischnitzer S. *Outline of Human Anatomy*. Springfield, IL: Charles C. Thomas; 1972.

Appendix

Average Permanent Teeth Dimensions as Recorded by Dr. Russell C. Wheeler

	Length of Crown	Length of Root	Mesiodistal Diameter of Crown*	Mesiodistal Diameter at Cervix	Labio- or Buccolingual Diameter	Labio- or Buccolingual Diameter at Cervix	Curvature of Cervical Line (Mesial)	Curvature of Cervical Line (Distal)
Maxillary Teeth								
Central incisor	10.5[†]	13.0	8.5	7.0	7.0	6.0	3.5	2.5
Lateral incisor	9.0[†]	13.0	6.5	5.0	6.0	5.0	3.0	2.0
Canine	10.0[†]	17.0	7.5	5.5	8.0	7.0	2.5	1.5
First premolar	8.5[†]	14.0	7.0	5.0	9.0	8.0	1.0	0.0
Second premolar[‡]	8.5[†]	14.0	7.0	5.0	9.0	8.0	1.0	0.0
First molar	7.5[†]	B 12 L 13	10.0	8.0	11.0	10.0	1.0	0.0
Second molar	7.0[†]	B 11 L 12	9.0	7.0	11.0	10.0	1.0	0.0
Third molar	6.5[†]	11.0	8.5	6.5	10.0	9.5	1.0	0.0
Mandibular Teeth								
Central incisor	9.0[†]	12.5	5.0	3.5	6.0	5.3	3.0	2.0
Lateral incisor	9.5[†]	14.0	5.5	4.0	6.5	5.8	3.0	2.0
Canine	11.0[†]	16.0	7.0	5.5	7.5	7.0	2.5	1.0
First premolar	8.5[†]	14.0	7.0	5.0	7.5	6.5	1.0	0.0
Second premolar	8.0[†]	14.5	7.0	5.0	8.0	7.0	1.0	0.0
First molar	7.5[†]	14.0	11.0	9.0	10.5	9.0	1.0	0.0
Second molar	7.0[†]	13.0	10.5	8.0	10.0	9.0	1.0	0.0
Third molar	7.0[†]	11.0	10.0	7.5	9.5	9.0	1.0	0.0

Wheeler RC. *A Textbook of Dental Anatomy and Physiology*, ed. 4. Philadelphia: WB Saunders; 1965.

*The sum of the mesiodistal diameters, both right and left, which gives the arch length, is maxillary 128 mm, mandibular 126 mm.

[†]Lingual measurement is approximately 0.5 mm longer.

[‡]Maxillary second premolar crown is usually slightly shorter than the maxillary first premolar, and its buccal cusp usually is more rounded giving the appearance of being more worn down.

Nerve Supply of Oral Cavity

	Mucosa	Teeth	Sinus
Maxillary Division (V$_2$)			
Posterior superior alveolar	Buccal; maxillary gingiva	Maxillary molars	Maxillary sinus
Middle superior alveolar	—	Maxillary premolars and mesiobuccal root of first molar	Maxillary sinus
Anterior superior alveolar	Labial gingiva of maxilla	Maxillary anteriors	
Infraorbital (superior labial)	Labial gingiva of maxilla	—	—
Nasopalatine	Lingual gingiva of maxillary incisors	—	—
Descending palatine			
Greater palatine	All hard palate except lingual gingiva of maxillary incisors	—	—
Lesser palatine	Soft palate	—	—
Mandibular Division (V$_3$)			
Inferior alveolar	—	All mandibular teeth	—
Mental	Facial gingivae from mandibular premolar to central incisor, mucosa, and skin of lower lip	—	—
Lingual	All mandibular lingual gingivae, floor of mouth, and anterior two-thirds of tongue	—	—
Buccal	Cheek and mandibular buccal gingivae from first premolar on back	—	—
Facial Nerve (VII)			
Chorda tympani	Taste in anterior two-thirds of tongue	—	—
Glossopharyngeal Nerve (IX)	Taste and sensation to posterior third of tongue	—	—

Glossary

A band Dark microscopic band in the middle of a muscle sarcomere. The A band contains the myosin and parts of the actin myofilaments.

abducens Sixth cranial nerve (VI); related to eye movement.

abrasion Mechanical wearing away of teeth by abnormal stresses. Can result from abnormal tooth brushing habits or other abnormal stresses on the teeth.

accessional Permanent teeth that do not replace deciduous teeth but rather become an accession (an addition) to the deciduous or succedaneous teeth or to both types.

accessory nerve Eleventh cranial nerve (XI); supplies motor control to the trapezius and sternomastoid muscles in the neck as well as to the muscles of the pharynx, larynx, and soft palate.

accessory root canals Extra openings into the pulp; usually located on the sides of the roots or in the bifurcations.

accidental grooves Tertiary grooves that occur on third molars; smaller than primary or secondary grooves and occurring with no uniformity.

acellular cementum Cementum in which no cells are trapped.

acetylcholine A neuron-produced substance that aids in the transmission of impulses from one neuron to another and from many neurons to muscles in contraction.

acini Bulbous or tubular secretion-producing end-pieces of a gland; pronounced a-sin-I.

acquired Pertaining to something obtained by oneself rather than inherited.

acquired occlusion *See* centric occlusion.

acquired centric occlusion *See* centric occlusion.

acromegaly Disease resulting from an excess of growth hormone, which causes some bones in the body to continue growing after normal growth has completed.

actin One of the myofilaments in muscle; it is thinner than myosin and located in the I band and part of the A band. It is also found as a component of microfilaments in cell cytoskeleton.

action Function of a muscle; the work accomplished when a muscle contracts or shortens.

adduct To move toward the midline, as in muscle movement of extremities.

adipocyte A fat cell found as a component of connective tissue. These cells increase or decrease in number as fat is accumulated or depleted.

adrenalin A substance produced primarily by the adrenal gland that increases activity of the heart and lungs.

afferent A type of nerve fiber carrying sensory messages to the brain.

afunctional Not performing a purpose or action.

agranulocytes White blood cells without granules in their cytoplasm; lymphocytes and monocytes.

ala Latin for *wing;* referring to the sides of the nostrils; plural *alae*.

alignment How the teeth are arranged in a row mesially, distally, facially, and lingually.

allergenic Capable of producing an allergic reaction.

allergic reaction Body's reaction to an allergen, as in hives.

alpha-tubulin One of two major protein components of microtubules; helps make up the cytoskeleton.

alveolar bone Bone that forms the sockets for the teeth.

alveolar bone proper *See* cribriform plate.

alveolar crest Highest part of the alveolar bone closest to the cervical line of the tooth.

alveolar crest group Alveolodental fibers running from the cementum to the alveolar crest of bone.

alveolar eminences Bulges on the facial surface of alveolar bone that outline the position of the roots.

alveolar mucosa Mucosa between the mucobuccal fold and gingiva.

alveolar process Part of the bone in the maxillae and mandible that forms the sockets for the teeth. *See* alveolar bone.

alveolodental fibers Periodontal fibers that run between the tooth and the alveolar bone.

alveolus (alveoli) Cavity or socket in the alveolar process in which the root of the tooth is held.

ameloblast Enamel-forming cell that arises from oral ectoderm.

amelogenesis imperfecta A hereditary form of enamel hypocalcification.

amylase Digestive enzyme that breaks starch into simpler compounds.

anatomic crown The part of the tooth covered by enamel.

anemia Deficiency of red blood cells or hemoglobin to carry oxygen.

angle of the mandible Point at the lower border of the mandible body where it turns up onto the ramus.

Angle's classification System of dental classifications based primarily on the relationship of the permanent first molars to each other and to a lesser degree on the relationship of the permanent canines to each other.

ankyloglossia *See* tongue-tie.

ankylosis Fusion of the cementum of a tooth with alveolar bone.

anodontia No teeth at all are present in the jaw.

anomaly Any noticeable difference or deviation from that which is ordinary or normal.

antagonists Having an opposing action to something else.

antegonial notch Notched in area on the inferior border of the mandible.

anterior Situated in front of; a term commonly used to denote the incisor and canine teeth or the area toward the front of the mouth.

anterior auricular muscle Muscle of facial expression that extends from in front of the ear into the skin of the ear.

anterior coupling The touching of the anterior teeth during centric occlusion.

anterior cranial fossa The anterior part of the cranial cavity that houses the frontal lobes of the brain.

anterior ethmoidal nerve The branch of the nasociliary nerve of V_1 that passes through the anterior ethmoidal foramen into the anterior ethmoid air cells and sends a branch to the external nose.

anterior ethmoid sinus Frontmost group of ethmoid air cells.

anterior nasal spine Small projection of the maxillae at the bottom of the nasal aperture.

anterior pillar Fold of tissue extending down in front of the tonsil.

anterior superior alveolar artery Branch of the infraorbital artery to the maxillary incisors, canines, and premolars.

anterior superior alveolar nerve Branch of the infraorbital nerve that serves the maxillary incisors and canines.

antibodies Defensive proteins, called immunoglobulins, produced by cells such as lymphocytes and plasma cells.

antihistamine Drug that controls the body's histamine reaction, which causes congestion of tissues.

aorta Large vessel carrying oxygenated blood from the heart to the remainder of the body.

A-P film Anterior-posterior film that is taken with a radiograph source in front and film behind.

apatite crystals Small crystals of mineral deposits.

apex (apices) Endpoint or farthest tip, as of the tooth root.

apical end of a cell Narrow end of a pyramidal cell forming the lumen of a duct.

apical foramen Aperture or opening at or near the apex of a tooth root through which the blood and nerve supply of the pulp enters the tooth.

apical group Alveolodental fibers that attach from the base of the alveolus to the apex of the tooth.

apposition Addition, as to the surface of bone or any hard substance. One of the processes that takes place in bone growth and remodeling.

appositional growth The process of adding to the surface of bone or any hard substance. *See* apposition.

arch, dental *See* dental arch.

arthritis Inflammation of body joints.

articular disc Fibrous disc between the condyle and the mandibular fossa.

articular eminence Slope of temporal bone in front of the mandibular fossa.

atrophic Pertaining to the wasting away of a tissue, organ, or part from disease, defective nutrition, or lack of use.

atrophy Wasting away of a tissue, organ, or part from disease, defective nutrition, or lack of use.

attached gingiva Tightly adherent gingiva that extends from free gingiva to alveolar mucosa.

attachment apparatus *See* attachment unit.

attachment epithelium The cells that attach the gingiva to the tooth. These originally are cells of the reduced enamel epithelium.

attachment unit Subdivision of the periodontium: cementum, periodontal ligament, and alveolar bone.

attrition Process of normal wear on the crown.

auditory tube *See* pharyngotympanic tube.

auriculotemporal nerve Branch of the third division of the trigeminal nerve that supplies the skin over the ear and the parotid gland.

autonomic nervous system Automatic nervous system of the body that is not willfully controlled. It controls the functions of the glands and smooth and cardiac muscle.

axon Process of the neuron that carries the message from the cell body to the next neuron.

B

balancing side Term used in denture construction to denote the side of the denture that must be balanced to prevent the denture from tipping. In natural dentition it occurs when the buccal cusps of the mandibular teeth are located directly under the lingual cusps of the maxillary teeth. These cusps actually touch.

basal end of cell Broad outer end of a pyramidal cell forming a duct; end of any tall cell resting on a basement membrane.

basal layer Bottom layer in multiple-layered epithelium; layer that undergoes cell division.

basement membrane Ultrastructural layer of connective tissue on which epithelial cells rest; they rest on the side of the cell farthest from the free cell surface.

basophils White granulocyte blood cells that play a role in phagocytosis and possible allergic reactions.

bell stage Third stage of enamel organ formation in which the crown form is established.

beta-tubulin One of two major protein components of microtubules, which help make up the cytoskeleton.

biconcave discs Discs that have a depression in the middle on both sides.

bicuspid *See* premolars.

biofilm A dental plaque substrate that adheres to teeth.

bifurcation Division into two parts or branches, as any two roots of a tooth.

bisecting angle technique Technique of taking radiographs that slightly compromises the accuracy of the image.

blastocyst Hollow ball of cells that results from division of a fertilized ovum. It becomes the outer and inner cell mass of an embryo.

B-lymphocyte A cell of connective tissue that, when antigenically stimulated, becomes plasma cell–producing antibodies.

body of the mandible Horizontal portion of the mandible, excluding the alveolar process.

bolus of food A ball of food that has been chewed and mixed with saliva and is ready to be swallowed.

bone Hard connective tissue that forms the framework of the body. The hardness is attributable to the hydroxyapatite crystal.

brachiocephalic artery Branch of the aorta that carries blood to the right arm and right side of the head.

brachiocephalic veins Paired veins that drain the right and left arms and sides of the head. These two veins unite to form the superior vena cava.

branchial arches *See* pharyngeal arches.

bruxism Abnormal grinding of the teeth.

bucca Latin word for *cheek.*

buccal Pertaining to the cheek; toward the cheek or next to the cheek. Also called *facial.*

buccal branch Branch of the maxillary artery that goes to the cheek and buccal gingiva.

buccal contour Posterior teeth; *see* facial contours.

buccal developmental groove Groove that separates the buccal cusps on a buccal surface.

buccal embrasure *See* embrasure.

buccal glands Small minor salivary glands in the cheek.

buccal nerve Branch of the third division of the trigeminal nerve that supplies the skin and mucosa of the cheek and buccal gingiva.

buccinator Muscle of facial expression that extends from the back buccal portion of the maxillae, mandible, and pterygomandibular raphe forward in the cheek to the corner of the mouth.

buccopharyngeal membrane Membrane that separates the stomodeum from the foregut.

bud stage First stage of development of the enamel organ. It develops from the dental lamina.

bundle bone Extra thickness of bone added to the cribriform plate.

C

calcification Process by which organic tissue becomes hardened by a deposit of calcium salts within its substance. The term, in a liberal sense, connotes the deposition of any mineral salts that contribute to the hardening and maturation of hard tissue.

canal Long tubular opening through a bone.

cancellous bone *See* spongy bone.

canine eminence Extra bulk of bone on the labial aspect of the maxillae; it overlies the roots of the canine teeth.

canine fossa Depression in the maxillae below the infraorbital foramen.

canine rise During lateral excursion, the only teeth to touch are the maxillary and mandibular canines on the side toward which the jaw is moving.

canines Third teeth from the midline, at the corner of the mouth; used for grasping; also called *cuspids.*

cap stage Second stage of enamel organ development.

capsule Fibrous sheet of tissue surrounding a joint.

cardiac muscle Striped, involuntarily controlled muscle of the heart.

carotene A yellow pigment that is found in varying amounts in the skin.

carotid canal Canal in the base of the skull for the passage of the internal carotid artery.

carotid sheath A fibrous sheath that surrounds the carotid arteries, internal jugular vein, and vagus nerve.

cartilage Type of firm connective tissue that gives form to different parts of the body, such as the ears, trachea, and larynx.

CAT scan Computer assisted tomography. A scan of all or part of the body that allows the information to be digitally stored and reconstructed to give virtually any view.

cell Basic functioning component of the body; capable of reproducing itself in most instances. Tissues are made up of groups of cells.

cell body Central part of a neuron containing the nucleus.

cell membrane Wall surrounding the cell.

cellular cementum Cementum in which cells are trapped.

cellular inclusions Storage products in a cell not actually used to maintain the cell under normal circumstances.

cementoblasts Cells that form cementum.

cementocytes Cementoblasts that have become entrapped in cementum.

cementoenamel junction (CEJ) Junction of enamel of the crown and cementum of the root. This junction forms the cervical line around the tooth.

cementoma Cementum tumor at root tip that destroys surrounding bone.

cementum Layer of bonelike tissue covering the root of the tooth.

central developmental groove Developmental groove that crosses the occlusal surface of a tooth from the mesial to the distal side; divides the tooth into buccal and lingual parts.

central developmental pit Pit that occurs in the central fossa.

central fossa Fossa that occurs in the center of the central groove.

central groove *See* central developmental groove.

central nervous system Brain and spinal cord.

central occlusion A system of classifying the occlusion based on the relationship of the mandibular teeth to the maxillary teeth.

centric occlusion Relationship of the occlusal surfaces of one arch to those of the other when the jaws are closed and the teeth are in maximum intercuspation.

centric relation Arch-to-arch relationship of the maxillae to the mandible when the condyles are in their most upward position, the mandible is in its most posterior position, and the jaw is most braced by its musculature.

cephalometric film Film of skull taken from a side view so that cephalometric tracings can be done for orthodontic evaluation.

cervical That portion of a tooth near the junction of the crown and root. Pertaining to the neck region (e.g., nerves of the neck).

cervical crest Gingival tissue located near the cervical line of the tooth.

cervical embrasure Embrasure or spillway located cervical to the contact area of the teeth.

cervical line Line formed by the junction of the enamel and cementum on a tooth.

cervical loop The deepest part of the inner and outer enamel epithelium seen in the bell stage; there is no interposing stellate reticulum or stratum intermedium; aids in root formation.

cervical third That portion of the crown or root of a tooth at or near the cervical line.

cervicoenamel ridge Any prominent ridge of enamel immediately near the cervical line on the crown of a tooth.

cervix Constricted structure; the narrow region at the junction of the crown and root of the tooth.

choana Region at the posterior end of the nasal septum where it opens into the nasal pharynx; means "funnel."

chondroblasts Cells that form cartilage.

chondrocytes Cartilage-forming cells that have surrounded themselves with their secretory product.

chorda tympani Branch of the facial nerve (VII) that joins with the lingual nerve to carry taste sensations from the anterior two thirds of the tongue and secretomotor fibers to the submandibular and sublingual glands.

cilia Movable, hairlike structures on the apical end of a columnar cell that help to move substances over the surface of the cells.

cingulum Lingual lobe of anterior teeth.

circumferential lamellae Growth layers in bone around the outermost portion of the bone.

circumvallate papillae Large V-shaped row of papillae lying on the posterior dorsum of the tongue.

class I occlusal relationship Normal relationship between maxillary and mandibular molars.

class II occlusal relationship Condition when a mandibular molar is posterior to its normal position.

class III occlusal relationship Condition when a mandibular molar is anterior to its normal position.

cleft lip Gap in the upper lip occurring during development.

cleft palate Lack of joining together of the hard or soft palates.

clinical crown That part of the tooth protruding out of the gingiva.

clinical root That part of the tooth embedded in the gingiva and socket.

coalescence Joining of two lobes of a tooth.

coccygeal Relating to the tailbone area; a single pair of nerves in the tailbone region.

col Area of an interdental papilla that lies cervical to the interproximal contact of the tooth.

collagen Nonelastic, primary fiber of connective tissue.

common carotid artery Main blood vessel on either side of the neck that supplies most of the head.

compound tubuloalveolar gland Glandular arrangement that has a branching duct system with secreting cells at the ends of the ducts arranged like tubes with a bulbous endpiece.

compressor naris Muscle in flared part of nostrils that closes them.

concavity Depression in a surface.

concha Shelf projecting from lateral nasal wall.

concrescence Two adjacent teeth or roots that fuse by their cementum.

condylar neck Constricted part of the ramus of the mandible, just below the condyle.

condyloid process The portion of the mandible formed from both the neck and the head of the condyle.

congenital Occurring at or before birth; may or may not be hereditary.

congenitally missing Condition of having never been developed.

conical tooth A supernumerary tooth that is cone shaped.

connective tissue One of the four basic tissues made up of cells, fibers, ground substance (glue), and sometimes crystal. Bone, cartilage, and blood are special types of connective tissue.

contact area Area of contact of one tooth with another in the same arch.

contact point Specific point at which a tooth from one arch occludes with another tooth from the opposing arch.

contour Shape of a tooth.

convenience occlusion *See* centric occlusion.

convexity Bulge in a surface.

copula Pharyngeal-arch structure that forms the posterior third of the tongue.

coronal suture Suture between the frontal bone and the two parietal bones; also called the *frontoparietal suture.*

coronoid notch Notch in the upper surface of the body of the mandible just anterior to the where the ramus joins the body and the alveolar process.

coronoid process Bony projection at the upper anterior ramus of the mandible; point of attachment for the temporal muscle.

corrugator Muscle from the bridge of the nose to the lateral part of the eyebrow.

cortical plate Dense bone on the buccal and lingual surfaces of the alveolar bone.

cortisone An anti-inflammatory drug.

cranial nerves Twelve pairs of nerves originating from the brain.

craniofacial deformities Abnormal development of the head and face region.

craniosacral outflow Another name for the parasympathetic nervous system.

cribriform plate Bone that forms the actual wall of the tooth socket.

cribriform plate of ethmoid Small perforations of ethmoid bone beside the crista galli that provide passages for olfactory nerves from the nasal to the cranial cavity.

cristae The inner leaflike projections of a mitochondrion; enzymes attached to them enhance cellular activity.

crista galli Small bony projection of ethmoid bone in the anterior cranial fossa; helps attach the dura mater covering of the brain.

crossbite Condition in which the cusps of a tooth in one arch exceed the cusps of a tooth in the opposing arch, buccally or lingually.

cross section Cutting through a tooth perpendicular to the long axis.

cross-over effect The overlap of enervation caused by terminal nerve fibers from adjacent nerve trunks intermixing with each other.

crown The part of the tooth covered with enamel.

crypt Term used to describe the early tooth socket.

curve of Spee Anatomic line beginning at the tip of the canines and following the buccal cusps of premolars and molars when viewed from the buccal aspect of the first molars.

curve of Wilson Curve that follows the cusp tips, as seen from a frontal view.

cusp Major pointed or rounded eminence on or near the occlusal surface of a tooth.

cusp of Carabelli Fifth lobe of a maxillary first molar.

cyst Epithelium-lined sac of fluid that may grow to varying sizes.

cytoplasm Fluid substance of cells.

D

dead tracts Empty dentinal tubules resulting from death of odontoblasts and their processes in that area.

debrided Having already accomplished the removal (debridement) of nerve tissue and other debris from the pulp cavity to leave a surgically cleaned area.

deciduous That which will be shed; specifically, the first dentition of human or animal.

deep petrosal nerve Sympathetic nerve from the carotid plexus that supplies blood vessels to glands in the palate, nose, and lacrimal gland.

deep bite When the teeth close together in a way that the relationship between the maxilla and mandible is closer together than in the normal bite, often due to the teeth being intruded farther than usual in alveolar bone.

deglutition Action of swallowing.

dendrite Single process or multiple processes of a neuron that picks up impulses from other neurons and carries them to the cell body of its neuron.

dens in dente An invagination of the outer surface of the tooth crown turning inward on itself.

dental arch All the teeth in either the maxillary or mandibular jaw that form an arch.

dental classification A system of classifying the relationship of the upper teeth to the lower teeth.

dental follicle *See* dental sac.

dental lamina Embryonic downgrowth of oral epithelium that is the forerunner of the tooth germ.

dental papilla Mesodermal structure partially surrounded by the inner enamel epithelial cells. The dental papilla forms the dentin and pulp.

dental sac Several layers of flat mesodermal cells partially surrounding the dental papilla and enamel organ; forms the cementum, periodontal ligament, and some alveolar bone.

dentin (formerly dentine) Hard calcified tissue forming the inside body of a tooth, underlying the cementum and enamel and surrounding the pulpal tissue.

dentinal tubule Space in the dentin occupied by odontoblastic process.

dentinocemental junction Location in the root where the dentin joins the cementum.

dentinoenamel junction Line marking the junction of the dentin and the enamel.

dentinogenesis imperfecta Hereditary, imperfect dentin formation.

dentition General character and arrangement of the teeth, taken as a whole, as in carnivorous, herbivorous, and omnivorous dentitions. Primary dentition refers to the deciduous teeth; secondary dentition to the permanent teeth. Mixed dentition refers to a combination of permanent and deciduous teeth in the same dentition.

depression Lowering of the mandible or opening of the mouth.

depressor anguli oris Muscle of facial expression that extends from the lower border of the mandible at the canine area up to the corner of the lower lip.

depressor labii inferioris Muscle that goes from the chin area up into the middle part of the lower lip.

descending palatine artery Branch of the maxillary artery that supplies the hard and soft palates.

descending palatine nerve Branch of the second division of the trigeminal nerve to the hard and soft palates.

desmosome Ultrastructural part of a cell next to the cell wall that helps hold cells together.

developmental depression Noticeable concavity on the formed crown or root of a tooth; occurs at the junction of two lobes, as on the mesial surface of maxillary first premolars, or at the furcation of roots.

developmental grooves Fine depressed lines in the enamel of a tooth that mark the union of the lobes of the crown.

developmental lines *See* developmental grooves.

developmental lobes Major growth centers of a tooth.

developmental pit Small hole formed by the junction of two or more developmental lines.

diaphysis The central shaft of a developing long bone.

diastema Any spacing between teeth in the same arch. Plural *diastemae.*

digastric fossae Two small depressions on the inferior surface of the mandible at the midline.

digastric muscle Suprahyoid muscle extending from the mastoid process area to the midline of the mandible; retracts and lowers the mandible; raises hyoid bone.

dilacerated Said of developing tooth roots that become bent and crooked because of developmental problems.

dilacerated tooth Tooth with sharply bent roots.

dilaceration A sharp bend in the root or crown of the tooth.

dilator naris Muscle that goes over the tip of the nose and opens the nostrils.

diploë Thin layer of cancellous bone between the outer and inner plates of skull bones.

disc derangement When there is damage and displacement to the articular disc of the temporomandibular joint.

distal Distant; farthest from the median line of the face or from the origin of a structure.

distal contact area *See* contact area.

distal marginal groove Groove that crosses the distal marginal ridge.

distal oblique groove Groove that separates the distolingual cusp from the remainder of the occlusal surface of an upper molar.

distal pit Pit found in the distal fossa.

distal proximal surface Proximal surface on the posterior side of a tooth.

distal step The mandibular molars are more posterior than the maxillary molars.

distal third Viewed from the facial or lingual surface; the third of a surface farthest from the midline.

distobuccal developmental groove Developmental groove that extends on the buccal surface of a lower first or third molar between the distobuccal and distal cusps.

distoclusion *See* class II occlusal relationship.

distolingual cusp Most distal of the lingual cusps.

distolingual groove, distolingual developmental groove *See* distal oblique groove.

distomolars Fourth molars.

DNA Deoxyribonucleic acid; the substance in a cell nucleus that builds the genetic information to enable the cell to build a duplicate of itself or control products produced by the cell.

dorsal primary ramus Dorsal branch of the mixed spinal nerve that goes to the midline of the back.

dorsal root Sensory root of a spinal nerve entering the spinal cord.

dorsal root ganglion Cell bodies of sensory nerves to the spinal cord. A ganglion is located in the dorsal root of a spinal nerve.

dorsum of the tongue Top surface of the tongue.

dwarfed roots Tooth with very short roots in comparison with the crown.

E

ectoderm Outer embryonic germ layer that forms skin, salivary glands, hair, sweat glands, sebaceous glands, nerves, and so on.

ectodermal dysplasia A pathologic condition in which all structures developing from embryonic ectoderm have their growth interrupted. This involves skin, hair, sebaceous glands, sweat glands, salivary glands, and enamel of teeth.

edema Swelling of tissue.

edge, incisal *See* incisal edge.

edentulous An area without the presence of teeth.

efferent Refers to a nerve fiber carrying motor messages from the brain.

elastic cartilage Type of cartilage that has a large number of elastic fibers in it; for example, the ear.

elastic fiber Fiber of connective tissue that has elastic properties. Many of these are found in the walls of large arteries.

elastin Major component of elastic fibers of connective tissue.

elevation Raising the mandible, or closing the mouth.

embrasure Open space between the proximal surfaces of two teeth where they diverge buccally, labially, or lingually and occlusally from the contact area.

enamel Hard, calcified tissue that covers the dentin of the crown portion of a tooth.

enamel cuticle Nasmyth's membrane; a thin membrane that covers the crown of a tooth at eruption.

enamel dysplasia Abnormality of enamel growth.

enamel fluorosis A form of enamel hypocalcification where enamel is discolored because of an excess of fluoride in the tooth structure.

enamel hypocalcification Enamel that is not as dense as regular enamel.

enamel hypoplasia Enamel that is thin or pitted.

enamel lamellae Imperfections or cracks in enamel formed by trauma or imperfect enamel formation.

enamel organ Ectodermal epithelial structure that leads to the formation of tooth enamel.

enamel pearls Small, rounded elevations of enamel, usually developing in the bifurcations or trifurcations of teeth; considered abnormal structures.

enamel rod Individual pillars of enamel formed by multiple ameloblasts.

enamel spindle Odontoblastic process trapped in enamel at the dentinoenamel junction.

enamel tuft Area of hypocalcified enamel at the dentinoenamel junction.

endochondral bone formation Bone that forms by replacing a hyaline cartilage model.

endocrine Gland or type of secretion that is carried away from the producing cells by blood vessels; the secretion is used in other parts of the body to control certain functions; has no duct system.

endoplasmic reticulum Tubular system in a cell related to the cell's production of secretions such as protein. There are two types depending on the presence or absence of RNA on its surface wall, a rough or a smooth endoplasmic reticulum.

endosteal Inside bone; in the center marrow area.

endosteal lamellae Layers of bone lining the walls of the marrow cavity of the bone.

endosteum See endosteal.

endothelial cells Simple squamous cells lining blood vessels, lymph vessels, and the inside and outside of the heart.

entoderm Inner germ layer of an embryo that forms the epithelial lining of organs such as the digestive tract, liver, lungs, and pancreas.

enzyme A protein that aids in increasing the speed of reaction in many types of cells and systems of the body.

eosinophils White granulocyte cells that have some phagocytosing properties and allergic properties.

epicranius Muscle of facial expression in the scalp region extending from front to back.

epiglottis Cartilage that helps cover the laryngeal opening.

epinephrine Substance produced either synthetically or by the body and that causes many reactions; in dentistry it is used to constrict blood flow in tissues; see also *adrenalin.*

epiphyseal plate Block of cartilage between the diaphysis and epiphysis in long bones; allows for longitudinal growth.

epiphysis The end components of growing bone found in long bones.

epithelial Pertaining to epithelium.

epithelial attachment The substance produced by the reduced enamel epithelium that helps secure the attachment epithelium at the base of the gingival sulcus to the tooth.

epithelial diaphragm Deep part of the epithelial root sheath that is turned horizontally.

epithelial rests Cells from the epithelial root sheath that remain in the periodontal space and cells that remain at areas of embryonic fusion.

epithelial rests of Malassez *See* epithelial rests.

epithelial root sheath Downgrowth of the inner and outer enamel epithelium that outlines the shape and number of the roots.

epithelium Layer or layers of cells that cover the surface of the body or line the tubes or cavities inside the body; one of the four basic tissues.

equilibrium Sense of balance.

eruption Movement of the tooth as it emerges through surrounding tissue so that the clinical crown gradually appears longer.

eruptive stage Period of eruption from the completion of crown formation until the teeth come into occlusion.

ethmoid air cells Small, interconnecting bony compartments in the lateral nasal wall that form the ethmoid sinuses.

ethmoid bone Bone that forms a very small part of the anterior neurocranium, part of the medial wall of the orbit, and a large part of the nasal cavity.

ethmoid bulla Oblong bulge in the middle meatus above the hiatus semilunaris, onto which open the middle ethmoid air cells.

ethmoid sinus Group of small air cavities in the bone of the lateral wall of the nasal cavity.

excretory duct Duct that is surrounded by connective tissue between the lobules of a gland or is outside the gland and carrying the salivary fluid to the surface without changing it.

exfoliation Shedding or loss of a primary tooth.

exocrine Gland or type of secretion that is carried away from the producing cells by a duct system.

exostoses Small extra growths of bone on a bone surface; usually seen on the buccal cortical plate.

external auditory meatus Opening of the ear on the side of the skull.

external carotid artery Branch of the common carotid artery that supplies most of the head except the inside of the skull.

external jugular vein Vein that drains the superficial structures of the neck and flows eventually into the subclavian vein in the neck.

external nasal nerve Branch of the anterior ethmoidal nerve of V_1 that supplies the upper bridge of the nose.

external oblique line The bony ridge running downward from the anterior border of the ramus of the mandible and out onto the lateral alveolar process and body.

extracellular fluid Fluid between cells; consists primarily of blood plasma.

extrinsic Originating outside a structure.

extrinsic factors External factors.

F

facial Term used to designate the outer surfaces of the teeth collectively (buccal or labial).

facial artery Branch of the external carotid artery that supplies the superficial face area.

facial contours Curvature of the facial surface of a tooth.

facial embrasure *See* embrasure.

facial nerve Seventh cranial nerve (VII), which serves the muscles of facial expression as well as most taste and salivary gland control.

facial surface *See* facial.

facial third From a proximal view, the third of the surface closest to the facial side.

familial tendency When an anomaly occurs more frequently than usual in one family.

fascia Connective tissue covering muscles and separating muscle layers.

fascial spaces Potential spaces between layers of muscles or layers of connective tissue.

fat cell *See* adipocyte.

fauces Space between the left and right palatine tonsils.

FDI system The Federation Dentaire Internationale (International Dental Federation) system for tooth identification.

fibroblast Basic cell of connective tissue that produces the collagen fiber.

fibrocartilage Type of cartilage containing large quantities of collagen fibers.

fifth-cusp developmental groove Groove that separates the cusp of Carabelli from the lingual surface on an upper molar.

fight-or-flight mechanism Another term for the reactions of the sympathetic nervous system.

filiform papillae Small, pointed projections that heavily cover most of the dorsum of the anterior two-thirds of the tongue. No taste buds.

fissure Deep cleft; developmental line fault usually found in the occlusal or buccal surface of a tooth; commonly the result of the imperfect fusion of the enamel of the adjoining dental lobes.

flange Projecting edge; the edge of a denture.

flexion A bend or a twist in the root only, not involving the crown.

fluorosis Discolored enamel resulting from excessive fluoride intake while the crown is developing.

flush terminal plane The mandibular and maxillary second molars are even, with neither being anterior or posterior.

foliate papillae Poorly developed papillae that appear as small vertical folds in the posterior part of the sides of the tongue.

foramen Short, circular opening through a bone (plural often foramina).

foramen cecum Depression in the tongue two-thirds of the way back that marks the beginning point of development of the thyroid gland; means "blind aperture."

foramen lacerum A jagged opening in the base of the skull that is part of the anterior floor of the carotid canal. In life, this foramen is filled with a piece of cartilage and nothing of any importance passes through it.

foramen magnum Large foramen in the base of the occipital bone.

foramen ovale Oval-shaped foramen in the sphenoid bone at the base of the skull. Transmits V_3.

foramen rotundum Foramen in the front part of the middle cranial fossa that opens into the pterygopalatine fossa behind and below the eye. Transmits V_2.

foramen spinosum Small opening in base of the skull just posterior to the foramen ovale; it transmits the middle meningeal artery to the covering of the brain.

Fordyce granules Misplaced sebaceous glands in the lips, cheek, or retromolar pad area.

foregut Front end of the gastrointestinal tube in the early developing embryo.

fossa Round, wide, relatively shallow depression in the surface of a tooth as seen commonly in the lingual surfaces of the maxillary incisors or between the cusps of molars; also a shallow depression in bone.

fovea palatinae Small depressions in mucosa on either side of the posterior nasal spine, indicating the junction of the hard and soft palates.

free gingiva Gingiva that forms the gingival sulcus.

free gingival groove The line in the gingiva that separates free gingiva from attached gingiva.

frenulum Little frenum or fold of tissue.

frontal bone Bone that forms the forehead.

frontal nerve One of the three main branches of the ophthalmic division of the trigeminal nerve.

frontal prominence Bulge in the forehead region that forms the upper facial area in the embryo.

frontal sinus Air sinus in the frontal bone above the eye that opens into the hiatus semilunaris in the middle meatus.

frontalis muscle The front belly of the epicranius muscle.

frontooccipitalis *See* occipitofrontalis.

frontoparietal suture *See* coronal suture.

functional eruptive stage *See* posteruptive stage.

fungiform papillae Small circular papillae scattered throughout the anterior two-thirds of the dorsum of the tongue.

fusion Two teeth that fuse at their dentin while they are developing. Also, a term used for the process of formation of the hard and soft palates.

G

ganglion An accumulation of nerve cell bodies outside of the brain or spinal cord.

gemination A tooth that partially or fully divides into two teeth while developing.

genial tubercles Small projections for muscle attachment on the lingual surface of the mandible at the midline.

genioglossus Extrinsic tongue muscle running from the superior genial tubercles up into the tongue.

geniohyoid muscle Suprahyoid muscle that extends from the inferior genial tubercles to the hyoid bone.

germinative layer *See* basal layer.

gingiva Part of the gum tissue that immediately surrounds the teeth and alveolar bone.

gingival crest Most occlusal or incisal extent of gingiva.

gingival crevice Subgingival space that, under normal conditions, lies between the gingival crest and the epithelial attachment.

gingival crevicular fluid The fluid that is found in the gingival sulcus between the free gingiva and the tooth.

gingival embrasure *See* cervical embrasure.

gingival fibers Periodontal fibers in the gingiva.

gingival papillae That portion of the gingiva found between the teeth in the interproximal spaces gingival to the contact area; also called *interdental papillae*.

gingival sulcus Space between the free gingiva and the tooth surface.

gingival tissue *See* gingiva.

gingival unit Subdivision of the periodontium.

gingivitis Inflammation involving the gingival tissues only.

glands of von Ebner Small, minor, serous salivary glands (lingual glands) that open into the crypts of the vallate papillae.

globulomaxillary cyst Cyst that forms between the maxillary lateral incisor and canine.

glossitis Inflammation of the tongue wherein the tongue is red and smooth.

glossopharyngeal glands Small minor salivary glands in the tonsillar pillars.

glossopharyngeal nerve Ninth cranial nerve (IX), serving a muscle of the pharynx, taste, general sensation, and salivary glands.

glycogen Form of starch that by enzymes makes glucose (body sugar) or is made from glucose, depending on bodily needs; stored as a cellular inclusion and readily available as instant energy.

glycoproteins One of the two main classes of proteins found in the ground substance of connective tissue.

goblet cells Single-celled glands that secrete mucus; found in the epithelium of respiratory and digestive tracts from the stomach through the gastrointestinal tract.

Golgi apparatus Flat saclike layers in a cell that "package" the cell products for transportation outside the cell.

granular layer of Tomes Interglobular dentin in the root.

granulocytes White blood cells that have small or large granules in their cytoplasm; neutrophils, basophils, and eosinophils.

gray matter Central portion of the spinal cord containing cell bodies of motor and sensory neurons.

greater auricular nerve Branch of the cervical plexus from C2-C3 that innervates the skin over the angle of the jaw.

greater palatine artery Branch of the descending palatine artery to the hard palate.

greater palatine foramen Foramen on either side of the hard palate between the maxillae and palatine bones.

greater palatine nerve Branch of the descending palatine nerve that serves the hard palate.

greater palatine nerve block An anesthetic deposited into the greater palatine foramen causing regional anesthesia that anesthetizes the lingual soft tissue of the palate distal to the canines on either side.

greater petrosal nerve A parasympathetic branch of the VII (facial) cranial nerve that supplies all glands from the hard palate, nasal cavity, and the lacrimal gland.

greater wing of the sphenoid Part of the sphenoid bone projecting onto the side of the skull behind the zygomatic bone as well as the posterior part of orbit.

ground substance Gluelike substance that serves as the background for connective tissue, including cartilage and bone; composed of a substance known as a mucopolysaccharide.

group function During lateral excursion, several teeth, not just a solitary canine, touch simultaneously. Usually the maxillary canine and the first and second premolars touch at the same time.

gubernacular canal A small canal in the alveolar bone of a mixed dentition individual, located just lingual to its primary tooth. This canal was occupied by the successional lamina of the permanent tooth.

H

habitual occlusion *See* centric occlusion.

hamular process *See* pterygoid hamulus.

hard tissue Calcified or mineralized tooth tissues or bone.

hairy tongue A condition wherein the filiform papillae on the tongue have elongated, giving the tongue a hairy appearance.

hare lip A midline cleft of the upper lip that resembles the upper lip of a rabbit. Very rare.

haversian lamellae Concentric layers of bone around blood vessels in bone.

Haversian system System of blood vessels located within the bones to provide them with nourishment.

hematoma Escape of blood from an injured blood vessel into tissue spaces.

hemoglobin Component in red blood cells that carries oxygen.

hereditary Inherited through the genes of parents.

Hertwig's epithelial root sheath *See* epithelial root sheath.

hiatus of the maxillary sinus The opening from the middle meatus of the nasal cavity into the maxillary sinus.

hiatus semilunaris Curving depression beneath the middle nasal concha in the middle meatus. It has openings in it for the frontal, anterior ethmoid, and maxillary sinuses.

hindgut The lower third of the embryonic gut tube that forms the lower part of the large intestine from the descending colon to the anus.

histamine Substance produced by some cells that causes swelling or edema of the tissues.

holocrine Method of secretion wherein the cell dies and releases its products.

horizontal group Group of alveolodental fibers.

hormones Chemical substances produced by the body that have certain effects on other organs or glands of the body.

Hutchinson's incisors Notched central incisors that develop as a result of congenital syphilis.

hyaline cartilage Type of cartilage that is very firm; sometimes replaced by bone. The larynx and trachea are examples of hyaline cartilage.

hydroxyapatite (sometimes spelled hydroxylapatite) The crystal that is found in hard substances of the body such as bone, cementum, dentin, and enamel.

hyoglossus Extrinsic tongue muscle running from the hyoid bone up into the lateral border of the tongue.

hyoid Horseshoe-shaped bone in the neck between the mandible and larynx.

hyoid arch Second pharyngeal arch, which forms some of the structures in the neck.

hyoid muscles Muscles that attach to the free-floating hyoid bone in the neck.

hypercementosis Increased thickness of cementum, usually seen at the apex of the root.

hyperdontia More than the usual number of teeth.

hyperemia Congestion of blood seen in pulp.

hypocalcified enamel Condition in which there is either an insufficient number of enamel crystals or insufficient growth of the crystals.

hypoglossal nerve Twelfth cranial nerve (XII); supplies motor control to most of the tongue muscles.

hypophyseal fossa Saddle-shaped depression on the body of the sphenoid bone located in the middle cranial fossa containing the pituitary gland.

hypoplastic enamel Thin enamel; may be hypocalcified as well.

I

I band Light microscopic band at either end of the sarcomere. The I band contains only actin myofilaments.

imbrication lines Horizontal lines best seen on the labial surfaces of anterior teeth. These are surface manifestations of the striae of Retzius.

immunity Body's resistance to certain organisms or diseases.

impacted Describing teeth not completely erupted that are fully or partially covered by bone or soft tissue.

incisal edge Edge formed at the labioincisal line angle of an anterior tooth after an incisal ridge has worn down.

incisal embrasure *See* embrasure.

incisal ridge Rounded ridge formed of the incisal portion of an anterior tooth.

incisal third From a proximal, lingual, or labial view of an anterior tooth, the third of the surface closest to the incisal edge.

incisive foramen Foramen at the midline of the anterior palate region.

incisive nerve block Anesthesia resulting from anesthetic being deposited into the mental foramen.

incisive papilla Small, rounded, oblong mound of tissue directly behind or lingual to the maxillary central incisors and lying over the incisive foramen.

incisors Four center teeth in either arch; essential for cutting.

inferior alveolar branch or artery Branch of the maxillary artery that supplies the lower teeth.

inferior alveolar nerve Branch of the third division (V_3) of the trigeminal nerve.

inferior alveolar nerve block Local anesthetic that anesthetizes the mandibular teeth, their associated periodontium, and lingual soft tissue for one side of the mandible to the midline.

inferior border of mandible Lower edge of the lower jaw.

inferior meatus Area sheltered by the inferior nasal conchae.

inferior nasal conchae Small bones that project from the lower lateral walls of the nasal cavity.

inferior orbital fissure Groovelike opening in the inferior lateral part of the orbit.

inferior pharyngeal constrictor muscle Lowest of three muscles that form the throat wall and help move food down into the esophagus.

inner cell mass Inner thickened layer of a blastocyst that becomes an embryo.

inflammatory reaction Body's mechanism to combat harmful organisms by bringing more plasma and blood cells to an injured area.

infrahyoid muscles Muscles below the hyoid bone that attach to it.

infraorbital artery Termination of the maxillary artery that passes out of the floor of the orbit through the infraorbital foramen; supplies the skin of the lower eyelid, upper lip, and side of the nose.

infraorbital block Local anesthetic deposited into infraorbital foramen that anesthetizes the anterior and middle superior alveolar nerves

infraorbital foramen Foramen just below the lower rim of the orbit in the maxillary bone.

infraorbital nerve Termination of the second division of the trigeminal nerve that supplies the skin of the lower eyelid, nose, and upper lip.

infratemporal fossa Area on the side of the skull immediately below the temporal fossa; pterygoid muscles and the maxillary artery are located there.

infratrochlear nerve A branch of the ophthalmic division of the trigeminal nerve that supplies the skin in the lower medial corner of the eye.

infraorbital verve block A local anesthetic block that covers the anterior and middle superior alveolar nerve by depositing anesthetic into the infraorbital foramen.

inherited Passed on from parents or grandparents.

inner cell mass The clump of cells on the inside of an embryonic blastocyst that forms the three germinal layers.

inner enamel epithelium (IEE) Group of epithelial cells in the enamel organ that eventually form the enamel of the crown.

inorganic matrix Hydroxyapatite crystals in the early matrix.

inorganic matter Mineral deposits such as calcium or phosphorus.

insertion End of a muscle attached to a more movable structure.

intercalated ducts Short, small ducts that carry saliva from acini to striated ducts.

intercuspal position (ICP) *See* centric occlusion.

intercuspation Relationship of the cusps of the premolars and molars of one jaw to those of the opposing jaw during any of the occlusal relationships.

interdental Located between the teeth.

interdental papilla Projection of gingiva between the teeth.

interdental space Space between the teeth.

interglobular dentin Areas of hypocalcified dentin between normal areas of dentin; found in both crown and root dentin.

interlobular ducts Ducts between lobules of glands.

intermaxillary suture Suture between the maxillae. It is seen below the nasal cavity and in the front portion of the hard palate.

internal acoustic meatus Opening in the lateral part of the posterior cranial fossa for the facial and statoacoustic cranial nerves.

internal carotid artery Branch of the common carotid artery that supplies the brain and inside of the skull.

internal jugular vein Main vein that drains the brain and deep structures of the head and neck; flows into the brachiocephalic vein.

interparietal suture *See* sagittal suture.

interproximal Between the proximal surfaces of adjoining teeth in the same arch.

interproximal space Triangular space between adjoining teeth; the proximal surfaces of the teeth form the sides of the triangle; the alveolar bone, the base, and the contact area of the teeth form the apex.

interstitial growth Growth from within, as seen in cartilage formation when chondrocytes divide and enlarge.

interstitial lamellae Parts of old bone layers found between newly formed layers of bone.

intertubular dentin All dentin that is not tubular or peritubular.

intralobular ducts Ducts surrounded by acini in a gland. Some of them help change the saliva before it leaves the gland.

intramembranous bone formation Bone formed directly from mesenchymal cells that become osteoblasts.

intrinsic Lying entirely inside a structure.

intrinsic factors Internal factors.

involuntary muscle Not voluntary; unable to be willfully controlled.

J

jugular foramen *See* jugular fossa.

jugular fossa Depression in the base of the skull with an opening for the passage of the internal jugular vein and the IX, X, and XI cranial nerves from the skull.

junctional epithelium Epithelium that functions to hold mucosa in the base of the gingival sulcus to the tooth.

K

keratin Substance that makes up the surface cells of skin, hair, and nails.

keratinized cells Dead cells of the stratum corneum.

keratinized stratified squamous epithelium Multilayered epithelium, like skin; upper layers are dead cells; makeup is similar to the composition of hair.

keratohyalin granules Granules in the stratum granulosum that help produce the dead layer of cells on the skin surface.

L

labia Latin word for lips; singular labium.

labial Of or pertaining to the lips; toward the lips.

labial frenum Fold of tissue that attaches the lip to the labial mucosa at the midline of the lips.

labial glands Small minor salivary glands in the lips.

lacrimal bone Small bone at the inner front of the orbit, forming part of the canal from the eye to the nose.

lacrimal groove Groove in the lacrimal bone for the lacrimal duct.

lacrimal nerve Branch of the ophthalmic division of the trigeminal nerve that provides sensation for the lacrimal gland and for skin lateral to and above the eye.

lambdoid suture Inverted V-shaped suture between the occipital and parietal bones; also known as the parietooccipital suture.

lamina dura Radiographic term denoting the cribriform plate and bundle bone.

laryngeal pharynx That part of the common pathway of the respiratory and digestive systems from the base of the tongue to the opening of the larynx.

larynx Voice box; trachea begins just below it.

lateral excursion Movement of the jaws sideways.

lateral head film *See* cephalometric film.

lateral lingual swellings Paired structures arising from the internal pharyngeal arches and forming the anterior two-thirds of the tongue.

lateral nasal process Embryologic structure that forms the side of the nose and the area beneath the medial corner of the eye.

lateral pharyngeal space Area or fascial space beside the throat wall.

lateral pterygoid muscle Muscle that extends from the pterygoid plate and the infratemporal crest of sphenoid to the condyle and protrudes the mandible.

lateral pterygoid plate Thin wall of bone projecting back from the pterygoid process on the lateral side.

leeway space The difference between the sum of the mesiodistal measurements of the deciduous canines and the deciduous molars compared with the mesiodistal measurements of the permanent canines and premolars in any one quadrant.

lesser palatine artery Branch of the descending palatine artery that goes to the soft palate.

lesser palatine foramen Foramen at the posterior end of the hard palate that transmits the lesser palatine nerve and artery to the soft palate.

lesser palatine nerve Branch of the descending palatine nerve that supplies the soft palate.

lesser petrosal nerve Branch of the glossopharyngeal nerve (IX) that carries secretomotor function to the parotid gland via the auriculotemporal nerve.

lesser wing of sphenoid Projection of the sphenoid bone that forms the posterior border of the anterior cranial fossa.

leukemia Cancer of white blood cells that chokes out red blood cell production.

levator anguli oris Muscle that goes from beneath the eye to the corner of the upper lip.

levator labii superiors Muscle that extends from below the eye to the middle part of the upper lip.

levator palpebri superioris Muscle inside the eye that is supplied by the oculomotor nerve that elevates the upper eyelid.

levator veli palatini Muscle of the soft palate that helps pull it back against the throat wall.

ligament Regularly arranged group of collagen fibers that attach bone to bone.

line angle Angle formed by two surfaces, for example, mesial and lingual; the junction is called the mesiolingual line angle.

lingual Pertaining to or affecting the tongue; next to or toward the tongue.

lingual artery Branch of the external carotid artery that supplies the tongue and floor of the mouth.

lingual contours Curvature of the lingual surface of a tooth.

lingual crest of curvature Most convex or widest portion of the lingual surface of a tooth.

lingual developmental groove Groove on the lingual surface that separates two lingual cusps; *see* lingual groove.

lingual embrasure *See* embrasure.

lingual frenum Fold of tissue that attaches the undersurface of the tongue to the floor of the mouth.

lingual glands Minor salivary glands of the tongue.

lingual groove Developmental groove that occurs on the lingual side of the tooth.

lingual nerve Branch of the third division (V3) of the trigeminal nerve that supplies general sensation to the anterior two-thirds of tongue and floor of the mouth.

lingual surface *See* lingual.

lingual third From a proximal view, the third of a surface closest to the lingual side.

lingual thyroid A thyroid gland that does not descend to the neck in development. It is found on the surface of the tongue posterior to the circumvallate papillae.

lingual tonsils Tonsil tissue on the dorsum of the posterior part of the tongue.

lingula Small projection of bone just in front of the mandibular foramen.

lining mucosa Mucosa of the soft palate, lips, cheeks, vestibule, and floor of the mouth.

lipid Fatty substance found in cells as an inclusion; used as a reserve source of energy.

lobe Part of a tooth formed by any one of the major developing centers that begin the calcification of the tooth.

lobe of Carabelli *See* cusp of Carabelli.

long buccal nerve Lower branch of the buccal nerve that supplies the mandibular buccal gingiva.

lower deep cervical Group of lymph nodes in the lower lateral neck beneath the sternomastoid muscle.

Ludwig's angina Infection in the fascial spaces beneath the chin.

lumbar Relating to the lower back, for example, vertebrae or nerves of the lower back.

lumen Inside of a tube or duct; inside diameter of the opening.

lymph nodes Small bean-shaped structures connected to one another by very small tubules. They combat infections in the body.

lymphadenopathy Enlarged lymph glands or nodes; may be seen or felt when one has a sore throat, infected ears, and so on.

lymphatic vessels Small tubes throughout the body that carry fluid from between the cells back into the vascular system via lymph nodes.

lymphocytes Kind of agranulocyte; active in the inflammatory process.

lymphoid tissue Tissues made up of lymphocytes, which fight infections.

lysosomes Small membrane-bound structures in a cell that act as a "garbage can" for the nonusable or harmful substances that find their way inside the cell.

M

macrodontia Teeth that are too large for the jaw.

macrophage Cell of connective tissue that destroys other cells, usually from outside the body.

malocclusion Abnormal occlusion of the teeth.

mamelon One of the three rounded protuberances of the incisal surface of a newly erupted incisor tooth.

mandible Lower jaw.

mandibular Pertaining to the lower jaw.

mandibular arch First pharyngeal arch that forms the area of the mandible and maxillae; the lower dental arch.

mandibular condyle Rounded top of the mandible that articulates with the mandibular fossa.

mandibular division Third part of the trigeminal nerve (V); frequently represented as V3.

mandibular foramen Opening on the medial surface of the ramus of the mandible for the entrance of nerves and blood vessels to the lower teeth.

mandibular fossa Depression on the inferior surface of the skull in the temporal bone that articulates with the condyle of the mandible.

mandibular nerve block Local anesthetic that anesthetizes the third division (V3) of the trigeminal nerve.

mandibular notch Notch in the mandibular ramus between the condyloid process and the coronoid process.

mandibular process That portion of the mandibular pharyngeal arch that forms the mandible.

mandibular tori Bony growths on the lingual cortical plate of bone opposite the mandibular canines; also called *torus mandibularis*.

marginal developmental groove *See* marginal groove.

marginal gingiva *See* free gingiva.

marginal groove Groove that crosses a marginal ridge.

marginal ridge Ridge or elevation of enamel forming the margin of the surface of a tooth; specifically, at the mesial and distal margins of the occlusal surfaces of premolars and molars and at the mesial and distal margins of the lingual surfaces of incisors and canines.

marrow cavity Hollow center of bone responsible for blood cell production and, later in life, for fat storage.

masseter muscle Muscle on the lateral surface of the mandible that elevates it.

masseteric branch Branch of the maxillary artery or nerve to the masseter muscle.

mast cells White blood cells in connective tissue that release histamines.

mastication Act of chewing or grinding.

masticatory mucosa Mucosa of the hard palate and gingiva.

mastoid process Large projection of temporal bone behind the ear.

matrix Framework for a material; the framework for hard-tissue formation.

maturation stage The stage of hard-tissue development where the crystals that have been deposited grow in size.

maxillae Paired main bones of the upper jaw.

maxillary Pertaining to the upper arch.

maxillary arch Upper dental arch.

maxillary artery Major branch of the external carotid artery that supplies the teeth, gingiva, cheeks, palate, and several other areas.

maxillary division Second part of the trigeminal nerve (V); usually represented as V2.

maxillary process Upper portion of the mandibular pharyngeal arch that forms the maxillae.

maxillary sinus Largest of the paired paranasal sinuses; located in the maxillae.

maxillary tuberosity Bulging posterior surface of the maxillae posterior to the third molar region.

meatus Space beneath the shelter of each of the nasal conchae.

medial nasal processes Embryologic structures that form the bridge of the nose, the middle part of the upper lip, part of the nasal septum, and part of the anterior hard palate.

medial pterygoid muscle Muscle that runs between the mandible and pterygoid process and elevates the mandible.

medial pterygoid plate Thin wall of bone projecting back from the pterygoid process on the medial side.

median line Vertical (central) line that divides the body into right and left; the median line of the face.

median palatine cyst Cyst that forms along lines of fusion of palatal shelves of maxillae.

median palatine suture Suture that goes down the middle of the hard palate. The anterior part of the suture may also be called part of the intermaxillary suture.

median raphe A midline joining of the left and right pharyngeal constrictor muscles in the posterior throat wall; runs from the base of the skull above to the esophagus below.

megakaryocyte Large cell in marrow that is the forerunner of white blood cells.

melanin Brown pigment in the skin. An increase in the amount of pigment is seen after sunburn and is produced by the melanocytes.

melanocytes Pigment-producing cells located below the basal layer of epithelium. The pigment granules are incorporated into the basal cells and move up through the layers to the surface.

mental artery Branch of the inferior alveolar artery that supplies the lower lip and gingiva adjacent to the lip.

mental branch *See* mental artery.

mental foramen Foramen on the lateral side of the mandible, below the premolars.

mental nerve Branch of the inferior alveolar nerve that supplies the skin and mucosa of the lower lip and labial gingiva.

mental nerve block Anesthetic deposited at the mental foramen, anesthetizing the facial soft tissue anterior to the mental foramen on one side of the mandible to the midline.

mental protuberance Point of the chin on the anterior inferior surface of the midline of the mandible.

mental spines *See* genial tubercles.

mentalis Muscle that extends from the bone on the chin into the skin of the chin.

merocrine Method of secretion wherein the droplets pass out of the cell by fusing with the cell membrane, eliminating the possibility of damage to the cell.

mesenchymal cell Primitive cell of the mesodermal embryonic layer. This cell has the ability to form a number of different tissues. Some of these cells are available throughout life.

mesial Toward or situated in the middle, for example, toward the midline of the dental arch.

mesial contact area *See* contact area.

mesial developmental depression Indented area on the mesial surface of a tooth.

mesial drift Phenomenon of permanent molars continuing to move mesially after eruption.

mesial marginal developmental groove *See* mesial marginal groove.

mesial marginal groove Developmental groove that crosses the mesial marginal ridge.

mesial pit Pit found in the mesial fossa.

mesial proximal surface Proximal surface closest to the midline.

mesial step The mandibular molars are more anterior than the maxillary molars.

mesial third From a facial or a lingual view, third of the surface closest to the midline.

mesiobuccal developmental groove Developmental groove that runs on the buccal surface of a lower first or third molar between the mesiobuccal and distobuccal cusps.

mesioclusion See class III occlusal relationship.

mesiodens Supernumerary teeth arising in the midline of the maxilla between central incisors.

mesiolingual cusp Most mesial of the lingual cusps.

mesiolingual developmental groove Lingual developmental groove that separates the mesiolingual and distolingual cusps.

mesiolingual groove See mesiolingual developmental groove.

mesoderm Middle germ layer of the embryo that forms connective tissue, muscle, bone, cartilage, blood, and so on.

mesothelial cells Simple squamous cells lining the pleural cavity of the chest, the peritoneal cavity of the abdomen, and covering of the digestive tract, as well as the inside of the pericardial sac surrounding the heart.

metabolism Building up or breaking down of food accompanied by the production or use of energy.

microdontia Teeth that are too small for the jaw.

microfilament The ultrastructural solid filament that is part of the cytoskeleton. Composed of actin.

microtubule The hollow ultrastructural filament of cytoskeleton; usually associated with motility of cilia or flagella.

microvilli Ultrastructural elongations of the surface of epithelial cells that absorb; for example, the gut, which increases the surface area of the cell so that it can absorb more.

middle cranial fossa The middle concavity in the floor of the skull that houses the temporal lobes and base of brain.

middle ethmoid sinus Middlemost group of ethmoid air cells.

middle meatus Area sheltered by the middle nasal concha.

middle meningeal artery Branch of the first part of the maxillary artery that is the main blood supply to the meninges of the brain.

middle nasal concha Small projection of thin bone from the middle of the lateral nasal wall.

middle pharyngeal constrictor muscle The middle of three muscles that form the throat wall and help move food down into the esophagus.

middle superior alveolar nerve Branch of the infraorbital nerve that supplies the maxillary premolars and usually the mesiobuccal root of the maxillary first molar.

middle third See mesial third.

midgut That part of the early digestive tract that will develop from the mid duodenum to the left colic flexure of the large intestine.

midline Imaginary line that divides the body into right and left halves.

midsagittal plane Divides the body vertically into right and left halves.

migration (movement) The flow of connective tissue in the upper lip that aids in the formation of the lip.

mineralization stage The stage in which hydroxyapatite crystals are laid down in developing hard tissue.

mitochondria Small organelles in a cell that produce energy and control the metabolism of the cell; singular, mitochondrion.

mitotic division Process of cell division that leads to the development of two cells from one.

mixed dentition State of having primary and permanent teeth in the dental arches at the same time.

molars Large posterior teeth used for grinding.

monocytes White agranulocytes that have phagocytic properties.

mortality rate Death rate; the number of deaths in a certain population for a certain reason; usually measured in a percentage, or may be the number of deaths per 1,000, 10,000, 100,000, and so on.

mottled enamel Enamel that has been discolored by excess fluorides in naturally fluoridated water or by excessive fluoride intake.

MRI scan A computer-generated body scan using magnetic fields instead of ionizing radiation.

mucocele A traumatized minor salivary gland, usually in the lip, that causes a blister-like lesion; generally will rupture and heal.

mucogingival junction Point at which the alveolar mucosa becomes gingiva.

mucosa Moist epithelial linings of the oral cavity and the respiratory and digestive systems.

mucous Pertaining to mucus, the thick viscous secretion of a gland.

mucous acini Salivary unit that produces viscous saliva.

mulberry molars Molars with multiple cusps; caused by congenital syphilis.

multiple root Root with more than one branch.

muscle One of the four basic tissues; has the properties of contraction or shortening of fibers and accomplishes work. There are three types of muscle: skeletal, cardiac, and smooth.

muscle of uvula The small muscular projection that extends down from the posterior of the soft palate.

myelin sheath Covering around axons or dendrites of some nerves.

myelinated Covered with myelin; a nerve that has a myelin sheath.

mylohyoid line Diagonal line on the medial surface of the mandible for attachment of the mylohyoid muscle.

mylohyoid muscle Suprahyoid muscle that forms the floor of the mouth.

mylohyoid nerve Branch of the inferior alveolar nerve to the mylohyoid muscle and anterior belly of the digastric muscle.

myoepithelial cell An epithelial-like cell that is found around glands and can contract like a muscle to help squeeze the secretions out of the ducts of the glands.

myofiber Single muscle fiber or muscle cell.

myofibril Component of muscle fiber; when grouped together, myofibrils make up a myofiber.

myofilaments Smallest thick and thin filaments in a myofibril that are responsible for contraction.

myosin One of the myofilaments located in the A band; thicker than actin.

N

nasal aperture Opening of the nasal cavity in the skull.

nasal bone Bones that form the bridge of the nose.

nasal pharynx That part of the nasal region from the posterior end of the nasal septum down to the level of the soft palate.

nasal pits Depressions in the developing facial area that deepen into the nasal passages.

nasal septum Wall between the left and right sides of the nasal cavity; made up of the ethmoid and vomer bones.

nasalis Nasal muscle of facial expression; divided into dilator naris and compressor naris.

Nasmyth's membrane See primary enamel cuticle.

nasociliary nerve Branch of the first division of the trigeminal nerve that supplies the ethmoid air sinuses, the skin in the lower medial corner of the eye, the cornea, and the bridge of the nose.

nasopalatine nerve Continuation of the sphenopalatine nerve that supplies the nasal septum and lingual gingiva of the maxillary incisors.

nasopalatine nerve block Anesthesia resulting from anesthetic being deposited in the nasopalatine foramen that anesthetizes the lingual soft tissue between the maxillary right and left canines

nervous tissue One of the four basic tissues. Groups of cells (neurons) carry messages to and from the brain and perform many other tasks.

neurocranium Part of the skull that surrounds the brain.

neuron Nerve cell.

neutroclusion See class I occlusal relationship.

neutrophils Granulocytes whose granules do not stain brightly. This is one of the major cell groups involved in the inflammatory process.

nodular Characterized by nodes or knotlike swellings.

nonkeratinized Lack of any keratinization.

nonsuccedaneous Permanent teeth that do not succeed or replace deciduous teeth.

nonworking side Opposite side from which the mandible is moved.

nucleolus Circular, dense area within the nucleus that contains most of the RNA within the nucleus.

nucleus Control center of the cell. DNA and RNA are found here to control cell division and production.

O

oblique groove See distolingual groove.

oblique group Group of alveolodental fibers.

oblique ridge Ridge running obliquely across the occlusal surface of the upper molars. It is formed by the union of the triangular ridge of the distobuccal cusp with the distal portion of the triangular ridge of the mesiolingual cusp.

occipital bone Bone of the base and back of the skull. The foramen magnum is found in the basal portion.

occipital condyles Thick, smooth surfaces on the basal part of the occipital bone just lateral to the foramen magnum. They articulate with the cervical vertebrae.

occipitofrontalis See epicranius.

occluding Contacting, opposing teeth.

occlusal Articulating or biting surface.

occlusal embrasure See embrasure.

occlusal plane Side view of the occlusal surfaces.

occlusal relationship Way in which the maxillary and mandibular teeth touch one another.

occlusal stress Pressures on the occlusal surfaces of teeth.

occlusal surface See occlusal.

occlusal table As seen from an occlusal view, the area bordered by the cusp tips and marginal ridges.

occlusal third From a proximal, lingual, or buccal view of a posterior tooth, the third of a surface closest to the occlusal surface.

occlusal trauma Injury brought about by one tooth prematurely hitting another during closure of the jaws.

occlusion Relationship of the mandibular and maxillary teeth when closed or during excursive movements of the mandible; when the teeth of the mandibular arch come into contact with the teeth of the maxillary arch in any functional relationship.

oculomotor nerve Third cranial nerve (III); aids in the movement of the eye.

odontoblast Dentin-forming cell that originates from the dental papilla.

odontoblastic process Cellular extension of the odontoblast, which is located along the full width of the dentin.

odontoma A tumor made up of enamel, dentin, cementum, and pulp.

olfactory epithelium Modified respiratory epithelium found in the superior nasal cavity containing nerves that allow the sensation of smell.

olfactory nerve First cranial nerve (I); transmits sensations of smell.

omohyoid muscle Infrahyoid muscle that extends from the shoulder blade to the hyoid bone.

opaque Not easily able to transmit light.

open bite Space left between the teeth when the jaws close.

open contact Space between adjacent teeth in the same arch; an interproximal opening instead of a contact area where the teeth touch.

ophthalmic division First part of the trigeminal nerve (V); usually represented as V_1.

optic foramen Opening into the posterior orbit that contains the optic nerve.

optic nerve Second cranial nerve (II); conducts visual stimuli.

oral cavity proper That area of the oral cavity bounded anteriorly and laterally by the teeth and posteriorly by the palatine tonsil.

oral epithelium Lining membrane of the oral cavity; stratified squamous epithelium.

oral pharynx The area behind the oral cavity that runs from the palatine tonsils to the back wall of the throat.

orbicularis oculi Muscle that goes around the eye and eyelid.

orbicularis oris Muscle that encircles the mouth; has many muscles running into it and blending with it.

orbit Bony opening for the eye in the skull.

organelles Means "little organs"; the functioning components in cells; they aid in the vital functions of the cells.

organic matrix Noncalcified framework in which crystals grow.

orifice An opening, such as an opening into a root canal or even the mouth as an opening of the body.

origin End of a muscle that is attached to the less movable structure.

ossicles Small bones of the middle ear.

osteoblasts Cells that form bone.

osteoclast Multinucleated cell that is responsible for destroying bone as well as cementum and dentin.

osteocyte Osteoblast that has surrounded itself with bone and becomes relatively inactive.

ostium of the maxillary sinus Opening of the maxillary sinus into the nasal cavity beneath the middle nasal concha.

otic ganglion Parasympathetic ganglion from the ninth cranial nerve (IX) that is attached to the medial side of the mandibular division of the trigeminal nerve and helps provide parasympathetic innervation to the parotid gland.

outer cell mass That outer layer of a blastocyst that becomes part of the membranes surrounding an embryo and fetus and helps form the placenta.

outer enamel epithelium (OEE) Outer epithelial layer of the enamel organ; serves as a protection for the developing enamel.

overbite Relationship of the teeth in which the incisal ridges of the maxillary anterior teeth extend below the incisal edges of the mandibular anterior teeth when the teeth are placed in a centric occlusal relationship.

overhanging restoration Excess of filling material extending past the confines of the tooth preparation; an overextension of filling material.

overjet Relationship of teeth in which the incisal ridges or buccal cusp ridges of the maxillary anterior teeth extend facially to the incisal ridges or buccal cusp ridges of the mandibular teeth when the teeth are in a centric occlusal relationship.

P

P-A films Radiographs taken with the ionizing source in the posterior position and the film in the anterior position.

palatal Pertaining to the palate or roof of the mouth.

palatal process of the maxillae Part of the maxillae that forms the anterior part of the hard palate.

palatal process of palatine bone Horizontal part of palatine bone that forms the posterior part of the hard palate.

palatal root Lingual root on any maxillary multi-rooted tooth.

palatal shelves Projections of the maxillary processes that form the hard and soft palates.

palatine bone Bone that forms the posterior part of the hard palate and the lateral nasal cavity.

palatine glands Minor salivary glands in the hard and soft palates.

palatine tonsils Normally just called *tonsils;* found at the side of the throat opposite the back of the tongue.

palatoglossal arch *See* anterior pillar.

palatoglossal fold *See* anterior pillar.

palatoglossus muscle Muscle that extends from the soft palate down into the sides of the tongue. The mucosa over this muscle forms the anterior pillar of the throat.

palatomaxillary suture *See* transverse palatine suture.

palatopharyngeal arch *See* posterior pillar.

palatopharyngeal fold *See* posterior pillar.

palatopharyngeal muscle Muscle that extends from the soft palate down into the lateral pharyngeal wall. The mucosa over this muscle forms the posterior pillar of the throat.

Palmer notation system System of coding the teeth, using brackets, numbers, and letters.

palpebral Referring to the eyelids.

pancreas Organ in the abdominal cavity behind the stomach that produces many enzymes necessary for the digestion of food as well as insulin and glucagon.

papillary gingiva Gingiva that forms the interdental papillae.

parakeratinized layer Stratum corneum where some cells are dead and some are still alive.

parakeratinized stratified squamous epithelium Multilayered epithelium in which top layers of cells are not completely dead.

paralleling technique Method of taking radiographs that supposedly gives the most accurate representation of proper tooth dimensions; requires the use of special film holders.

paramolar Small supernumerary tooth located buccally or lingually to a molar.

paranasal sinuses Four pairs of cavities in the bones around the nasal cavity.

parapharyngeal *See* lateral pharyngeal.

parasympathetic nervous system Part of the autonomic (automatic) nervous system that originates from some of the cranial nerves and some of the sacral nerves. It controls a number of functions, including stimulation of the salivary glands.

parathyroid gland Small gland embedded in the thyroid gland that helps control calcium metabolism in the body.

parietal bone Pair of bones that forms the upper lateral part of the skull.

parietooccipital suture *See* lambdoid suture.

parotid gland Large salivary gland on the side of the face in front of the ear.

passive eruption Condition in which the tooth does not move but the gingival attachment moves farther apically.

peg-shaped lateral Poorly formed maxillary lateral incisor with a cone-shaped crown.

periapical Around the tip of a tooth root.

pericardial cavity Space between heart wall and sac surrounding the heart.

pericardium Sac that surrounds the heart and allows it to contract without irritation of heart muscle.

perichondrium The fibrous and cellular covering of cartilage; provides new cells for appositional growth.

pericoronitis The swelling and infection of the gum tissue surrounding a wisdom tooth.

periodontal Surrounding a tooth.

periodontal membrane or ligament Collagen fibers attached to the teeth roots and alveolar bone and serving as an attachment of the tooth to the bone.

periodontium Supporting tissues surrounding the teeth, including cementum, alveolar process, and periodontal ligament.

periosteum Fibrous and cellular layer that covers bones and contains cells that become osteoblasts.

peripheral nervous system Made up of the nerves originating from the spinal cord and brain (spinal and cranial nerves).

periphery Circumferential boundary; outer border.

peristaltic contractions The rhythmic waves of contraction of the smooth muscle of the gut wall that moves the food through the digestive tract.

peritoneal cavity Space between abdominal wall and digestive tract.

peritubular dentin Dentin immediately surrounding the tubule; slightly more calcified than the rest of the dentin.

petrous temporal bone The hard portion of the temporal bone that houses the middle and inner ear and separates the middle from the posterior cranial fossa.

phagocytes Cells that destroy various microorganisms.

pharyngeal Relating to the pharynx or throat.

pharyngeal arches Development tissue in the upper throat areas from which a number of structures in that region develop.

pharyngeal grooves or clefts The exterior grooves in the neck region of a developing embryo between the pharyngeal arches.

pharyngeal plexus of nerves Fibers of the glossopharyngeal (IX), vagus (X), and accessory (XI) cranial nerves that supply the pharyngeal or throat wall with both motor and sensory.

pharyngeal pouches The internal grooves in the embryonic neck region between the pharyngeal arches.

pharyngotympanic tube Bony and cartilaginous tube that leads from the middle ear into the posterior-lateral nasal pharynx.

pharynx Throat area, from the nasal cavity to the larynx.

pheresis Process of removing platelets from a blood donor and then pumping the collected blood, minus the platelets, back into the donor.

philtrum Small depression at the midline of the upper lip.

pillars Folds of tissue appearing in front of and behind the palatine tonsils.

pinocytosis The procedure wherein cells take in fluids without losing cytoplasm.

piriform aperture *See* nasal aperture.

pit Small, pointed depression in dental enamel, usually at the junction of two or more developmental grooves; a small hole anywhere on the crown.

pituitary gland Master controlling endocrine gland located in the middle cranial fossa.

plasma Fluid part of the blood without the cells.

plasma cell One of the cells that helps produce antibodies.

platysma Broad muscle in the neck going from the mandible down into the upper chest region.

pleural cavity The space in the chest between the lungs and the inner chest wall.

point angles Meeting of three surfaces at a point to form a corner; angles formed by the junction of three surfaces, for example, the mesiolingual occlusal point angle.

posterior Situated toward the back, as premolars and molars.

posterior auricular muscle Muscle extending from behind the ear into the back of the ear.

posterior cranial fossa The posterior depression in the cranial cavity, behind the petrous temporal bone. It houses the cerebellum and part of the brainstem.

posterior ethmoidal nerve Branch of the nasociliary nerve of V_1 that passes through the posterior ethmoidal foramen and supplies the posterior ethmoid air cells.

posterior ethmoid sinus Posterior-most group of ethmoid air cells.

posterior mediastinum Space in the chest behind the heart and between the lungs.

posterior nasal aperture See choana.

posterior nasal spine Pointed bony projection at the posterior end of the hard palate.

posterior pillar Folds of tissue behind the tonsil that contain the palatopharyngeus muscle.

posterior superior alveolar artery Branch of the maxillary artery that enters the maxillary tuberosity and supplies the maxillary molars.

posterior superior alveolar nerve Part of the second division of the trigeminal nerve that enters the maxillary tuberosity and supplies the maxillary molars, generally excluding the mesiobuccal root of the first molar.

posterior teeth Teeth of either jaw to the rear of the incisors and canines.

posteruptive stage Period of eruption from the time the teeth occlude until they are lost and characterized by occlusal wear of teeth and compensating eruption.

potential spaces Areas between two layers of tissue that are normally closed but may be spread apart, as in a tissue space infection.

preameloblast Cell in the intermediate stage between an inner enamel epithelial cell and an ameloblast.

preeruptive stage Period when the crown of the tooth is developing.

prefunctional eruptive stage See eruptive stage.

premature contact area The area where an upper and a lower tooth touch and hit each other before the rest of the teeth occlude together.

premaxilla Bony area of the upper jaw that includes the alveolar ridge for the incisors and the area immediately behind it.

premolars Permanent teeth that replace the primary molars.

preventive considerations Ideas relating to the prevention of dental disease rather than the treatment of the disease after it occurs.

primary anatomy Refers to the basic arrangement and number of developmental and triangular grooves on a tooth.

primary attachment epithelium Remains of reduced enamel epithelium that provides for the initial attachment of mucosa at the base of the gingival sulcus.

primary dentin Dentin formed from the beginning of calcification until tooth eruption.

primary dentition First set of teeth; baby teeth; milk teeth; deciduous teeth.

primary enamel cuticle Keratin-like covering on the surface of the enamel; the final product of the ameloblast.

primary nodes First group of lymph nodes to be involved in the spread of infection.

primary palate The early developing part of the hard palate that comes from the medial nasal process and forms a V-shaped wedge of tissue that runs from the incisive foramen forward and laterally between the lateral incisors and canines of the maxilla.

primary teeth See deciduous.

primate spaces The diastema present mesial to the maxillary canine and distal to the mandibular canine. A characteristic usually present in primates such as apes, monkeys, and humans.

Primitive streak A rod-shaped, downward growth into the middle of the embryo.

procerus Muscle going from the bridge of the nose to the medial part of the eyebrow.

prognathic A more anterior positioning of the lower jaw in relation to the upper jaw and the rest of the skull.

prosthetic appliance Any constructed appliance that replaces a missing part.

protein One of the basic components of many foodstuffs and much of the body. Proteins are made up of small units known as amino acids strung together in long chains.

proteoglycans One of two classes of carbohydrates and proteins that are found in the ground substance of connective tissue.

protrude See protrusion.

protrusion Condition of being thrust forward, referring to the teeth being too far labial; the forward movement of the mandible.

proximal Nearest, next, immediately adjacent to; distal or mesial.

proximal contact areas Proximal area on a tooth that touches an adjacent tooth on the mesial or distal side.

proximal surface See proximal.

pseudostratified columnar epithelium Single layer of cells appearing as many layers because the cells have various heights; found primarily in the respiratory tract.

pterygoid branches Branches of the maxillary artery that supply the medial and lateral pterygoid muscles.

pterygoid fossa Depression between the medial and lateral pterygoid plates.

pterygoid hamulus Small curving process projecting down from the medial pterygoid plate of the sphenoid bone.

pterygoid plexus of veins Meshwork of veins behind the maxillary tuberosity that flows into the maxillary veins.

pterygoid processes Large downward projections of the sphenoid bone behind the maxillae.

pterygomandibular raphe Band of connective tissue of the tendon that connects the posterior end of the buccinator muscle with the anterior end of the superior constrictor of the pharynx.

pterygomaxillary fissure Elongated opening between the maxillary tuberosity and the pterygoid process of the sphenoid bone. The third part of the maxillary artery enters the pterygopalatine fossa through this opening.

pterygopalatine artery Branch of the maxillary artery for the nasal cavity that joins the greater palatine artery in the anterior hard palate.

pterygopalatine fossa Space behind and below the orbit; location of the maxillary nerve and the last part of the maxillary artery.

pterygopalatine ganglion Parasympathetic ganglion associated with the seventh cranial nerve (VII), but attached to the maxillary part of the fifth cranial nerve (V). It supplies the glands of the palate and nasal cavity and lacrimal gland.

pterygopalatine nerves Two small branches of the second division of the trigeminal nerve that attaches the pterygopalatine ganglion to the main part of the maxillary division of V.

pulmonary artery Blood vessel that carries blood from the heart to the lungs to pick up oxygen.

pulmonary veins Blood vessels that carry blood back to the heart from the lungs.

pulp canal Canal in the root of a tooth that leads from the apex to the pulp chamber. Under normal conditions it contains dental pulp tissue.

pulp cavity Entire cavity within the tooth, including the pulp canal and pulp chamber.

pulp chamber Cavity or chamber in the center of the crown of a tooth that normally contains the major portion of the dental pulp. The pulp canals lead into the pulp chambers.

pulp, dental Highly vascular and innervated connective tissue contained within the pulp cavity of the tooth. The dental pulp is composed of arteries, veins, nerves, connective tissues and cells, lymph tissue, and odontoblasts.

pulp horn (horn of pulp) Extension of pulp tissue into a thin point of the pulp chamber in the tooth crown.

pulp stones Small dentin-like calcifications in pulp.

Purkinje's fibers Specialized heart muscle fibers that carry nerve impulses.

pyramidal cells Cuboidal cells in smaller ducts that are pushed into a pyramid shape because of the smaller diameter of the inside (lumen) versus the outside.

Q

quadrants One-fourth of the dentition. The four quadrants are divided into right and left, maxillary and mandibular.

R

radiopacities Whitish region on a radiograph.

ramus of the mandible Vertical portion of the mandible.

raphe Term generally used to refer to the fusion of paired muscles at the middle; it is actually a collagenous union.

Rathke's pouch Outpouching in the embryonic oral cavity that becomes part of the pituitary gland.

recession Migration of the gingival crest in an apical direction, away from the crown of the tooth.

red blood cells Most numerous of the blood cells; responsible for carrying oxygen to the rest of the body; erythrocytes.

reduced enamel epithelium Fusion of the ameloblast layer with the outer enamel epithelium.

referred pain Pain that seems to originate in one area but actually originates in another area.

reflex arc Sensory message that goes to the spinal cord and meets with a motor nerve to cause an action. The reflex action occurs without the messages first reaching the brain to voluntarily cause the action.

reparative dentin Localized formation of dentin in response to local trauma such as occlusal trauma or caries.

resorption Physiologic removal of tissues or body products, as of the roots of deciduous teeth or of some alveolar process after the loss of the permanent teeth.

respiratory epithelium Pseudostratified columnar ciliated epithelium that is found in the nose and most of the rest of the respiratory tract.

rete peg formation Development of interdigitation between the epithelium and the underlying connective tissue.

reticular fiber Smaller collagen-like fiber that forms the framework for a number of organs.

retrodiscal pad Vascular and nerve tissue behind the disc of the temporomandibular joint.

retrognathic A more posterior positioning of the lower jaw in relation to the upper jaw and the rest of the skull.

retromandibular vein Vein lying behind the mandible. It drains the side of the head and sends blood to both the external and internal jugular veins.

retromolar pad Pad of tissue behind the mandibular third molars found in retromolar triangle.

retromolar triangle Triangular area of bone just behind the mandibular third molars.

retropharyngeal Group of lymph nodes behind the posterior throat wall; refers to the area behind the pharynx.

retropharyngeal nodes *See* retropharyngeal.

retropharyngeal space Space behind the pharynx and in front of the cervical vertebrae.

retrusion Act or process of retraction or moving back, as when the mandible is placed in a posterior relationship to the maxillae.

ribosomes Small granules of RNA found free in the cytoplasm of cells or attached to endoplasmic reticulum.

ridge Long narrow elevation or crest, as on the surface of a tooth or bone.

risorius Small muscle that lies on the surface of and parallel to the buccinator muscle.

RNA Ribonucleic acid; the substance in the cell nucleus and cytoplasm that carries the DNA "message" to build other cells or cell products.

rod sheath Material surrounding the enamel rod. It is slightly more organic than the enamel rod.

root That portion of a tooth embedded in the alveolar process and covered with cementum.

root canal *See* pulp canal.

root planing Process of smoothing the cementum of the root of a tooth.

root trunk That portion of a multirooted tooth found between the cervical line and the points of bifurcation or trifurcation of roots.

rudimentary lobe Small, underdeveloped lobe of a tooth; less than a minor lobe.

rugae Small ridges of tissue extending laterally across the anterior of the hard palate.

S

sacral Relating to the hip region; for example, sacral nerves and vertebrae.

sagittal suture Suture that extends along the middle of the top of the skull between the parietal bones.

salpingopharyngeal muscle Muscle that runs from the end of the auditory tube in the nasal pharynx down into the lateral wall of the pharynx and helps elevate it in the swallowing process.

sarcomere Smallest functional unit of a striated muscle fiber, composed of an A band with half of an I band at either end and running from Z line to Z line.

sclerotic dentin Condition in which the tubules have been filled in with dentin because of damage to the odontoblast.

sebaceous glands Small, oil-producing glands that are usually connected to hairs to lubricate them.

secondary anatomy Extra grooves and pits in addition to the main primary anatomy on a tooth.

secondary attachment epithelium Epithelium of free gingiva that produces mucosal attachment at the base of the gingival sulcus.

secondary dentin Dentin formed throughout the pulp chamber and pulp canal from the time of eruption.

secondary dentition Permanent dentition.

secondary enamel cuticle Mucopolysaccharide-cementing substance secreted by the reduced enamel epithelium that functions in cementing the base of the gingival sulcus to the tooth.

secondary groove *See* supplemental groove.

secondary nodes Second group of lymph nodes involved in the spread of infection.

seromucous Pertaining to a mixture of serum- and mucus-secreting cells in the same gland.

seromucous acini Glandular acini that have both mucous and serous cells.

serotonin Compound that can affect blood flow in different parts of the body.

serous Pertaining to a thin watery type of glandular secretion; serum.

serous acini Glandular cells that produce watery secretion.

serous demilunes Cluster of serous salivary cells that sits like a cap or half-moon on a mucous acinus. This acinus therefore secretes both mucus and serum.

Sharpey's fibers Part of the periodontal ligament; embedded in cementum or alveolar bone.

short palate Palate of insufficient length to meet the back wall of the throat.

sickle cell anemia Disease in which the red blood cells are defective and cannot properly carry oxygen.

simple columnar epithelium Single layer of tall cells found lining the digestive tract and other ducts of the body.

simple cuboidal epithelium Single layer of square or cubelike cells that line many of the ducts of the body.

simple squamous epithelium Single layer of flat cells that are found lining blood vessels, chest and abdominal cavities, and many other areas.

single root Root with one main branch.

skeletal classification A system of classifying bones based on the position of the maxilla in relation to that of the mandible. This classification does not pertain to the teeth.

skeletal muscle Striped, voluntarily controlled muscle that allows for body movement.

sleep apnea A condition in which an individual ceases breathing for 20 or more seconds many times per hour.

slough Loss of dead cells from the surface of tissue.

sluiceway Pathways to allow the dissipation of occlusal forces, escape of food debris, and pressure caused by the teeth occluding.

smooth muscle Unstriped, involuntarily controlled muscle found in the digestive tract and other organs; helps move food along the digestive tract.

soft tissue Noncalcified tissues, such as epithelium, nerves, arteries, veins, and connective tissue.

spasm Constant contraction of muscle.

specialized mucosa Mucosa found on the top or dorsum of the tongue that includes the papillae and taste buds.

sphenoethmoidal recess Most posterosuperior area of the nasal cavity.

sphenoid bone Large bone that helps form the base of the skull in front of the occipital bone and part of the side of the skull.

sphenoid sinus One of the paired paranasal sinuses located in the body of the sphenoid bone.

sphenomandibular ligament Ligament running from the spine of the sphenoid to the lingula of the mandible.

sphenooccipital synchondrosis Area of endochondral bone growth between the sphenoid and occipital bones that allows for growth of the cranial base and helps determine future occlusion.

sphenopalatine artery *See* pterygopalatine artery.

sphenopalatine nerve Branch of the second division of the trigeminal nerve that goes to the mucosa of the nasal cavity and anterior hard palate.

sphere of Monson Imaginary sphere that theoretically could rest on the mandibular arch.

spillway Escape pathways for food crushed between occluding teeth.

spinal accessory nerve Another name for the eleventh cranial nerve (XI). *See* accessory nerve.

spinal nerve The joining together of the dorsal and ventral roots to form a mixed spinal nerve.

spinal nerves Thirty-one pairs of nerves that exit from the spinal cord at each vertebral level.

spongy bone Less dense bone in the middle of a bone, frequently referred to as the marrow area. In alveolar bone, the layer between the cribriform plate and the cortical plate.

squamosal suture Suture between the temporal and parietal bones.

stapedius muscle Small muscle in the middle ear supplied by the seventh cranial nerve (VII) that is attached to the stapes bone and protects the inner ear from loud sounds.

statoacoustic nerve Eighth cranial nerve (VIII); related to hearing and balance.

stellate reticulum Ectodermally and epithelially derived middle layer of the enamel organ. It serves as a cushion for the developing enamel.

sternocleidomastoid muscle Muscle extending from the mastoid process down and forward in the lateral neck to the sternum and clavicle.

sternohyoid muscle Infrahyoid muscle from the sternum to the hyoid bone.

sternomastoid muscle *See* sternocleidomastoid muscle.

sternothyroid muscle Muscle that goes from the sternum to the thyroid cartilage of the larynx.

stolarized molar The permanent maxillary first molar is tipped mesially so that the distal marginal ridge of the upper first molar touches the mesial marginal ridge of the lower second molar.

stomodeum Depression in the facial region of the embryo that is the beginning of the oral cavity.

stratified columnar epithelium Epithelium that is rather rare but, when seen in large ducts, consists of two, or more, rows of columnar cells.

stratified cuboidal epithelium *See* stratified columnar epithelium.

stratified squamous epithelium Most common of the multiple-layered epithelia; found as skin and mucosa.

stratum basale Bottom layer of stratified squamous epithelium; *see also* basal layer.

stratum corneum Top layer of stratified squamous epithelium.

stratum granulosum Layer above the stratum spinosum in stratified squamous epithelium. Granules in this layer indicate the beginning of cell death.

stratum intermedium Fourth developing layer of the enamel organ; responsible for aiding ameloblast nourishment.

stratum lucidum Clear layer of epithelial cells found between stratum granulosum and stratum corneum in thick skin such as palms of hands and soles of feet.

stratum spinosum Layer immediately above the basal layer in stratified squamous epithelium. The cells produced in the basal layer move up into the spinous layer.

striae of Retzius Incremental growth lines seen in sections of enamel.

striated ducts Salivary intralobular and interlobular ducts that look as if they have stripes at the base of the cells because of infolding of basal cell membrane and mitochondria trapped in between the infoldings.

styloglossus muscle Extrinsic tongue muscle running from the styloid process into the tongue.

stylohyoid muscle Suprahyoid muscle going from the styloid process to the hyoid bone.

styloid process Small, pointed projection of bone that points down and forward from the base of the skull just behind the mandible.

stylomastoid foramen Small foramen between the mastoid and styloid process. The facial nerve exits from the skull here.

stylopharyngeal muscle Muscle that runs from the styloid process down into the lateral wall of the pharynx; helps elevate and dilate the pharynx in the swallowing process.

subclavian vein Vein that drains blood from the arm. It joins with the internal jugular vein to form the brachiocephalic vein.

sublingual caruncle Small elevation of soft tissue at the base of the lingual frenum that is the opening for the submandibular duct.

sublingual fold Fold of tissue extending backward on either side of the floor of the mouth; duct of the submandibular gland lies below it.

sublingual fossa Depression for the sublingual gland on the medial surface of the mandible above the mylohyoid line in the canine region.

sublingual gland Major salivary gland that lies in the floor of the mouth adjacent to the mandibular canines.

subluxation Dislocation of the mandible.

submandibular Referring to the region below the mandible; a group of lymph nodes around the submandibular gland.

submandibular fossa Depression for the submandibular gland on the medial surface of the mandible below the mylohyoid line in the molar region.

submandibular ganglion Parasympathetic ganglion of the seventh nerve (VII) suspended from the lingual nerve. Postganglionic nerves go to the submandibular and sublingual glands.

submandibular gland Large major salivary gland that lies beneath the mandible near the angle of the mandible.

submandibular nodes *See* submandibular.

submaxillary gland *See* submandibular gland.

submental Area below the chin; a group of lymph nodes beneath the chin.

submental nodes *See* submental.

submucosa Supporting layer of loose connective tissue under a mucous membrane; may contain fat or minor salivary glands.

succedaneous Permanent teeth that succeed or take the place of the deciduous teeth after the latter have been shed—that is, the incisors, canines, and premolars.

successional lamina Lingual growth of the dental lamina that forms permanent incisors, canines and premolars.

sulcus Long V-shaped depression or valley in the surface of a tooth between the ridges and the cusps. A sulcus has a developmental groove at the apex of its V. Sulcus also refers to the trough around the teeth formed by the gingiva.

sulfites A form of preservative, usually bisulfites, in local anesthetics designed to increase the shelf life of anesthetics.

superior alveolar block A local anesthetic given to one of the three branches of the superior alveolar nerve; the anterior, middle, or posterior. Each block covers a large area of hard, soft, and plural tissues and involves several teeth since the anesthetic is deposited close to the nerve trunk.

superior auricular muscle Muscle extending from above the ear down into the upper part of the ear.

superior constrictor muscle Uppermost of the three pharyngeal constrictor muscles.

superior lateral nasal nerves Branch of the sphenopalatine nerve that supplies the superior and lateral parts of the nasal cavity.

superior nasal concha Small projection of ethmoid bone from the upper lateral nasal wall.

superior nuchal line Horizontal line on the external surface of the occipital bone for the attachment of neck muscles.

superior orbital fissure Elongated opening in the upper lateral part of the orbit between the greater and lesser wings of the sphenoid.

superior pharyngeal constrictor muscle The upper of three muscles that forms the throat wall and helps move food down into the esophagus. Part of the muscle joins anteriorly with the buccinator muscle of the cheek.

superior vena cava Vein that drains blood from the head and arms into the heart.

supernumeraries Extra teeth in the jaw.

supplemental canal *See* accessory root canals.

supplemental groove Shallow linear groove in the enamel of a tooth. It differs from a developmental groove in that it does not mark the junction of lobes; it is a secondary or smaller groove.

supplemental tooth Supernumerary tooth that resembles a regular tooth.

supraeruption Eruption of a tooth beyond the occlusal plane.

suprahyoid muscles Muscles above the hyoid bone that attach to it.

supraorbital foramen Supraorbital notch when it has a small projection of bone extending across it.

supraorbital nerve Branch of the ophthalmic division of V; innervates the skin of the forehead.

supraorbital notch Small notch in the upper rim of the orbit.

supraperiosteal Tissue lying on the surface of bone.

supraperiosteal injection A local anesthetic injection into a region containing large terminal nerve branches, providing anesthesia to the hard, soft, and pulpal tissues involving one tooth.

supratrochlear nerve Branch of the frontal nerve that innervates the skin in the upper medial corner of the eye.

surfaces Four sides and the top of a tooth.

suture Line where two bones join.

sympathetic system Part of the autonomic (automatic) nervous system that originates from the thoracic and lumbar levels of the spinal cord.

synovial cavity Epithelium-lined space that secretes tiny amounts of fluid and synovia and is found in joints that are free moving.

synovial fluid Thin, watery fluid secreted in joints that lubricate articulating surfaces.

T

taste buds Small structures primarily found in vallate, fungiform, and foliate papillae that detect taste.

temporal bone Bone that forms part of the side of the skull, including the ear area.

temporal branches Branches of the maxillary artery that serve the temporal muscle.

temporal fossa Large, flattened area on the side of the skull that is the origin of the temporal muscle.

temporal muscle Muscle on the side of the head attached to the mandible; elevates and pulls the mandible back.

temporalis muscle *See* temporal muscle.

temporomandibular joint Jaw joint between the temporal bone and mandible.

temporomandibular ligament Thickened part of the temporomandibular joint (TMJ) capsule on the lateral side.

tendon Regularly arranged group of collagen fibers that connects skeletal muscle to bone.

tensor tympani muscle Small muscle in the middle ear attached to the malleus bone and supplied by the mandibular division of V. Dampens loud sounds and protects the inner ear.

tensor veli palatini Muscle that runs from the auditory tube region down, forward, and around the lateral side of the hamular process and then turns medially into the anterior part of the soft palate. As its name indicates, when it contracts, it tenses the soft palate in swallowing and speech.

tertiary anatomy Very shallow and numerous grooves, pits, and lines often seen in third molars, giving them a wrinkled appearance.

tertiary grooves *See* accidental grooves.

tertiary nodes Third group of lymph nodes involved in the spread of infection.

tetracycline staining Discolored teeth that result when an expectant mother or a young child takes the antibiotic tetracycline while tooth crowns are still developing.

therapeutic considerations Treating diseased teeth.

thoracolumbar outflow Another name for the sympathetic nervous system.

thorax (thoracic) Chest region; pertaining to nerves of the chest.

thymus Gland in the chest above the heart that is responsible for early establishment of immune cells to protect the body.

thyrohyoid muscle Muscle going from the thyroid cartilage of the larynx to the hyoid bone.

thyroid gland Gland in the neck that controls much of the body's metabolic rate.

T-lymphocyte Type of lymphocyte that multiplies in the thymus and fights virus-infected cells, tumors, and tissue and organ grafts.

Tomes's process *See* odontoblastic process.

Tomes's resorbing organ Osteoclastic tissue that dissolves bone and root and aids in the eruption process.

tongue-tie, tongue-tied Condition in which the lingual frenum is short and attached to the tip of the tongue, making normal speech difficult.

tonsillar pillars The vertical folds of tissue that lie in front of and behind the palatine tonsils in the lateral throat wall.

tooth germ Soft tissue that develops into a tooth.

tooth migration Movement of the tooth through the bone and gum tissue.

torus palatinus Large bony growth in the hard palate.

trabeculae Interlacing meshwork that makes up the cancellous bony framework.

transitional epithelium Multiple rows of epithelial cells that seem to change in thickness when stretched or relaxed; found in the ureters, urinary bladder, and part of the urethra.

transparent dentin *See* sclerotic dentin.

transseptal fibers Periodontal fibers that extend from the cementum of one tooth to the cementum of the adjacent tooth.

transverse groove of oblique ridge *See* oblique groove.

transverse palatine suture Suture that runs across the posterior part of the hard palate between the maxillae and the palatine bones.

transverse ridge Ridge formed by the union of two triangular ridges, traversing the surface of a posterior tooth from the buccal to the lingual side.

trapezius Muscle at the back of the neck that goes down and out to the lateral part of the clavicle and scapula.

trauma Wound; bodily injury or damage.

triangular fossa Depression formed by the triangular groove between the triangular ridge and the marginal ridge.

triangular ridge Any ridge on the occlusal surface of a posterior tooth that extends from the point of a cusp to the central groove of the occlusal surface.

trifurcation Division of three tooth roots at their point of junction with the root trunk.

trigeminal nerve Fifth cranial nerve (V); supplies motor control to the muscles of mastication and sensation to the teeth, oral cavity, and face.

trochlear nerve Fourth cranial nerve (IV); aids in movements of the eye.

tubercle Overcalcification of enamel resulting in a small cusplike elevation on some portion of a tooth crown.

tubercle tooth Very small rudimentary supernumerary tooth.

tuberculum impar Structure from the first pharyngeal arch that forms the midline of the tongue about one-half to two-thirds of the way back.

Turner's teeth Hypocalcification of a single tooth.

type I collagen The type of collagen fiber found most frequently in irregular and regular connective tissue.

U

ultraviolet radiation One of the wavelengths in the electromagnetic spectrum; found in sunlight and produced by sunlamps.

united oral epithelium Joining of the reduced enamel epithelium with the oral epithelium.

Universal system, Universal Code System of coding teeth using the numbers 1 to 32 for permanent teeth and the letters A to T for the deciduous teeth.

upper deep cervical Group of lymph nodes in the upper lateral neck beneath the sternomastoid muscle.

uvula Small hanging fold of tissue in the back of the soft palate.

V

V₁ First or ophthalmic division of the trigeminal nerve.

V₂ Second or maxillary division of the trigeminal nerve.

V₃ Third or mandibular division of the trigeminal nerve.

vagus nerve Tenth cranial nerve (X); controls the muscles of the larynx and pharynx, muscles and glands of the digestive tract, and muscle of the heart.

vallate papillae *See* circumvallate papillae.

vascular Relating to blood supply.

vasoconstrictor Substance that constricts blood vessels.

ventral primary ramus The major branch of a spinal nerve, which we recognize as a nerve.

ventral root Motor root of spinal nerve.

vermilion zone Red part of the lip where the lip mucosa meets the skin.

vestibule Space between the lips or cheeks and the teeth.

visceral Referring to the organs of the body and the structures supplied by involuntary muscle, such as the heart and digestive tract.

viscerocranium Facial part of the skull.

Volkmann's canals Blood vessel canal in bone that runs into bone from the outside.

voluntary muscle Muscle able to be willfully controlled by the person or organism.

vomer Bone that forms the lower part of the nasal septum.

W

white blood cells Least numerous of the blood cells; responsible for the inflammatory process and other protective functions of the body; leukocytes.

white matter The whitish appearing peripheral part of the spinal cord made up of myelinated axons of motor and sensory nerves.

working side Side to which the mandible is moved.

Z

Z line Junction between two sarcomeres in skeletal and cardiac muscle.

zygomatic arch Arch of bone on the side of the face or skull formed by the zygomatic bone and temporal bone.

zygomatic bone Bone that forms the cheek area.

zygomatic nerve Branch of the maxillary division of V that innervates the skin of the cheek bone and temple and also carries parasympathetic fibers from VII to the lacrimal gland.

zygomaticoalveolar crest Heavy ridge of maxilla and zygomatic bone that forms a heavy supporting ridge running up from the alveolar process of the maxillary premolar-molar region.

zygomaticus major Muscle that extends from the cheek to the corner of the upper lip.

zygomaticus minor Muscle that extends from the cheek toward the middle part of the upper lip.

Index

Page numbers followed by "*f*" indicate figures, "*t*" indicate tables, and "*b*" indicate boxes.

Chapter 1

Oral Cavity

True-False Questions

_____ 1. The buccinator is a muscle of the cheek.

_____ 2. The red margin of the lip is known as the muco-gingival junction.

_____ 3. Small bony growths that may be found on the buc-cal mandible or maxilla arc known as *endostoses*.

_____ 4. A cleft lip would form at the lateral junction of the philtrum.

_____ 5. The incisive papilla is the anterior part of the hard palate.

Multiple-Choice Questions

6. The _____ is posterior to the last mandibular molar.
   a. Retromolar pad
   b. Rugae
   c. Sublingual caruncle
   d. Mandibular tori

7. Another name for the inside of the cheek is the:
   a. Alveolar mucosa
   b. Buccal mucosa
   c. Mucobuccal fold
   d. Vestibule

8. Yellowish spots on the buccal and labial mucosa are most often:
   a. Fovea palatine
   b. Traumatic lesions
   c. Salivary ducts
   d. Sebaceous glands

9. Which structure could cause difficulty in constructing a denture?
   a. Uvula
   b. Palatine tonsils
   c. Torus palatinus
   d. Posterior nasal spine

10. The _____ is a pathway to the respiratory and digestive systems.
    a. Oral pharynx
    b. Laryngeal pharynx
    c. Nasal pharynx
    d. Tonsillar pillars
    e. Both a and b

11. The _____ is a structure that can make it difficult to take maxillary posterior radiographs as well as maxillary impressions.
    a. Mucobuccal fold
    b. Zygomatic arch
    c. Coronoid process
    d. Condyloid process

12. The transverse ridges of epithelial and connective tissue in the hard palate area are known as:
    a. Rugae
    b. Incisive papilla
    c. Incisive foramen
    d. Torus palatinus

13. The opening for the submandibular salivary gland is known as the:
    a. Lingual mucosa
    b. Lingual frenulum
    c. Sublingual fold
    d. Sublingual caruncle

14. The anterior pillar is located:
    a. Anterior to the uvula
    b. Anterior to the palatine tonsil
    c. Posterior to the palatopharyngeal fold
    d. On either side of the sublingual fold

15. The oral cavity can manifest symptoms of:
    a. Measles
    b. Kaposi's sarcoma
    c. Childhood cancer
    d. Vitamin deficiencies
    e. All of the above

Case Study

Use the following information to answer questions 16 to 18.

An 8-year-old boy was brought to the dental office. His mother made the appointment because her son had "a large space" forming between his maxillary front teeth. An oral examination confirmed a diastema between his maxillary central incisors.

16. What is the probable reason for the separation of maxillary central incisors?
    a. A sports injury
    b. Newly erupted teeth
    c. A firm labial frenum
    d. Use of pacifiers when an infant

17. What immediate corrective procedure can be performed to allow normal contact between teeth?
    a. Fabricate a mouthguard
    b. Provide orthodontic treatment
    c. Wait until all permanent teeth erupt
    d. Surgical cutting of the frenum
    e. Both b and d

18. This condition would _____ be seen on the mandibular central incisors.
    a. Never
    b. Seldom
    c. Often
    d. Also

Chapter 2

The Tooth: Functions and Terms

True-False Questions

_____ 1. The cervical third portion of the root is covered with enamel.

_____ 2. Dentin is contained within both the crown and the root of a tooth.

_____ 3. Cementum does not have the ability to reproduce itself.

_____ 4. Pulp tissue contains odontoblasts.

_____ 5. An alveolus is a bony tooth socket.

_____ 6. The mandibular alveolar process surrounds mandibular teeth.

_____ 7. The mesiodistal angle is an example of a line angle.

_____ 8. The biting area of a posterior tooth is called the _occlusal surface_.

_____ 9. Mesiobuccal is an example of an anterior line angle.

_____ 10. The labio-bucco-incisal angle is an example of a point angle.

_____ 11. There are four anterior point angles.

_____ 12. A transverse ridge is two triangular ridges joined together.

_____ 13. All teeth have at least one cusp.

_____ 14. Both anterior and posterior teeth have triangular ridges.

_____ 15. A cingulum is an elevation on the lingual surface of an anterior tooth.

Matching

Match each tooth with its functions.

_____ 16. Cutting food
_____ 17. Shoveling food into the mouth
_____ 18. Holding food
_____ 19. Grinding food
_____ 20. Tearing food
_____ 21. Holding and crushing food
_____ 22. Resisting lateral forces of displacement

a. Incisors
b. Canines
c. Premolars
d. Molars

Match the descriptions with the corresponding line and point angles.

_____ 23. Distolabial
_____ 24. Disto-occlusal
_____ 25. Disto-labio-incisal
_____ 26. Disto-linguo-occlusal
_____ 27. Mesiolingual
_____ 28. Linguoincisal

a. Anterior tooth line angle
b. Anterior tooth point angle
c. Posterior tooth line angle
d. Posterior tooth point angle

Multiple-Choice Questions

29. Enamel is thickest at the:
    a. cementoenamel junction (CEJ)
    b. lateral borders of the tooth
    c. incisal edge
    d. middle third of the tooth

30. If a molar has three roots it would have _____ pulp chamber(s).
    a. zero
    b. one
    c. two
    d. three

31. The pulp contains all the following, except:
    a. blood vessels
    b. nerves
    c. lymph vessels
    d. ameloblasts

32. _____ is composed of 70% inorganic matter.
    a. Enamel
    b. Dentin
    c. Cementum
    d. Pulp

33. Which of the following is _not_ a depression?
    a. fossa
    b. pit
    c. groove
    d. oblique ridge

34. Which tooth is formed from more than four lobes?
    a. maxillary central incisor
    b. mandibular canine
    c. maxillary first premolar
    d. mandibular first molar

35. A small elevation of enamel that may be found on tooth surfaces is a:
    a. cusp
    b. tubercle
    c. sulcus
    d. fossa

36. How many marginal ridges are on a tooth?
    a. one
    b. two
    c. four
    d. varies per tooth

Case Study

Mr. Allen reported that he was bothered by a lateral incisor that hurt whenever he ate certain foods or beverages, particularly hot or cold ones. He said that his tooth could feel temperature changes that were different from regular pain.

37. What sensation did Mr. Allen's pulp actually transmit?
   a. heat
   b. cold
   c. pain
   d. both a and b

38. Mr. Allen's lateral incisor had some root exposure as a result of gingival recession. The entire visible portion of his tooth is the:
   a. clinical crown
   b. anatomic crown
   c. cementoenamel junction
   d. exposed crown

39. Identify the following structures:
   a. _____
   b. _____
   c. _____

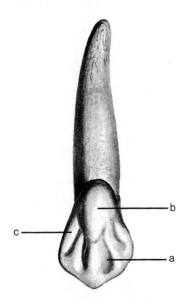

Maxillary right canine, lingual view. (From Zeisz RC, Nuckolls J. *Dental Anatomy.* St. Louis, MO: Mosby; 1949.)

40. Identify the following structures:
   a. _____
   b. _____
   c. _____
   d. _____

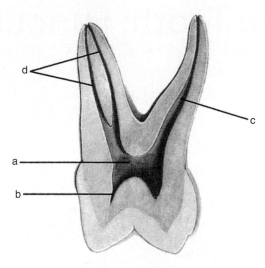

Pulp cavity of maxillary right first molar, linguobuccal section, mesial view. (From Zeisz RC, Nuckolls J. *Dental Anatomy.* St. Louis, MO: Mosby; 1949.)

41. Identify the following structures:
   a. _____
   b. _____

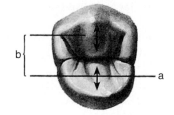

Chapter 3

Fundamental and Preventative Curvatures: Proximal Alignment of the Teeth and Protection of the Periodontium

True-False Questions

_____ 1. Teeth that are well aligned with adequate self-cleansing characteristics will be resistant to dental caries.

_____ 2. The lingual embrasure spaces are wider than the buccal embrasure spaces.

_____ 3. The distal height of curvature of the cervical line is greater than the mesial height of curvature of the cervical line.

_____ 4. Cementum is part of the periodontium.

_____ 5. The interdental space is the same as the interproximal space.

_____ 6. The curvature of the CEJ is usually 1 mm greater mesially than distally.

_____ 7. Anterior teeth show greater curvature of the CEJ than posterior teeth.

Matching

Place the terms in the column below with the appropriate phrases 8 through 14.

_____ 8. Gingiva that covers the interdental papilla

_____ 9. Fills the interproximal space in the ideal situation

_____ 10. Void that is cervical to the contact area

_____ 11. Spillways that help dissipate occlusal forces

_____ 12. The same as height of curvature

_____ 13. Causes understimulation of tissue

_____ 14. Causes food impaction

a. Open contacts

b. Embrasures

c. Papillary gingiva

d. Crest of curvature

e. Interdental papilla

f. Cervical embrasure

g. Overcontouring of restorations

Multiple-Choice Questions

15. An open contact between the maxillary central incisors would change the contour of the
    a. cingulum.
    b. CEJ curvature.
    c. interdental papilla.
    d. clinical crown.

16. Mandibular anterior teeth that are crowded would affect all the following *except:*
    a. CEJ curvatures.
    b. contact areas.
    c. contact points.
    d. interdental papilla.

17. Which of the following does *not* affect the interproximal space?
    a. alignment of teeth
    b. amount of interproximal bone loss
    c. infrequent brushing and flossing
    d. deep pits and fissures

18. Which of the following surfaces is a contact area?
    a. buccal
    b. mesial
    c. lingual
    d. occlusal

19. Which of the following is a contact point?
    a. the proximal contact area
    b. the contact area itself
    c. the point where the occlusal cusp of one tooth touches the occlusal portion of another
    d. An area between two interproximally adjacent teeth

20. Where is the distal contact area of the maxillary canine?
    a. closer to the incisal edge than the middle of the tooth
    b. in the middle of the tooth
    c. apical to the middle of the tooth
    d. in the incisal third of the tooth

21. The location of the _____ remains at the same anatomic location throughout the life of the tooth.
    a. CEJ
    b. interdental papilla
    c. gingival crest
    d. alveolar bone

Case Study

Use the information below to answer questions 22 and 23.

A 54-year-old woman has recently lost a mandibular lateral incisor to a traumatic injury. She plans to get an implant to replace the missing tooth.

22. If the patient waits several years before having the implant surgically placed, what can occur in the area of the missing tooth?
    a. alveolar bone loss
    b. changes in tooth alignment
    c. loss of interdental papillae
    d. all of the above

23. If the tooth is replaced by an implant, which is the most important factor in restoring its natural function?
    a. Increase brushing and flossing because of the artificial tooth requiring more care.
    b. Restore the appropriate contour and function of the implant tooth.
    c. Create a cervical embrasure to allow for preventive spillways.
    d. Do not provide proximal contact areas for implants or dental restorations.

Chapter 4

Dentition

True-False Questions

_____ **1.** The permanent first molar replaces the deciduous first molar.

_____ **2.** A 3-year-old child will have mixed dentition.

_____ **3.** The deciduous dentition does not include premolars.

_____ **4.** There are a total of eight incisors in the deciduous dentition.

Fill-In-the-Blanks

Give the codes for the following **permanent teeth**:

	Universal	FDI	Palmer notation
5. Maxillary right canine			
6. Mandibular left second premolar			
7. Maxillary right second molar			
8. Mandibular right central			
9. Maxillary left canine			

Give the codes for the following **deciduous teeth**:

10. Maxillary right canine

11. Mandibular left second molar

12. Mandibular right first molar

13. Maxillary left lateral incisor

Name the system of each code and the tooth it represents.

14. 2 _____

15. 9 _____

16. R _____

17. L _____

18. 48 _____

19. 55 _____

20. 7⌋ _____

21. ⌐C _____

Multiple-Choice Questions

22. Permanent molars are succedaneous teeth. They replace deciduous molars.
   a. Both statements are true.
   b. Both statements are false.
   c. The first statement is true; the second is false.
   d. The first statement is false; the second is true.

23. The permanent right maxillary arch has _____ teeth.
   a. 5
   b. 6
   c. 8
   d. 16

24. After the first permanent tooth erupts, a child has a _____ dentition.
   a. primary
   b. mixed
   c. permanent
   d. succedaneous

25. A 46-year-old patient has a deciduous mandibular left canine. Her dentition would be classified as _____.
   a. primary
   b. mixed
   c. permanent
   d. succedaneous

26. What separates the two quadrants in each dental arch?
   a. maxilla and mandible
   b. midline
   c. anterior and posterior
   d. palate

27. There are _____ nonsuccedaneous teeth.
   a. 8
   b. 12
   c. 20
   d. 32

28. What is referenced by the first number in the FDI system?
   a. quadrant
   b. deciduous dentition
   c. permanent dentition
   d. all of the above

29. Which of the following notations do not refer to a central incisor?
   a. P
   b. 8
   c. 24
   d. 5

Chapter 5

Development, Form, and Eruption

True-False Questions

_____ 1. The primary dentin begins to form in the alveolar crypt.

_____ 2. The cingulum will develop into the lingual cusp of posterior teeth.

_____ 3. Lobes are centers of formation that develop into teeth.

_____ 4. Premolars are considered bicuspids because they all have two cusps.

_____ 5. Third molars show great variation in size and shape.

_____ 6. Permanent teeth begin to calcify at birth.

_____ 7. Permanent maxillary first molars typically erupt before permanent mandibular first molars.

_____ 8. Permanent mandibular first molars typically erupt before permanent central incisors.

_____ 9. Permanent maxillary canines typically erupt before maxillary first premolars.

_____ 10. Teeth erupt bilaterally in right and left pairs.

_____ 11. The permanent maxillary central incisors erupt around ages 7 to 8 years.

_____ 12. Deciduous canines typically erupt after deciduous first molars.

Multiple-Choice Questions

13. Deciduous tooth germs begin to grow and develop by
    a. the sixth week of fetal life
    b. the sixth month of fetal life
    c. birth
    d. 6 weeks of age

14. Deciduous root calcification is completed by what age?
    a. 3 months
    b. 6 months
    c. 2 years
    d. 3 to 4 years

15. Which of the following clinical signs does not refer to lobe fusion?
    a. coalescence
    b. developmental grooves
    c. root bifurcation
    d. mamelons

16. Which molar is most likely to have a cusp of Carabelli?
    a. mandibular first
    b. mandibular second
    c. maxillary first
    d. maxillary second

17. A 20-month-old child would have all of the following deciduous teeth *except*
    a. mandibular lateral incisors
    b. maxillary canines
    c. maxillary first molars
    d. mandibular second molars

18. A 10-year-old child would have all of the following teeth *except*
    a. deciduous second molars
    b. deciduous maxillary canine
    c. permanent maxillary lateral incisors
    d. permanent maxillary first molars
    e. none of the above

19. Which of the following is *not* a factor in causing tooth movement?
    a. mesial drift
    b. curve of Spee
    c. eruption
    d. lingual forces of tongue

20. Which of the following could occur when parents do not have the proper knowledge of their child's tooth eruption patterns?
    a. a 5-year-old with no primate space
    b. an 8-year-old with missing permanent molars
    c. a 10-year-old with crowded mandibular incisors
    d. a 13-year-old with unerupted molars

21. Root resorption of deciduous teeth begins
    a. immediately after eruption
    b. soon after eruption
    c. 1 year after root completion
    d. 1 or 2 years before exfoliation

22. A 7-year-old child enters the office with only six permanent teeth. Which of the following is *most* likely true?
    a. Four of the permanent teeth are incisors.
    b. The child has delayed eruption.
    c. Two permanent teeth have been extracted.
    d. Four of the permanent teeth are first molars.

23. Based on the eruption pattern, what age is the child?

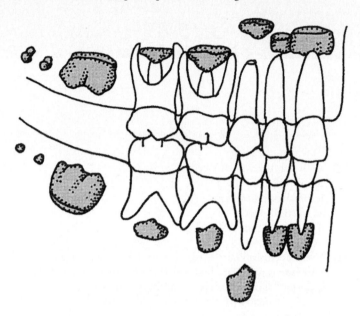

25. Based on the eruption pattern, what age is the child?

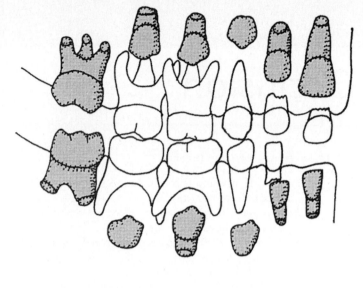

24. Based on the eruption pattern, what age is the child?

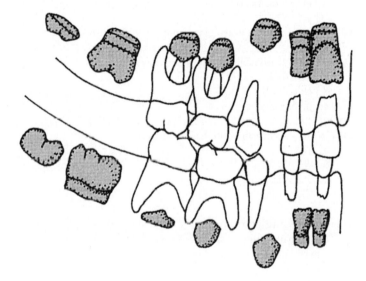

Chapter 6

Occlusion

True-False Questions

_____ 1. Class II, division II malocclusion is often associated with a deep overbite.

_____ 2. An open bite can exist even if the anterior incisors are touching edge to edge.

_____ 3. An overjet is often the result of severely protruded maxillary incisors.

_____ 4. Retruded teeth are inclined lingually.

_____ 5. Occlusion cannot be determined if permanent first molars are missing.

_____ 6. In patients with acromegaly, the maxilla grows faster and more than the mandible.

Matching

Match the terms in the column below with the corresponding phrases:

a. leeway space   **d.** primate space
b. occlusion   **e.** alignment
c. diastemas   **f.** centric occlusion

_____ 7. The arrangement of teeth in a row

_____ 8. The extra space that the deciduous canines and molars occupy and that saves room for the eruption of permanent teeth

_____ 9. The diastemas next to deciduous canines

_____ 10. The spaces between teeth

_____ 11. The relationship of maxillary teeth to mandibular teeth when they are closed together

_____ 12. Affords the greater interdigitation of teeth when jaws are closed

Multiple-Choice Question

13. A class II, division II occlusion often has
    a. a deep overbite
    b. crowded maxillary incisors
    c. a normal overjet
    d. disto-occlusion
    e. all of the above

14. A class III occlusion is associated with
    a. a retrognathic mandibular jaw
    b. a prognathic mandibular jaw
    c. a prognathic maxillary jaw
    d. crowded maxillary anterior teeth

15. An overbite can be described as a(n):
    a. openbite
    b. horizontal overlap
    c. vertical overlap
    d. cusp-to-cusp bite

16. What occlusion occurs when the mesiobuccal cusp of the permanent maxillary first molar is directly over the buccal groove of the permanent mandibular first molar?
    a. class I malocclusion
    b. class II malocclusion
    c. class III malocclusion
    d. mesio-occlusion

17. What occlusion is associated with a retrognathic profile?
    a. class I
    b. class II division I
    c. class II division II
    d. class III
    e. both b and c

18. Which occlusion is the least common?
    a. class I
    b. class II
    c. class III
    d. they occur equally (about 33% each)

19. What occlusion occurs when the distal surface of the permanent mandibular canine is mesial to the mesial surface of a permanent maxillary canine by at least a width of one tooth?
    a. class I
    b. class II
    c. class III
    d. none of the above

20. What occurs when permanent mandibular molars are buccal to permanent maxillary molars?
    a. crossbite
    b. overbite
    c. overjet
    d. retrusion

21. Which of these teeth occlude in the ideal centric occlusion?
    a. posteriors
    b. anteriors
    c. lingual cusps of the mandibular posteriors
    d. canines

22. Which teeth touch in the ideal protrusive movement?
    a. anteriors
    b. anteriors and posteriors
    c. canines
    d. canines and posteriors

23. When the premolars occlude in lateral excursion, it is called a(n)
    a. working side
    b. balancing side
    c. group function
    d. interference

Case Study

Use the information below to answer questions 24 and 25.

Five-year-old Jenny and 3-year-old Holly, who are sisters, have appointments for dental examinations and prophylaxis. Jenny has spaces between several of her teeth, and Holly has slightly protruded maxillary anterior teeth and an anterior open bite.

24. Jenny's spaces are indicative of
    a. distal steps that are normal for a child of her age
    b. diastemas that allow for the eruption of permanent teeth
    c. excessive development of the maxilla and the mandible
    d. future malocclusion of the permanent dentition

25. Holly's anterior teeth are characteristic of
    a. excessive leeway space
    b. retrusion of mandibular anterior teeth
    c. malocclusion of permanent dentition
    d. a habit of tongue thrusting

Match the letter of each illustration with the corresponding description below.

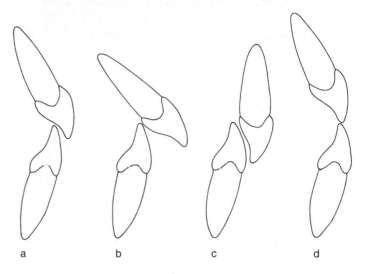

a   b   c   d

_____ 26. overbite
_____ 27. severe overjet
_____ 28. open bite
_____ 29. normal anterior bite

30. Which dental arch is most likely to have a diastema between central incisors?

31. Name the spaces indicated by the arrows.

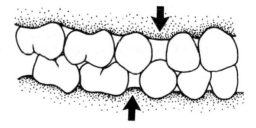

Chapter 7

Dental Anomalies

True-False Questions

_____ 1. Dental anomalies are deviations of hard or soft dental tissue.

_____ 2. Dental anomalies can be caused by intrinsic or extrinsic factors.

_____ 3. Hereditary causes of dental anomalies are the same as familial tendencies.

_____ 4. Teeth with gemination have a divided crown, a root, and a pulp.

_____ 5. Developmental anomalies occur while a structure is in the beginning stages of formation.

_____ 6. Hereditary conditions can become evident many years after birth.

_____ 7. Most supernumerary teeth are found in the mandible.

_____ 8. Paramolars are usually associated with premolars.

_____ 9. Enamel dysplasia is a disturbance in enamel formation.

_____ 10. Dilaceration is a sharp bend in the root or the crown of a tooth.

_____ 11. Macrodontia are teeth that are smaller than normal.

_____ 12. Maxillary canines often have accessory roots.

_____ 13. An odontoma is a cancerous tumor.

_____ 14. Dens in dente occurs when two tooth roots have fused together and are connected by dentin.

_____ 15. Congenital syphilis may lead to the presence of Turner's tooth.

_____ 16. If primary teeth do not develop, succedaneous permanent teeth will also not develop.

_____ 17. Nutritional deficiencies can cause a variety of tooth anomalies.

Matching

_____ 18. Macrodontia
_____ 19. Hyperdontia
_____ 20. Anodontia
_____ 21. Microdontia
_____ 22. Mesiodens
_____ 23. Developmental anomaly
_____ 24. Familial tendency
_____ 25. Hereditary
_____ 26. Paramolar
_____ 27. Fusion
_____ 28. Concrescence

a. very small teeth
b. tendency of condition to occur within a small genetic population
c. very large teeth
d. contains supernumerary teeth
e. no teeth or too few teeth
f. caused from genetic condition that could become evident before or after birth
g. supernumeraries found in midline or maxilla
h. small, rudimentary teeth found buccally or lingually to a molar
i. fusion of roots of two teeth after the teeth have formed
j. two tooth germs fuse at dentin
k. occurs while a structure is forming
l. most common type of supernumerary tooth

Matching

Match the terms in the list below with the appropriate descriptive statements. More than one answer is possible.

_____ 29. The most common supernumeraries
_____ 30. Forms after the root has been formed; occurs most frequently at the apex
_____ 31. Small masses of enamel often found in trifurcations
_____ 32. Hypoplasia of the enamel of a single tooth
_____ 33. Form of hypercementosis associated with localized bone destruction
_____ 34. Occurs when two different teeth join at dentin during formation
_____ 35. Can be caused by prenatal syphilis

a. cementoma
b. enamel pearls
c. fusion
d. hypercementosis
e. mesiodens
f. Turner's tooth
g. Hutchinson's incisors
h. mulberry molars

Multiple-Choice Questions

Check all that apply.

36. Which of the following might be caused by prenatal syphilis?
    a. Hutchinson's incisors
    b. mulberry molars
    c. screwdriver incisors
    d. notched incisors

37. Which of the following affects only the root of the tooth?
    a. concrescence
    b. hypercementosis
    c. fusion
    d. dilaceration
    e. flexion
    f. cementoma

38. Which of the following is a manifestation of inhibited enamel development?
    a. fluorosis
    b. hypocalcification
    c. hypoplasia
    d. enamel pearl

39. Which of the following discolors teeth?
    a. enamel fluorosis
    b. mottled enamel
    c. tetracycline staining
    d. amelogenesis imperfecta
    e. dentinogenesis imperfecta
    Select **only one** answer.

40. Which of the following does *not* refer to a supernumerary tooth?
    a. distomolar
    b. paramolar
    c. mulberry molar
    d. mesiodens

41. Which anomaly is clinically visible in the oral cavity?
    a. concrescence
    b. fusion
    c. flexion
    d. enamel pearl

42. Accessory cusps or tubercles are *most* commonly found on
    a. maxillary lateral incisors
    b. maxillary canines
    c. mandibular premolars
    d. maxillary molars

Case Study

Use the information below to answer questions 43 and 44.

A 7-year-old child is scheduled for a dental prophylaxis. His health history indicates no illnesses or medications except for an ear infection when he was 6 years old for which tetracycline had been prescribed. He takes fluoride supplements and brushes his teeth with a fluoridated toothpaste. His permanent teeth have white opaque flecks as well as some slightly darker discolorations. The dental prophylaxis does not affect the appearance of his teeth.

43. The appearance of the child's teeth suggests that he has
    a. tetracycline staining
    b. fluorosis
    c. amelogenesis imperfecta
    d. dental caries

44. Which follow-up questions should be asked of the mother?
    a. Does the child use an excessive amount of fluoridated toothpaste on his toothbrush?
    b. Did the mother take any antibiotics during her pregnancy?
    c. Did the child have a fever or illness during his infancy?
    d. Does the family use well water as their primary drinking source?
    e. all of the above

Chapter 8

Supporting Structures: The Periodontium

True-False Questions

_____ **1.** The dimpled texture of the attached gingiva is caused by rete peg formation.

_____ **2.** Free gingiva is nonmobile because of the lamina propria below it.

_____ **3.** Sharpey's fibers are embedded in bundle bone.

_____ **4.** Healthy free gingiva appears stippled.

_____ **5.** There are no fibroblast cells in the periodontal ligament.

_____ **6.** Oblique fibers are those periodontal fibers running between the roots of multirooted teeth.

Fill-in-the-Blank

Complete each statement with a term from the list below. Some terms may be used more than once.

Bundle bone	Interradicular
Cellular cementum	Lamina dura
Cementocytes	Sharpey's fibers
Fibroblasts	Supraperiosteal

7. Collagen fibers are formed by _____.

8. Periodontal fibers embedded in bone are called _____.

9. Periodontal fibers embedded in cementum are called _____.

10. When viewed on a radiograph, the compact alveolar bone that surrounds a tooth is called _____.

11. Blood is supplied to gingival tissue by the _____ vessels.

12. Cementoblasts trapped in their own cementum are called _____.

13. The periodontal fibers between the roots of multirooted teeth belong to the _____ periodontal ligament group.

14. The type of cementum found at the apex that can add onto itself is _____.

15. The bony thickening of the alveolar wall caused by numerous additions of bone with Sharpey's fibers is called _____.

Multiple-Choice Questions

Select all that apply for questions 16 to 19.

16. Which of the following is *not* true of the attached gingiva?
    a. It is composed of thick epithelial tissue.
    b. It displays a texture like an orange peel.
    c. It is keratinized.
    d. It has no rete peg formation.

17. Which of the following are true of the alveolar mucosa?
    a. It is movable.
    b. It is smooth.
    c. It is reddish.
    d. It has rete peg formation.

18. Which of the following are true about cementum?
    a. It grows by the apposition of new layers.
    b. It contains collagen fibers.
    c. It is surrounded by alveolar mucosa.
    d. It is formed by cementoblasts.

19. Which of the following are true of the attached gingiva?
    a. It is covered with stratified squamous epithelium.
    b. It has rete peg formation.
    c. It has a stippled texture.
    d. It can contain melanin.

Select only the best answer for questions 20 to 25.

20. Which of the following is *not* one of the formative functions of the periodontal ligament?
    a. Activating the apposition of bone
    b. Activating osteoclasts
    c. Regenerating periodontal fibers
    d. Initiating cementoblast activation

21. Which of the following is *not* true about the nutritive function of the periodontal ligament?
    a. It supplies nutrients to cementum.
    b. It provides vascularity to the periodontal ligament.
    c. It senses pressure on the tooth.
    d. It provides nutrition to bone.

22. How can the root canal tooth tell pressure, pain, and temperature change?
    a. The root canal still has some nerve tissue in it.
    b. The periodontal ligament has resorptive abilities.
    c. The periodontal ligament has sensory capabilities.
    d. The attached gingiva does all the tooth's sensory gathering.
    e. The nerve remains active in the tooth after root canal therapy.

23. In normal healthy tissue the free gingiva should be:
    a. Firmly attached to cementum
    b. Slightly separated from the tooth
    c. Covered with lining mucosa
    d. About 3.5 mm within the gingival sulcus

24. The interradicular group of periodontal fibers is found on the:
    a. Maxillary central incisor
    b. Maxillary canine
    c. Mandibular first premolar
    d. Mandibular first molar

25. Which type of force can cause mobility in a tooth with little or no bone remodeling?
    a. Active eruption
    b. Masticatory occlusal forces
    c. Orthodontic corrective forces
    d. Traumatic occlusal forces

26. Name the five periodontal ligament **fiber** groups:
    a. _____
    b. _____
    c. _____
    d. _____
    e. _____

27. Label the parts of the gingival unit.

a. _____   d. _____
b. _____   e. _____
c. _____   f. _____

Chapter 9

Clinical Considerations

True-False Questions

_____ 1. The primary cause of periodontal disease and dental caries is bacteria living in the oral cavity.

_____ 2. Placing a wooden wedge interproximally during tooth restoration procedures can prevent an overhang.

_____ 3. Occlusal pits and fissures with noncarious but deep anatomy should be filled with amalgam to create a smooth surface.

_____ 4. Overcontoured buccal and lingual surfaces can force food and plaque into the gingival sulcus.

_____ 5. Occlusal trauma can result when there is premature contact between two opposing teeth.

_____ 6. Inflammation within the pulp cavity can lead to a widening of the apical foramen.

_____ 7. Tooth migration can occur within 24 hours of loss of contact with an antagonist tooth.

_____ 8. Hypersensitivity can be experienced when dentin is exposed.

_____ 9. If the mandibular first premolar is missing, the mandibular second premolar will move in a distal direction.

Multiple-Choice Questions

10. Root planing promotes smooth roots that discourage bacterial and plaque accumulation. Cementum that is irregular or rough should be planed or reduced to create an even surface.
    a. Both statements are true.
    b. Both statements are false.
    c. The first statement is true; the second is false.
    d. The first statement is false; the second is true.

11. Which of the following is *least likely* to cause a periodontal problem?
    a. an open contact
    b. a large diastema
    c. an overhang on the distal surface of a first molar
    d. poor oral hygiene

12. Which of the following situations is *not* acceptable?
    a. In lateral excursion, only the canines hit.
    b. In protrusion, only the incisors hit.
    c. In centric occlusion, one or two teeth slightly hit before the rest.
    d. In lateral excursion, no teeth on the balancing side hit.

13. Which teeth would move mesially if the tooth in front of them was extracted?
    a. deciduous first molars
    b. deciduous second molars
    c. permanent first molars
    d. permanent second premolars

14. Which of these tissues can be affected by occlusal trauma?
    a. temporomandibular joint tissue
    b. enamel of the offending tooth
    c. periodontal ligament tissue
    d. alveolar bone tissue
    e. all of the above

15. Why can a tooth still feel pressure, temperature extremes, and pain after it has had a root canal?
    a. The root canal tooth no longer has pain response, but the surrounding bone, gingiva, and periodontal ligament tissues do.
    b. The surrounding periodontal ligament feels pressure, so it only seems like the tooth can feel pressure.
    c. The surrounding gingiva can feel temperature changes, even though the tooth no longer can.
    d. all of the above

16. When can tooth migration occur?
    a. when a restoration comes off a tooth and is left off for more than 2 days
    b. when periodontal disease causes bone loss
    c. when a tooth is severely fractured
    d. when a tooth is under constant pressure from mechanical forces, such as braces
    e. all of the above

Case Study

Use the following information to answer question 17.

A 7-year-old patient has an exposed nerve. The dentist performs a pulpectomy, taking out most of the live pulp tissue and putting in a nerve treatment dressing. The tooth has a very large opening at its apex; the apical foramen did not have a chance to close because of the patient's age. The dentist changes the dressing for several months, and the apical foramen finally closes.

17. What mechanism is responsible for this?
    a. The tooth has regenerated a new nerve.
    b. Cementocytes, independent of the pulp, continued to lay down cellular cementum.
    c. Bone and the periodontal ligament have filled it in.
    d. Secondary dentin has been produced, and it has closed off the apical foramen.

Case Study

Use the following information to answer questions 18 and 19.

Mr. Willis has fractured and lost the distobuccal third of his permanent right mandibular first molar. The dentist has advised Mr. Willis that he will need a crown. Mr. Willis does not plan to begin the dental treatment for at least several months.

18. If Mr. Willis delays having the crown made for about 6 months, which of the following would be the *least* likely to occur?
  a. open contact
  b. tooth migration
  c. an abscess
  d. gingival changes

19. What would be the best option for Mr. Willis while he delays having the crown made?
  a. He can eat on the left side.
  b. The dentist can make a temporary crown.
  c. The tooth can be extracted to avoid further fracture.
  d. The fractured area can be filled in with a temporary restoration material.

Case Study

Use the following information to answer questions 20 and 21.

A patient complains of frequent pain in the mandibular left premolar region. Radiographs do not reveal bone loss or dental caries. Clinically, there is some buccal gingival recession and smooth dentin in the premolar area. The patient reports that she brushes vigorously with a hard-bristled toothbrush about five times daily.

20. What factor(s) could be leading to the patient's pain?
  a. frequent aggressive brushing
  b. use of the hard-bristled toothbrush
  c. gingival recession
  d. exposed dentin
  e. all of the above

21. Which procedure should be performed immediately to relieve the patient's pain?
  a. Cover the exposed dentin with a dentin-desensitizing varnish.
  b. Instruct the patient to brush only twice a day.
  c. Instruct the patient to use a soft-bristled toothbrush.
  d. Schedule a topical fluoride treatment.

Group Exercise

22. Study the figure and identify as many problems as you can. Meet with a study group of classmates to discuss your findings.

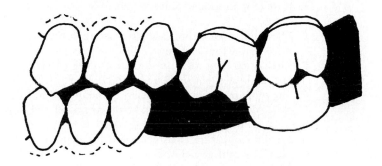

Chapter 10

Tooth Identification

True-False Questions

_____ **1.** If there is a root curvature, it generally is to the distal.

_____ **2.** Mandibular teeth show a slight wearing down on the linguoincisal surface.

_____ **3.** *Tertiary anatomy* refers to the numerous grooves, pits, and lines that third molars often have.

_____ **4.** The more posterior the position of the molar, the closer together the roots will be to each other.

_____ **5.** All anterior teeth have a biting edge.

_____ **6.** Mandibular central incisors are smaller than maxillary central incisors.

_____ **7.** Molars have between two and five cusps.

_____ **8.** The maxillary molars have small distobuccal cusps.

Fill-in-the-Blank

9. The distal cusp of the permanent mandibular first molar is on the _____ (buccal or lingual) surface of the tooth.

10. The _____ cusp is the cusp on which Carabelli's cusp is found.

11. The permanent mandibular premolar with a groove in its mesial marginal ridge is the _____.

12. The _____ premolar often has three cusps.

13. The _____ canine has a well-developed cingulum.

14. The _____ canine has a smoother, less-developed lingual surface.

15. The _____ molars have four almost equally divided cusps.

16. Anterior teeth have a more rounded marginal ridge on the _____ (mesial or distal) side.

Case Study

Use the information below to answer questions 17 and 18.

A 14-year-old boy, Jonathan, has had an orthodontic appliance for 2 years. He had four premolars extracted to alleviate the crowding in both arches. He asks if it is possible to tell whether his existing teeth are first or second premolars.

17. The maxillary premolars have a buccal cusp that is almost the same height as the lingual cusp. The occlusal surface has numerous short grooves that connect to the central groove; there are no obvious proximal marginal developmental grooves or depressions. Which premolar is this?

18. The mandibular premolars have a prominent buccal cusp and a shorter lingual cusp; the lingual cusp has a lingual groove that slightly separates the linguo-occlusal surface into two lingual cusps; there is a central pit but there is no transverse ridge. Which premolar is this?

Identification of Teeth

19. Mandibular anterior teeth have their contact areas closer to the distal and mesial marginal ridges. Which of the anterior teeth in the illustration are mandibular and which are maxillary?

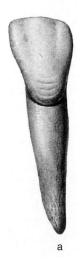
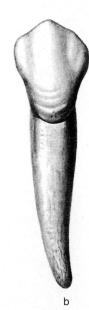
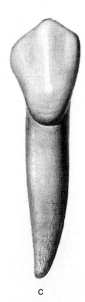

a

b

c

20. Which of the premolars in the illustration are maxillary, and which are mandibular?

22. In the illustration, which tooth is *c*?

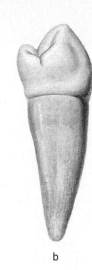

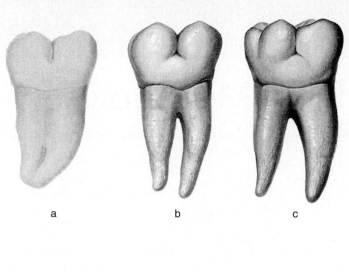

a   b

a   b   c

21. In the illustration, which tooth is *a*?

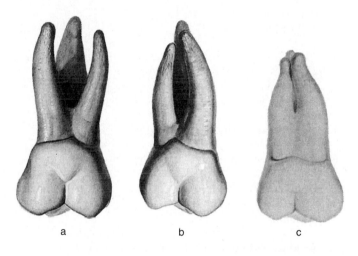

a   b   c

Chapter 11

Root Morphology

True-False Questions

_____ **1.** A healthy tooth will exhibit slight mobility when pressure is applied.

_____ **2.** The removal of carbon dioxide from the pulp canal through the apical foramen is called *anoxia*.

_____ **3.** If there is an infection within a tooth, harmful gases can cause the root canal to expand.

_____ **4.** Furcations are closer to the CEJ on mandibular molars than on maxillary molars.

_____ **5.** A central incisor is better able to resist displacement forces compared with a canine.

Matching

Match the usual number of pulp canals with the appropriate tooth.

_____ **6.** Maxillary first premolar   **a.** One canal

_____ **7.** Mandibular first premolar   **b.** Two canals

_____ **8.** Mandibular first molar   **c.** Two or three canals

_____ **9.** Maxillary first molar   **d.** Three or four canals

Multiple-Choice Questions

10. Which can elicit a pain response?
   a. air stimulus
   b. temperature extremes
   c. chemical agents
   d. sweets
   e. all of the above may elicit a pain response

11. Calculus formation is likely if roots have
   a. grooves
   b. roughness
   c. a prominent CEJ
   d. furcations
   e. all of the above

12. Which tooth is most likely to have two pulp canals?
   a. maxillary central
   b. maxillary lateral
   c. mandibular central
   d. mandibular canine
   e. both a and b

13. Canines can have two root canals. One canal is mesial and one is distal.
   a. Both statements are true.
   b. Both statements are false.
   c. First statement is true; the second is false.
   d. The first statement is false; the second is true.

14. Which of the following may *not* cause dentin tubules to be opened and exposed to sensory stimulus?
   a. hot foods
   b. root decay
   c. root abrasion
   d. bleaching agents

15. Which will not favorably affect the stability and anchorage of a tooth within the periodontium?
   a. root length
   b. root ridges
   c. number of roots
   d. direction of periodontal fibers

16. Which is not a characteristic of hypercementosis?
   a. cementoma
   b. cellular cementum formation
   c. acellular cementum formation
   d. trauma

17. Which would not be a result of consistent pressure on a tooth?
   a. bone resorption
   b. bone remodeling
   c. periodontal ligament (PDL) tension and compression
   d. periodontal fiber regeneration

18. Identify the items in the figure below:

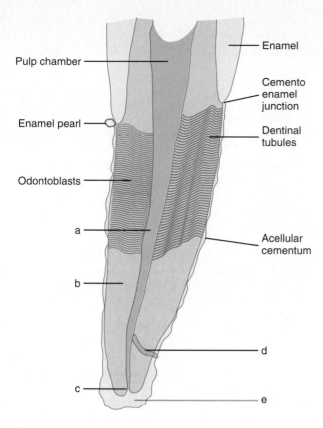

Enamel

Pulp chamber

Cemento enamel junction

Enamel pearl

Dentinal tubules

Odontoblasts

a

Acellular cementum

b

d

c

e

a. _____
b. _____
c. _____
d. _____
e. _____

Chapter 12

Incisors

True-False Questions

_____ 1. If there is a root curvature on incisors, it is generally toward the mesial surface.

_____ 2. Mandibular incisors show slight attrition (or wearing down) on the labioincisal surface.

_____ 3. The pulp cavity will decrease in size with the age of the tooth.

_____ 4. All permanent mandibular lateral incisors have a prominent lingual pit.

_____ 5. All anterior teeth have a ridge-like biting edge.

_____ 6. A mandibular central incisor is the smallest of the incisors.

_____ 7. Because of their longer roots, maxillary lateral incisors have a greater root-to-crown ratio compared with maxillary centrals.

_____ 8. Maxillary central and lateral incisors are wider labiolingually than they are mesiodistally.

Matching

Match the teeth in the list below with the appropriate characteristics in questions 9 to 14.

a. Maxillary central incisor   **c.** Mandibular central incisor
b. Maxillary lateral incisor   **d.** Mandibular lateral incisor

_____ 9. Sharp mesioincisal angle

_____ 10. Rounded incisal edge

_____ 11. Crown appears rotated on root

_____ 12. Bilaterally symmetric crown

_____ 13. Most likely to have a lingual pit

_____ 14. Root-to-crown ratio is relatively close

Multiple-Choice Questions

15. Which anomaly is *not* characteristic of a maxillary central incisor?
    a. gemination
    b. microdont
    c. long crown
    d. short root

16. Which is *not* true of the mandibular central incisors?
    a. smallest teeth in the mouth
    b. contact one antagonist only
    c. often have lingual pit
    d. incisal edge wears on labial surface

17. When does the mandibular lateral incisor erupt?
    a. 6–7 years
    b. 7–8 years
    c. 8–9 years
    d. none of the above

18. Which of the anterior teeth listed below are wider mesiodistally than faciolingually?
    a. maxillary incisors
    b. mandibular incisors
    c. canines
    d. none of the above
    e. both a and b

19. Which teeth are *most* likely to have a proximal groove in the roots?
    a. maxillary centrals
    b. maxillary laterals
    c. mandibular laterals
    d. both a and b

20. Which incisors are tipped lingually in a class II, division II malocclusion?
    a. maxillary central incisors
    b. maxillary lateral incisors
    c. maxillary laterals and mandibular incisors
    d. mandibular incisors only

21. Which teeth might be protruded in a class II, division II malocclusion?
    a. maxillary centrals
    b. maxillary laterals
    c. mandibular centrals
    d. mandibular laterals

Case Study

Use the following information to answer questions 22 and 23.

A 10-year-old boy, Michael Davis, is brought into the office. His mother feels that Michael's teeth "look unbalanced, as if the teeth on one side don't match with those on the other side." You agree with Mrs. Davis's observation Michael's maxillary left lateral is small and somewhat pointed; the maxillary right lateral is appropriately shaped. Mrs. Davis also mentions that about 2 years ago, Michael lost a mandibular incisor in a bicycle accident. The dental team will develop a treatment plan for Michael that balances esthetics and occlusion, but first the teeth in question must be identified.

22. With regard to the maxillary left lateral, what is the logical explanation of its appearance?
    a. It could be a deciduous lateral.
    b. Michael's mixed dentition is typical; teeth appear to have disproportionate sizes and shapes until permanent teeth erupt.
    c. It is a peg lateral.
    d. It is a supernumerary tooth.

23. How would you identify Michael's missing mandibular incisor? Select all that apply.
    a. Compare the widths of the three incisors.
    b. Compare the heights of the three incisors.
    c. Compare the contact areas.
    d. Assess if mamelons are present.

24. Identify the following incisors:

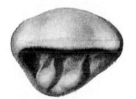

a. _____

b. _____

c. _____

d. _____

25. Identify the following incisors:

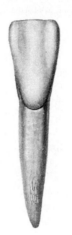

a. _____

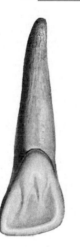

b. _____

Chapter 13

Canines

True-False Questions

_____ 1. Both canines show evidence of calcification beginning at 6 months of age.
_____ 2. Mandibular canines erupt 1 year before maxillary canines.
_____ 3. Canines do not have mamelons.
_____ 4. The maxillary canine is wider mesiodistally than the mandibular canine.
_____ 5. Longitudinal grooves on the roots of mandibular canines often signify that there are two root canals.
_____ 6. The labial surfaces of both canines are more convex from the cervical line to the cusp tip than any other tooth.

Multiple-Choice Questions

7. Which of these anterior teeth is most likely to be bifurcated?
   a. maxillary central
   b. maxillary lateral
   c. mandibular canine
   d. mandibular lateral
   e. maxillary canine

8. Which of the following statements is true?
   a. The maxillary canine is the last anterior tooth to erupt.
   b. The mandibular canine develops from three lobes.
   c. The mandibular canine root is completed at age 12 years.
   d. Both a and c.
   e. Both b and c.

9. The mesial contact area of the maxillary canine is located
   a. slightly cervical to the middle of the crown
   b. at the junction of the middle and incisal thirds
   c. within the incisal third of the crown
   d. at the center of the middle of the crown

10. Which of the following teeth might have a cervicoincisal crown length as long as or longer than a maxillary canine?
    a. maxillary lateral
    b. mandibular canine
    c. mandibular lateral
    d. none of the above

11. Which of the following might have a root as long as or longer than a maxillary canine?
    a. maxillary central
    b. mandibular canine
    c. maxillary lateral
    d. none of the above

12. The lingual surface of a mandibular canine *most* resembles the lingual surface of which tooth?
    a. mandibular lateral
    b. maxillary lateral
    c. maxillary canine
    d. maxillary central

13. Which tooth has the *most* prominent cingulum?
    a. maxillary central incisor
    b. maxillary lateral incisor
    c. maxillary canine
    d. mandibular canine

14. Maxillary canines have certain unique characteristics that contribute to their stability and their self-cleansing properties. Which of the following does not meet these criteria?
    a. smooth, rounded contours
    b. long, thick root
    c. position in the arch
    d. thin, flat lingual surface

Match the following terms with the corresponding labels on the figure below:

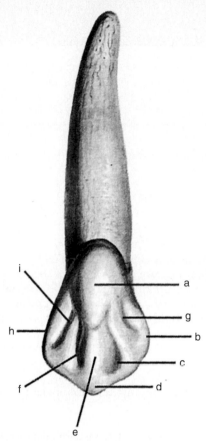

_____ **15.** Mesial fossa
_____ **16.** Distal fossa
_____ **17.** Cingulum
_____ **18.** Mesial marginal ridge
_____ **19.** Distal marginal ridge
_____ **20.** Lingual cusp ridge
_____ **21.** Cusp tip
_____ **22.** Mesial marginal groove
_____ **23.** Distal marginal groove

Chapter 14

Premolars

True-False Questions

_____ 1. The buccal cusps of premolars are always larger than their lingual cusps.

_____ 2. The "Y"-grooved premolar could have up to three occlusal pits.

_____ 3. The mandibular first premolar is usually the first premolar to erupt.

_____ 4. The maxillary first premolar can be identified by the mesial marginal groove that crosses the marginal ridge.

_____ 5. All the premolars will have erupted by age 12 years.

_____ 6. The mesial developmental depression is a characteristic of maxillary premolars.

_____ 7. Both maxillary premolars have cusp tips centered over their roots.

_____ 8. Mandibular premolars have functional lingual cusps.

Matching

Place **A** for maxillary first premolar and **B** for maxillary second premolar.

_____ 9. Rounded occlusal outline

_____ 10. Two root canals

_____ 11. Buccal and lingual cusps are nearly the same height

_____ 12. Has more occlusal supplemental grooves

_____ 13. Facially, resembles canine

_____ 14. Distinct mesial marginal groove

Place **A** for mandibular first premolar and **B** for mandibular second premolar.

_____ 15. High marginal ridges

_____ 16. Mesiolingual developmental groove

_____ 17. Two to three pulp horns

_____ 18. Occlusal surface slopes lingually

_____ 19. Least developed lingual cusp

_____ 20. Has two lingual cusps

Multiple-Choice Questions

21. A triangular ridge extends from the cusp tip to the
    a. opposite cusp tip
    b. mesial and distal triangular fossae
    c. marginal ridges
    d. central groove

22. Which premolar erupts at ages 11 to 12 years of age?
    a. maxillary first premolar
    b. maxillary second premolar
    c. mandibular first premolar
    d. mandibular second premolar

23. Which groove pattern is *most* common in mandibular second premolars?
    a. "U"
    b. "H"
    c. "Y"
    d. "W"

24. Which of the following has the deepest longitudinal groove?
    a. the mesial surface of a maxillary second premolar
    b. the mesial surface of a maxillary first premolar
    c. the mesial surface of a mandibular first premolar
    d. the distal surface of a maxillary first premolar

25. Which tooth in Fig. 14.1 is a maxillary first premolar?

_____

26. Which tooth in Fig. 14.1 is a mandibular first premolar?

_____

27. Which tooth in Fig. 14.1 is a mandibular second premolar?

_____

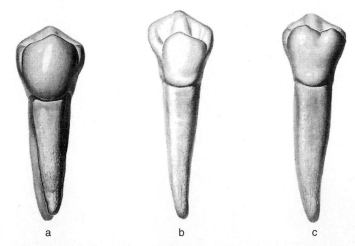

• **Figure 14.1.** (From Zeisz RC, Nuckolls J. *Dental Anatomy*. St. Louis, MO: Mosby; 1949.)

28. What type of ridge is between the lines in Fig. 14.2?

_____

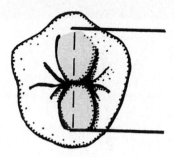

• **Figure 14.2.**

Chapter 15

Molars

True-False Questions

_____ 1. First molars are the largest permanent teeth.

_____ 2. Permanent mandibular first molars are the first permanent teeth to erupt.

_____ 3. Permanent maxillary third molars vary more in form than any other maxillary teeth.

_____ 4. Maxillary second molars are the most likely molars to have buccal pits.

_____ 5. Maxillary first molars are wider faciolingually than mesiodistally.

_____ 6. The distal cusp of the mandibular first molar is the same height as the mesiobuccal cusp.

_____ 7. The cusp of Carabelli is found on the lingual surface of the mesiolingual cusp of the maxillary first molar.

_____ 8. Lingual cusps on mandibular molars are shorter than buccal cusps.

_____ 9. Mandibular third molars resemble mandibular second molars.

_____ 10. Maxillary first molars have mesial, distal, and palatal roots.

Matching

Place **A** for maxillary first molar and **B** for maxillary second molar.

_____ 11. Begins calcification at birth

_____ 12. Develops from four lobes

_____ 13. Somewhat heart-shaped occlusal outline

_____ 14. Roots closer together

_____ 15. Has one supplemental cusp

Place **A** for mandibular first molar and **B** for mandibular second molar.

_____ 16. Has five cusps

_____ 17. Has a distobuccal developmental groove

_____ 18. Roots are completed at ages 14 to 15 years

_____ 19. Occlusal outline is rectangular

_____ 20. Y-shaped occlusal pattern

Multiple-Choice Questions

21. Which mandibular first molar root is the longest and strongest?
    a. mesial
    b. palatal
    c. distal
    d. mesiobuccal

22. When is the root formation complete in a third molar?
    a. 11 to 13 years
    b. 12 to 13 years
    c. 14 to 18 years
    d. 18 to 25 years

23. Which molars have only one antagonist?
    a. maxillary third
    b. maxillary second
    c. mandibular third
    d. mandibular first

24. Which is the smallest cusp on all maxillary molars?
    a. mesiobuccal
    b. mesiolingual
    c. distobuccal
    d. distolingual

25. The relationship of the _____ molars is evaluated to assess occlusion.
    a. maxillary first
    b. maxillary second
    c. mandibular third
    d. mandibular second

26. Which landmark is not found on the mandibular first molar?
    a. buccal pit
    b. oblique ridge
    c. triangular ridge
    d. lingual groove

27. Which is a significant factor in occlusal caries?
    a. pits and fissures
    b. triangular ridges
    c. position in the arch
    d. age at eruption

28. Mandibular second molars erupt at ages _____ years.
    a. 6–7
    b. 7–8
    c. 9–11
    d. 11–13

29. Third molars that are prevented from erupting because of an obstruction are _____.
    a. congenitally missing
    b. impeded
    c. impacted
    d. partial anodontia

30. Which root rarely has two root canals?
    a. mesiobuccal root of maxillary first molar
    b. mesiobuccal root of maxillary second molar
    c. mesial root of mandibular first molar
    d. mesial root of mandibular second molar

Match the terms below with their correct locations in the figure:

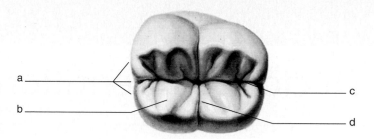

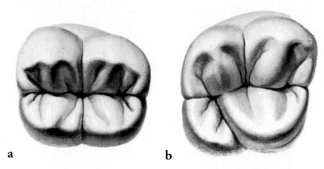

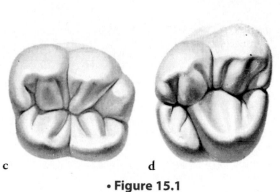

a   b

c   d

• **Figure 15.1**

_____ **35.** Lingual groove
_____ **36.** Mesiolingual triangular ridge
_____ **37.** Mesial marginal ridge
_____ **38.** Distal triangular fossa

31. Which tooth in Fig. 15.1 is a maxillary first molar?

    _____

32. Which tooth in Fig. 15.1 is a maxillary second molar?

    _____

33. Which tooth in Fig. 15.1 is a mandibular first molar?

    _____

34. Which tooth in Fig. 15.1 is a mandibular second molar?

    _____

Chapter 16

Deciduous Dentition

True-False Questions

_____ 1. Deciduous maxillary first molars are the smallest deciduous molars mesiodistally.

_____ 2. Deciduous second molars erupt next after the deciduous first molars.

_____ 3. The mesial root of deciduous mandibular first molars has two root canals.

_____ 4. The occlusal table of permanent teeth is narrower than that of deciduous teeth.

_____ 5. Deciduous maxillary first molars are wider mesio-distally than permanent first premolars.

_____ 6. Deciduous maxillary first molars have only two major cusps.

_____ 7. The lingual height of contour of deciduous molars is at the cervical third.

_____ 8. The facial height of contour of deciduous teeth is at the cervical third.

_____ 9. Deciduous molar roots are flared to accommodate permanent teeth.

_____ 10. Roots of all deciduous molars are bifurcated closely to the cervical line.

Multiple-Choice Questions

11. The molar *most* likely to have three cusps is the
    a. deciduous mandibular second molar
    b. deciduous maxillary second molar
    c. deciduous maxillary first molar
    d. permanent maxillary second molar

12. Which deciduous molars are wider mesiodistally than they are faciolingually?
    a. mandibular first molars
    b. maxillary second molars
    c. mandibular second molars
    d. both a and c
    e. both b and c

13. What is the *most* distinguishing feature of the deciduous mandibular first molars?
    a. root length
    b. presence of lingual pit
    c. buccocervical ridge
    d. distal cusp

14. Which deciduous molars most resemble permanent first molars?
    a. maxillary first molars
    b. second molars
    c. mandibular first molars
    d. both a and c

15. All deciduous teeth have a prominent
    a. linguocervical ridge
    b. Carabelli's cusp
    c. bucco-occlusal ridge
    d. faciocervical ridge

16. The occlusal surface of the deciduous mandibular second molar resembles the occlusal surface of which permanent teeth?
    a. mandibular first premolars
    b. mandibular second premolars
    c. mandibular first molars
    d. it does not resemble the occlusal surface of any other tooth

17. Which two cusps are the largest on deciduous maxillary first molars?
    a. mesiobuccal and distobuccal
    b. Carabelli's and distal
    c. mesiobuccal and mesiolingual
    d. lingual and distal

18. Which deciduous tooth is wider than its cervicoincisal length?
    a. maxillary central incisor
    b. maxillary lateral incisor
    c. mandibular central incisor
    d. mandibular lateral incisor

19. Which is *not* a characteristic of deciduous teeth compared with permanent teeth?
    a. thicker dentin between pulp and enamel
    b. smaller in crown height
    c. whiter in color
    d. shorter root trunk

20. Which deciduous teeth are *most* likely to have mamelons?
    a. maxillary central incisors
    b. maxillary lateral incisors
    c. mandibular central incisors
    d. mandibular lateral incisors

21. Deciduous mandibular lateral incisors are
    a. rotated on their roots
    b. distally inclined at the incisal ridge
    c. rounded at the mesioincisal angle
    d. slightly narrower than deciduous mandibular central incisors

22. Which is *not* a characteristic of the deciduous maxillary canine?
    a. It has one lingual fossa.
    b. It has a lingual ridge.
    c. It is bulkier than other deciduous anterior teeth.
    d. It has a root that is about twice as long as its crown.

23. Which *best* describes the appearance of the deciduous maxillary first molar?
    a. It resembles the permanent maxillary first molar.
    b. It resembles the permanent maxillary second molar.
    c. It resembles the deciduous maxillary second molar.
    d. It does not resemble any other molar.

24. Compared with the permanent maxillary first molar, what is *not* true of the deciduous maxillary second molar?
    a. It has Carabelli's cusp.
    b. The mesiolingual cusp is the largest cusp.
    c. The lingual root is by far the longest root.
    d. It has a small distolingual cusp.

25. Which characteristic of the deciduous mandibular second molar is different from that of the permanent mandibular first molar?
    a. The mesial root has two canals.
    b. The distal cusp is the same size as the two buccal cusps.
    c. The occlusal surface has a "Y" shape.
    d. It is the largest molar.

Case Study

Use the following information to answer questions 26 to 29.

There are four siblings in the dental reception room; two of them have appointments with the dental hygienist, and two have appointments with the dentist. You inform them that you are the dental assistant and tell them that they will be seen shortly. While they are in the waiting room, one of them says, "I bet you can't guess my age!" You reply that you can guess all of their ages (within 1 year) by looking at their teeth. The children are very eager to open their mouths and play this guessing game. You chart the teeth that are present and make your best guess:

26. Beth has 20 deciduous teeth, and her permanent mandibular first molars have partially erupted. Her age is _____ years.

27. Julia has her deciduous mandibular molars and canines. She has her permanent incisors and first molars. Her age is _____ years.

28. Kevin has his deciduous maxillary canines and second molars. He has permanent incisors, mandibular canines, maxillary and mandibular first premolars, and first molars. His age is _____ years.

29. Alexander has his permanent incisors, mandibular canines, maxillary canines (partially erupted), maxillary first and second premolars, mandibular first and second premolars (partially erupted), and permanent first molars. His age is _____ years.

30. Which tooth in Fig. 16.1 is a deciduous maxillary first molar? _____

31. Which tooth in Fig. 16.1 is a deciduous maxillary second molar? _____

32. Which tooth in Fig. 16.1 is a deciduous mandibular first molar? _____

33. Which tooth in Fig. 16.1 is a deciduous mandibular second molar? _____

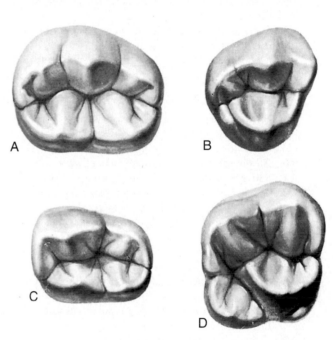

• Figure 16.1

Chapter 17

Basic Tissues

True-False Questions

_____ 1. *Pinocytosis* refers to a "drinking in."

_____ 2. Ribosomes are made up of deoxyribonucleic acid (DNA).

_____ 3. Lipid droplets and glycogen are two examples of cell organelles.

_____ 4. The nucleolus is a repository for nuclear ribonucleic acid (RNA).

_____ 5. Lysosomes are scavengers, destroying substances foreign to the cell.

_____ 6. Cells may assume different shapes depending on the pressure around them.

_____ 7. Melanocytes that cause pigmenting of the skin are found between the stratum basale and the stratum spinosum.

_____ 8. The star shape of the stratum spinosum cells results from the presence of desmosomes.

_____ 9. Endocrine glands develop as the epithelium grows down into the underlying connective tissue.

_____ 10. All glands develop from epithelial layers.

_____ 11. Salivary glands produce only serous secretions.

_____ 12. The arrangement of blood vessels and osteocytes inside bones is called the *marrow cavity.*

_____ 13. The nutrient arteries that bring blood back to the inside of the bone are called *Volkmann's canals.*

_____ 14. Every cubic millimeter of blood contains 4 to 6 million red blood cells.

_____ 15. Collagen is the most common fiber in connective tissue.

_____ 16. A tendon is an example of a regular connective tissue, but a ligament is irregular connective tissue.

_____ 17. Calcium crystals are the substance that makes bone hard.

_____ 18. Bone grows interstitially.

_____ 19. Bone marrow is lined with periosteum.

_____ 20. Purkinje fibers are specialized muscle cells found in smooth muscle.

_____ 21. Skeletal muscles may have hundreds of nuclei in a cell, whereas cardiac muscles only have one or two nuclei per cell.

_____ 22. Smooth muscle is found in the digestive tract, blood vessels, and lungs.

_____ 23. The myelin sheath plays a significant role in regeneration of damaged nerves.

_____ 24. In a sensory nerve, the wave of depolarization of a neuron travels from the axon to the cell body and finally to the dendrite.

_____ 25. If a nerve axon in the peripheral nervous system is damaged, the neuron will usually die.

_____ 26. Acetylcholine and epinephrine are the chemical substances that allow nerves to communicate with each other.

Multiple-Choice Questions

27. Which of the following is *not* true about cell membranes?
    a. Their function is to keep cytoplasm inside the cell and foreign substances outside.
    b. Many can selectively take in water through the process of pinocytosis.
    c. Many are able to accomplish merocrine secretion.
    d. None of the above.

28. Which organelle is responsible for cellular energy production?
    a. Organelles
    b. Mitochondria
    c. Endoplasmic reticulum
    d. Microfilaments

29. What granules appear on the rough endoplasmic reticulum?
    a. Cristae
    b. Lysosomes
    c. Cellular inclusions
    d. Ribosomes

30. Which is the storage form of cellular energy?
    a. Ribosomes
    b. Glycogen
    c. Cytoplasm
    d. Lysosomes

31. Goblet cells are found in the _____.
    a. Epidermis
    b. Respiratory tract
    c. Urinary tract
    d. Cardiovascular system

32. _____ epithelium lines the oral cavity.
    a. Stratum corneum
    b. Pseudostratified columnar
    c. Stratified squamous
    d. Stratified columnar

33. A stratum granulosum will be found in _____ stratified squamous epithelium.
a. Nonkeratinized
b. Parakeratinized
c. Keratinized
d. Both b and c

34. Where is stratum lucidum found?
a. Mucous membranes of the cheek
b. Skin of the cheek
c. Skin of the back of the hand
d. Skin of the palm of the hand

35. Which structure functions as a cushioning substance?
a. Elastic cartilage
b. Hyaline cartilage
c. Fibrocartilage
d. Endosteum

36. The cell frequently found in connective tissue that has the *most* potential for forming numerous other cell types is the:
a. Fibroblast
b. Lymphocyte
c. Mesenchymal cell
d. Macrophage

37. Which of the following is *not* true of blood?
a. All blood cells have nuclei.
b. The cellular part of blood is made up of red blood cells, white blood cells, and platelets.
c. Anemia is a condition in which there is a decrease in the amount of red blood cells.
d. Most extracellular body fluids come from blood plasma.

38. Histamine is found in mast cells and _____.
a. Neutrophils
b. Basophils
c. Eosinophils
d. Lymphocytes

39. Which muscle's movement is voluntary?
a. Skeletal
b. Cardiac
c. Smooth
d. All of the above

40. Which of these types of muscles are striated or striped?
a. Smooth
b. Cardiac
c. Skeletal
d. Both b and c
e. All of the above

41. Which of the following muscle components has the smallest diameter?
a. Myosin
b. Myofibril
c. Actin
d. Myofiber

42. What is the functional unit of skeletal muscle?
a. A-band
b. I-band
c. M-band
d. None of the above

Case Study

Use the information below to answer questions 43 and 44.

A young Caucasian patient is scheduled for their recall hygiene appointment. They appear to have lost weight and report that they have been tired and under a great deal of stress. On examination, their oral tissues appear pale pink.

43. What is the most likely diagnosis, with respect to their pallor and weight loss?
a. Infection
b. Anemia
c. Allergy symptoms
d. Sickle cell disease

44. The dentist will probably refer them to their physician for a(n):
a. Prescription for antibiotics
b. Complete blood count
c. Allergy test
d. Screening for sickle cell disease

45. Identify the following cell structures:

a._____
b._____
c._____
d._____

46. In the cross section, identify the following bone structures:

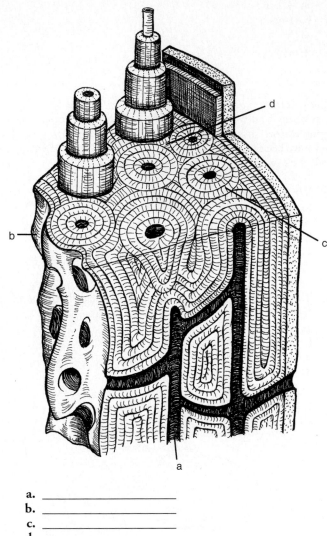

a. _____

b. _____

c. _____

d. _____

47. Identify the following structures:

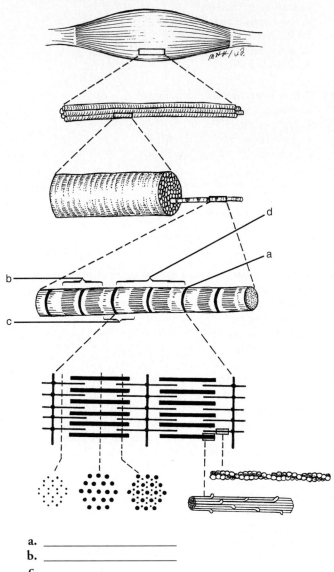

a. _____

b. _____

c. _____

d. _____

Chapter 18

Development of Orofacial Complex

True-False Questions

_____ 1. There are six pharyngeal arches that start developing, but two of them disappear.

_____ 2. The primitive oral cavity is known as the *stomodeum*.

_____ 3. The cardiac bulge is located beneath the pharyngeal arches.

_____ 4. The maxillary lip forms because connective tissues migrate into the lip between the maxillary processes.

_____ 5. The epithelial rest cells in the midline of the palate may cause cysts later in life.

_____ 6. A globulomaxillary cyst is found between the maxillary central and lateral incisors.

_____ 7. For the palatal shelves to come into contact with each other and the nasal septum, the tongue must move up and out of the way.

_____ 8. The first pharyngeal arch forms the mandibular and maxillary processes.

_____ 9. A bilateral cleft palate occurs when neither palatal process is in contact with the nasal septum.

_____ 10. One in every 2500 babies is born with a cleft palate.

_____ 11. Hereditary factors are the only known cause for cleft defects.

Matching

Match each pharyngeal arch with the cranial nerve that innervates it.

_____ 12. Fourth–sixth arch   a. Cranial nerve III
_____ 13. First arch   b. Cranial nerve X (XI)
_____ 14. Third arch   c. Cranial nerve VII
_____ 15. Second arch   d. Cranial nerve V
       e. Cranial nerve VIII
       f. Cranial nerve IX

Multiple-Choice Questions

16. The embryonic stage is from weeks _____.
    a. 2 to 4
    b. 3 to 6
    c. 3 to 8
    d. 4 to 9

17. The foregut is located between the:
    a. Throat region and the stomach
    b. Throat region and the duodenum
    c. Esophagus and the duodenum
    d. Esophagus and jejunum

18. During which embryonic week does the oropharyngeal membrane disintegrate?
    a. Week 3
    b. Week 4
    c. Week 6
    d. Week 7

19. The critical timing for face and lip development is the:
    a. Third to the sixth embryonic week
    b. Third to the eighth embryonic week
    c. Fourth to the seventh embryonic week
    d. Fourth to the eighth embryonic week

20. The maxillary lip is formed from the:
    a. Medial and lateral nasal processes
    b. Maxillary and lateral nasal processes
    c. Maxillary and medial nasal processes
    d. Left and right maxillary processes

21. The nasal pits develop from the:
    a. Medial and lateral processes
    b. Lower end of the frontal prominence
    c. Two medial nasal processes
    d. Two lateral nasal processes

22. The external auditory meatus originates from the _____ pharyngeal groove.
    a. First
    b. Second
    c. Third
    d. Fourth

23. The malleus and incus bones of the ear are formed by the _____ pharyngeal arch(es).
    a. First
    b. Second
    c. Third
    d. Fourth through sixth

24. The hyoid bone originates from the _____ pharyngeal arch.
    a. First
    b. Second
    c. Third
    d. Both a and b
    e. Both b and c

25. Muscles of facial expression originate from the _____ pharyngeal arch.
    a. First
    b. Second
    c. Third
    d. Both a and b

26. The palatine tonsils arise from the _____ pharyngeal pouch.
    a. First
    b. Second
    c. Third
    d. Fourth

Case Study

Use the information below to answer questions 27 to 29.

A 6-week-old infant is brought into the office. The infant has bilateral cleft lips, but the hard and soft palate are normal. The child is sent to oral surgery for surgical correction of the cleft lips.

27. Bilateral cleft lips are caused by the:
    a. Failure of the palatal shelves to fuse
    b. Lack of fusion between the maxillary process and the medial nasal process
    c. Lack of fusion between the lateral nasal process and nasal septum
    d. Lack of fusion between the palatal process and the nasal septum

28. At what point in development did the cleft lips develop?
    a. Week 6
    b. Week 7
    c. 3 to 6 months
    d. At any embryonic stage

29. Which is the best treatment for cleft lips?
    a. Speech therapy
    b. A prosthetic device
    c. Surgery
    d. Both b and c

30. Identify the following structures:

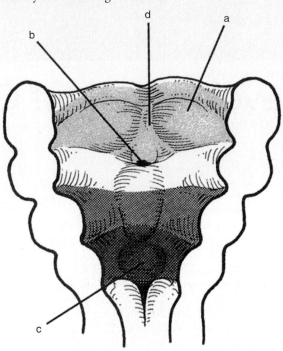

a. _____

b. _____

c. _____

d. _____

Chapter 19

Dental Lamina and Enamel Organ

True-False Questions

_____ **1.** In each dental arch, there are 16 localized downgrowths of the dental lamina into the underlying connective tissue that will form the primary dentition.

_____ **2.** Poor development of structures, such as enamel, skin, and salivary glands, is known as *dental dysplasia*.

_____ **3.** The bud stage of the enamel organ arises from the mesoderm.

_____ **4.** There are two components of the cap stage: outer enamel epithelium and inner enamel epithelium.

_____ **5.** The inner and outer enamel epithelium layers are continuations of one another.

_____ **6.** The successional lamina forms permanent molars.

_____ **7.** The successional lamina goes through the three stages of the enamel organ.

_____ **8.** The vestibular lamina is a lingual thickening of the oral epithelium that splits to form the sublingual fold.

_____ **9.** The dental papilla forms the dentin and cementum of the tooth.

_____ **10.** The dental sac forms the pulp.

_____ **11.** The dental papilla and the dental sac both develop from the mesoderm.

_____ **12.** The dental papilla contacts the inner enamel epithelial cells.

Matching

Match the following parts of the bell stage with their functions:

_____ **13.** Outer enamel epithelium (OEE)

_____ **14.** Stellate reticulum

_____ **15.** Inner enamel epithelium (IEE)

_____ **16.** Stratum intermedium

a. Forms ameloblasts
b. Protective layer
c. Aids in nourishing ameloblast
d. Cushioning layer
e. Forms dental pulp

Multiple-Choice Questions

17. Which of the following statements about dental lamina is *not* true?
a. It is a thickening of embryonic oral epithelium that pushes up into the oral cavity.
b. It starts forming during week six of embryonic development, and the posterior portions of it may be seen many years later.
c. It will further the development of tooth enamel.
d. It is derived from the ectoderm.

18. The dental sac consists of several rows of flat cells. They surround part of the enamel organ.
a. Both statements are true.
b. Both statements are false.
c. The first statement is true; the second is false.
d. The first statement is false; the second is true.

19. Identify the following components of the bell stage:

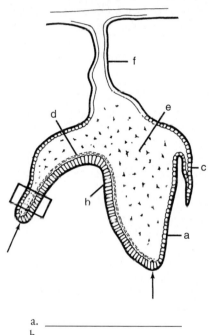

a. _____
b. _____
c. _____
d. _____
e. _____
f. _____

Chapter 20

Enamel, Dentin, and Pulp

True-False Questions

_____ 1. The Tomes' process is responsible for the direction of the crystals in the rod.

_____ 2. Mineralization is the laying down of the crystals in the enamel matrix.

_____ 3. Hypocalcified enamel results if an insufficient number of crystals are laid down in the matrix or if the crystals do not grow sufficiently.

_____ 4. Secondary dentin is not formed by the same odontoblasts that lay down regular dentin.

_____ 5. The dental pulp develops from mesenchymal tissue.

_____ 6. An enamel spindle is an odontoblast trapped in enamel at the dentinoenamel junction (DEJ).

_____ 7. Imbrication lines develop from the striae of Retzius.

_____ 8. Secondary dentin starts being formed at the time of tooth eruption.

_____ 9. Primary dentin is as calcified as enamel.

_____ 10. Dead tracts have empty dentin tubules.

_____ 11. True pulp stones look like an onion cut in cross section.

_____ 12. Fibroblasts and macrophages are not present in healthy pulpal tissue.

_____ 13. As the pulp ages, odontoblasts replace damaged cells.

_____ 14. Dentin lays down crystals, which begin to calcify.

_____ 15. Preameloblasts cannot change their polarity.

_____ 16. Pulpal tissue consists of blood vessels, lymphatic vessels, nerves, and only one kind of connective tissue.

_____ 17. Odontoblasts secrete the dentin matrix.

_____ 18. Ameloblasts lay down fibers which begin to calcify and form dentin.

_____ 19. Ameloblasts secrete the enamel matrix which then becomes calcified.

_____ 20. Enamel tufts can easily be seen clinically and can cause plural erosion.

Multiple-Choice Questions

21. The dental papilla originates from:
   a. mesenchymal cells
   b. ameloblasts
   c. odontoblasts
   d. none of the above

22. As enamel organ cells go from mesenchymal cells into dental papilla cells, they look:
   a. more rounded and condensed
   b. more pointed and condensed
   c. more rounded and diffuse
   d. more pointed and diffuse

23. Which of the statements about enamel is *not* true?
   a. It is the hardest substance of the body.
   b. Its basic unit of structure is the rod.
   c. It mainly consists of hydroxyapatite.
   d. Enamel is mostly organic in composition.

24. Which of these statements about enamel rods is *not* true?
   a. They are parallel to the DEJ.
   b. They contain an organic substance in the rod sheath.
   c. They are (each) formed by more than one ameloblast.
   d. They have a key-hole shape.

25. Which of these statements about ameloblasts is *not* true?
   a. It forms Nasmyth's membrane.
   b. It produces the primary enamel cuticle.
   c. The reduced enamel epithelium produces the secondary enamel cuticle.
   d. It has no part in the production of the epithelial attachment.

26. Cracks in the enamel caused by trauma are known as:
   a. enamel tufts
   b. enamel lamellae
   c. hypocalcified enamel
   d. hypoplastic enamel

27. Which of the following is *not* true of dentin?
   a. It is the second-hardest tissue in the body.
   b. It is made up of about 50% hydroxyapatite.
   c. It is microscopically made up of intertubular dentin, dentin tubules, and peritubular dentin.
   d. Clinically, it appears solid.

28. Which statement below is *not* true?
   a. Nasmyth's membrane is also called the *primary enamel cuticle.*
   b. Secondary enamel cuticle is the same as epithelial attachment.
   c. Reparative dentin may be formed in response to occlusal trauma.
   d. Nasmyth's membrane helps hold the attached gingiva against the tooth.

29. Which of these statements about pulp is *not* true?
    a. It is derived from mesodermal tissue.
    b. It has sensory nerve fibers that transmit only pain sensation.
    c. It cannot form new odontoblasts as the old ones are damaged.
    d. It is more cellular and less fibrous when it is young.

30. Which of the following is *not* true about pulp stones?
    a. They are found in about 80% of older adults.
    b. Most are true pulp stones.
    c. They are made up of free, attached, or embedded stones.
    d. They are generally not dangerous to the health of the pulpal tissue.

31. Mineralization is the initial laying down of the crystals in the enamel matrix. Maturation is the growth of the crystals to their full size.
    a. Both statements are true.
    b. Both statements are false.
    c. The first statement is true; the second statement is false.
    d. The first statement is false; the second statement is true.

Chapter 21

Root Formation and Attachment Apparatus

True-False Questions

_____ **1.** How the horizontal part of the root sheath grows inward determines how many roots will be formed.

_____ **2.** The dental papilla and the dental sac are on the inside of the epithelial root sheath.

_____ **3.** The first cementum laid down is cellular cementum at the CEJ.

_____ **4.** As cementum is deposited, it always overlaps enamel.

_____ **5.** Cellular cementum is seen more in the apical area of teeth than in the region of the cervical line.

_____ **6.** Trauma to a tooth may manifest on radiographs as a thickened lamina dura.

_____ **7.** The cribriform plate is an area of avascular bone.

_____ **8.** Sharpey's fibers are the attached part of the periodontal ligament.

_____ **9.** The fibers of the periodontal ligament are elastic fibers.

Matching

Place the steps of the development of the epithelial root sheath, root dentin, cementum, and the periodontal ligament in the proper developmental stage. Assign numbers **1** to **10** to the steps, 1 being the earliest step and 10 being the last step.

_____ **10.** The root sheath turns horizontally to form the epithelial diaphragm.

_____ **11.** The inner dental sac cells differentiate, forming cementoblasts, which migrate to the dentinal root surface.

_____ **12.** The epithelial rests are formed.

_____ **13.** The periodontal ligament fibers start organizing.

_____ **14.** The root sheath completely separates from the dentinal surface in that area.

_____ **15.** The bell stage is completed.

_____ **16.** The epithelial root sheath begins to break up.

_____ **17.** The middle layer of the dental sac forms fibroblasts, which form collagen.

_____ **18.** The cervical loop is formed from the inner enamel epithelium (IEE) and the outer enamel epithelium (OEE).

_____ **19.** The dental papilla cells are stimulated to form root dentin.

Matching

Match each function with a particular group of fibers.

_____ **20.** Gingival

_____ **21.** Transseptal

_____ **22.** Oblique

_____ **23.** Apical

_____ **24.** Horizontal

a. Resists occlusal trauma

b. Resists tooth being pulled out of the socket

c. Supports relationship between tooth and the surrounding epithelium

d. Aids in maintaining interproximal contact

e. Resists horizontal movement of tooth

Multiple-Choice Questions

25. Which of the following is *not* true about the formation of the cervical loop?
  a. It originates from the enamel organ.
  b. It contains all four layers from the bell stage of the enamel organ.
  c. Its turned-inward portion is the epithelial diaphragm.
  d. It forms the epithelial root sheath.

26. Enamel pearls originate from the
  a. epithelial root sheath cells
  b. epithelial rests of Malassez
  c. epithelial diaphragm
  d. cementoblasts

27. Hypercementosis may occur as a response to tooth trauma. Excess cementum could be deposited anywhere but in the apical area of the root.
  a. Both statements are true.
  b. Both statements are false.
  c. The first statement is true; the second is false.
  d. The first statement is false; the second is true.

28. Acellular and cellular cementum differ in that
  a. they are formed from different types of cells
  b. a cellular cementum has cementocytes trapped in it
  c. cellular cementum if present forms at the apex of the root
  d. cellular cementum is more common than acellular cementum
  e. both b and c

29. Which of the following is *not* true about the alveolar bone proper (cribriform plate)?
    a. Radiographically it is called lamina dura.
    b. It is derived from the mesoderm.
    c. It is a solid wall of compact bone with no blood vessels.
    d. It is covered by a normal periosteum.

30. The fibers of the periodontal ligament
    a. contain nerves that can only transmit impulses of pain
    b. can run to or from the cementum, alveolar bone, and/or gingiva
    c. all run parallel to the root
    d. are divided into four main groups, which have subgroups
    e. both a and b.

31. Which of the following is true about bone remodeling?
    a. Teeth may be moved bodily or tilted.
    b. A tilted tooth will show resorption on one side and apposition on the other.
    c. For every area of resorption there must be an area of apposition.
    d. Both a and b.
    e. All of the above.

32. Identify the following groups of alveolodental fibers:

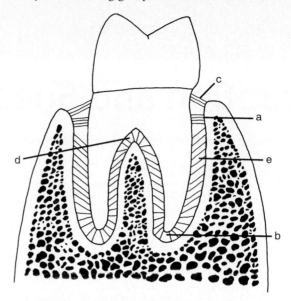

a. _____
b. _____
c. _____
d. _____
e. _____

Chapter 22

Eruption and Shedding of Teeth

True-False Questions

_____ 1. The posteruptive stage goes on for the life of the tooth or the life of the patient.

_____ 2. The eruptive stage begins with the development of the root.

_____ 3. The gubernacular canal was formed by the presence of the successional lamina from the original dental lamina.

_____ 4. If interproximal contact between molars is lost, attempts at reestablishment are made through mesial drift.

_____ 5. Supraeruption is not considered as a part of the eruptive stages.

_____ 6. A retained primary tooth in an adult only occurs when there is no permanent successor.

_____ 7. Retained root fragments result when the root tip is not in the pathway of the erupting permanent tooth.

_____ 8. Osteoblasts resorb roots of primary teeth.

Multiple-Choice Questions

9. Which of the following along with the gubernacular canal aid in the eruption of the teeth?
   a. macrophages
   b. osteoclasts
   c. enzymes
   d. all of the above

10. Which of these statements is *not* true about the eruptive stage of tooth eruption?
    a. Osteoclastic activity may deepen the crypt while the root is growing.
    b. Alveolar bone growth keeps pace with eruption for a while but then slows down.
    c. As the tooth approaches the surface, the reduced enamel epithelium fuses with the oral epithelium to form what is sometimes called the *united oral epithelium.*
    d. All of the above are true.

11. The dental sac (or dental follicle) plays a role in forming all of the following *except:*
    a. cementum
    b. periodontal ligament
    c. alveolar bone
    d. all of the above

12. During the eruptive stage the primary and permanent dentition erupts in an occlusal and facial position. The permanent dentition may sometimes erupt to the lingual of the anterior deciduous teeth.
    a. Both statements are true.
    b. Both statements are false.
    c. The first statement is true; the second is false.
    d. The first statement is false; the second is true.

Case Study

Use the following information to answer questions 13 and 14.

A parent brings their 7-year-old child into the dental office. They say that the child has "two sets of lower front teeth," and upon examination two sets of mandibular central incisors are found. One set is located immediately lingual to the other set; the teeth in front seem to be a bit smaller than the ones behind.

13. Which teeth are located lingually?
    a. primary teeth
    b. permanent teeth
    c. some primary and some permanent teeth
    d. impossible to determine without a radiograph

14. Which statement *best* explains the presence of two sets?
    a. There was no resorption of primary roots.
    b. Primary and permanent incisors erupted at the same time.
    c. The permanent teeth erupted too early in the eruptive process.
    d. The primary incisors are ankylosed.

Chapter 23

Oral Mucosa

True-False Questions

_____ 1. Specialized mucosa is found on all surfaces of the tongue.

_____ 2. Masticatory mucosa is found on the hard palate, the gingiva, and the alveolar mucosa.

_____ 3. Lining mucosa can be found on the floor of the mouth.

_____ 4. In keratinized epithelium, the stratum corneum is made up of dead cells.

_____ 5. The stratum corneum of lining mucosa displays cells without nuclei.

_____ 6. Lining mucosa is a stiff, tight tissue.

_____ 7. The col is located on the interdental papilla.

_____ 8. The attached gingival groove separates the free gingiva from the attached gingiva.

_____ 9. Lining mucosa is generally found in protected areas or less-stimulated areas.

_____ 10. Based on the degree of stimulation, the col and the gingival sulcus are two areas of the thinnest lining mucosa.

_____ 11. Submucosa usually contains connective tissue, nerves, and blood vessels.

_____ 12. Passive eruption is the apical movement of the attachment epithelium on the tooth and has nothing to do with the movement of the tooth itself.

_____ 13. Stage IV of passive eruption may be pathologic.

_____ 14. The health of the gingival tissue can be determined by the level of the attachment epithelium.

_____ 15. The layers of whitened epithelium that tend to increase in thickness are the stratum corneum and the stratum granulosum.

Multiple-Choice Questions

16. Which of the following *best* describes stage III of passive eruption?
    a. The attachment epithelium is totally on cementum.
    b. The attachment epithelium is on the CEJ and cementum.
    c. The attachment epithelium is totally on enamel.
    d. The attachment epithelium is on enamel and cementum.

17. What is the turnover rate of the attachment epithelium at the base of the gingival sulcus?
    a. 2 to 3 days
    b. 3 to 5 days
    c. 7 to 10 days
    d. 10 to 14 days
    e. 14 to 21 days

18. Which of the following is not a general sign of inflammation?
    a. edema
    b. whiteness
    c. pain
    d. heat

19. Sebaceous glands are frequently found on the
    a. alveolar mucosa
    b. submucosa
    c. buccal mucosa
    d. mucosa of soft palate

20. Stippling is a characteristic of the
    a. free gingiva
    b. attached gingiva
    c. alveolar mucosa
    d. labial mucosa

Chapter 24

The Tongue

True-False Questions

_____ 1. The epithelium of the tongue is derived from all three embryonic germ layers.

_____ 2. General sensation is carried to the anterior two-thirds of the tongue via cranial nerve (CN) VII.

_____ 3. The root of the tongue develops from the copula.

_____ 4. There are four sets of intrinsic muscles in the tongue.

_____ 5. If the tongue decreases in size in one dimension, it must increase in size in another dimension.

_____ 6. The lingual tonsils are located on the posterior third of the ventral surface of the tongue.

_____ 7. The lingual tonsils are one of three pairs of tonsillar tissue situated in the throat area that help combat infections.

_____ 8. The tongue is covered with stratified squamous epithelium.

_____ 9. The tiny, round, red raised spots on the tongue are the filiform papillae.

Multiple-Choice Questions

10. Which of the following is part of the embryonic origin of the anterior two-thirds of the tongue?
    a. Tuberculum impar
    b. Hypobranchial eminence
    c. Copula
    d. Lateral lingual swellings
    e. Both a and d

11. Which of the following CNs do not have a general sensory supply to the epithelium of the tongue?
    a. CN V
    b. CN VII
    c. CN IX
    d. CN X

12. If a patient is not able to pull the sides of the tongue downward, which of the following muscles is not functioning?
    a. Styloglossus
    b. Genioglossus
    c. Hyoglossus
    d. Stylohyoid

13. Which of these muscles could help pull the base of the tongue back and up?
    a. Palatoglossus
    b. Styloglossus
    c. Genioglossus
    d. Both a and b

14. The inability to protrude the tongue basically results from the loss of which muscle?
    a. Palatoglossus
    b. Genioglossus
    c. Geniohyoid
    d. Longitudinal intrinsic group

15. If the longitudinal group of muscles contract, the tongue will become:
    a. Wider
    b. Thicker
    c. Longer
    d. Shorter
    e. a, b, and d

16. Which of the following papillae are positioned between the anterior two-thirds and the posterior third of the dorsum of the tongue?
    a. Filiform
    b. Fungiform
    c. Circumvallate
    d. Foliate

17. Which of these papillae is only for general sensation and not for taste?
    a. Filiform
    b. Fungiform
    c. Foliate
    d. Circumvallate

18. Von Ebner's glands are minor salivary glands. They are located in the foliate papilla.
    a. Both statements are true.
    b. Both statements are false.
    c. The first statement is true; the second is false.
    d. The first statement is false; the second is true.

Case Study

Use the following information to answer questions 19 and 20.

A 30-year-old patient is having an oral examination. They are a heavy smoker with poor oral hygiene. Their tongue has dark-colored, distended papillae, and the lateral borders in the area of the foliate papillae appear to be irritated.

19. The distended papillae are probably a characteristic of:
    a. A vitamin deficiency
    b. Glossitis
    c. Hairy tongue
    d. Oral cancer

20. The lateral border irritation could indicate:
    a. A vitamin deficiency
    b. Glossitis
    c. Hairy tongue
    d. Oral cancer

Chapter 25

Histology of the Salivary Glands

True-False Questions

_____ 1. Serous demilunes are found in pure serous glands.

_____ 2. Mucous secretions release an enzyme that helps break down carbohydrates.

_____ 3. The contraction of myoepithelial cells, which surround individual serous and mucous cells, causes these cells to secrete.

_____ 4. Myoepithelial cells have characteristics of nervous tissue.

_____ 5. In striated ducts, an infolding with trapped mitochondria at the apical end of the cell causes striations.

_____ 6. Connective tissue septa, which run into the salivary gland from the capsule, break the gland up into lobules.

_____ 7. In merocrine secretion, the salivary droplets have a membrane placed around them by the cell membrane.

_____ 8. Saliva buffers the pH of the oral cavity.

_____ 9. Saliva helps in combating caries and periodontal disease.

_____ 10. Salivary flow is mainly controlled by the sympathetic nervous system.

_____ 11. Lysozymes are present in saliva.

Multiple-Choice Questions

12. Which of the following is true about the origin of the salivary glands?
    a. They originate as a downgrowth of the oral epithelium.
    b. They are ectodermally derived.
    c. They start out as a cord of cells and then form a duct.
    d. Both a and b.
    e. All of the above.

13. Which of the following is *not* descriptive of mucous acini?
    a. A rounded nucleus lying near the base of the cell
    b. Large lumen
    c. Frothy apical granules
    d. A fairly distinct cell membrane

14. Which of the following may be interlobular ducts?
    a. Excretory ducts
    b. Striated ducts
    c. Intercalated ducts
    d. Both a and b
    e. All of the above.

15. Which of the following are small, cuboidal intralobular ducts that carry secretions to the next set of ducts?
    a. Intercalated ducts
    b. Striated ducts
    c. Acini
    d. Excretory ducts
    e. Both b and d

16. Ducts that add electrolytes to salivary secretions are known as:
    a. Intercalated
    b. Striated
    c. Interlobular
    d. Both b and c

17. Mucous secretions are highly viscous. They are composed of 90% water.
    a. Both statements are true.
    b. Both statements are false.
    c. The first statement is true; the second is false.
    d. The first statement is false; the second is true.

18. Which of the following is *not* true of intercalated ducts?
    a. They do not have nuclei.
    b. They drain the acini.
    c. They may be short or long ducts.
    d. They carry secretions to the next set of ducts.

Chapter 26

Osteology of the Skull

True-False Questions

_____ **1.** Genial tubercles are found on the lingual midline, just above the inferior border of the mandible.

_____ **2.** The mylohyoid ridge separates the submandibular fossa from the sublingual fossa.

_____ **3.** The mandibular lingula lies just posterior to the mandibular foramen.

_____ **4.** The rim of the orbit is made up of the frontal, maxillary, and zygomatic bones.

_____ **5.** The alveolar processes form the tooth sockets.

_____ **6.** The zygomatic process is formed from three bones: the maxilla, zygomatic, and temporal bones.

_____ **7.** The transverse palatine suture marks the articulation of the right and left palatine processes.

_____ **8.** The ethmoid bone forms most of the lateral wall of the orbit.

_____ **9.** The foramen ovale is located in the sphenoid bone.

_____ **10.** A maxilla is a single bone.

_____ **11.** There are 14 bones of the neurocranium.

_____ **12.** The coronoid notch is the depression between the coronoid process and the condyle.

_____ **13.** The mandible is made up of a body and four processes

Multiple-Choice Questions

14. Which of the following is *not* a bone of the neurocranium?
 a. Frontal
 b. Ethmoid
 c. Parietal
 d. Sphenoid
 e. They are all bones of the neurocranium.

15. Which of the following is *not* a bone of the viscerocranium?
 a. Sphenoid
 b. Maxilla
 c. Vomer
 d. Nasal
 e. They are all part of the viscerocranium.

16. The sella turcica is part of the:
 a. Styloid process
 b. Sphenoid bone
 c. Zygomatic process of mandible
 d. Posterior palatine process

17. Which of the following is *not* a process of the maxilla?
 a. Frontal
 b. Zygomatic
 c. Coronoid
 d. Alveolar

18. Another name for the chin is the mental spine. Posterior to the chin (bilaterally) is the mental foramen.
 a. Both statements are true.
 b. Both statements are false.
 c. The first statement is true; the second is false.
 d. The first statement is false; the second is true.

19. The mandibular foramen is located on the:
 a. Medial ramus of mandible
 b. Medial angle of mandible
 c. Floor of mandible
 d. Depression on lateral border of angle of mandible

20. Identify the following landmarks on the palatal view of the maxillae and palatine bones:

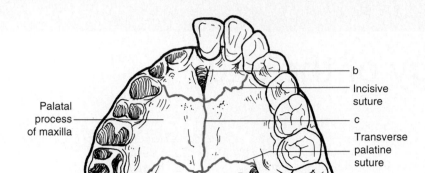

a. _____

b. _____

c. _____

d. _____

e. _____

21. Identify the following landmarks on the lateral view of the mandible:

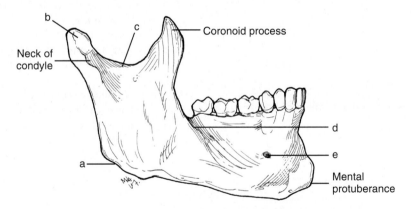

a. _____

b. _____

c. _____

d. _____

e. _____

Chapter 27

Nose, Nasal Cavity, and Paranasal Sinuses

True-False Questions

_____ 1. To view the paranasal sinuses (on a skull), one should first identify the nasal conchae.

_____ 2. The maxillary sinus can enlarge and expand after maxillary molars are extracted.

_____ 3. The sphenoid sinuses have numerous clusters of air cells.

_____ 4. The cribriform plate is a part of the ethmoid bone.

_____ 5. The respiratory epithelium has goblet cells with hairlike projections.

_____ 6. The three nasal conchae on each side of the nasal cavity all arise from ethmoid bone.

_____ 7. The choana is the area at the posterior end of the nasal septum.

_____ 8. The epithelium of the nasal cavity comprises only pseudostratified columnar epithelium.

_____ 9. The frontal and sphenoid sinuses cross over the midline.

_____ 10. The opening for the maxillary sinus is at the posteroinferior end of the hiatus semilunaris.

Multiple-Choice Questions

11. Which of these statements is *not* true about the paranasal sinuses?
    a. They enlarge with age.
    b. They are lined with respiratory epithelium.
    c. They help to warm the air entering the nasal cavity.
    d. They help to make bone lighter.

12. The maxilla and ethmoid bones meet in the lateral wall of the nasal cavity. There is a medial projection where the bones meet called the superior nasal conchae.
    a. Both statements are true.
    b. Both statements are false.
    c. The first statement is true; the second is false.
    d. The first statement is false; the second is true.

13. Each of the following can indicate a maxillary sinus infection. Which one is the exception?
    a. fluid-filled sinus space
    b. closed-off sinus openings
    c. periodontal pocketing surrounding maxillary molars
    d. pain in maxillary molar area
    e. congestion or clogging in the nose and ear

14. The _____ and ethmoid bones form the main part of the nasal septum.
    a. maxilla
    b. sphenoid
    c. vomer
    d. posterior nasal spine

15. The nasolacrimal duct is located within the
    a. inferior meatus
    b. hiatus semilunaris
    c. middle nasal conchae
    d. choana

16. Which of these is true about the middle nasal concha?
    a. The middle meatus lies beneath the middle nasal concha.
    b. The middle ethmoid air cells are located in their base.
    c. Both a and b.
    d. The middle meatus is part of the ethmoid bone.
    e. all of the above

17. The maxillary sinus
    a. is the largest of the paranasal sinuses
    b. opens into the hiatus semilunaris
    c. extends down around the maxillary root tips
    d. all of the above

18. Which of the following sinuses, if infected, could cause a pain response in maxillary teeth?
    a. frontal sinus
    b. maxillary sinus
    c. neither a nor b
    d. both a and b

Muscles of Mastication, Hyoid Muscles, and Sternocleidomastoid and Trapezius Muscles

True-False Questions

_____ 1. The temporalis muscle is the only muscle of mastication that retrudes the mandible.

_____ 2. The masseter muscle inserts into the medial side of the angle of the mandible.

_____ 3. All of the infrahyoid muscles are innervated by cervical nerves.

_____ 4. The temporalis muscle is fan shaped.

_____ 5. The slinglike muscle that has an anterior and posterior belly is the digastric muscle.

_____ 6. The sternothyroid muscle originates on the thyroid cartilage and inserts on the sternum.

_____ 7. Retrusion of the mandible is a side-to-side movement.

_____ 8. The hyoid bone is connected to other bones only by muscles.

_____ 9. The sternocleidomastoid (SCM) muscle elevates the shoulders in the shrugging movement.

_____ 10. The SCM inserts into the mastoid process of the temporal bone.

Multiple-Choice Questions

11. Which muscle takes a small part of its origin from the maxillary tuberosity?
    a. Masseter
    b. Temporal
    c. Medial pterygoid
    d. Lateral pterygoid

12. Which of the following muscles has more than one site of origin?
    a. Masseter
    b. Medial pterygoid
    c. Lateral pterygoid
    d. Both b and c
    e. All of the above

13. Which of these muscles do *not* function to elevate the mandible and close the mouth?
    a. Masseter
    b. Temporal
    c. Medial pterygoid
    d. Lateral pterygoid

14. Which muscle has fibers that primarily run horizontally?
    a. Masseter
    b. Temporal
    c. Medial pterygoid
    d. Lateral pterygoid

15. Which muscle is *not* a suprahyoid muscle?
    a. Geniohyoid
    b. Stylohyoid
    c. Thyrohyoid
    d. Digastric

16. Which muscle does *not* aid in pulling down on the hyoid bone?
    a. Omohyoid
    b. Sternothyroid
    c. Sternohyoid
    d. Thyrohyoid
    e. All function to pull down the hyoid bone

17. Which infrahyoid muscle functions to elevate the larynx?
    a. Sternothyroid
    b. Sternohyoid
    c. Omohyoid
    d. Thyrohyoid

18. If there is a deviation of the mandible to one side during protrusion, which muscle is *not* functioning properly?
    a. Masseter
    b. Lateral pterygoid
    c. Medial pterygoid
    d. Temporal

19. Which muscle has two origins on the zygomatic arch?
    a. Masseter
    b. Lateral pterygoid
    c. Medial pterygoid
    d. Temporal

20. Which muscle forms the floor of the mouth?
    a. Mylohyoid
    b. Geniohyoid
    c. Digastric
    d. Stylohyoid

Chapter 29

Temporomandibular Joint

True-False Questions

_____ **1.** One of the major treatments of bruxism is prescription tranquilizers.

_____ **2.** Arthritis may affect the disc of the temporomandibular joint (TMJ).

_____ **3.** The upper posterior lamina is collagenous and prevents the disc from being pulled too far forward.

_____ **4.** The articular disc is tightly attached to the medial and lateral poles of the condyle.

_____ **5.** The thickest region of the disc is the anterior band.

_____ **6.** In the chewing motion, the mandible moves downward, and then shifts toward the nonchewing side.

_____ **7.** Irregular movements of the disc may make popping sounds.

_____ **8.** There are synovial cavities above and below the articular disc.

_____ **9.** The central portion of the disc has numerous pain fibers.

Matching

Match the symptoms on the right with the diagnosis on the left.

10. Referred pain   **a.** Attrition
11. Arthritis   **b.** Inability to close mouth
12. Bruxism   **c.** Neck spasms; TMJ pain
13. Subluxation   **d.** Torn lateral pole attachment
14. Disc derangement   **e.** Grinding sensation in TMJ

Multiple-Choice Questions

15. Which of these statements is true about the movements of the TMJ?
  a. The movements of the TMJ are rotational and gliding.
  b. Each synovial cavity is primarily involved in one type of movement.
  c. The upper synovial cavity is involved in rotational movement.
  d. Both a and b.
  e. All of the above.

16. Which of the following is true about lateral excursions of the jaw?
  a. They are controlled by the upper head of the lateral pterygoid.
  b. They are controlled by the lower head of the lateral pterygoid.
  c. The jaw moves toward the side on which the lateral pterygoid contracts.
  d. If the jaw moves to the right, the condyle on the other side moves posteriorly.
  e. All of the above.

17. Which is _not_ a structure of the temporal bone?
  a. Articular eminence
  b. Mandibular fossa
  c. Posterior tubercle
  d. Articular disc

18. Which structure(s) prevents the condyle from moving too far anteriorly?
  a. Pterygoid muscles
  b. TMJ capsule
  c. Lower collagenous lamina
  d. Temporomandibular ligament
  e. Both b and c

19. The condyle of the mandible articulates with the _____ of the temporal bone.
  a. Articular eminence
  b. Coronoid fossa
  c. Mandibular fossa
  d. Temporal fossa
  e. None of the above

20. Identify the following labeled structures:

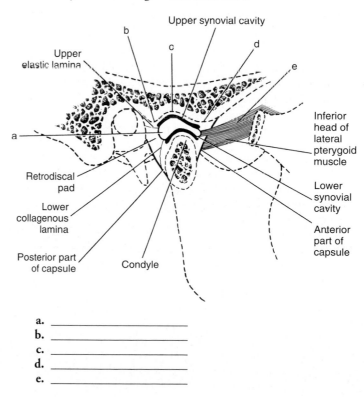

  a. _____
  b. _____
  c. _____
  d. _____
  e. _____

Chapter 30

Muscles of Facial Expression

True-False Questions

_____ 1. The auricular muscles are more functional in lower mammals.

_____ 2. The epicranius muscle aids in expressing surprise or disappointment.

_____ 3. The platysma muscle inserts into the skin over the sternum.

_____ 4. All of the facial expression muscles are innervated by CN VII.

_____ 5. The epicranius has a flat, intermediate tendon between its two bellies.

_____ 6. The procerus muscle pulls the lateral corner of the eyebrow down laterally.

_____ 7. The compressor naris flares the nostrils.

_____ 8. The buccinator muscle is an accessory muscle of mastication.

_____ 9. The levator anguli oris originates from just above the infraorbital foramen.

_____ 10. The mentalis muscle aids in depressing the mandibular lip.

Multiple-Choice Questions

11. Which of these muscles is used in frowning?
    a. occipitofrontalis
    b. corrugator
    c. procerus
    d. both a and b
    e. all of the above

12. Which of these muscles has an insertion in the area above the eyes?
    a. occipitofrontalis
    b. corrugator
    c. procerus
    d. both a and b
    e. all of the above

13. Which of these muscles would _not_ be involved in smiling?
    a. risorius
    b. zygomaticus major
    c. zygomaticus minor
    d. mentalis

14. Which muscle does _not_ insert into the orbicularis oris?
    a. zygomaticus major
    b. zygomaticus minor
    c. buccinator
    d. risorius
    e. All insert into the orbicularis oris.

15. The facial muscles greatly influence all of the following _except_
    a. speech
    b. appearance
    c. swallowing
    d. mastication

Case Study

Use the information below to answer questions 16 to 17.

Mr. Green has been slowly recovering from a stroke. His speech is slightly slurred, and the left side of his face shows little expression. Mr. Green complains that he cannot drink from a straw and cannot clean certain areas of his teeth as well as he used to.

16. Which muscles are preventing Mr. Green from compressing his lips to hold onto a straw?
    a. levator labii superioris
    b. depressor labii inferioris
    c. depressor anguli oris
    d. orbicularis oris

17. On examination of Mr. Green's mandibular left posterior teeth, more plaque and food residue are observed, as Mr. Green had implied. The paralysis of which muscle contributes to this situation?
    a. buccinator
    b. mentalis
    c. levator labii superioris
    d. levator anguli oris

18. Identify the following muscles of facial expression.

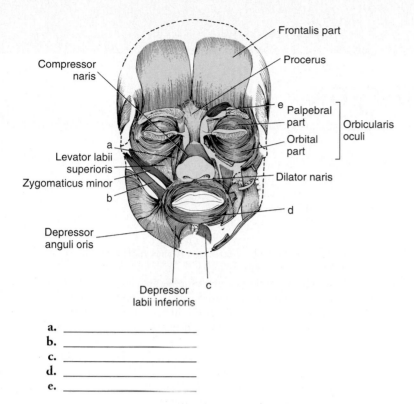

a. _____

b. _____

c. _____

d. _____

e. _____

Chapter 31

Soft Palate and Pharynx

True-False Questions

_____ 1. The palatoglossal muscle forms the posterior tonsillar pillar.

_____ 2. When the uvula contracts, it becomes elongated.

_____ 3. There are six pairs of soft palate muscles.

_____ 4. The tensor veli palatini originates from the medial pterygoid plate and the auditory tube.

_____ 5. The soft palate separates the oral pharynx from the nasal pharynx.

_____ 6. The salpingopharyngeus originates from the bony end of the Eustachian tube.

_____ 7. All of the pharyngeal muscles are innervated by the XI cranial nerve.

_____ 8. As food is moved to the posterior part of the tongue, it is important to close off the oral and nasal pharynxes from one another.

_____ 9. The overlapping of the pharyngeal constrictor muscles adds thickness and strength to the middle part of the pharyngeal wall.

_____ 10. During swallowing, the bolus of food passes through the larynx.

Multiple-Choice Questions

11. Which of the following muscles functions to dilate the pharynx?
    a. palatoglossus
    b. palatopharyngeus
    c. tensor veli palatini
    d. stylopharyngeus

12. Which muscle "tenses" the anterior portion of the soft palate?
    a. tensor veli palatini
    b. levator veli palatini
    c. faucial pillars
    d. palatoglossal muscle

13. The palatopharyngeal muscle originates from the anterolateral part of the soft palate. It narrows the fauces and elevates the pharynx.
    a. Both statements are true.
    b. Both statements are false.
    c. The first statement is true; the second is false.
    d. The first statement is false; the second is true.

14. Which of these muscles does *not* elevate the pharynx?
    a. salpingopharyngeus
    b. palatopharyngeus
    c. stylopharyngeus
    e. They all elevate the pharynx.

15. The pharyngeal constrictor muscles have a role in all of the following functions *except:*
    a. moving food into the esophagus
    b. compressing the upper part of the oral pharynx
    c. promoting elevation and dilation of the pharynx
    d. all of the above are functions

16. Which pharyngeal constrictor muscle inserts into the median raphe?
    a. superior pharyngeal constrictor
    b. middle pharyngeal constrictor
    c. inferior pharyngeal constrictor
    d. all of the above

17. Voluntary control of swallowing ends in the _____ third of the esophagus.
    a. upper
    b. middle
    c. lower

18. Identify the following muscles in this view of the pharynx:

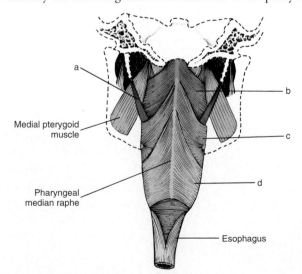

    a. _____
    b. _____
    c. _____
    d. _____

Chapter 32

Arterial Supply and Venous Drainage

True-False Questions

_____ **1.** The right side of the heart carries oxygenated blood; the left side carries deoxygenated blood.

_____ **2.** The common carotid artery divides into the superior and inferior carotid branches.

_____ **3.** The internal carotid artery does not supply the oral cavity.

_____ **4.** The first posterior branch off of the external carotid artery is the posterior auricular artery.

_____ **5.** Both the masseter artery and the mental artery are branches of the inferior alveolar artery.

_____ **6.** The infraorbital artery is the most anterior branch of the maxillary artery.

_____ **7.** Veins of the face usually have the same names as the arteries that travel with them.

_____ **8.** The anterior retromandibular vein and the facial vein form the internal jugular vein.

Multiple-Choice Questions

9. Which of the following is a branch of the maxillary artery?
   a. Lower inferior alveolar artery
   b. Masseter artery
   c. Buccal artery
   d. All of the above

10. Which of these is *not* a branch of the maxillary artery in the infratemporal fossa?
   a. Pterygoid artery
   b. Buccal branch of maxillary artery
   c. Deep temporal artery
   d. Masseteric artery
   e. They are all branches of the maxillary artery.

11. The _____ artery supplies blood to the maxillary molars.
   a. Posterior superior alveolar
   b. Pterygopalatine
   c. Maxillary
   d. Infraorbital

12. The _____ artery has a branch that supplies maxillary anterior teeth and maxillary premolars.
   a. Greater palatine artery
   b. Anterior superior alveolar
   c. Posterior superior alveolar
   d. Infraorbital

13. After blood travels through the pulmonary veins it goes to the:
   a. Aorta
   b. Left atrium
   c. Pulmonary valve
   d. Lungs

14. A pressure point for facial bleeding is found on the lower border of the mandible. This is the point where the facial artery and the facial vein cross the mandible.
   a. Both statements are true.
   b. Both statements are false.
   c. The first statement is true; the second is false.
   d. The first statement is false; the second is true.

15. The pterygoid plexus of veins flows directly into the:
   a. Superficial temporal vein
   b. External jugular vein
   c. Internal jugular vein
   d. Maxillary vein

Case Study

Use the following information to answer question 16.

A young woman comes into the office as a new patient with a dental emergency. She has a large purplish bruise and some swelling under her eye and across the upper cheek to her nose. She states that she had a "deep cavity" and that her dentist gave her an injection and filled the tooth (#6). Her dentist is away on vacation, and she is worried that she may have an infection.

16. You suspect that the lesion is:
   a. The result of an assault
   b. A cavernous sinus infection
   c. A hematoma
   d. An allergic reaction to anesthesia

Chapter 33

Salivary Glands

True-False Questions

_____ 1. Mumps become more painful when the parotid gland decreases its secretion.

_____ 2. The submandibular salivary gland provides about 25% of the resting salivary volume.

_____ 3. The duct for the parotid gland is located opposite the maxillary second premolar.

_____ 4. The parasympathetic nervous system controls salivary gland secretion.

_____ 5. Major salivary glands are compound tubuloalveolar glands.

_____ 6. Most minor salivary glands are purely or mostly mucous in nature.

_____ 7. von Ebner's glands are found around the base of the fungiform papillae.

Matching

Match one choice from the right column with each gland on the left. Choices (a, b, c) can be used more than once.

_____ 8. Submandibular gland   a. Purely serous

_____ 9. Sublingual gland   b. Mostly mucous

_____ 10. Parotid gland   c. Mostly serous

_____ 11. von Ebner's glands

_____ 12. Anterior lingual gland

Multiple-Choice Questions

13. The _____ gland is located lateral, posterior, and medial to the ramus.
    a. Parotid
    b. Submandibular
    c. Sublingual
    d. Lingual

14. The submandibular gland is also called the _____ gland.
    a. Submaxillary
    b. Mandibular
    c. Sublingual
    d. Lingual

15. The opening of the duct for the parotid gland is in the _____ muscle.
    a. Lateral pterygoid
    b. Zygomatic
    c. Masseter
    d. Buccinator

16. Where does the submandibular duct open into the mouth?
    a. Lingual to the mandibular first molar
    b. Along the sublingual fold
    c. Onto the sublingual caruncle
    d. Opposite the mandibular second molar

17. Which structure does _not_ have minor salivary glands?
    a. Tongue
    b. Anterior hard palate
    c. Labial mucosa
    d. Buccal mucosa

18. Which of the following is _not_ true of minor salivary glands?
    a. Less branching
    b. Short ducts
    c. Fewer glands have individual duct openings.
    d. Help keep mucous membranes moist

Chapter 34

Nervous System

True-False Questions

_____ **1.** There are 12 pairs of cervical nerves.

_____ **2.** Gray matter is made up of motor and sensory neurons.

_____ **3.** Afferent nerves send impulses from the periphery to the central nervous system.

_____ **4.** If the ventral root of a spinal nerve was damaged, it would cause a loss of sensory function.

_____ **5.** Visceral nerves provide innervation to the internal organs.

_____ **6.** The autonomic nervous system is one that is not willfully controlled.

_____ **7.** Spinal nerves are formed by the fusion of the dorsal and ventral root.

_____ **8.** Increasing the blood flow to the digestive system is a parasympathetic nervous system response.

_____ **9.** The three divisions of the trigeminal nerve are: ophthalmic, maxillary, and mandibular.

_____ **10.** There are 30 pairs of spinal nerves.

Matching

Match the cranial nerve (CN) numbers in the right column with the functions in the left column. Only use one CN for each function (only eight nerves will be used).

_____ **11.** Controls heart rate

_____ **12.** Sense of smell

_____ **13.** Vision

_____ **14.** Constricts pupil

_____ **15.** Hearing

_____ **16.** Muscles of facial expression

_____ **17.** Sensation to face

_____ **18.** Parotid gland secretion

a. I
b. II
c. III
d. IV
e. V
f. VI
g. VII
h. VIII
i. IX
j. X
k. XI
l. XII

Multiple-Choice Questions

19. The sympathetic nervous system functions in all _except:_
a. Increasing respiration
b. Increasing heart rate
c. Increasing salivary flow
d. Dilating pupils

20. Which nerve does _not_ innervate the gingiva?
a. Nasopalatine
b. Infraorbital
c. Posterior superior alveolar
d. Facial

21. Following a local anesthesia injection, a portion of the tongue becomes numb. Which nerve has been anesthetized?
a. Posterior superior alveolar
b. Middle superior alveolar
c. Lingual
d. Chorda tympani

22. The muscles of mastication are innervated by CN _____.
a. V
b. VII
c. IX
d. X

23. The maxillary division of the trigeminal nerve exits the skull through the:
a. Foramen ovale
b. Superior orbital fissure
c. Gasserian ganglion
d. Foramen rotundum

24. Which nerve supplies taste sensation to the posterior one-third of the tongue?
a. CN V
b. CN VII
c. CN IX
d. CN XI

25. The _____ nerve innervates the anterior mucosa of the hard palate.
a. Posterior superior alveolar
b. Descending palatine
c. Pterygopalatine
d. Nasopalatine

26. The long buccal nerve innervates the:
a. Buccal side of the posterior mandibular gingiva
b. Pulp of posterior mandibular teeth
c. Mucosa of the posterior cheek
d. Both a and c
e. All of the above

27. The nerve that is responsible for causing numbness of the mandibular lip and chin during local anesthesia is the _____ nerve.
    a. Mandibular
    b. Lingual
    c. Mental
    d. Mylohyoid

28. Four different nerves are involved in the functions of the tongue. Three of these nerves provide the taste sensation.
    a. Both statements are true.
    b. Both statements are false.
    c. The first statement is true; the second is false.
    d. The first statement is false; the second is true.

29. The nasopalatine nerve branches through the:
    a. Incisive foramen
    b. Nasopalatine foramen
    c. Pterygopalatine canal
    d. None of the above

30. The _____ nerve provides sensation to the maxillary premolars.
    a. Posterior superior alveolar
    b. Middle superior alveolar
    c. Buccal
    d. Mental

31. All mandibular teeth in one quadrant are innervated by the _____ nerve.
    a. Second division of the trigeminal
    b. Inferior alveolar
    c. Buccal
    d. Long buccal

32. The posterior superior alveolar nerve innervates:
    a. The maxillary arch
    b. Maxillary molars
    c. Maxillary third and second molars and two roots of the first molars
    d. Maxillary posterior teeth

Case Study

Use the following information to answer questions 33 and 34.

Mrs. Graystone is a 78-year-old woman, who has been in good health. When she walks into the treatment room, she loses her balance for a moment but regains it quickly. You also notice that she is wearing a hearing aid. You ask Mrs. Graystone if there has been any other change in her health, and she mentions that she has a slight twitch at the corner of her mouth and cheek area.

33. Assuming that there is no systemic illness, Mrs. Graystone's loss of balance and hearing difficulty could be attributed to a deterioration of the _____ nerve.
    a. Abducens
    b. Facial
    c. Statoacoustic
    d. Accessory

34. The facial twitch may be caused by malfunction of the _____ nerve.
    a. Oculomotor
    b. Trigeminal
    c. Abducens
    d. Facial

35. Label the branches of the trigeminal nerve:

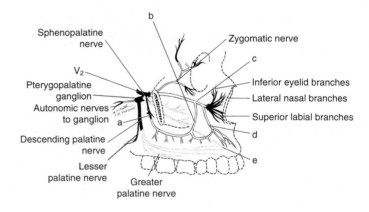

    a. _____
    b. _____
    c. _____
    d. _____
    e. _____

Chapter 35

Lymphatics and the Spread of Dental Infection

True-False Questions

_____ **1.** Lymphatic vessels in the head and neck eventually drain into the junction of the internal jugular and subclavian veins.

_____ **2.** All lymph nodes are connected by lymphatic ducts or tubules.

_____ **3.** An abscess of mandibular premolars would drain into the submental nodes.

_____ **4.** The tooth pulp has lymph vessels.

_____ **5.** In a throat infection at the posterior wall, the upper deep cervical nodes will be tender and enlarged.

_____ **6.** A buccal abscess of a mandibular molar usually drains into the buccal vestibule.

_____ **7.** Ludwig's angina is an infection in the sublingual space.

_____ **8.** The submandibular lymph nodes drain the parotid glands.

Matching

Trace the progress of a mandibular molar fascial infection as it advances in severity from **a** to **d**.

_____ **9.** First site   **a.** Submental space
_____ **10.** Second site   **b.** Posterior mediastinum
_____ **11.** Third site   **c.** Lateral pharyngeal space
_____ **12.** Fourth site   **d.** Retropharyngeal space

Multiple-Choice Questions

13. Which of these sites of oral cancer would tend to have the highest mortality rate?
    a. root of the tongue
    b. hard palate
    c. midline of the mandibular lip
    d. floor of mouth

14. Where would the secondary nodes of involvement be in a posterior throat wall infection?
    a. submandibular
    b. submental
    c. upper deep cervical
    d. lower deep cervical

15. Which of the following is *not* primarily drained by the upper deep cervical nodes?
    a. third molars
    b. hard palate
    c. soft palate
    d. base of tongue
    e. tonsils

16. Drainage of the mandibular incisors is accomplished by the submandibular nodes. The submandibular nodes also drain the floor of the mouth.
    a. Both statements are true.
    b. Both statements are false.
    c. The first statement is true; the second is false.
    d. The first statement is false; the second is true.

17. If you see a patient with an eye that is swollen because of a dental infection, which tooth is most likely involved?
    a. mandibular canine
    b. maxillary canine
    c. maxillary first molar
    d. mandibular first molar

Case Study

Use the following information to answer questions 17 and 18.

A new patient, a 65-year-old man, comes into the office with a medical history that indicates 40 years of heavy pipe smoking. The intraoral examination evidences a small white lesion in the foliate papillary area of the tongue. A biopsy determines that the lesion is oral cancer.

18. Which are the primary nodes of invasion for this lesion?
    a. lower cervical nodes
    b. upper cervical nodes
    c. submental nodes
    d. submandibular nodes

19. Which are the tertiary nodes of invasion?
    a. lower cervical nodes
    b. upper cervical nodes
    c. submental nodes
    d. submandibular nodes

Chapter 36

Anatomic Considerations of Local Anesthesia

True-False Questions

_____ 1. Local infiltrations can be given in the interdental papilla, free gingiva, and attached gingiva.

_____ 2. Maxillary supraperiosteal injections are given in the attached vestibular tissue at the height of the mucobuccal fold.

_____ 3. All mandibular teeth are innervated by the inferior alveolar nerve.

_____ 4. Mandibular supraperiosteal injections are more effective in children than in adults.

_____ 5. Maxillary nerve blocks anesthetize portions of the fourth cranial nerve.

_____ 6. Both the nasopalatine and greater palatine nerve blocks require the use of pressure anesthesia.

_____ 7. The lingula just above the mandibular canal is the target location for the inferior alveolar nerve block.

_____ 8. Bilateral mandibular nerve blocks should be avoided because the patient could bite through his mandibular lip.

_____ 9. To achieve anesthesia of mandibular anterior teeth during an incisive block, the anesthetic should be deposited close to the mental foramen and massaged with pressure into the foramen.

_____ 10. Nerves and anatomic landmarks are always found at their expected location.

Multiple-Choice Questions

11. The posterior superior alveolar nerve, artery, and vein are all located together within the
   a. pterygopalatine fossa
   b. coronoid notch
   c. incisive canal
   d. infraorbital foramen

12. Which of the following is an anatomic consideration when administering both palatal nerve blocks?
   a. Both injection sites are covered by tissue that is firmly bound to bone.
   b. A plexus can form between the greater palatine and nasopalatine nerves causing crossover.
   c. Neither of the injections affects maxillary teeth.
   d. all of the above

13. Which of the following statements about the inferior alveolar nerve block is *not* true?
   a. The target area for the injection is the mandibular canal.
   b. The injection path is 6 to 10 mm above the coronoid notch.
   c. It will anesthetize all hard and soft tissues of one entire mandibular quadrant.
   d. The injection will anesthetize both inferior alveolar and lingual nerves.

14. Which tissues are anesthetized by the middle superior alveolar nerve block?
   a. maxillary premolars
   b. mesial buccal root of the maxillary first molar
   c. buccal periodontium of maxillary premolars
   d. buccal gingival of the maxillary premolars
   e. a, c, and d only
   f. all of the above

15. Which nerve is *not* affected by the Vazirani-Akinosi nerve block?
   a. inferior alveolar nerve
   b. auriculotemporal nerve
   c. lingual nerve
   d. mylohyoid nerve
   e. incisive nerve
   f. All are affected by this nerve block.

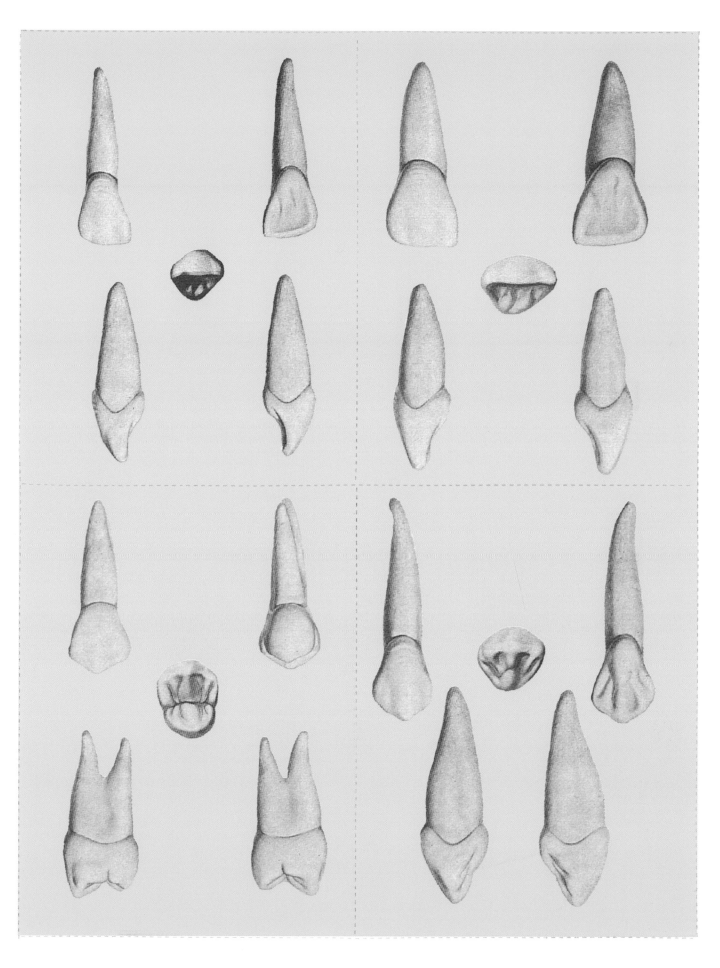

Permanent Maxillary

Right Central Incisor

Eruption: 7–8 years
Root Completed: 10 years

	RIGHT
Universal Code	8
International Code	11
Palmer notation	1⌋
Number of roots	1
Number of pulp horns	3
Number of developmental lobes	4

Location of proximal contact areas
MESIAL: Incisal third

DISTAL: Junction of incisal and middle thirds

Height of contour
FACIAL: Cervical third, 0.5 mm
LINGUAL: Cervical third, 0.5 mm

Identifying characteristics: These incisors are the largest and most prominent incisors. The distoincisal is more rounded than the mesioincisal angle. The lingual surface has a prominent cingulum, broad lingual fossa, and distinct marginal ridges. The pulp cavity is one large single chamber and root canal.

Permanent Maxillary

Right Lateral Incisor

Eruption: 8–9 years
Root Completed: 11 years

	RIGHT
Universal Code	7
International Code	12
Palmer notation	2⌋
Number of roots	1
Number of pulp horns	1 to 3
Number of developmental lobes	4

Location of proximal contact areas
MESIAL: Junction of incisal and middle thirds
DISTAL: Middle third

Height of contour
FACIAL: Cervical third, 0.5 mm
LINGUAL: Cervical third, 0.5 mm

Identifying characteristics: The lingual anatomical features are similar to those of the central incisors, but are more highly developed and have more prominent marginal ridges and deeper lingual fossae. Lateral incisors are more likely to have a lingual pit. The cingulum may be smaller, almost absent. The labial surface resembles that of a central incisor except that the labial surface is more convex. The crown-to-root ratio is less than in a central incisor because the crown is usually smaller, whereas the root is almost as long. In all other ways the lateral incisors appear as smaller, more rounded versions of the central incisors.

Permanent Maxillary

Right Canine

Eruption: 11–12 years

Root Completed: 13–15 years	RIGHT
Universal Code	6
International Code	13
Palmer notation	3⌋
Number of roots	1
Number of pulp horns	1
Number of cusps	1
Number of developmental lobes	4

Location of proximal contact areas
MESIAL: Junction of incisal and middle thirds
DISTAL: Middle third

Height of contour
FACIAL: Cervical third, 0.5 mm
LINGUAL: Cervical third, 0.5 mm

Identifying characteristics: The maxillary canines are the longest teeth in the mouth. They have a single cusp, with mesial and distal ridges forming an incisal edge. A prominent facial ridge is off-center toward the mesial. Cingulum is prominent. The prominent mesiofacial lobe forms this facial ridge of the cusp. The centrofacial lobe forms the lingual ridge of the cusp. This lingual ridge divides the mesial and distal fossae. The distofacial ridge is longer and more rounded than the mesiofacial's.

Permanent Maxillary

Right First Premolar

Eruption: 10–11 years

Root Completed: 12–13 years	RIGHT
Universal Code	5
International Code	14
Palmer notation	4⌋
Number of roots	2
Number of pulp horns	2
Number of cusps	2
Number of developmental lobes	4

Location of proximal contact areas
MESIAL AND DISTAL: Just cervical to the junction of occlusal and middle thirds

Height of contour
FACIAL: Cervical third, 0.5 mm
LINGUAL: Middle third, 0.5 mm

Identifying characteristics: These premolars have bifurcated roots. A longitudinal groove is present on the root. The mesial surface shows a developmental fossa. The mesial marginal groove crosses the mesial marginal ridge and extends onto the mesial surface. The facial cusp is wider and longer than the lingual cusp. The mesial ridge of the facial cusp may have a slight concavity.

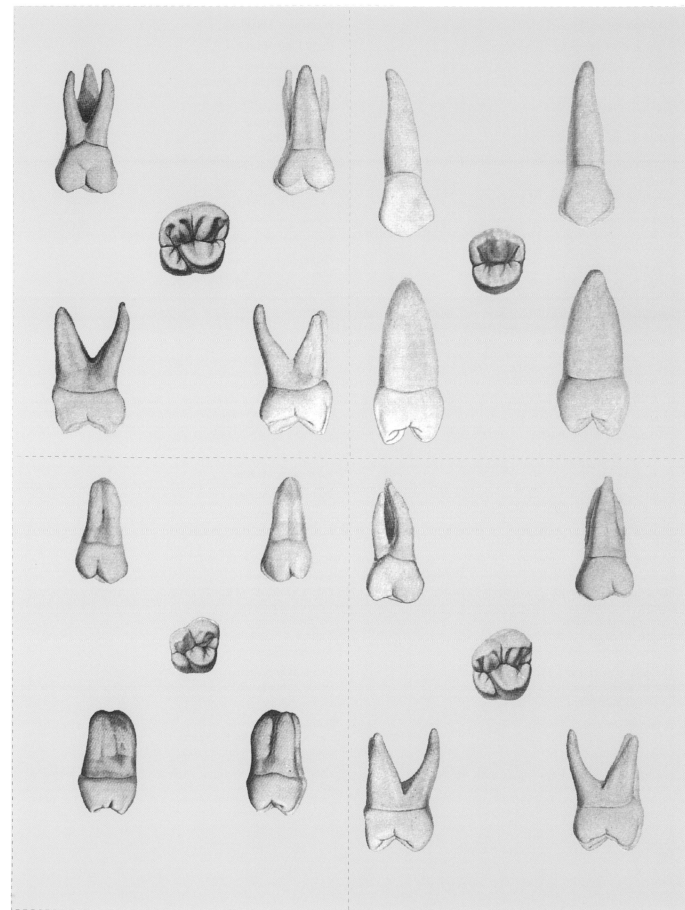

Permanent Maxillary

Right Second Premolar

Eruption: 10–12 years
Root Completed: 12–14 years

	RIGHT
Universal Code	4
International Code	15
Palmer notation	5⌋
Number of roots	1
Number of pulp horns	2
Number of cusps	2
Number of developmental lobes	4

Location of proximal contact areas
MESIAL AND DISTAL: Just cervical to the junction of occlusal and middle thirds

Height of contour
FACIAL: Cervical third, 0.5 mm
LINGUAL: Middle third, 0.5 mm

Identifying characteristics: These premolars usually have a single root that is slightly longer than that of the first premolar. The buccal and lingual cusps are nearly equal in length. The buccal cusp is shorter than that of a first premolar. The entire crown, especially the occlusal outline, is less angular and more rounded. The occlusal surface has more supplemental grooves. The occlusal developmental grooves are shorter, shallower, and more irregular. There is no developmental depression on the mesial surface of the crown.

Permanent Maxillary

Right First Molar

Eruption: 6–7 years
Root Completed: 9–10 years

	RIGHT
Universal Code	3
International Code	16
Palmer notation	6⌋
Number of roots	3
Number of pulp horns	4
Number of cusps	4
	5 (including cusp of Carabelli)
Number of developmental lobes	5

Location of proximal contact areas
MESIAL: Middle third
DISTAL: Middle third

Height of contour
FACIAL: Cervical third, 0.5 mm
LINGUAL: Middle third, 0.5 mm

Identifying characteristics: A cusp of Carabelli may be present. The occlusal outline is square or rhomboidal rather than triangular. The distolingual cusp is well developed. There is a prominent oblique ridge and distal facial and lingual grooves. The crown is nearly as wide mesiodistally as buccolingually. The three roots are widely separated.

Permanent Maxillary

Right Second Molar

Eruption: 12–13 years
Root Completed: 14–16 years

	RIGHT
Universal Code	2
International Code	17
Palmer notation	7⌋
Number of roots	3
Number of pulp horns	4
Number of cusps	4
Number of developmental lobes	4

Location of proximal contact areas
MESIAL: Middle third
DISTAL: Middle third

Height of contour
FACIAL: Cervical third, 0.5 mm
LINGUAL: Middle third, 0.5 mm

Identifying characteristics: These teeth are similar to maxillary first molars except that the fifth cusp is usually absent and the distolingual, cusp is less well developed. The oblique ridge is less prominent. The crown is shorter occlusocervically and narrower mesiodistally. It is just as wide buccolingually. The occlusal outline of the crown is rhomboidal to heart shaped. The three roots are less separated.

Permanent Maxillary

Right Third Molar

Eruption: 17–22 years
Root Completed: 18–25 years

	RIGHT
Universal Code	1
International Code	18
Palmer notation	8⌋
Number of roots	1 to 4
Number of pulp horns	1 to 4
Number of cusps	3 to 5
Number of developmental lobes	4

Location of proximal contact areas
MESIAL: Middle third
DISTAL: None

Height of contour
FACIAL: Cervical third, 0.5 mm
LINGUAL: Middle third, 0.5 mm

Identifying characteristics: These teeth vary more in form than any others. They usually do not have a distolingual cusp. The occlusal outline is heart shaped, with three cusps. The roots, usually three, have a tendency to be very close together or to fuse with an extreme distal inclination.

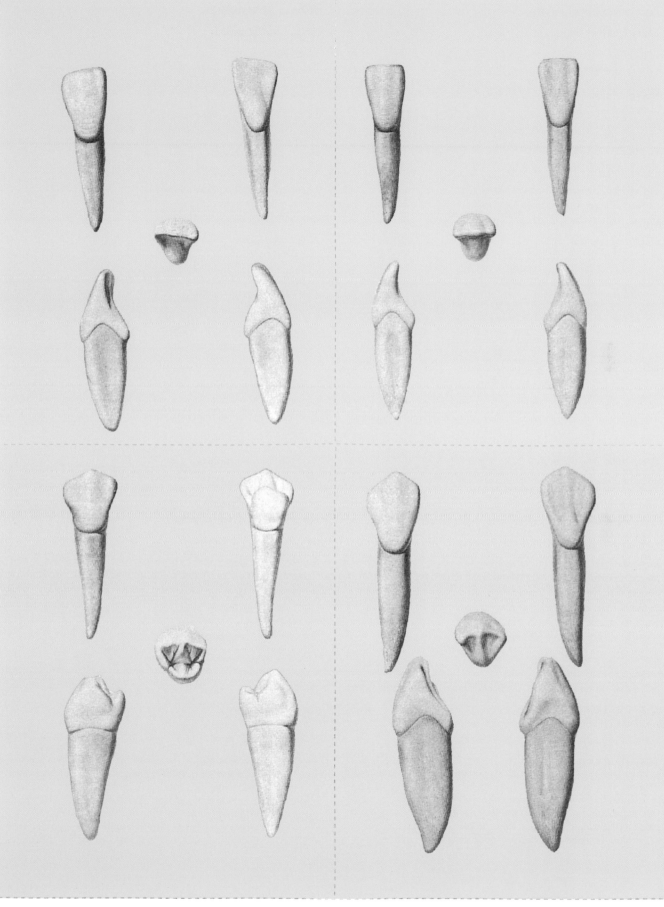

Permanent Mandibular

Right Central Incisor

Eruption: 6–7 years
Root Completed: 9 years

	RIGHT
Universal Code	25
International Code	41
Palmer notation	1⌋
Number of roots	1
Number of pulp horns	3
Number of developmental lobes	4

Location of proximal contact areas
MESIAL: Incisal third
DISTAL: Incisal third

Height of contour
FACIAL: Cervical third, less than 0.5 mm
LINGUAL: Cervical third, less than 0.5 mm

Identifying characteristics: The distoincisal and mesioincisal angles are nearly identical. The lingual surface is shallow, with no prominent features. The crown is wider faciolingually than mesiodistally. The root is oval shaped in cross-section. The incisal edge shows wear on the facioincisal edge. From a proximal view, the incisal edge appears to be tilted toward the lingual side. Smallest permanent tooth.

Permanent Mandibular

Right Lateral Incisor

Eruption: 7–8 years
Root Completed: 10 years

	RIGHT
Universal Code	26
International Code	42
Palmer notation	2⌋
Number of roots	1
Number of pulp horns	3
Number of developmental lobes	4

Location of proximal contact areas
MESIAL: Incisal third
DISTAL: Incisal third

Height of contour
FACIAL: Cervical third, less than 0.5 mm
LINGUAL: Cervical third, less than 0.5 mm

Identifying characteristics: The crown is similar to that of the mandibular central incisors. The distal lobe is more highly developed than the mesial. The distal incisal ridge angles toward the lingual, as if rotating on the root axis. The crown and the root are slightly larger than those of the central incisors.

Permanent Mandibular

Right Canine

Eruption: 9–10 years
Root Completed: 12–14 years

	RIGHT
Universal Code	27
International Code	43
Palmer notation	3⌋
Number of roots	1 or 2
Number of pulp horns	1
Number of cusps	1
Number of developmental lobes	4

Location of proximal contact areas
MESIAL: Incisal third
DISTAL: Just cervical to the junction of incisal and middle thirds

Height of contour
FACIAL: Cervical third, less than 0.5 mm
LINGUAL: Cervical third, less than 0.5 mm

Identifying characteristics: The crown is similar to the crown of the maxillary canines, but narrower and smoother. It has less prominent lingual features. From a proximal view, the cusp tip is inclined to the lingual. From an incisal view, the distal end of the incisal edge is rotated to the lingual. They have the longest roots in the mandibular arch, longitudinal grooves on the roots, most likely mandibular anterior tooth to have 2 root canals.

Permanent Mandibular

Right First Premolar

Eruption: 10–12 years
Root Completed: 12–13 years

	RIGHT
Universal Code	28
International Code	44
Palmer notation	4⌋
Number of roots	1
Number of pulp horns	1 or 2
Number of cusps	2
Number of developmental lobes	4

Location of proximal contact areas
MESIAL AND DISTAL: Just cervical to junction of occlusal and middle thirds

Height of contour
FACIAL: Cervical third, 0.5 mm
LINGUAL: Middle third, 1 mm

Identifying characteristics: These premolars have two cusps, one large buccal and one small lingual. The buccal cusps are centered directly over the root. The lingual cusps are centered lingual to the root and are afunctional and nonoccluding. The occlusal surface slopes sharply lingual in a cervical direction. The mesiobuccal cusp ridge is shorter than the distobuccal cusp ridge. It has a mesiolingual developmental groove and one root.

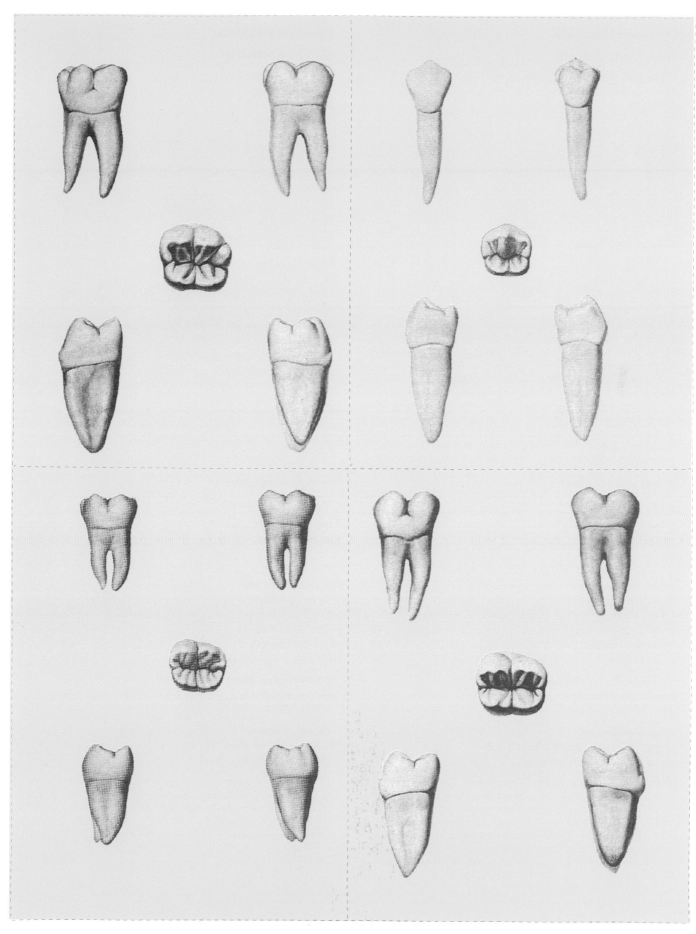

Permanent Mandibular

Right Second Premolar

Varies in number of developmental lobes: 4 or 5
Eruption: 11–12 years
Root Completed: 13–14 years

	RIGHT	
Universal Code	29	
International Code	45	
Palmer notation	5⌐	
Number of roots		1
Number of pulp horns		2 or 3
Number of cusps		2 or 3
Number of development lobes		4 or 5

Location of proximal contact areas
MESIAL AND DISTAL: Just cervical to junction of occlusal and middle thirds

Height of contour
FACIAL: Cervical third, 0.5 mm
LINGUAL: Middle third, 1 mm

Identifying characteristics: These premolars have two or three cusps. The buccal cusp is very large. If two lingual cusps are present, the mesiolingual is the larger. Although the lingual cusps are larger than on a first premolar, they are afunctional and do not occlude with the maxillary teeth. A second premolar has more secondary anatomical features and more variation than any other tooth except a third molar. The two-cusp form has a U- or H-groove pattern. A mesiolingual groove is rare and is poorly developed if present. The three-cusp form has a lingual developmental groove between the two lingual cusps. The single root is longer and larger than that of a first premolar.

Permanent Mandibular

Right First Molar

Eruption: 6–7 years
Root Completed: 9–10 years

	RIGHT	
Universal Code	30	
International Code	46	
Palmer notation	6⌐	
Number of roots		2
Number of pulp horns		5
Number of cusps		5
Number of developmental lobes		5

Location of proximal contact areas
MESIAL: Middle third
DISTAL: Middle third

Height of contour
FACIAL: Cervical third, 0.5 mm
LINGUAL: Middle third, 1 mm

Identifying characteristics: The five cusps make these the largest mandibular teeth. They are wider mesiodistally than buccolingually. The crown converges lingually and slightly distally. The three buccal cusps are separated by two buccal grooves. The two lingual cusps are separated by one lingual groove. These three grooves converge to form a Y pattern. There are two roots, a mesial and a distal, and three root canals (the mesial root has two root canals).

Permanent Mandibular

Right Second Molar

Eruption: 12–13 years
Root Completed: 14–16 years

	RIGHT	
Universal Code	31	
International Code	47	
Palmer notation	7⌐	
Number of roots		2
Number of pulp horns		4
Number of cusps		4
Number of developmental lobes		4

Location of proximal contact areas
MESIAL: Middle third
DISTAL: Middle third

Height of contour
FACIAL: Cervical third, 0.5 mm
LINGUAL: Middle third, 1 mm

Identifying characteristics: These molars have four cusps of nearly equal size. The crown is smaller in all dimensions and has less lingual convergence. There is only one buccal groove and one lingual groove, which join together on the occlusal surface as they bisect the central developmental groove. The groove pattern is therefore a cross (+). The two roots are closer together and incline slightly distally. There is one root canal in the distal root. The mesial root can have one or two root canals.

Permanent Mandibular

Right Third Molar

Eruption: 18–24 years
Root Completed: 18–25 years

	RIGHT	
Universal Code	32	
International Code	48	
Palmer notation	8⌐	
Number of roots		2 (fused into 1)
Number of pulp horns		4 or 5
Number of cusps		4 or 5
Number of developmental lobes		4 or 5

Location of proximal contact areas
MESIAL: Middle third
DISTAL: Middle third

Height of contour
FACIAL: Cervical third, 0.5 mm
LINGUAL: Middle third, 1 mm

Identifying characteristics: These are the most variable mandibular teeth in form. They usually resemble the mandibular second molars, with four cusps and a shallower, smaller central fossa, with more secondary and tertiary grooves. A five-cusp form is not unusual. The two roots (mesial and distal) are often fused and inclined toward the distal side.

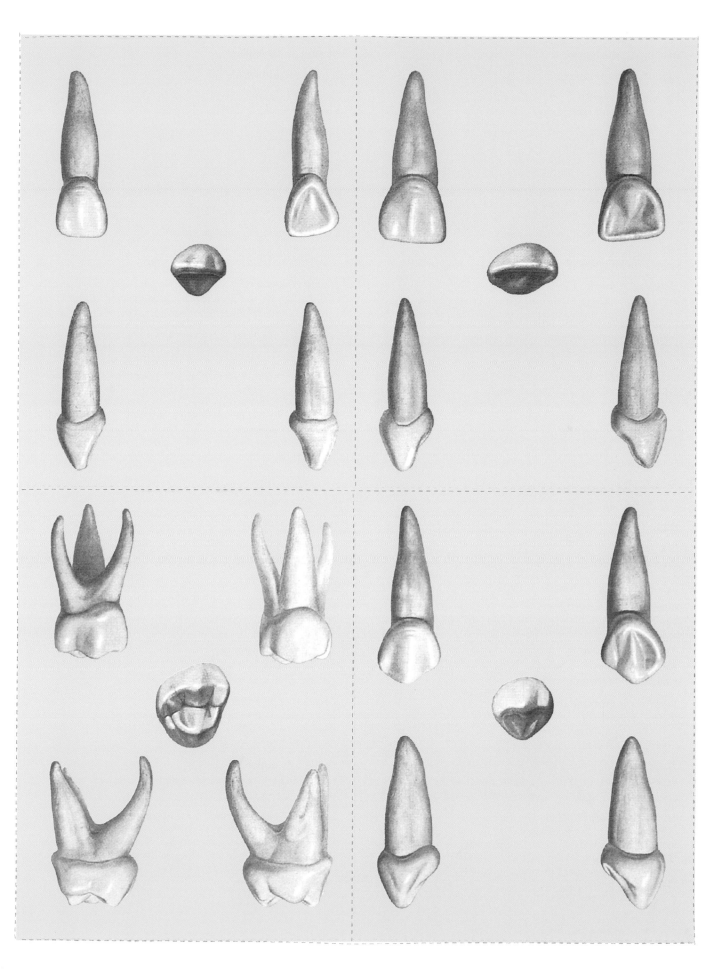

Deciduous Maxillary

Right Central Incisor

Eruption: 10 months
Root Completed: 1 1/2 years

	RIGHT
Universal Code	E
International Code	51
Palmer notation	A⌋
Number of roots	1
Number of pulp horns	3
Number of developmental lobes	4

Location of proximal contact areas
MESIAL: Incisal third toward incisal angle
DISTAL: Incisal third toward middle third

Height of contour
FACIAL: Cervical third (more accentuated than permanent teeth)
LINGUAL: Cervical third (more accentuated than permanent teeth)

Identifying characteristics: Crown is wider mesiodistally than longer cervicoincisally. It is more rounded and more bulbous than the permanent central. It is also smaller and constricts more at the cementoenamel junction. Lingual features are more distinct. The facial and lingual height of contours are more convex than the permanent incisors. The pulp horn is larger in relation to the permanent teeth.

Deciduous Maxillary

Right Lateral Incisor

Eruption: 11 months
Root Completed: 2 years

	RIGHT
Universal Code	D
International Code	52
Palmer notation	B⌋
Number of roots	1
Number of pulp horns	3
Number of developmental lobes	4

Location of proximal contact areas
MESIAL: Incisal third toward incisal angle
DISTAL: Incisal third toward middle third

Height of contour
FACIAL: Cervical third (more accentuated than permanent teeth)
LINGUAL: Cervical third (more accentuated than permanent teeth)

Identifying characteristics: The crown is longer cervicoincisally than wider mesiodistally. The crown is smaller and narrower mesiodistally. It is more slender than the primary centrals. The lateral is less squat and resembles the permanent incisors more closely than the primary maxillary centrals. In proportion to the primary maxillary central, the root is much longer. The lingual features are less distinctive, and the cervical constriction is greater.

Deciduous Maxillary

Right Canine

Eruption: 19 months
Root Completed: 3 1/4 years

	RIGHT
Universal Code	C
International Code	53
Palmer notation	C⌋
Number of roots	1
Number of pulp horns	3
Number of cusp	1
Number of developmental lobes	4

Location of proximal contact areas
MESIAL: Incisal part of middle third

DISTAL: Incisal part of middle third

Height of contour
FACIAL: Cervical third (more accentuated than the incisors)
LINGUAL: Cervical third (more accentuated than the incisors)

Identifying characteristics: The cusp tip is in the center of the crown from the proximal view. The mesial slope is indented incisally, and the distal slope is more rounded (obtuse). The crown is much wider labiolingually than the incisors. The root of the primary canine is proportionally longer than the root of the secondary maxillary canine. The root of the primary canine is long, slender, and tapering and is more than twice the crown length.

Deciduous Maxillary

Right First Molar

Eruption: 16 months
Root Completed: 2 1/2 years

	RIGHT
Universal Code	B
International Code	54
Palmer notation	D⌋
Number of roots	3
Number of pulp horns	3
Number of cusps	3–4
Number of developmental lobes	4

Location of proximal contact areas
MESIAL: Junction of middle and occlusal third
DISTAL: Middle third

Height of contour
FACIAL: Extremely prominent mesiobuccal cervical bulge
LINGUAL: Cervical convexity

Identifying characteristics: Resembles a premolar and a molar. This is a three-cusped molar. The mesiolingual cusp is the largest and sharpest. The most characteristic thing about this tooth is the well-pronounced convexity on the mesiobuccal outline in the cervical third. Three roots—two buccal and one lingual root.

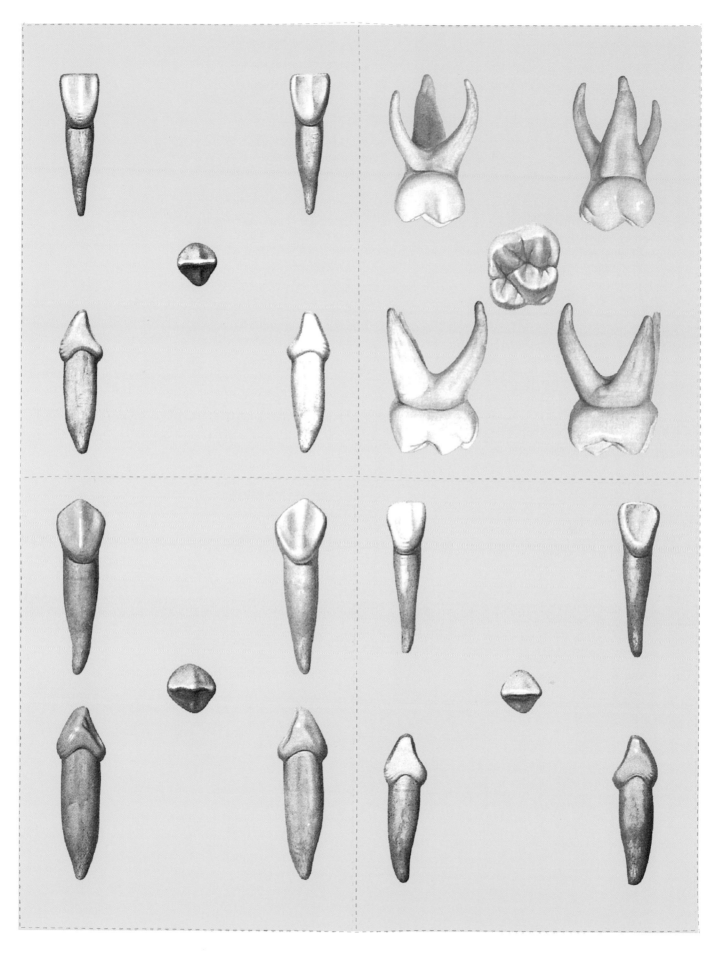

Deciduous Maxillary

Right Second Molar

Eruption: 29 months
Root Completed: 3 years

	RIGHT
Universal Code	A
International Code	55
Palmer notation	E⌋
Number of roots	3
Number of pulp horns	5 or 4
Number of cusps	5 or 4
Number of developmental lobes	5

Location of proximal contact areas
MESIAL: Junction of occlusal and middle third
DISTAL: Middle third

Height of contour
FACIAL: Junction of occlusal and middle third
LINGUAL: Junction of occlusal and middle third

Identifying characteristics: Resembles permanent maxillary first molar, even has prominent oblique ridge. Three roots—two buccal and one lingual. Roots are long, slender, and flared widely apart. The faciolingual measurement of the crown is greater than the mesiodistal.

Deciduous Mandibular

Right Central Incisor

Eruption: 8 months
Root Completed: 1 1/2 years

	RIGHT
Universal Code	P
International Code	81
Palmer notation	A⌋
Number of roots	1
Number of pulp horns	3
Number of developmental lobes	4

Location of proximal contact areas
MESIAL: Incisal angle
DISTAL: Incisal angle

Height of contour
FACIAL: Cervical of crown
LINGUAL: Cervical of crown

The prominences of the facial and lingual at the cervical are as pronounced as any other deciduous teeth and more so than the permanent mandibular incisors.

Identifying characteristics: The incisal ridge is straight from an incisal view. From a facial view the crown is flat. The distal and mesial are almost identical. The crown is wide in proportion to its length in comparison with its permanent successor. The root is long and tapered. It is almost twice as long as the crown.

Deciduous Mandibular

Right Lateral Incisor

Eruption: 13 months
Root Completed: 1 1/2 years

	RIGHT
Universal Code	Q
International Code	82
Palmer notation	B⌋
Number of roots	1
Number of pulp horns	3
Number of developmental lobes	4

Location of proximal contact areas
MESIAL: Near incisal angle
DISTAL: Slightly lower than mesial

Height of contour
FACIAL: Cervical third
LINGUAL: Cervical third

As all anterior deciduous teeth, they exhibit pronounced cervical prominences.

Identifying characteristics: The incisal ridge runs slightly toward the distal. The lateral is longer and larger than the mandibular primary central incisor and the root is also longer. The lateral has a more rounded (obtuse) distoincisal angle.

Deciduous Mandibular

Right Canine

Eruption: 20 months
Root Completed: 3 1/4 years

	RIGHT
Universal Code	R
International Code	83
Palmer notation	C⌋
Number of roots	1
Number of pulp horns	3
Number of cusps	1
Number of developmental lobes	4

Location of proximal contact areas
MESIAL: Junction of middle third and incisal third
DISTAL: Junction of middle third and incisal third

Height of contour
FACIAL: Distinct cervical bulge
LINGUAL: Distinct cervical bulge

Identifying characteristics: Similar to primary maxillary canine, except it is slightly shorter and much narrower labiolingually. The mandibular canine also has a shorter root.

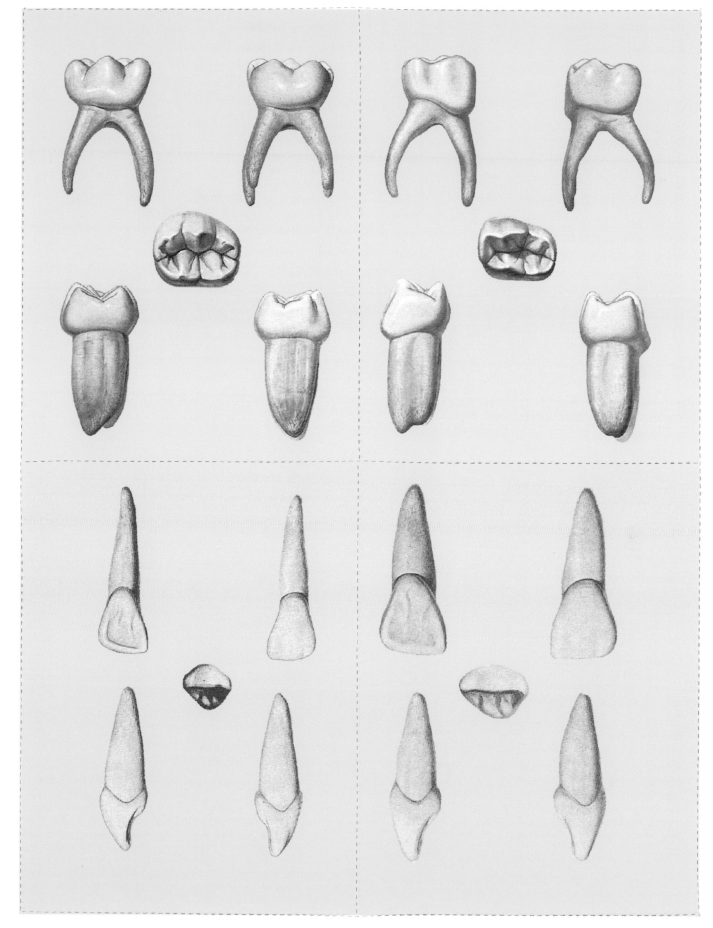

Deciduous Mandibular

Right First Molar

Eruption: 16 months
Root Completed: 2 1/2 years

	RIGHT
Universal Code	S
International Code	84
Palmer notation	D⌋
Number of roots	2
Number of pulp horns	4
Number of cusps	4
Number of developmental lobes	4

Location of proximal contact areas
MESIAL: Middle third
DISTAL: Middle third

Height of contour
FACIAL: An extremely bulbous curvature on the mesiobuccal cervical third
LINGUAL: Middle third

Identifying characteristics: This tooth does not resemble any of the other teeth, deciduous or permanent. This tooth varies so much it appears strange and primitive. The mesial root is much larger than the distal, and the mesial half of the crown is much larger than the distal. The most characteristic thing about this tooth is the extreme convexity on the mesiobuccal at the cervical third. There are two roots, a mesial and a distal.

Deciduous Mandibular

Right Second Molar

Eruption: 27 months
Root Completed: 3 years

	RIGHT
Universal Code	T
International Code	85
Palmer notation	E⌋
Number of roots	2
Number of pulp horns	5
Number of cusps	5
Number of developmental lobes	5

Location of proximal contact areas
MESIAL: Junction of occlusal and middle third
DISTAL: Middle third

Height of contour
FACIAL: Buccal cervical ridge
LINGUAL: Middle third

Identifying characteristics: Resembles the permanent mandibular first molar. There are three buccal cusps and two lingual cusps and two roots, a mesial and a distal. The roots are longer than the deciduous first molars and flared far apart.

Permanent Maxillary

Left Central Incisor

Eruption: 7–8 years
Root Completed: 10 years

	LEFT
Universal Code	9
International Code	21
Palmer notation	⌊1
Number of roots	1
Number of pulp horns	3
Number of developmental lobes	4

Location of proximal contact areas
MESIAL: Incisal third

DISTAL: Junction of incisal and middle thirds

Height of contour
FACIAL: Cervical third, 0.5 mm
LINGUAL: Cervical third, 0.5 mm

Identifying characteristics: These incisors are the largest and most prominent incisors. The distoincisal is more rounded than the mesioincisal angle. The lingual surface has a prominent cingulum, broad lingual fossa, and distinct marginal ridges. The pulp cavity is one large single chamber and root canal.

Permanent Maxillary

Left Lateral Incisor

Eruption: 8–9 years
Root Completed: 11 years

	LEFT
Universal Code	10
International Code	22
Palmer notation	⌊2
Number of roots	1
Number of pulp horns	1 to 3
Number of developmental lobes	4

Location of proximal contact areas
MESIAL: Junction of incisal and middle thirds
DISTAL: Middle third

Height of contour
FACIAL: Cervical third, 0.5 mm
LINGUAL: Cervical third, 0.5 mm

Identifying characteristics: The lingual anatomical features are similar to those of the central incisors but are more highly developed and have more prominent marginal ridges and deeper lingual fossae. Lateral incisors are more likely to have a lingual pit. The cingulum may be smaller, almost absent. The labial surface resembles that of a central incisor except that the labial surface is more convex. The crown-to-root ratio is less than in a central incisor, because the crown is usually smaller, whereas the root is almost as long. In all other ways the lateral incisors appear to be smaller, more rounded versions of the central incisors.

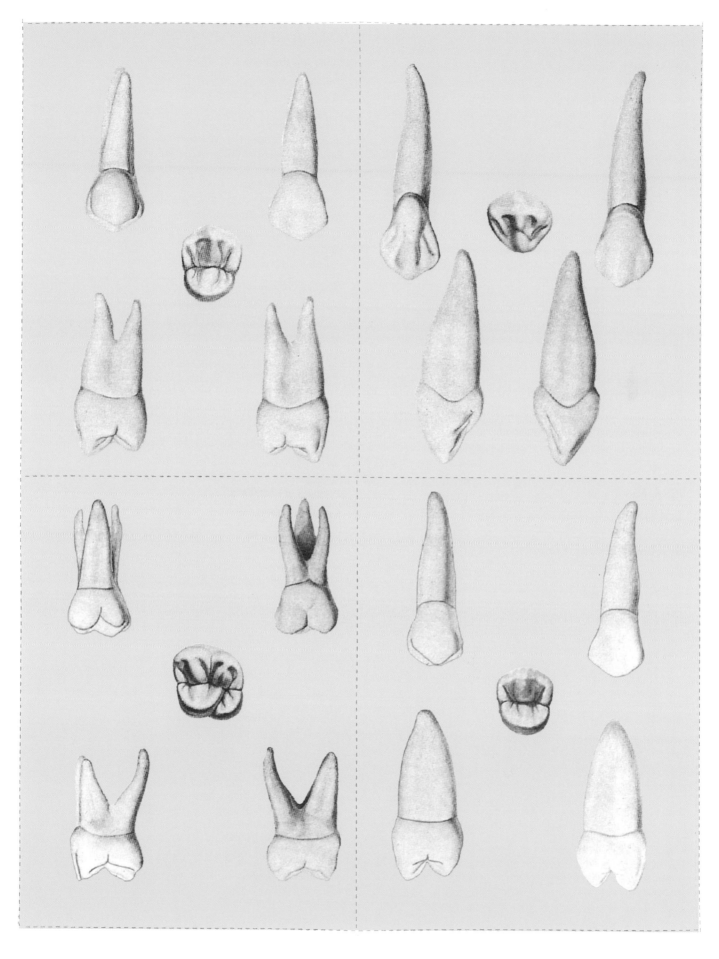

Permanent Maxillary

Left Canine

Eruption: 11–12 years
Root Completed: 13–15 years

	LEFT
Universal Code	11
International Code	23
Palmer notation	3⌋
Number of roots	1
Number of pulp horns	1
Number of cusps	1
Number of developmental lobes	4

Location of proximal contact areas
MESIAL: Junction of incisal and middle thirds
DISTAL: Middle third

Height of contour
FACIAL: Cervical third, 0.5 mm
LINGUAL: Cervical third, 0.5 mm

Identifying characteristics: The maxillary canines are the longest teeth in the mouth. They have a single cusp with mesial and distal ridges forming an incisal edge. A prominent facial ridge is off-center toward the mesial. Cingulum is prominent. The prominent mesiofacial lobe forms this facial ridge of the cusp. The centrofacial lobe forms the lingual ridge of the cusp. This lingual ridge divides the mesial and distal fossae. The distofacial ridge is longer and more rounded than the mesiofacial.

Permanent Maxillary

Left First Premolar

Eruption: 10–11 years
Root Completed: 12–13 years

	LEFT
Universal Code	12
International Code	24
Palmer notation	4⌋
Number of roots	2
Number of pulp horns	2
Number of cusps	2
Number of developmental lobes	4

Location of proximal contact areas
MESIAL AND DISTAL: Just cervical to the junction of occlusal and middle thirds

Height of contour
FACIAL: Cervical third, 0.5 mm
LINGUAL: Middle third, 0.5 mm

Identifying characteristics: These premolars have bifurcated roots. A longitudinal groove is present on the root. The mesial surface shows a developmental fossa. The mesial marginal groove crosses the mesial marginal ridge and extends onto the mesial surface. The facial cusp is wider and longer than the lingual cusp. The mesial ridge of the facial cusp may have a slight concavity.

Permanent Maxillary

Left Second Premolar

Eruption: 10–12 years
Root Completed: 12–14 years

	LEFT
Universal Code	13
International Code	25
Palmer notation	5⌋
Number of roots	1
Number of pulp horns	2
Number of cusps	2
Number of developmental lobes	4

Location of proximal contact areas
MESIAL AND DISTAL: Just cervical to the junction of occlusal and middle thirds

Height of contour
FACIAL: Cervical third, 0.5 mm
LINGUAL: Middle third, 0.5 mm

Identifying characteristics: These premolars usually have a single root that is slightly longer than that of the first premolar. The buccal and lingual cusps are nearly equal in length. The buccal cusp is shorter than that of a first premolar. The entire crown, especially the occlusal outline, is less angular and more rounded. The occlusal surface has more supplemental grooves. The occlusal developmental grooves are shorter, shallower, and more irregular. There is no developmental depression on the mesial surface of the crown.

Permanent Maxillary

Left First Molar

Eruption: 6–7 years
Root Completed: 9–10 years

	LEFT
Universal Code	14
International Code	26
Palmer notation	6⌋
Number of roots	3
Number of pulp horns	4
Number of cusps	4
	5 (including cusp of Carabelli)
Number of developmental lobes	5

Location of proximal contact areas
MESIAL: Middle third
DISTAL: Middle third

Height of contour
FACIAL: Cervical third, 0.5 mm
LINGUAL: Middle third, 0.5 mm

Identifying characteristics: A cusp of Carabelli may be present. The occlusal outline is square or rhomboidal rather than triangular. The distolingual cusp is well developed. There is a prominent oblique ridge and distal facial and lingual grooves. The crown is nearly as wide mesiodistally as buccolingually. The three roots are widely separated.

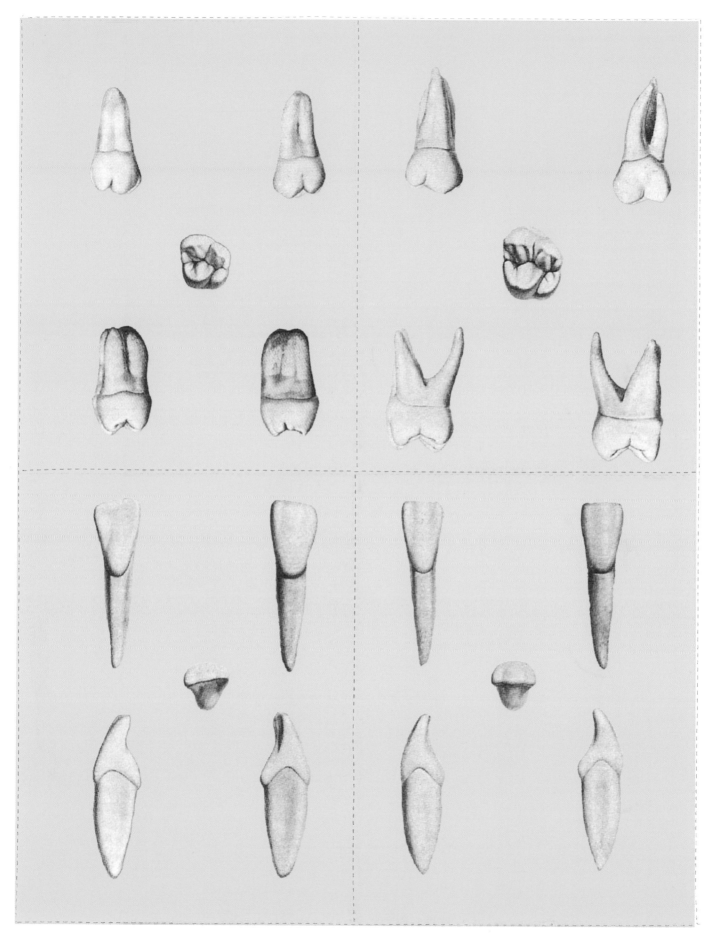

Permanent Maxillary

Left Second Molar

Eruption: 12–13 years
Root Completed: 14–16 years

	LEFT
Universal Code	15
International Code	27
Palmer notation	|7
Number of roots	3
Number of pulp horns	4
Number of cusps	4
Number of developmental lobes	4

Location of proximal contact areas
MESIAL: Middle third
DISTAL: Middle third

Height of contour
FACIAL: Cervical third, 0.5 mm
LINGUAL: Middle third, 0.5 mm

Identifying characteristics: These teeth are similar to maxillary first molars except that the fifth cusp is usually absent and the distolingual cusp is less developed. The oblique ridge is less prominent. The crown is shorter occlusocervically and narrower mesiodistally. It is just as wide buccolingually. The occlusal outline of the crown is rhomboidal to heart shaped. The three roots are less separated.

Permanent Maxillary

Left Third Molar

Eruption: 17–22 years
Root Completed: 18–25 years

	LEFT
Universal Code	16
International Code	28
Palmer notation	|8
Number of roots	1 to 4
Number of pulp horns	1 to 4
Number of cusps	3 to 5
Number of developmental lobes	4

Location of proximal contact areas
MESIAL: Middle third
DISTAL: None

Height of contour
FACIAL: Cervical third, 0.5 mm
LINGUAL: Middle third, 0.5 mm

Identifying characteristics: These teeth vary more in form than any others. They usually do not have a distolingual cusp. The occlusal outline is heart shaped, with three cusps. The roots, usually three, have a tendency to be very close together or to fuse with an extreme distal inclination.

Permanent Mandibular

Left Central Incisor

Eruption: 6–7 years
Root Completed: 9 years

	LEFT
Universal Code	24
International Code	31
Palmer notation	|1
Number of roots	1
Number of pulp horns	3
Number of developmental lobes	4

Location of proximal contact areas
MESIAL: Incisal third
DISTAL: Incisal third

Height of contour
FACIAL: Cervical third, less than 0.5 mm
LINGUAL: Cervical third, less than 0.5 mm

Identifying characteristics: The distoincisal and mesioincisal angles are nearly identical. The lingual surface is shallow, with no prominent features. The crown is wider faciolingually than mesiodistally. The root is oval shaped in cross-section. The incisal edge shows wear on the facioincisal edge. From a proximal view the incisal edge appears to be tilted toward the lingual side. Smallest of all permanent teeth.

Permanent Mandibular

Left Lateral Incisor

Eruption: 7–8 years
Root Completed: 10 years

	LEFT
Universal Code	23
International Code	32
Palmer notation	|2
Number of roots	1
Number of pulp horns	3
Number of developmental lobes	4

Location of proximal contact areas
MESIAL: Incisal third
DISTAL: Incisal third

Height of contour
FACIAL: Cervical third, less than 0.5 mm
LINGUAL: Cervical third, less than 0.5 mm

Identifying characteristics: The crown is similar to that of the mandibular central incisors. The distal lobe is more highly developed than the mesial. The distal incisal ridge angles toward the lingual as if rotating on the root axis. The crown and the root are slightly larger than those of the central incisors.

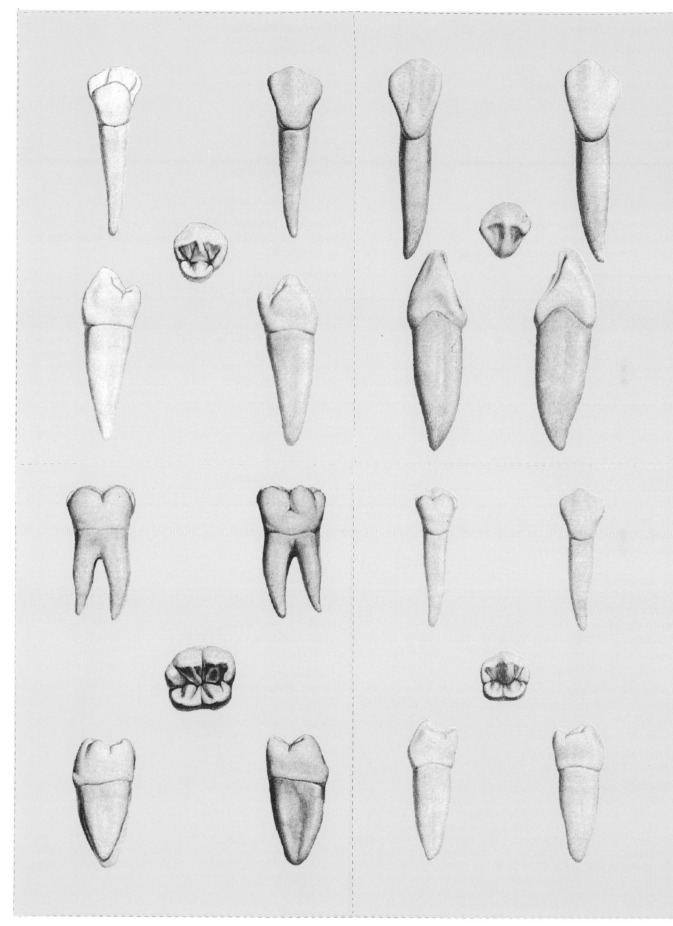

Permanent Mandibular

Left Canine

Eruption: 9–10 years
Root Completed: 12–14 years

	LEFT
Universal Code	22
International Code	33
Palmer notation	3⌋
Number of roots	1 or 2
Number of pulp horns	1
Number of cusps	1
Number of developmental lobes	4

Location of proximal contact areas
MESIAL: Incisal third
DISTAL: Just cervical to the junction of incisal and middle thirds

Height of contour
FACIAL: Cervical third, less than 0.5 mm
LINGUAL: Cervical third, less than 0.5 mm

Identifying characteristics: The crown is similar to the crown of the maxillary canines., but narrower and smoother. It has less prominent lingual features. From a proximal view, the cusp tip is inclined to the lingual. From an incisal view, the distal end of the incisal edge is rotated to the lingual. They have the longest roots in the mandibular arch, with longitudinal grooves on the root, most likely mandibular with 2 root canals.

Permanent Mandibular

Left First Premolar

Eruption: 10–12 years
Root Completed: 12–13 years

	LEFT
Universal Code	21
International Code	34
Palmer notation	4⌋
Number of roots	1
Number of pulp horns	1 or 2
Number of cusps	2
Number of developmental lobes	4

Location of proximal contact areas
MESIAL AND DISTAL: Just cervical to junction of occlusal and middle thirds

Height of contour
FACIAL: Cervical third, 0.5 mm
LINGUAL: Middle third, 1 mm

Identifying characteristics: These premolars have two cusps, one large buccal and one small lingual. The buccal cusps are centered directly over the root. The lingual cusps are centered lingual to the root and are afunctional and nonoccluding. The occlusal surface slopes sharply lingual in a cervical direction. The mesiobuccal cusp ridge is shorter than the distobuccal cusp ridge. It has a mesiolingual developmental groove and one root.

Permanent Mandibular

Left Second Premolar

Varies in number of developmental lobes: 4 or 5
Eruption: 11–12 years
Root Completed: 13–14 years

	LEFT
Universal Code	20
International Code	35
Palmer notation	5⌋
Number of roots	1
Number of pulp horns	2 or 3
Number of cusps	2 or 3
Number of development lobes	4–5

Location of proximal contact areas
MESIAL AND DISTAL: Just cervical to junction of occlusal and middle thirds

Height of contour
FACIAL: Cervical third, 0.5 mm
LINGUAL: Middle third, 1 mm

Identifying characteristics: These premolars have two or three cusps. The buccal cusp is very large. If two lingual cusps are present, the mesiolingual is larger. Although the lingual cusps are larger than on a first premolar, they are afunctional and do not occlude with the maxillary teeth. A second premolar has more secondary anatomical features and more variation than any other tooth except a third molar. The two-cusp form has a U- or H-groove pattern. A mesiolingual groove is rare and is poorly developed if present. The three-cusp form has a lingual developmental groove between the two lingual cusps. The single root is longer and larger than that of a first premolar.

Permanent Mandibular

Left First Molar

Eruption: 6–7 years
Root Completed: 9–10 years

	LEFT
Universal Code	19
International Code	36
Palmer notation	6⌋
Number of roots	2
Number of pulp horns	5
Number of cusps	5
Number of development lobes	5

Location of proximal contact areas
MESIAL: Middle third
DISTAL: Middle third

Height of contour
FACIAL: Cervical third, 0.5 mm
LINGUAL: Middle third, 1 mm

Identifying characteristics: The five cusps make these the largest mandibular teeth. They are wider mesiodistally than buccolingually. The crown converges lingually and slightly distally. The three buccal cusps are separated by two buccal grooves. The two lingual cusps are separated by one lingual groove. These three grooves converge to form a Y pattern. There are two roots, a mesial and a distal, and three root canals (the mesial root has two root canals).

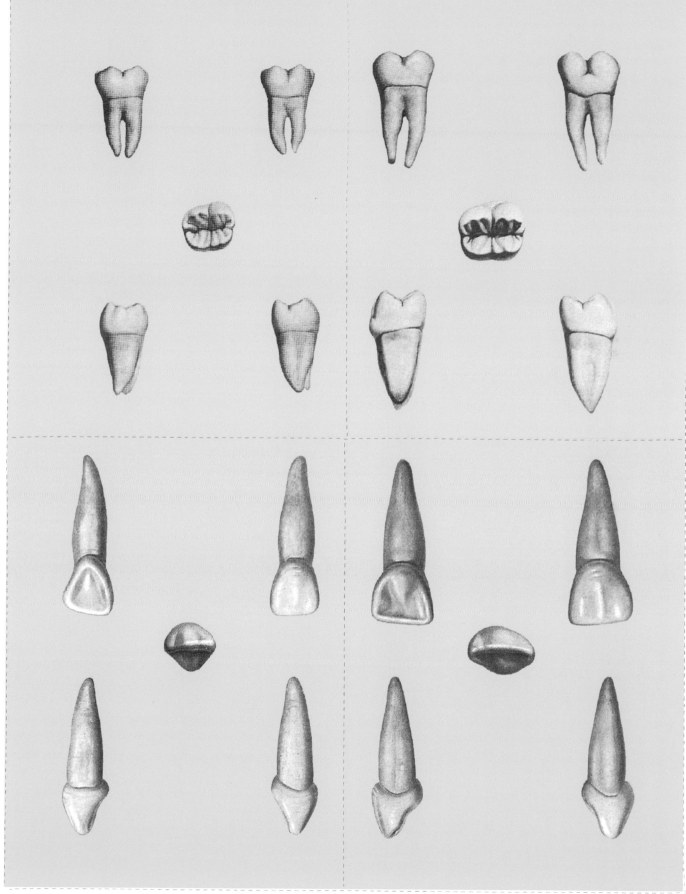

Permanent Mandibular

Left Second Molar

Eruption: 12–13 years
Root Completed: 14–16 years

	LEFT
Universal Code	18
International Code	37
Palmer notation	$\overline{7|}$
Number of roots	2
Number of pulp horns	4
Number of cusps	4
Number of developmental lobes	4

Location of proximal contact areas
MESIAL: Middle third
DISTAL: Middle third

Height of contour
FACIAL: Cervical third, 0.5 mm
LINGUAL: Middle third, 1 mm

Identifying characteristics: These molars have four cusps of nearly equal size. The crown is smaller in all dimensions and has less lingual convergence. There is only one buccal groove and one lingual groove, which join together on the occlusal surface as they bisect the central developmental groove. The groove pattern is therefore a cross (+). The two roots are closer together and incline slightly distally. There is one root canal in the distal root. The mesial root can have one or two root canals.

Permanent Mandibular

Left Third Molar

Eruption: 18–24 years
Root Completed: 18–25 years

	LEFT
Universal Code	17
International Code	38
Palmer notation	$\overline{8|}$
Number of roots	2 (fused into 1)
Number of pulp horns	4 or 5
Number of cusps	4 or 5
Number of developmental lobes	4 or 5

Location of proximal contact areas
MESIAL: Middle third
DISTAL: Middle third

Height of contour
FACIAL: Cervical third, 0.5 mm
LINGUAL: Middle third, 1 mm

Identifying characteristics: These are the most variable mandibular teeth in form. They usually resemble the mandibular second molars, with four cusps and a shallower, smaller central fossa, with more secondary and tertiary grooves. A five-cusp form is not unusual. The two roots (mesial and distal) are often fused and inclined toward the distal side.

Deciduous Maxillary

Left Central Incisor

Eruption: 10 months
Root Completed: 1 1/2 years

	LEFT
Universal Code	F
International Code	61
Palmer notation	$\underline{|A}$
Number of roots	1
Number of pulp horns	3
Number of developmental lobes	4

Location of proximal contact areas
MESIAL: Incisal third toward incisal angle

DISTAL: Incisal third toward middle third

Height of contour
FACIAL: Cervical third (more accentuated than permanent teeth)
LINGUAL: Cervical third (more accentuated than permanent teeth)

Identifying characteristics: Crown is wider mesiodistally than longer cervicoincisally. It is more rounded and more bulbous than the permanent central. It is also smaller and constricts more at the cementoenamel junction. Lingual features are more distinct. The facial and lingual height of contours are more convex than the permanent incisors. The pulp horn is larger in relation to the permanent teeth.

Deciduous Maxillary

Left Lateral Incisor

Eruption: 11 months
Root Completed: 2 years

	LEFT
Universal Code	G
International Code	62
Palmer notation	$\underline{|B}$
Number of roots	1
Number of pulp horns	3
Number of developmental lobes	4

Location of proximal contact areas
MESIAL: Incisal third toward incisal angle
DISTAL: Incisal third toward middle third

Height of contour
FACIAL: Cervical third (more accentuated than permanent teeth)
LINGUAL: Cervical third (more accentuated than permanent teeth)

Identifying characteristics: The crown is longer cervicoincisally than wider mesiodistally. The crown is smaller and narrower mesiodistally. It is more slender than the primary centrals. The lateral is less squat and resembles the permanent incisors more closely than the primary maxillary centrals. In proportion to the primary maxillary central the root is much longer. The lingual features are less distinctive, and the cervical constriction is greater.

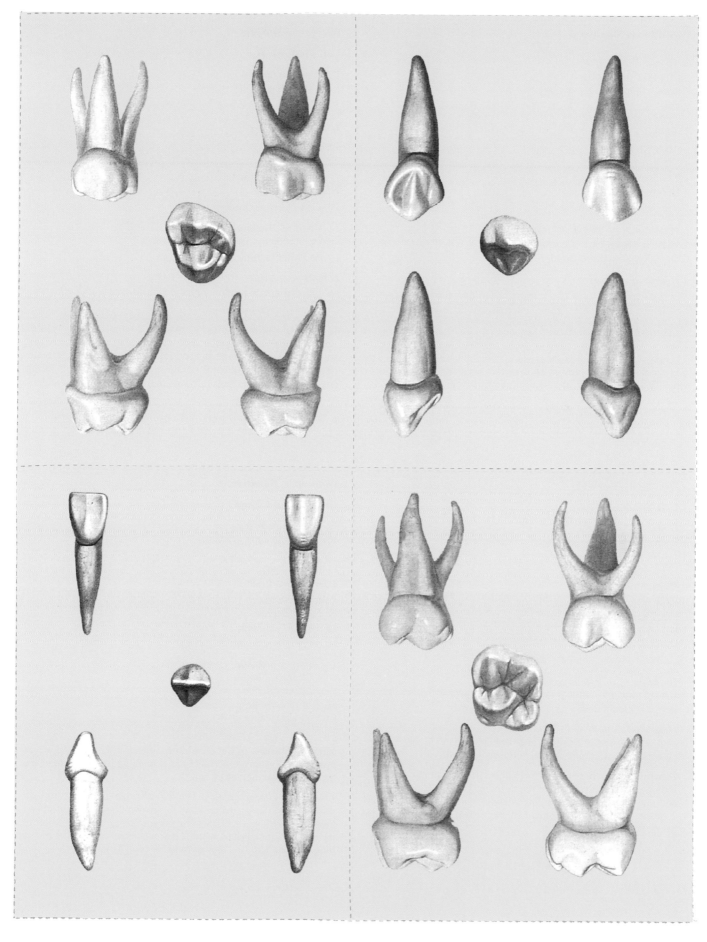

Deciduous Maxillary

Left Canine

Eruption: 19 months
Root Completed: 3 1/4 years

	LEFT
Universal Code	H
International Code	63
Palmer notation	$\underline{\text{C}}$
Number of roots	1
Number of pulp horns	3
Number of cusp	1
Number of developmental lobes	4

Location of proximal contact areas
MESIAL: Incisal part of middle third
DISTAL: Incisal part of middle third

Height of contour
FACIAL: Cervical third (more accentuated than the incisors)
LINGUAL: Cervical third (more accentuated than the incisors)

Identifying characteristics: The cusp tip is in the center of the crown from the proximal view. The mesial slope is indented incisally, and the distal slope is more rounded (obtuse). The crown is much wider labiolingually than the incisors. The root of the primary canine is proportionally longer than the root of the secondary maxillary canine. The root of the primary canine is long, slender, and tapering and is more than twice the crown length.

Deciduous Maxillary

Left First Molar

Eruption: 16 months
Root Completed: 2 1/2 years

	LEFT
Universal Code	I
International Code	64
Palmer notation	$\underline{\text{D}}$
Number of roots	3
Number of pulp horns	3
Number of cusps	3–4
Number of developmental lobes	4

Location of proximal contact areas
MESIAL: Junction of middle and occlusal third
DISTAL: Middle third

Height of contour
FACIAL: Extremely prominent mesiobuccal cervical bulge
LINGUAL: Cervical convexity

Identifying characteristics: Resembles a premolar and a molar. This is a three-cusped molar. The mesiolingual cusp is the largest and sharpest. The most characteristic thing about this tooth is the well-pronounced convexity on the mesiobuccal outline in the cervical third. Three roots—two buccal and one lingual roots.

Deciduous Maxillary

Left Second Molar

Eruption: 29 months
Root Completed: 3 years

	LEFT
Universal Code	J
International Code	65
Palmer notation	$\underline{\text{E}}$
Number of roots	3
Number of pulp horns	5 or 4
Number of cusps	5 or 4
Number of developmental lobes	5

Location of proximal contact areas
MESIAL: Junction of occlusal and middle third
DISTAL: Middle third

Height of contour
FACIAL: Junction of occlusal and middle third
LINGUAL: Junction of occlusal and middle third

Identifying characteristics: Resembles permanent maxillary first molar, even has prominent oblique ridge. Three roots–two buccal and one lingual. Roots are long, slender, and flared widely apart. The faciolingual measurement of the crown is greater than the mesiodistal.

Deciduous Mandibular

Left Central Incisor

Eruption: 8 months
Root Completed: 1 1/2 years

	left
Universal Code	O
International Code	71
Palmer notation	$\overline{\text{A}}$
Number of roots	1
Number of pulp horns	3
Number of developmental lobes	4

Location of proximal contact areas
MESIAL: Incisal angle
DISTAL: Incisal angle

Height of contour
FACIAL: Cervical of crown
LINGUAL: Cervical of crown

The prominences of the facial and lingual at the cervical are as pronounced as any other deciduous teeth and more so than the permanent mandibular incisors.

Identifying characteristics: The incisal ridge is straight from an incisal view. From a facial view the crown is flat. The distal and mesial are almost identical. The crown is wide in proportion to its length in comparison with its permanent successor. The root is long and tapered. It is almost twice as long as the crown.

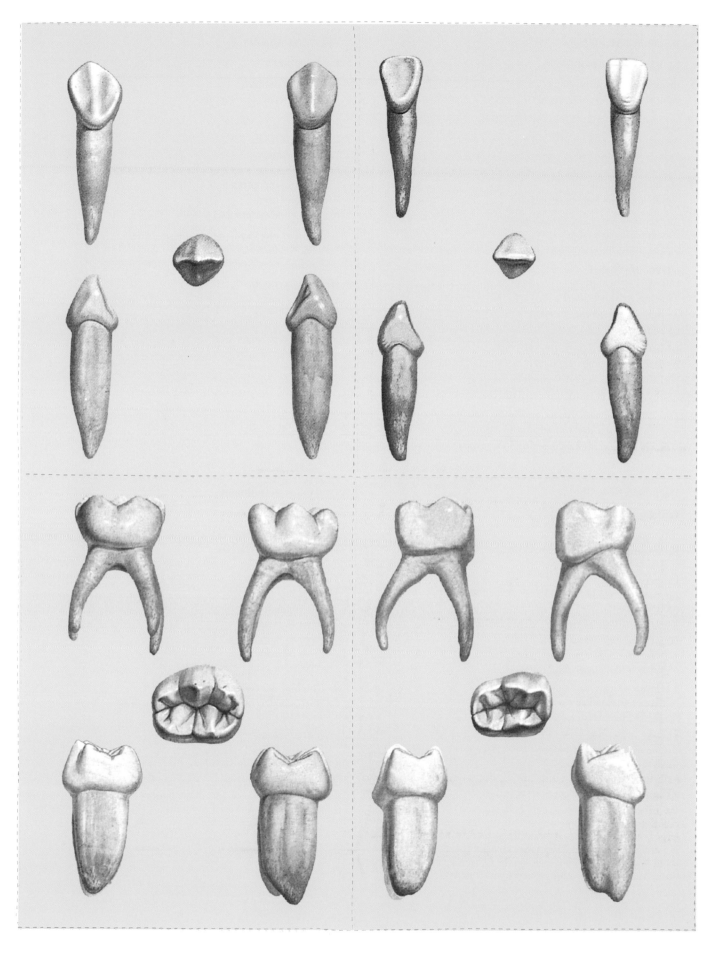

Deciduous Mandibular

Left Lateral Incisor

Eruption: 13 months
Root Completed: 1 1/2 years

	LEFT
Universal Code	N
International Code	72
Palmer notation	$\overline{B}$
Number of roots	1
Number of pulp horns	3
Number of developmental lobes	4

Location of proximal contact areas
MESIAL: Near incisal angle
DISTAL: Slightly lower than mesial

Height of contour
FACIAL: Cervical third
LINGUAL: Cervical third

As all anterior deciduous teeth, they exhibit pronounced cervical prominences.

Identifying characteristics: The incisal ridge runs slightly toward the distal. The lateral is longer and larger than the mandibular primary central incisor and the root is also longer. The lateral has a more rounded (obtuse) distoincisal angle.

Deciduous Mandibular

Left Canine

Eruption: 20 months
Root Completed: 3 1/4 years

	LEFT
Universal Code	M
International Code	73
Palmer notation	$\overline{C}$
Number of roots	1
Number of pulp horns	3
Number of cusps	1
Number of developmental lobes	4

Location of proximal contact areas
MESIAL: Junction of middle third and incisal third
DISTAL: Junction of middle third and incisal third

Height of contour
FACIAL: Distinct cervical bulge
LINGUAL: Distinct cervical bulge

Identifying characteristics: Similar to primary maxillary canine, except it is slightly shorter and much narrower labiolingually. The mandibular canine also has a shorter root.

Deciduous Mandibular

Left First Molar

Eruption: 16 months
Root Completed: 2 1/2 years

	LEFT
Universal Code	L
International Code	74
Palmer notation	$\overline{D}$
Number of roots	2
Number of pulp horns	4
Number of cusps	4
Number of developmental lobes	4

Location of proximal contact areas
MESIAL: Middle third
DISTAL: Middle third

Height of contour
FACIAL: An extremely bulbous curvature on the mesiobuccal cervical third
LINGUAL: Middle third

Identifying characteristics: This tooth does not resemble any of the other teeth, deciduous or permanent. This tooth varies so much it appears strange and primitive. The mesial root is much larger than the distal, and the mesial half of the crown is much larger than the distal. The most characteristic thing about this tooth is the extreme convexity on the mesiobuccal at the cervical third. There are two roots, a mesial and a distal.

Deciduous Mandibular

Left Second Molar

Eruption: 27 months
Root Completed: 3 years

	LEFT
Universal Code	K
International Code	75
Palmer notation	$\overline{E}$
Number of roots	2
Number of pulp horns	5
Number of cusps	5
Number of developmental lobes	5

Location of proximal contact areas
MESIAL: Junction of occlusal and middle third
DISTAL: Middle third

Height of contour
FACIAL: Buccal cervical ridge
LINGUAL: Middle third

Identifying characteristics: Resembles the permanent mandibular first molar. There are three buccal cusps and two lingual cusps; two roots, a mesial and a distal. The roots are longer than the deciduous first molars and flared far apart.

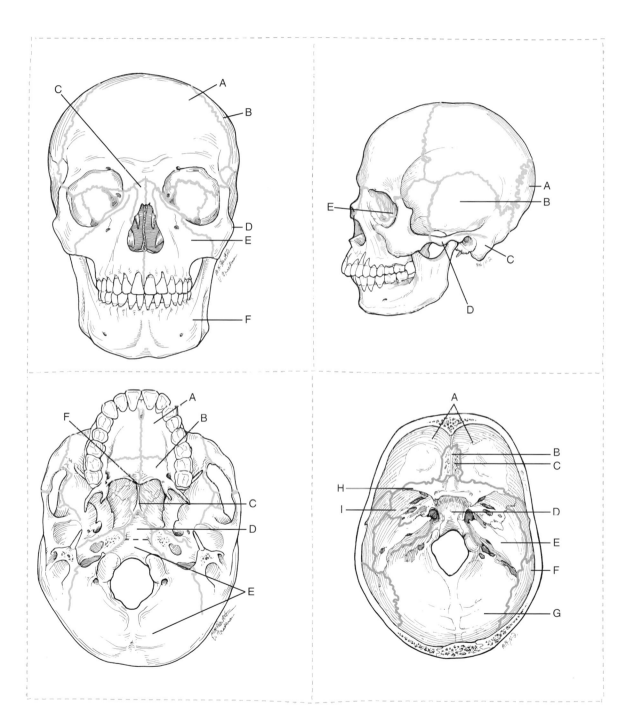

A. Occipital bone
B. Squamous part of temporal bone
C. Mastoid process of temporal bone
D. Zygomatic process
E. Ethmoid bone

A. Frontal bone
B. Parietal bone
C. Nasal bone
D. Zygomatic body
E. Maxilla
F. Mandible

A. Frontal bone
B. Crista galli
C. Cribriform plate
D. Sphenoid bone body
E. Temporal bone
F. Parietal bone
G. Occipital bone
H. Lesser wing of sphenoid
I. Greater wing of sphenoid

A. Palatal process of maxilla
B. Palatal process of palatine bone
C. Vomer
D. Sphenoid bone
E. Occipital bone
F. Posterior nasal spine

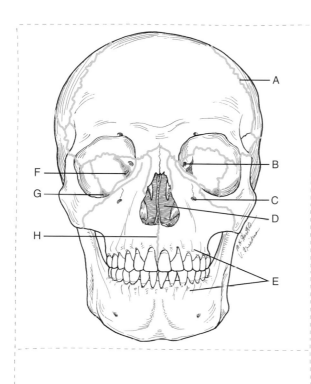

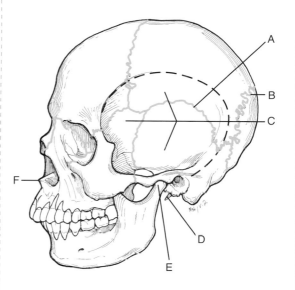

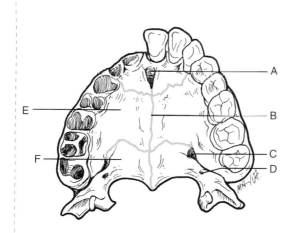

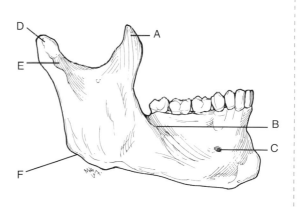

A. Squamosal suture
B. Lambdoid suture
C. Temporal fossa
D. Styloid process
E. Mandibular condyle
F. Anterior nasal spine

A. Coronal suture
B. Optic foramen
C. Infraorbital foramen
D. Nasal aperture
E. Alveolar processes
F. Superior orbital fissure
G. Inferior orbital fissure
H. Intermaxillary suture

A. Coronoid process
B. External oblique line
C. Mental foramen
D. Condyle
E. Neck of condyle
F. Angle of mandible

A. Incisive foramen
B. Median palatine suture
C. Greater palatine foramen
D. Lesser palatine foramen
E. Palatal process of maxilla
F. Palatal process of palatine bone

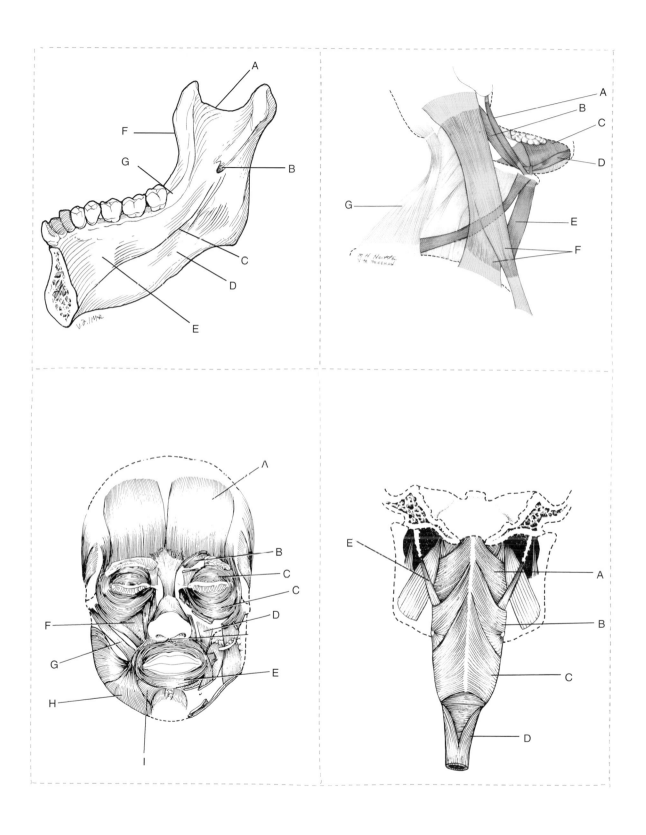

A. Stylohyoid muscle
B. Posterior digastric muscle
C. Mylohyoid muscle
D. Anterior digastric muscle
E. Sternohyoid muscle
F. Sternocleidomastoid muscle
G. Trapezius muscle

A. Coronoid notch
B. Mandibular foramen
C. Mylohyoid line
D. Submandibular fossa
E. Sublingual fossa
F. Anterior border of ramus
G. Retromolar triangle

A. Superior pharyngeal constrictor muscle
B. Middle pharyngeal constrictor muscle
C. Inferior pharyngeal constrictor muscle
D. Esophagus
E. Stylopharyngeus muscle

A. Frontalis muscle (occipitofrontalis)
B. Corrugator muscle
C. Orbicularis oculi muscle
D. Levator anguli oris muscle
E. Orbicularis oris muscle
F. Levator labii superioris muscle
G. Zygomaticus major muscle
H. Depressor anguli oris muscle
I. Depressor labii inferioris muscle